Intervention and Reflection

Intervention and Reflection
BASIC ISSUES IN MEDICAL ETHICS
Third Edition

Ronald Munson

University of Missouri—St. Louis

Wadsworth Publishing Company, Belmont, California
A division of Wadsworth, Inc.

Philosophy editor: Kenneth King
Production: Cece Munson, The Cooper Company
Manuscript editor: John N. Joyner
Cover designer: Albert Burkhardt
Print buyer: Ruth Cole
Compositor: TCSystems
Interior designers: Katie Michels and John Edeen
Signing Representative: George Weiss

Printed in the United States of America

2 3 4 5 6 7 8 9 10—92 91 90 89 88

ISBN 0-534-08088-X

Library of Congress Cataloging-in-Publication Data
Intervention and reflection.
  Bibliography: p.
  Includes index.
  1. Medical ethics.   I. Munson, Ronald, 1939–
R724.I57   1987   174'.2   86-28259
ISBN 0-534-08088-X

To Miriam
"Giver of bright rings"

CONTENTS

7. REPRODUCTIVE CONTROL: IN VITRO FERTILIZATION, ARTIFICIAL INSEMINATION, SURROGATE PREGNANCY, AND STERILIZATION

PREFACE

This is the third edition of this book, and the differences between it and the previous edition are significant. Yet before I discuss the changes, I want to say something about the character of the work itself, for that is one thing that has not changed.

In shaping this book, I have tried to capture both the intellectual excitement and the great seriousness that surround the field of medical ethics. I've done my best to convey both these aspects to students new to the field. In the choice of topics, in the introductions, and by other means, I have tried to familiarize readers with the issues and make them active participants in the enterprise. Whether someone is an undergraduate or graduate student, a nursing or medical student, with or without training in ethics, I think that she or he will find this a useful and engaging book.

The topics presented here are all fundamental ones in current medical ethics. They reflect the range and variety of problems that we now confront and involve the basic moral and social issues that have excited most concern. Each day's newspaper is likely to contain at least one story that focuses on a problem dealt with here. But more than this, the problems presented here are morally serious ones that lead people to turn hopefully to philosophical consideration in search of satisfactory resolutions.

The reading selections represent current thinking about the topics and show that such consideration can be worthwhile. All are readable and relatively non-technical, and several represent medical ethics at its very best. While some essays are published here for the first time, most of them have been chosen from the vast body of literature that has developed in the last five to ten years.

Although philosophers are strongly represented in the readings, the authors also include jurists, biologists, legal theorists, and practicing physicians. The moral problems of medicine almost always have scientific, social, legal, and economic aspects, and to deal with them sensibly we need the knowledge and perceptions of people from a variety of disciplines.

I have also opted for diversity in another way, for I have tried to see to it that opposing viewpoints are given for each major topic. Part of the intellectual excitement of medical ethics is generated by the hot controversies surrounding its issues, and to ignore those controversies would be misleading. Even worse, it would deny readers the opportunity of dealing directly with proposals and arguments that may be incompatible with their own views. The topics and readings are of crucial importance in a book of this kind. Yet I have also introduced several special features that I believe will be of particular help to students and will make the book more useful in class.

Most important, perhaps, is the general introduction. Here, among other things, I briefly sketch the principles of five major medical theories and indicate how they might be used to answer particular moral questions in medicine. The main purpose in doing this is to give students without a background in ethics the information they need to understand and evaluate the arguments in the readings. In this edition, with this same end in view, I have taken the suggestion of a number of people and added a section presenting and illustrating several major moral principles. These two sections are independent so that it is possible to read one without reading the other. Whether or not both sections are read, I hope that the introduction will help prepare students for independent inquiry in medical ethics.

In each of the nine chapters of the book I try to present in an introduction whatever factual information is needed to understand the moral issues that arise in actual medical practice and research. I also suggest ways in which the moral theories might be used to resolve some of the problems. These suggestions are offered merely as starting points in the search for a satisfactory answer. I have also included in each chapter a summary of the main line of argument in the selections and have indicated how the selections relate to one another. This should make it possible to identify the major themes that run through the chapter.

The Case Presentations are each based upon an actual event or situation. They are intended to provide a focus for discussion and to illustrate how genuine moral problems arise in ordinary life. Some of the cases are very well known, while others are quite obscure. Both types serve to remind us that in dealing with medical ethics we are not engaged in some purely intellectual abstract game.

The Social Context sections are intended to provide information relevant to understanding the current social and political situation in which various issues are being debated. Policies such as the now-rejected "Baby Doe" regulations, court decisions such as the recent one confirming the doctrine of *Roe* v. *Wade*, and requirements such as the use of diagnostic-related groups (DRGs) in Medicare constitute the social circumstances in which serious moral issues arise. A discussion of the issues in ignorance of the circumstances is possible and may be valuable. However, if we hope to raise the level of public discussion and genuinely inform the life of our society, then it is essential to have an understanding of the social facts as well as the scientific and medical ones.

At the end of each chapter, following the readings, are a number of Decision Scenarios. These are brief dramatic presentations of situations in which moral questions are crucial—in which ethical decisions have to be made. The scenarios are followed by questions that ask the reader to decide what the problems are and how they might be dealt with by a particular moral theory or by principles argued for in the readings. Thus, the Decision Scenarios are, in effect, exercises in medical ethics. Although almost all the scenarios have been dramatized, a great number of them are based on actual cases. (Should there be any doubt about whether a case is fictional, the answer is provided in the Notes and References section in the back of the book. Sources for the Case Presentations, Social Context sections, and Introductions are also listed there.)

Finally, I have included at the end of the book a quite extensive bibliography. It is arranged to correspond to the chapter divisions of the book, so that anyone who wants to do further reading on a particular topic should have no trouble locating appropriate works.

An inherent limitation of any book of this sort is the impossibility of including selections dealing with all the issues in a particular area. To compensate for this restriction, the chapter introductions raise and discuss more issues than are dealt with in the readings. My hope is that this will give readers a better sense of the scope and variety of issues in an area like informed consent or genetic engineering, even if little can be done to address the issues in a substantive way. I also hope that I have provided enough information to allow an instructor to discuss and develop the issues in class. In any case, I have done my best to make it possible for both students and instructors to go beyond the scope of the text.

Of course I could have touched on a larger number of issues in a more direct way had I used shorter selections. However, with few exceptions, I have chosen to include entire articles or chapters. I believe that most people who will use this book prefer to have the whole text of an article. An excerpt that includes the main argument may fairly represent a position, but the reader is deprived of participating in much of the dialectical process that is so crucial to arriving at a philosophically defensible conclusion.

The opportunity to prepare a third edition has allowed me to introduce a number of changes that I believe substantially improve both the philosophical and pedagogical character of the book. I shall merely list here, with little discussion, some of the more important alterations. For the sake of completeness, I will also include the few I mentioned earlier.

Nine Case Presentations have been added. The total is now eighteen, and previous ones have been revised and brought up to date where necessary. Because the Case Presentations focus on recent events, these changes increase the scope and relevance of the book.

Seven Social Context sections have been included. They offer the opportunity to connect discussions of ethical issues with current social policies, debates, and circumstances.

Over a dozen Decision Scenarios have been added. Previous ones have been revised where necessary, and questions have often been rewritten to tie the scenarios to the readings or to ethical principles. More actual cases have also been included in the scenarios, giving a greater sense of immediacy and relevance to the moral issues they raise.

The chapter introductions have been revised to take into account recent changes in policies, statistics, or relevant scientific or medical information. Statistics on abortion and on health-care costs and coverage of changes in Medicare, new in vitro fertilization techniques, new developments in gene therapy, and new prenatal tests are some of the examples of the changes made to provide current information.

The general Introduction, as mentioned earlier, has been substantially rewritten. Some discussion was eliminated and new material was added. Most important, a section discussing major moral principles has been included. This makes it possible for those who wish to deal with moral principles, either instead of basic ethical theories or in addition to them, in teaching or class discussion to do so without taking on the task of presenting the principles themselves.

In Chapter 1, "Abortion," the readings have been significantly changed. The new selections are more clearly written and represent a wider range of positions. The new Social Context section deals with the current political and social debate, which seems to have taken a nasty turn.

Chapter 2, "Treating or Terminating," includes a new Social Context section dealing with the controversy over the Baby Doe regulations and with recent Supreme Court decisions. A new article by John Arras has also been added.

Chapter 3, "Euthanasia," includes a new selection by Peter Singer and an excerpt from the court decision in the Conroy case, a case some see as being as significant in its impact as the Quinlan decision had been. A new Case Presentation focuses on Elizabeth Bouvia's demand that she be allowed to refuse food, while still receiving hospital care. In addition, a number of recent and controversial cases involving issues connected with euthanasia are dealt with in the Decision Scenarios.

Chapter 4, "Paternalism, Truth Telling, and Confidentiality," has been expanded to include both a Social Context section on AIDS and a new article on the topic written especially for this book. The issue of prediction of dangerousness and its connection with confidentiality and autonomy is discussed in a new Case Presentation dealing with the Juan Gonzalez affair. An article by Mark Siegler on the problem of protecting confidentiality in the modern medical setting has also been added.

Chapter 5, "Medical Experimentation and Informed Consent," includes a new Social Context section dealing with the issues surrounding the use of the artificial heart and a new Case Presentation that focuses on the case of Baby Fae, who received a baboon heart in a transplant. Two new articles dealing with these topics have also been included, and other recent cases are dealt with in the Decision Scenarios.

Chapter 6, "Genetics: Intervention, Control, and Research," has been altered to include a new Case Presentation on Huntington's Disease, an inherited disorder, and on the current status of gene therapy. The readings have been substantially altered to reflect some of the concerns with genetics and genetic engineering that have emerged during the last few years.

Chapter 7, "Reproductive Control," includes two new Case Presentations, one dealing with fertilized embryos and the other with surrogate pregnancy. The readings have been significantly changed to broaden the range of views, and a new essay on donor responsibility and artificial insemination appears here for the first time.

Chapter 8, "Allocating Scarce Medical Resources," has been expanded to include a new Social Context section dealing with the issues of securing and allocating transplant organs. An article by George J. Annas on the allocation issue has been added.

In Chapter 9, "The Claim to Health Care," the Social Context section presents information about recent health-care costs, policies, problems, and proposals that is relevant to understanding the way in which the present system functions. The selection of readings has been revised to focus on the issue of whether there is a right to health care and, if so, to what sort of care. Gene Outka's well-known essay on social justice and equal access has been added.

Finally, the Bibliography has been both expanded and brought up to date. Although not comprehensive, it is much more than a guide to further reading.

Like many others, I have had some experience in using this book to teach medical ethics. I have also had many discussions and some correspondence with others who have chosen it as a text. Perhaps then it would be appropriate to conclude my comments on this book with a few suggestions about its use in class.

The logic of the organization of the book remains unaltered in this edition. Roughly, the first topics presented (abortion, decisions about impaired infants, euthanasia, and so on) involve making individual moral decisions, while the later topics (such as genetic screening and rights to health care) require decisions about social goals and policies. But of course virtually all of the issues in medical ethics overlap and intertwine. (Abortion is a good example of this.)

For this reason, it seemed to me sensible to arrange the topics and write the introductions in a way that would make each chapter more or less independent of the others. Thus, the structure of the book does not have to be followed in teaching. Someone who wants to start with (say) informed consent or euthanasia may do so without being faced with text or selections that presuppose familiarity with preceding chapters.

In each chapter, I have placed the Case Presentation before the introductory text. My reason for doing so is that a case provides students with a concrete example and gives them the opportunity to appreciate the sorts of circumstances in which particular moral issues arise. Anyone who believes it is better to discuss cases after ethical issues have been talked about in a more abstract way may want to ask students to read the Case Presentation after the introductory text or the philosophical materials. The cases are written to stand alone, even when they are explicitly discussed in the selections.

The Social Context sections also appear before the introductions, and much of what I have said about the Case Presentations applies to them as well. Some may want their students to know something about the social and political aspects of an issue like organ transplantation before dealing with specific philosophical claims and arguments. Others may choose to focus exclusively on the philosophical issues and ignore the public aspects of the debate, on the grounds that students should make their own connections.

Finally, although the Decision Scenarios are most naturally considered after the reading selections, a strategy that has something to recommend it is to ask students to read the scenarios before the selections. The cases presented and the questions about them can then serve as guides in reading. Also, although time rarely permits it, if at least a few of the scenarios are discussed both before and after the selections are read, students are given a chance to see the ways in which their own views change. They are also sometimes in a better position to defend their initial views with relevant arguments.

I have tried to be helpful without being too intrusive. Anyone who teaches medical ethics wants enough flexibility to arrange a course in the way she or he sees fit. I have tried to offer that flexibility, while at the same time supplying students with the kind of information and support they need.

The third edition of this book, with its introductory materials and other appurtenances, continues to be more ambitious than any similar work currently available. The first two editions proved themselves generally useful, and I have been pleased by the responses of my colleagues. Even criticisms were tempered by a sympathetic understanding of the difficulty of producing a book of this scope that attempts to do so many things. I was able to make some important changes in this edition, but I am under no illusion that the book is now perfect. (If trying always meant succeeding, six-year-olds would be able to fly.) Accordingly, I would very much appreciate comments or suggestions from those who use the book and discover ways in which it can be improved.

By the time a book goes into a third edition, its list of debts has grown so long that the only possible response is to declare bankruptcy. In practical terms, this means that those who invested their help in this project have to settle for an acknowledgment that is less than they are rightly owed. My greatest debt on behalf of this book is to those authors who allowed their work to be printed here. I hope they will find no grounds for objecting to the way I have dealt with them.

I owe much to William E. Mann, Kirk Monfort, and John Arras, whose informed criticisms and suggestions were crucial in shaping the first edition. I am also indebted to my colleagues Lawrence H. Davis, Robert M. Gordon, James F. Doyle, David Conway, Paul Roth, and Stephanie Ross who all helped in various ways at various times.

I am similarly grateful to reviewers James R. Beattie, Jr., Xavier University; Sarah Ann Ketchum, Rollins College; Gareth B. Matthews, University of Massachusetts; William H. Oman, Slippery Rock University; Bruce Russell, Wayne State University; and George Sher, University of Vermont; for their criticisms and recommendations. John T. Wilcox's penchant for accuracy did much to save me from continuing to fall victim to my own carelessness and ignorance. I thank him for his efforts, even though it took a while to recover from the shock of receiving a multipaged, mimeographed handout entitled "Errors in Munson." (It's impossible not to wonder how many other such handouts are circulating in classes throughout the country.)

Kenneth King, Wadsworth's philosophy editor, has shown a steady faith in this book from its conception. This revision has been more extensive and more time-consuming than either of us anticipated, and I am grateful to him for his patience and his support. Working together, we have made this a better book than it would have been otherwise.

Miriam Grove Munson has endured, over the years, a continuing litany of sorrows and complaints connected with this book. Her patience has been unfailing, her sympathy unstinting, her encouragement unflagging. Her help has also been quite practical, for much of the introductory material has been improved by the exercise of her sharp critical judgment. Rebecca Grove Munson has constantly reminded me in a forceful fashion that there is more to life than the making of books.

I have had much help and advice, and like most human beings, I hate to acknowledge responsibility for errors. But the truth is that I sometimes refused to change direction even when warned I was walking into quicksand. If it swallows me up, it's my own fault.

Ronald Munson
University of Missouri—St. Louis, 1987

Intervention and Reflection

MORAL PRINCIPLES, ETHICAL THEORIES, AND MEDICAL DECISIONS: AN INTRODUCTION

"He's stopped breathing, Doctor," the nurse said. She sounded calm and not at all hysterical. By the time Dr. Sarah Cunningham had reached Mr. Sabatini's bedside, the nurse was already providing mouth-to-mouth resuscitation. But Mr. Sabatini still had the purplish blue color of cyanosis, caused by a lack of oxygen in his blood.

Dr. Cunningham knew that, if he was to survive, Mr. Sabatini would have to be given oxygen fast and placed on a respirator. But should she order this done?

Mr. Sabatini was an old man, almost ninety. So far as anyone knew, he was alone in the world and would hardly be missed when he died. His health was poor. He had congestive heart disease and was dying slowly and painfully from intestinal cancer.

Wouldn't it be a kindness to Mr. Sabatini to allow him this quick and painless death? Why condemn him to lingering on for a few extra hours or weeks?

The decision that Sarah Cunningham faces is a moral one. She has to decide whether she should take the steps that might prolong Mr. Sabatini's life or not take them and accept the consequence that he will almost surely die within minutes. She knows the medical procedures that can be employed, but she has to decide whether she should employ them.

This kind of case rivets our attention because of its immediacy and drama. But there are many other situations that arise in the context of medical practice and research that present problems that require moral decisions. Some are equal in drama to the problem facing Dr. Cunningham, while others are not so dramatic but are of at least equal seriousness. There are far too many to catalogue, but consider this sample: Is it right for a woman to have an abortion for any reason? Should children with serious birth defects be put to death? Do people have a right to die? Does everyone have a right to medical care? Should physicians ever lie to their patients? Should people suffering from a genetic disease be allowed to have children? Can parents agree to allow their children to be used as experimental subjects?

Most of us have little tolerance for questions like these. They seem so cold and abstract. Our attitude changes, however, when we find ourselves in a position in which *we* are the decision makers. It changes, too, when we are in a position in which we must advise those who make the decisions. Or when we are on the receiving end of the decision.

But whether we view the problems abstractly or concretely, we are inclined to ask the same question: Are there any rules, standards, or principles that we can use as guides when we are faced with moral decisions? If there are, then Dr. Cunningham need not be wholly unprepared to decide whether she should order steps taken to save Mr. Sabatini. Nor need we be unprepared to decide issues like those in the questions above.

1

The branch of philosophy concerned with principles that allow us to make decisions about what is right and wrong is called *ethics* or *moral philosophy*. *Medical ethics* is specifically concerned with moral principles and decisions in the context of medical practice, policy, and research. Moral difficulties connected with medicine are so complex and important that they require special attention. Medical ethics gives them this attention, but it remains a part of the discipline of ethics. Thus, if we are to answer our question as to whether there are any rules or principles to use when making moral decisions in the medical context, we must turn to general ethical theories and to a consideration of moral principles that have been proposed to hold in all contexts of human action.

In the first major part of this chapter, we will discuss five major ethical theories that have been put forward by philosophers. Each of these theories represents an attempt to supply basic principles that we can rely on in making moral decisions. We'll consider these theories and examine how they might be applied to moral issues in the medical context. We will discuss the reasons that have been offered to persuade us to accept each theory, but we will also point out some of the difficulties that each theory presents.

In the second major part of the chapter, we will examine and illustrate several moral principles that are of special relevance to medical research and practice. These principles are frequently appealed to in discussions of practical ethical problems and are sufficiently uncontroversial as to be endorsed in a general way by any of the ethical theories mentioned in the first section.

The two sections are not dependent on one another, and it is possible to profit from either without reading the other. (The price for this independence is a small amount of repetition.) Nevertheless, reading both is recommended. The discussions and arguments presented in the selections that make up the majority of this book can most easily be followed by someone who has at least some familiarity with basic moral theories. At the same time, some points in discussions turn upon questions about the applicability of certain familiar moral principles. Being acquainted with those principles makes it easier to understand and evaluate such discussions.

I. BASIC ETHICAL THEORIES

Ethical theories attempt to articulate and justify principles that can be employed as guides for making moral decisions and as standards for the evaluation of actions and policies. In effect, such theories define what it means to act morally, and in doing so they stipulate in a general fashion the duties or obligations that fall upon us.

Ethical theories also offer a means to explain and justify actions. If our actions are guided by a particular theory, then we can explain them by demonstrating that the principles of the theory required us to act as we did. In such cases, the explanation also constitutes a justification. We justify our actions by showing that, according to the theory, we had an obligation to do what we did. (In some cases, we may justify our actions by showing that the theory *permitted* our actions—that is, didn't require them, but didn't rule them out as wrong.)

Advocates of a particular ethical theory present what they consider to be good reasons and relevant evidence in its support. Their general aim is to show that the theory is one that any reasonable individual would find persuasive or would endorse as correct. Accordingly, appeals to religion, faith, or nonnatural factors are not considered to be either necessary or legitimate to justify the theory. Rational persuasion alone is regarded as the basis of justification.

In this section, we will briefly consider four general ethical theories and one theory of justice that has an essential ethical component. In each case, we will begin by examining the basic principles of the theory and the grounds offered for its acceptance. We will then explore some of the possibilities of applying the theory to problems that arise within the medical context. Finally, we will mention some of the practical consequences and conceptual difficulties that raise questions about the theory's adequacy or correctness.

UTILITARIANISM

The ethical theory known as utilitarianism was given its most influential formulation in the nineteenth century by the British philosophers Jeremy Bentham (1748–1832) and John Stuart Mill (1806–1873). Bentham and Mill did not produce identical theories, but both their versions have come to be spoken of as "classical utilitarianism." Subsequent elaborations and qualifications of utilitarianism are inevitably based on the formulations of Bentham and Mill, so their theories are worth careful examination.

The Principle of Utility

The foundation of utilitarianism is a single apparently simple principle. Mill calls it the "principle of utility" and states it this way: *"Actions are right in proportion as they tend to promote happiness, wrong as they tend to produce the reverse of happiness."*

The principle focuses attention on the *consequences* of actions, rather than upon some feature of the actions themselves. The "utility" or "usefulness" of an action is determined by the extent to which it produces happiness. Thus, no action is *in itself* right or wrong. Nor is an action right or wrong by virtue of the actor's hopes, intentions, or past actions. Consequences alone are important. Breaking a promise, lying, causing pain, or even killing a person may, under certain circumstances, be the right action to take. Un-

der other circumstances, the action might be wrong.

We need not think of the principle as applying to just one action that we are considering. It supplies the basis for a kind of cost-benefit analysis to employ in a situation in which several lines of action are possible. Using the principle, we are supposed to consider the possible results of each of the actions. Then we are to choose the one that produces the most benefit (happiness) at the least cost (unhappiness). The action we take may produce some unhappiness, but it is a balance of happiness over unhappiness that the principle tells us to seek.

Suppose, for example, that a woman in a large hospital is near death: she is in a coma, an EEG shows only minimal brain function, and a respirator is required to keep her breathing. Another patient has just been brought to the hospital from the scene of an automobile accident. His kidneys have been severely damaged, and he is in need of an immediate transplant. There is a good tissue match with the woman's kidneys. Is it right to hasten her death by removing a kidney?

The principle of utility would probably consider the removal justified. The woman is virtually dead, while the man has a good chance of surviving. It is true that the woman's life is threatened even more by the surgery. It may, in fact, kill her. But, on balance, the kidney transplant seems likely to produce more happiness than unhappiness. In fact, it seems better than the alternative of doing nothing. For in that case both patients are likely to die.

The principle of utility is also called the "greatest happiness principle" by Bentham and Mill. The reason for this name is clear when the principle is stated in this way: *Those actions are right that produce the greatest happiness for the greatest number of people.* This alternative formulation makes it obvious that in deciding how to act it is not just my happiness or the happiness of a particular person or group that must be considered. According to utilitarianism, every person is to count just as much as any other person. That is, when we are considering how we should act, everyone's interest must be considered. The right action, then, will be the one that produces the most happiness for the largest number of people.

Mill is particularly anxious that utilitarianism not be construed as no more than a sophisticated justification for crude self-interest. He stresses that in making a moral decision we must look at the situation in an objective way. We must, he says, be a "benevolent spectator" and then act in a way that will bring about the best results for all concerned. This view is summarized in a famous passage:

> The happiness which forms the utilitarian standard of what is right in conduct, is not the agent's own happiness, but that of all concerned. As between his own happiness and that of others, utilitarianism requires him to be as strictly impartial as a disinterested and benevolent spectator. In the golden rule of Jesus of Nazareth, we read the complete spirit of the ethics of utility. To do as you would be done by, and to love your neighbor as yourself, constitute the ideal perfection of utilitarian morality.

The key concept in both formulations of the principle of utility is "happiness." Bentham simply identifies happiness with pleasure—pleasure of any kind. The aim of ethics, then, is to increase the amount of pleasure in the world to the greatest possible extent. To facilitate this, Bentham recommends the use of a "calculus of pleasure and pain," in which characteristics of pleasure such as intensity, duration, and number of people affected are measured and assigned numerical values. To determine which of several possible actions is the right one, we need only determine which one receives the high-

est numerical score. Unfortunately, Bentham does not tell us what units to use nor how to make the measurements.

Mill also identifies happiness with pleasure, but he differs from Bentham in a major respect. Unlike Bentham, he insists that some pleasures are "higher" than others. Thus, pleasures of the intellect are superior to, say, purely sensual pleasures. This difference in the concept of pleasure can become significant in a medical context. For example, in the choice of using limited resources to save the life of a lathe operator or of an art historian, Mill's view might assign more value to the life of the art historian. That person, Mill might say, is capable of "higher pleasures" than the lathe operator. (Of course other factors would be relevant here for Mill.)

Both Mill and Bentham regard happiness as an intrinsic good. That is, it is something good in itself or for its own sake. Actions, by contrast, are good only to the extent to which they tend to promote happiness. Therefore, they are only instrumentally good. Since utilitarianism determines the rightness of actions in terms of their tendency to promote the greatest happiness for the greatest number, it is considered to be a *teleological* ethical theory. ("Teleological" comes from the Greek word "telos," which means "end" or "goal.") A teleological ethical theory judges the rightness of an action in terms of an external goal or purpose—"general happiness" or utility for utilitarianism. However, utilitarianism is also a *consequentialist* theory, for the outcomes or consequences of actions are the only considerations relevant to determining their moral rightness. Not all teleological theories are consequentialist.

Some more recent formulations of utilitarianism have rejected the notion that happiness, no matter how defined, is the sole intrinsic good that actions or policies must promote. Critics of the classical view have argued that the list of things we recognize as valuable in themselves should be increased to include ones such as knowledge, beauty, love, friendship, liberty, and health. According to this *pluralistic* view, in applying the principle of utility we must consider the entire range of intrinsic goods that an action is likely to promote. Thus, the right action is the one that can be expected to produce the greatest sum of intrinsic goods. In most of the following discussion, we will speak of the greatest happiness or benefit, but it is easy enough to see how the same points can be made from a pluralistic perspective.

Act and Rule Utilitarianism

All utilitarians accept the principle of utility as the standard for determining the rightness of actions. But they divide into two groups over the matter of the application of the principle.

Act utilitarianism holds that the principle should be applied to particular acts in particular circumstances. *Rule utilitarianism* maintains that the principle should be used to test rules, which can in turn be used to decide the rightness of particular acts. Let's consider each of these views and see how it works in practice.

Act utilitarianism holds that an act is right if, and only if, no other act could have been performed that would produce a higher utility. Suppose that a child is born with severe impairments. The child has an open spine, severe brain damage, and dysfunctional kidneys. What should be done? (We will leave open the question of who should decide.)

The act utilitarian holds that we must attempt to determine the consequences of the various actions that are open to us. We should consider, for example, these possibilities: (1) give the child only the ordinary treatment that would be given to a normal child, (2) give the child special treatment for its problems, (3) give the child no treatment—

allow it to die, (4) put the child to death in a painless way.

According to act utilitarianism, we must explore the potential results of each of these possibilities. We must realize, for example, that when such a child is given only ordinary treatment it will be worse off, if it survives, than if it had been given special treatment. Also, a child left alone and allowed to die is also likely to suffer more pain than one killed by a lethal injection. Furthermore, a child treated aggressively will have to undergo numerous surgical procedures of limited effectiveness. We must also consider the family of the child and judge the emotional and financial effects that each of the possible actions will have on them. Then, too, we must take into account such matters as the "quality of life" of a child with severe brain damage and multiple defects, the effect on physicians and nurses in killing the child or allowing it to die, and the financial costs to society in providing long-term care.

After these considerations, we should then choose the action that has the greatest utility. We should act in the way that will produce the most benefit for all concerned. Which of the possibilities we select will depend on the precise features of the situation: how impaired the child is, how good its chances are for living an acceptable life, the character and financial status of the family, and so on. The great strength of act utilitarianism is that it invites us to deal with each case as unique. When the circumstances of another case are different, we might, without being inconsistent, choose another of the possible actions.

Act utilitarianism shows a sensitivity to specific cases, but it is not free from difficulties. Some philosophers have pointed out that there is no way that we can be sure that we have made the right choice of actions. We are sure to be ignorant of much relevant information. Besides, we can't know with much certainty what the results of our actions will really be. There is no way to be sure, for example, that even a severely impaired infant will not recover enough to live a better life than we predict.

The act utilitarian can reply that acting morally doesn't mean being omniscient. We need to make a reasonable effort to get relevant information, and we can usually predict the probable consequences of our actions. Acting morally doesn't require any more than this.

Another objection to act utilitarianism is more serious. According to the doctrine, we are obligated to keep a promise only if keeping it will produce more utility than some other action. If some other action will produce the same utility, then keeping the promise is permissible but not obligatory. Suppose that a surgeon promises a patient that only he will perform an operation, then allows a well-qualified resident to perform part of it. Suppose that all goes well and the patient never discovers that the promise was not kept. The outcome for the patient is exactly the same as if the surgeon had kept the promise. From the point of view of act utilitarianism, there is nothing wrong with the surgeon's failure to keep it. Yet critics charge that there is something wrong, that in making the promise the surgeon took on an obligation. Act utilitarianism is unable to account for obligations engendered by such actions as promising and pledging, critics say, for such actions involve something other than consequences.

A third objection to act utilitarianism arises in situations in which virtually everyone must follow the same rules in order to achieve a high level of utility, but even greater utility can be achieved if a few people do not follow the rules. Consider the relationship between physicians and the Medicaid program. The program pays physicians for services provided to those poor enough to qualify for the program. The program would collapse if nearly all physicians were not honest in billing Medicaid for their services. Not only would many poor people suffer, but physicians themselves would lose a source of income.

Suppose that a particular physician believes that the requirements to qualify for Medicaid are too restrictive and that many who urgently need medical care cannot afford it. As an act utilitarian, he reasons that it is right for him to get money to open a free clinic under the program. He intends to bill for services he does not provide, then use that money to treat those not covered by Medicaid. His claims will be small compared to the entire Medicaid budget, so it is unlikely that anyone who qualifies for Medicaid will go without treatment. Since he will tell no one what he is doing, others are not likely to be influenced by his example and make false claims for similar or less worthy purposes. The money he is paid will bring substantial benefit to those in need of health care. Thus, he concludes, by violating the rules of the program, his actions will produce greater utility than would be produced by following the rules.

The physician's action would be morally right, according to act utilitarianism. Yet, critics say, we expect an action that is morally right to be one that is right for everyone in similar circumstances. If every physician in the Medicaid program acted in this way, however, the program would be destroyed and thus produce no utility at all. Furthermore, according to critics, the physician's action produces unfairness. While it is true that the patients he treats at his free clinic gain a benefit they would not otherwise have, similar patients must go without treatment. The Medicaid policy, whatever its flaws, is at least prima facie fair in providing benefits to all who meet its requirements. Once again, then, according to critics, more seems to be involved in judging the moral worth of an action than can be accounted for by act utilitarianism.

In connection with such objections, some

critics have gone so far as to claim that it is impossible to see how a society in which everyone were an act utilitarian could function. We could not count on promises being kept nor take for granted that people were telling us the truth. Social policies would be no more than general guides to action, and we could never be sure that people would regard themselves as obligated to adhere to their provisions. Decisions made by individuals about each individual action would not obviously lead to the promotion of the highest degree of utility. Indeed, some critics say, such a society might collapse, for communication among individuals would be difficult, if not impossible, social cohesion would be weakened, and general policies and regulations would have very uncertain effects.

The critics are not necessarily right, of course, and defenders of act utilitarianism have made substantial efforts to answer the criticisms we have presented. Some have denied that the theory has those implications and argued that some of our generally accepted moral perceptions should be changed. In connection with this last point, Carl Wellman provides an insight into the sort of conflict between moral feelings and rational judgment that the acceptance of act utilitarianism can produce. Concerning euthanasia, Wellman writes:

> Try as I may, I honestly cannot discover great hidden disutilities in the act of killing an elderly person suffering greatly from an incurable illness, provided that certain safeguards like a written medical opinion by at least two doctors and a request by the patient are preserved. In this case I cannot find any way to reconcile my theory with my moral judgment. What I do in this case is to hold fast to act-utilitarianism and distrust my moral sense. I claim that my condemnation of such acts is an irrational disapproval, a condemnation that will change upon further reasoning about the act. . . . That I feel wrong-

ness is clear, but I cannot state to myself any rational justification for my feeling. Hence, I discount this particular judgment as irrational.

Rule utilitarianism maintains that an action is right if it conforms to a rule of conduct that has been validated by the principle of utility as one that will produce at least as much utility as any other rule applicable to the situation. A rule like "Provide only ordinary care for severely brain-damaged newborns with multiple impairments," if it were established, would allow us to decide about the course of action to follow in situations like that of our earlier example.

The rule utilitarian is not concerned with assessing the utility of individual actions, but of particular rules. In practice, then, we do not have to go through the calculations involved in determining in each case whether a specific action will increase utility. All that we have to establish is that following a certain rule will, in general, result in a situation in which utility is maximized. Once rules are established, they can be relied on to determine whether a particular action is right.

The basic idea behind rule utilitarianism is that having a set of rules that are always observed produces the greatest social utility. Having everyone follow the same rule in each case of the same kind yields more utility for everybody in the long run. An act utilitarian can agree that having rules may produce more social utility than not having them. But the act utilitarian insists that the rules be regarded as no more than general guides to action, as "rules of thumb." Thus, for act utilitarianism it is perfectly legitimate to violate a rule if doing so will maximize utility in that instance. By contrast, the rule utilitarian holds that rules must generally be followed, even though following them may produce less net utility (more unhappiness than happiness) in a particular case.

Rule utilitarianism can endorse rules like "Keep your promises." Thus, unlike act utilitarianism, it can account for the general sense that in making promises we are placing ourselves under an obligation that cannot be set aside for the sake of increasing utility. If "Keep your promises" is accepted as a rule, then the surgeon who fails to perform all of an operation himself, when he has promised his patient he would do so, has not done the right thing, even if the patient never learns the truth.

Rule utilitarians recognize that circumstances can arise in which it would be disastrous to follow a general rule, even when it is true that *in general* greater happiness would result from following the rule all the time. Clearly we should not keep a promise to meet someone for lunch when we have to choose between keeping the promise and rushing a heart-attack victim to the hospital. It is consistent with the theory to formulate rules that include appropriate escape clauses. For example, "Keep your promises, unless breaking them is required to save a life" and "Keep your promises, unless keeping them would lead to a disastrous result unforeseen at the time the promise was made" are rules that a rule utilitarian might regard as more likely to lead to greater utility than "Always keep your promises no matter what the consequences may be." What a rule utilitarian cannot endorse is a rule like "Keep your promises, except when breaking a promise would produce more utility." This would, in effect, transform the rule utilitarian into an act utilitarian.

Of course, rule utilitarians are not committed to endorsing general rules only. It is compatible with the view to offer quite specific rules, and in fact there is no constraint on just how specific a rule may be. A rule utilitarian might, for example, establish a rule like "If an infant is born with an open spine, severe brain damage, and dysfunctional kidneys, then the infant should receive no life-sustaining treatment."

The possibility of formulating a large number of rules and establishing them separately opens this basic version of rule utilitarianism to two objections. First, some rules are likely to conflict when they are applicable to the same case, and basic rule utilitarianism offers no way to resolve such conflicts. What should a physician do when faced both with a rule like that above and with another that directs him to "Provide life-sustaining care to all who require it"? Rules which, when considered individually, pass the test of promoting utility, may when taken together express contradictory demands. A further objection to basic rule utilitarianism is that establishing rules to cover many different circumstances and situations results in such an abundance of rules that employing the rules to make moral decisions becomes virtually impossible in practice.

Partly because of such difficulties, rule utilitarians have taken the approach of establishing the utility of a *set* of rules or an entire moral code. The set can include rules for resolving possible conflicts, and an effort can be made to keep the rules few and simple to minimize the practical difficulty of employing them. Once again, as with individual actions or rules, the principle of utility is employed to determine which set of rules, out of the various sets considered, ought to be accepted.

In this more sophisticated form, rule utilitarianism can be characterized as the theory that an action is right when it conforms to a set of rules that has been determined to produce at least as much overall utility as any other set. It is possible to accept the present forms of social and economic institutions, such as private property and a market economy, as constraints, then argue for the set of rules that will yield the most utility under those conditions. However, it is also possible to be more radical and argue for a particular set of rules that would lead to the greatest possible utility, quite apart from present social forms. Indeed, such a set of rules might be proposed and defended in an effort to bring about changes in present society that are needed to increase the overall level of utility. Utilitarianism, whether act or rule, is not restricted to being a theory about individual moral obligation. It is also a social and political theory.

We have already seen that rule utilitarianism, unlike act utilitarianism, makes possible the sort of obligation we associate with making a promise. But how might rule utilitarianism deal with the case of the physician who files false Medicaid claims to raise money to operate a free clinic? An obvious answer, although certainly not the only one possible, is that any set of rules likely to be adopted by a rule utilitarian will contain at least one rule making fraud morally wrong. Without a rule forbidding fraud, no social program that requires the cooperation of its participants is likely to achieve its aim. Such a rule protects the program from miscalculations of utility that individuals may make for self-serving reasons, keeps the program focused on its goal, and prevents it from becoming fragmented. Even if some few individuals commit fraud, the rule against it is crucial in discouraging as many as possible. Otherwise, as we pointed out earlier, such a program would collapse. By requiring that the program operate as it was designed, rule utilitarianism also preserves prima facie fairness, because only those who qualify receive benefits.

The most telling objection to rule utilitarianism, according to some philosophers, is that it is inconsistent. The justification of a set of moral rules is that the rules maximize utility. If rules are to maximize utility, then it seems obvious that they must require that an act produce more utility than any other possible act in a particular situation. Otherwise, the maximum amount of utility would not result. But if the rules satisfy this demand, then they will justify exactly the same actions as act utilitarianism. Thus the rules will consider it right to break promises, make fraudu-

lent claims, and so on. When rule utilitarianism moves to block these possibilities by requiring that rules produce only the most utility overall, it becomes inconsistent: the set of rules is said to maximize utility, but the rules will require actions that do not maximize utility. Thus, rule utilitarianism seems both to accept and reject the principle of utility as the ultimate moral standard.

Preference Utilitarianism

Some philosophers have called into question the idea of using happiness or any other intrinsic value (knowledge or health, for example) as a criterion of the rightness of an action. The notion of an intrinsic value, they have argued, is too imprecise to be used as a practical guide. Furthermore, it is not at all clear that people share the same values, and even if they do, they are not committed to them to the same degree. Someone may value knowledge more than health, while someone else may value physical pleasure over knowledge or health. As a result, there can be no clear-cut procedure for determining what action is likely to produce the best outcome for an individual or group.

The attempt to develop explicit techniques (such as those of decision theory) to help resolve questions about choosing the best action or policy has led some thinkers to replace considerations of intrinsic value with considerations of actual preferences. What someone wants, desires, or prefers can be determined, in principle, in an objective way by consulting the person directly. In addition, people are often able to do more than merely express a preference. Sometimes they can rank their preferences from that which is "most desired" to that which is "least desired."

Such a ranking is of special importance in situations involving risk, for people can be asked to decide how much risk they are willing to take to attempt to realize a given preference. A young woman with a hip injury who is otherwise in good health may be willing to accept the risk of surgery to increase her chances of being restored to many years of active life. By contrast, an elderly woman in frail health may prefer to avoid surgery and accept the limitations that the injury imposes on her physical activities. For the elderly woman, not only are the risks of surgery greater because of her poor health, but even if the surgery is successful, she will have fewer years to benefit from it.

By contrast, the older woman may place such a premium on physical activity that she is willing to take the risk of surgery to improve her chances of securing even a few more years of it. Only she can say what is important to her and how willing she is to take the risk required to secure it.

These considerations about personal preferences can also be raised about social preferences. Statistical information about what people desire and what they are willing to forgo to see their desires satisfied becomes relevant to institutional and legislative deliberations about what policies to adopt. For example, a crucial question facing our own society is whether we are willing to provide everyone with at least a basic minimum of health care, even if this requires increasing taxes or reducing our support for other social goods, such as education and defense.

Employing the satisfaction of preferences as the criterion of the rightness of an action or policy makes it possible to measure some of the relevant factors in some situations. The life expectancy of infants with particular impairments at birth can be estimated by statistics; a given surgical procedure has a certain success rate and a certain mortality rate. Similarly, a particular social policy has a certain financial cost, and if implemented, the policy is likely to mean the loss of other possible benefits and opportunities.

Ideally, information of this kind should allow a rational decision maker to calculate the best course of action for an individual or group. The best action will be the one that best combines the satisfaction of preferences with other conditions (financial costs and risks, for example) that are at least minimally acceptable. To use the jargon of the theorists, the best action is the one that maximizes the utilities of the person or group.

A utilitarianism that employs preferences has the advantage of suggesting more explicit methods of analysis and rules for decision making than the classical formulation. It also has the potential for being more sensitive to the expressed desires of individuals. However, preference utilitarianism is not free from special difficulties.

Most prominent is the problem posed by preferences that we would generally regard as unacceptable. What are we to say about those who prefer mass murder, child abuse, or torturing animals? Obviously, subjective preferences cannot be treated equally, and we must have a way to distinguish acceptable from unacceptable ones. Whether this can be done by relying on the principle of utility alone is doubtful. In the view of some commentators, some other moral principle (or principles) is needed. (See the discussion of justice immediately following.)

Difficulties

Classical utilitarianism is open to a variety of objections. We shall concentrate on only one, however, for it seems to reveal a fatal flaw in the structure of the entire theory. This most serious of all objections is that the principle of utility appears to justify the imposition of great suffering on a few people for the benefit of many people.

Certain kinds of human experimentation forcefully illustrate this possibility. Suppose that an investigator is concerned with acquiring a better understanding of brain functions. He could learn a great deal by systematically destroying the brain of one person and carefully noting the results. Such a study would offer many more opportunities for increasing our knowledge of the brain than those studies that use as subjects people who have damage to their brains in accidental ways. We may suppose that the experimenter chooses as his subject a person without education or training, without family or friends, who cannot be regarded as making much of a contribution to society. The subject will die from the experiment, but it is not unreasonable to suppose that the knowledge of the human brain gained from the experiment will improve the lives of countless numbers of people.

The principle of utility seems to make such experiments legitimate because the outcome is a greater amount of good than harm. One or a few have suffered immensely, but the many have profited to an extent that far outweighs that suffering.

Clearly what is missing from utilitarianism is the concept of *justice*. It cannot be right to increase the general happiness at the expense of one person or group. There must be some way of distributing happiness and unhappiness and avoiding exploitation.

Mill was aware that utilitarianism needs a principle of justice, but most contemporary philosophers do not believe that such a principle can be derived from the principle of utility. In their opinion, utilitarianism as an ethical theory suffers severely from this defect. Yet some philosophers, while acknowledging the defect, have still held that utilitarianism is the best substantive moral theory available.

KANT'S ETHICS

For utilitarianism, the rightness of an action depends upon its consequences. In stark contrast to this view is the ethical theory formulated by the German philosopher Immanuel Kant (1724–1804) in his book *Fundamental Principles of the Metaphysics of Morals*. For Kant, the consequences of an action are mor-

ally irrelevant. Rather, an action is right when it is in accordance with a rule that satisfies a principle he calls the "categorical imperative." Since this is the basic principle of Kant's ethics, we can begin our discussion with it.

The Categorical Imperative

If you decide to have an abortion and go through with it, it is possible to view your action as involving a rule. You can be thought of as endorsing a rule to the effect "Whenever I am in circumstances like these, then I shall have an abortion." Kant calls such a rule a "maxim." In his view, all reasoned and considered actions can be regarded as involving maxims.

The maxims in such cases are personal or subjective, but they can be thought of as being candidates for moral rules. If they pass the test imposed by the categorical imperative, then we can say that such actions are right. Furthermore, in passing the test, the maxims cease to be merely personal and subjective. They gain the status of objective rules of morality that hold for everyone.

Kant formulates the categorical imperative in this way: Act only on that maxim which you can will to be a universal law. Kant calls the principle "categorical" to distinguish it from "hypothetical" imperatives. These tell us what to do if we want to bring about certain consequences—such as happiness. A categorical imperative prescribes what we ought to do without reference to any consequences. The principle is an "imperative" because it is a command.

The test imposed on maxims by the categorical imperative is one of generalization or "universalizability." The central idea of the test is that a moral maxim is one that can be generalized to apply to all cases of the same kind. That is, you must be willing to see your rule adopted as a maxim by everyone who is in a situation similar to yours. You must be willing to see your maxim universalized, even though it may turn out on some other occasion to work to your disadvantage.

For a maxim to satisfy the categorical imperative it is not necessary that we be agreeable in some psychological sense to see it made into a universal law. Rather, the test is one that requires us to avoid inconsistency or conflict in what we will as a universal rule.

Suppose, for example, that I am a physician and I tell a patient that he has a serious illness, although I know that he doesn't. This may be to my immediate advantage, for the treatment and the supposed cure will increase my income and reputation. The maxim of my action might be phrased as, "Whenever I have a healthy patient, I shall lie to him and say that he has an illness."

Now suppose that I try to generalize my maxim. In doing so, I will discover that I am willing the existence of a practice that has contradictory properties. If "Whenever any physician has a healthy patient, he shall lie to him and say he has an illness" is made a universal law, then every patient will be told that he has an illness. Trust in the diagnostic pronouncements of physicians will be destroyed, while my scheme depends on my patients' trusting me and accepting the truth of my lying diagnosis.

It is as if I were saying, "Let there be a rule of truth telling such that people can assume that others are telling them the truth, but let there also be a rule that physicians may lie to their patients when it is in the interest of the physician to do so." In willing both rules, I am willing something contradictory. Thus, I can will my action in a particular case, but I can't will that my action be universal without generating a logical conflict.

Kant claims that such considerations show that it is always wrong to lie. Lying produces a contradiction in what we will. On one hand, we will that people believe what we say—that they accept our assurances and promises. On the other hand, we will that

people be free to give false assurances and make false promises. Lying thus produces a self-defeating situation, for, when the maxim involved is generalized, the very framework required for lying collapses.

Similarly, consider the egoist who seeks only his self-interest and so makes "Never show love or compassion for others" the maxim of his actions. When universalized, this maxim results in the same kind of self-defeating situation that lying does. Since the egoist will sometimes find himself in need of love and compassion, if he wills the maxim of his action to be a universal law, then he will be depriving himself of something that is in his self-interest. Thus, in willing the abolition of love and compassion out of self-interest, he creates a logical contradiction in what he wills.

Another Formulation

According to Kant, there is only one categorical imperative, but it can be stated in three different ways. Each is intended to reveal a different aspect of the principle. The second formulation, the only other we shall consider, can be stated in this way: Always act so as to treat humanity, either yourself or others, always as an end and never as only a means.

This version illustrates Kant's notion that every rational creature has a worth in itself. This worth is not conferred by being born into a society with a certain political structure, nor even by belonging to a certain biological species. The worth is inherent in the sheer possession of rationality. Rational creatures possess what Kant calls an "autonomous, self-legislating will." That is, they are able to consider the consequences of their actions, make rules for themselves, and direct their actions by those self-imposed rules. Thus, rationality confers upon everyone an intrinsic worth and dignity.

This formulation of the categorical imperative perhaps rules out some of the standards that are sometimes used to determine who is selected to receive certain medical resources (such as kidney machines) when the demand is greater than the supply. Standards that make a person's education, accomplishments, or social position relevant seem contrary to this version of the categorical imperative. They violate the basic notion that each person has an inherent worth equal to that of any other person. Unlike dogs or horses, people cannot be judged on "show points."

For Kant, all of morality has its ultimate source in rationality. The categorical imperative, in any formulation, is an expression of rationality, and it is the principle that would be followed in practice by any purely rational being. Moral rules are not mere arbitrary conventions or subjective standards. They are objective truths that have their source in the rational nature of human beings.

Duty

Utilitarianism identifies the good with happiness or pleasure and makes the production of happiness the supreme principle of morality. But for Kant happiness is at best a conditional or qualified good. In his view, there is only one thing that can be said to be good in itself: a good will.

Will is what directs our actions and guides our conduct. But what makes a will a "good will"? Kant's answer is that a will becomes good when it acts purely for the sake of duty.

We act for the sake of duty (or from duty) when we act on maxims that satisfy the categorical imperative. This means, then, that it is the motive force behind our actions—the character of our will—that determines their moral character. Morality does not rest on results—such as the production of happiness—but neither does it rest on our feelings, impulses, or inclinations. An action is right,

for Kant, only when it is done for the sake of duty.

Suppose that I decide to donate one of my kidneys for transplanting. If my hope is to gain approval or praise or even if I am moved by pity and a genuine wish to reduce suffering, and this is the only consideration behind my action, then, although I have done the morally right thing, my action has no inner moral worth. By contrast, if I make the donation because I perceive it is my duty to do so, then my action is not only right, but has moral worth. In the first case, I may have acted *in accordance with duty* (done the same thing as duty would have required), but I did not act *from duty*.

This view of duty and its connection with morality captures attitudes we frequently express. Consider a nurse who gives special care to a severely ill patient. Suppose you learned that the nurse was providing such extraordinary care only because he hoped that the patient or her family would reward him with a special bonus. Knowing this, you would be unlikely to say that the nurse was acting in a morally outstanding way. We might even think the nurse was being greedy or cynical, and we would say that he was doing the right thing for the wrong reasons.

Kant distinguishes between two types of duties: perfect and imperfect. (The distinction corresponds to the two ways in which maxims can be self-defeating when tested by the categorical imperative.) A *perfect* duty is one we must always observe, while an *imperfect* duty is one that we must observe only on some occasions. I have a perfect duty not to injure another person, but I have only an imperfect duty to show love and compassion. I must sometimes show it, but when I show it and which people I select to receive it are entirely up to me.

My duties determine what others can legitimately claim from me as a right. Some rights can be claimed as perfect rights, while others cannot. Everyone can demand of me that I do him or her no injury. But no one can tell me that I must make him or her the recipient of my love and compassion. In deciding how to discharge my imperfect duties, I am free to follow my emotions and inclinations.

For utilitarianism, an action is right when it produces something that is intrinsically valuable (happiness). Because actions are judged by their contributions to achieving a goal, utilitarianism is a teleological theory. By contrast, Kant's ethics holds that an action has features in itself that make it right or in accordance with duty. These features are distinct from the action's consequences. Such a theory is called "deontological," a term derived from the Greek word for "duty" or "obligation."

Kant's Ethics in the Medical Context

Four features of Kant's ethics are of particular importance in dealing with issues in medical treatment and research:

1. No matter what the consequences may be, it is always wrong to lie.

2. We must always treat people (including ourselves) as ends and not as means only.

3. An action is right when it satisfies the categorical imperative.

4. Perfect and imperfect duties give a basis for claims that certain rights should be recognized.

We can present only two brief examples of how these features can be instrumental in resolving ethical issues, but these are suggestive of other possibilities.

Our first application of Kant's ethics bears on medical research. The task of medical investigators would be easier if they did not have to tell patients that they were going to be made part of a research program. Patients would then become subjects without

even knowing it, and more often than not the risk to them would be negligible. Even though no overt lying would be involved, on Kantian principles this procedure would be wrong. It would require treating people as a means only and not as an end.

Likewise, it would never be right for an experimenter to deceive a potential experimental subject. If an experimenter told a patient, "We would like to use this new drug on you because it might help you" and this were not really so, the experimenter would be performing a wrong action. Lying is always wrong.

Nor could the experimenter justify this deception by telling himself that the research is of such importance that it is legitimate to lie to the patient. On Kant's principles, good results never make an action morally right. Thus, a patient must give voluntary and informed consent to become a subject of medical experimentation. Otherwise, he or she is being deprived of autonomy and treated as a means only.

We may volunteer because we expect the research to bring direct benefits to us. But we may also volunteer even though no direct personal benefits can be expected. We may see participation in the research as an occasion for fulfilling an imperfect duty to improve human welfare.

But, just as Kant's principles place restrictions on the researcher, they place limits on us as potential subjects. We have a duty to treat ourselves as ends and act so as to preserve our dignity and worth as humans. Therefore, it would not be right for us to volunteer for an experiment that threatened our lives or threatened to destroy our ability to function as autonomous rational beings without first satisfying ourselves that the experiment was legitimate and necessary.

Our second application of Kant's ethics in a medical context bears on the relationship between people as patients and those who accept responsibility for caring for them. A physician, for example, has only an imperfect duty to accept me as a patient. He has a duty to make use of his skills and talents to treat the sick, but I cannot legitimately insist on being the beneficiary. How he discharges his duty is his decision.

If, however, I am accepted as a patient, then I can make some legitimate claims. I can demand that nothing be done to cause me pointless harm, because it is never right to injure a person. Furthermore, I can demand that I never be lied to or deceived. Suppose, for example, I am given a placebo (a harmless but inactive substance) and told that it is a powerful and effective medication. Or suppose that a biopsy shows that I have an inoperable form of cancer, but my physician tells me, "There's nothing seriously wrong with you." In both cases, the physician may suppose that he is deceiving me "for my own good": the placebo may be psychologically effective and make me feel better, and the lie about cancer may save me from useless worry. Yet, by being deceived, I am being denied the dignity inherent in my status as a rational being. Lying is wrong in general, and in such cases as these it also deprives me of my autonomy, of my power to make decisions and form my own opinions. As a result, such deception dehumanizes me.

As an autonomous rational being, a person is entitled to control over his or her own body. This means that medical procedures can be performed on me only with my permission. It would be wrong, for example, for my physician to have me held down and injected with a drug that I explicitly refused. It would be wrong even if the medication were needed for my "own good." I may voluntarily put myself under the care of a physician and submit to all that I am asked to, but the decision belongs to me alone.

In exercising control over my body, however, I also have a duty to myself. Suppose, for example, that I refuse to allow surgery to be performed on me, although I have been

told it is necessary to preserve my life. Since I have a duty to preserve my life, as does every person, my refusal is morally unjustifiable. Even here, however, it is not legitimate for others to force me to "do my duty." In fact, in Kantian ethics it is impossible to force another to do his or her duty because it is not the action but the maxim involved that determines whether or not one's duty has been done.

It is obvious even from our sketchy examples that Kantian ethics is a fruitful source of principles and ideas for working out some of the specific moral difficulties of medical experimentation and practice. The absolute requirements imposed by the categorical imperative can be a source of strength and even of comfort. By contrast, utilitarianism requires us to weigh alternative courses of actions by anticipating their consequences and deciding whether what we are considering doing can be justified by those results. Kant's ethics saves us from this kind of doubt and indecision; we know we must never lie, no matter what good may come of it. Furthermore, the lack of a principle of justice that is the most severe defect of utilitarianism is met by Kant's categorical imperative. When every person is to be treated as an end and never as only a means, the possibility of legitimately exploiting some for the benefit of others is wholly eliminated.

Difficulties

Kant's ethical theory is complex and controversial. It has problems of a theoretical sort that manifest themselves in practice and lead us to doubt whether the absolute rules determined by the categorical imperative can always provide a straightforward solution to our moral difficulties. We will limit ourselves to discussing just three problems.

First, Kant's principles supply no clear way of resolving cases in which there is a conflict of duties. I have a duty to keep my promises, and I also have a duty to help those in need. Suppose, then, that I am a physician and I have promised a colleague to attend a staff conference. Right before the conference starts, I am talking with a patient who lapses into an insulin coma. If I get involved in treating the patient, I'll have to break my promise to attend the conference. What should I do?

The answer is obvious: I should treat the patient. Our moral intuition tells us this. But Kant does not provide us with a clear way of answering this question. He does not rank duties. His view seems to be that a promise should never be broken—even when the promise concerns a relatively trivial matter and the consequences of keeping it are disastrous.

Another difficulty with the categorical imperative arises because we are free to choose how we formulate a maxim for testing. In all likelihood none of us would approve a maxim such as "Lie when it is convenient for you." But what about one like "Lie when telling the truth is likely to cause harm to another"? We would be more inclined to make this a universal law. Now consider the maxim "Whenever a physician has good reason to believe that a patient's life will be seriously threatened if he is told the truth about his condition, then the physician should lie." Virtually everyone would be willing to see this made into a universal law.

Yet these three maxims could apply to the same situation. Since Kant does not tell us how to formulate our maxims, it is clear that we can act virtually any way we choose if we are willing to describe the situation in detail. We might be willing to have everyone act just as we are inclined to act whenever they find themselves in *exactly* this kind of situation. The categorical imperative, then, does not seem to solve our moral problems quite so neatly as it first appears to.

A final problem arises from Kant's notion that we have duties to rational beings or persons. Ordinarily, we have little difficulty with

this commitment to persons, yet there are circumstances, particularly in the medical context, in which serious problems arise. Consider, for example, a fetus developing in its mother's womb. Is the fetus to be considered a person? The way this question is answered makes all the difference in deciding about the rightness or wrongness of abortion.

A similar difficulty is present when we consider how we are to deal with an infant with serious birth defects. Is it our duty to care for this infant and do all we can to see that it lives? If the infant is not a person, then perhaps we do not owe him the sort of treatment it would be our duty to provide a similarly afflicted adult. It's clear from these two cases that the notion of a person as an autonomous rational being is both too restrictive and arbitrary. It begs important moral questions.

Another difficulty connected with Kant's concept of a rational person is the notion of an "autonomous self-regulating will." Under what conditions can we assume that an individual possesses such a will? Does a child, a mentally retarded person, or someone in prison? Without such a will, in Kant's view, such an individual cannot legitimately consent to be the subject of an experiment or even give permission for necessary medical treatment. This notion is very much in need of development before Kant's principles can be relied on to resolve ethical questions in medicine.

The difficulties that we have discussed require serious consideration. This does not mean, of course, that they cannot be resolved or that because of them Kant's theory is worthless. As with utilitarianism, there are some philosophers who believe the theory is the best available, despite its shortcomings. That it captures many of our intuitive beliefs about what is right (not to lie, to treat people with dignity, to act benevolently) and supplies us with a test for determining our duties (the categorical imperative) recommends it strongly as an ethical theory.

ROSS'S ETHICS

The English philosopher W. D. Ross (b. 1877) presented an ethical theory in his book *The Right and the Good* that can be seen as an attempt to incorporate aspects of utilitarianism and aspects of Kantianism. Ross rejected the utilitarian notion that an action is made right by its consequences alone, but he was also troubled by Kant's absolute rules. He saw not only that such rules fail to show sensitivity to the complexities of actual situations, but also that they sometimes conflict with one another. Like Kant, Ross is a deontologist, but with an important difference. Ross believes it is necessary to consider consequences in making a moral choice, even though he believes that it is not the results of an action taken alone that make it right.

Moral Properties and Rules

For Ross there is an unbridgeable distinction between moral and nonmoral properties. There are only two moral properties—rightness and goodness—and these cannot be replaced by, or explained in terms of, other properties. Thus, to say that an action is "right" is not at all the same as saying that it "causes pleasure" or "increases happiness," as utilitarianism claims.

At the same time, however, Ross does not deny that there is a connection between moral properties and nonmoral ones. What he denies is the possibility of establishing an identity between them. Thus, it may be right to relieve the suffering of someone, but right is not identical with relieving suffering. (More exactly put, the rightness of the action is not identical with the action's being a case of relieving suffering.)

Ross also makes clear that we must often know many nonmoral facts about a situation before we can legitimately make a moral judgment. If I see a physician injecting someone, I cannot say whether she is acting rightly without determining what she is in-

jecting, why she is doing it, and so on. Thus, rightness is a property that depends partly on the nonmoral properties that characterize a situation. I cannot determine whether the physician is doing the right thing or the wrong thing until I determine what the nonmoral properties are.

Ross believes that there are cases in which we have no genuine doubt about whether the property of rightness or goodness is present. The world abounds with examples of cruelty, lying, and selfishness, and in these cases we are immediately aware of the absence of rightness or goodness. But the world also abounds with examples of compassion, reliability, and generosity in which rightness and goodness are clearly present. Ross claims that our experience with such cases puts us in a position to come to know rightness and goodness with the same degree of certainty as when we grasp the mathematical truth that a triangle has three angles.

Furthermore, according to Ross, our experience of many individual cases puts us in a position to recognize the validity of a general statement like "It is wrong to cause needless pain." We come to see such rules in much the same way that we come to recognize the letter A after having seen it written or printed in a variety of handwritings or typefaces.

Thus, our moral intuitions can supply us with moral rules of a general kind. But Ross refuses to acknowledge these rules as absolute. For him they can serve only as guides to assist us in deciding what we should do. Ultimately, in any particular case we must rely not only on the rules, but also on reason and our understanding of the situation.

Thus, even with rules, we may not recognize what the right thing to do is in a given situation. We recognize, he suggests, that there is always *some* right thing to do, but what it is may be far from obvious. In fact, doubt about what is the right way of acting may arise just because we have rules to guide us. We become aware of the fact that there are several possible courses of action, and all of them seem to be right.

Consider the problem of whether to lie to a terminally ill patient about her condition. Let us suppose that, if we lie to her, we can avoid causing her at least some useless anguish. But then aren't we violating her trust in us to act morally and to speak the truth?

In such cases, we seem to have a conflict in our duties. It is because of such familiar kinds of conflicts that Ross rejects the possibility of discovering absolute, invariant moral rules like "Always tell the truth" and "Always eliminate needless suffering." In cases like the one above, we cannot hold that both rules are absolute without contradicting ourselves. Ross says that we have to recognize that every rule has exceptions and must in some situations be overridden.

Actual Duties and Prima Facie Duties

If rules like "Always tell the truth" cannot be absolute, then what status can they have? When our rules come into conflict in particular situations, how are we to decide which rule applies? Ross answers this question by making use of a distinction between what is actually right and what is prima facie right. Since we have a duty to do what is right, this distinction can be expressed as one between *actual duty* and *prima facie duty.*

An actual duty is simply what my real duty is in a situation. It is the action that, out of the various possibilities, I ought to perform. More often than not, however, I may not know what my actual duty is. In fact, for Ross, the whole problem of ethics might be said to be the problem of knowing what my actual duty is in any given situation.

"Prima facie" literally means "at first sight," but Ross uses the phrase to mean something like "other things being equal." Accordingly, a prima facie duty is one that dictates what I should do when other rele-

vant factors in a situation are not considered. If I promised to meet you for lunch, then I have a prima facie duty to meet you. But suppose I am a physician and, just as I am about to leave for our appointment, the patient I am with suffers cardiac arrest. In such circumstances, according to Ross's view, I should break my promise and render aid to the patient. My prima facie duty to keep my promise doesn't make that act obligatory. It constitutes a moral reason for meeting you, but there is also a moral reason for not meeting you. I also have a prima facie duty to aid my patient, and this is a reason that outweighs the first one. Thus, aiding the patient is both a prima facie duty and, in this situation, my actual duty.

The notion of a prima facie duty permits Ross to offer a set of moral rules stated in such a way that they are both universal and free from exceptions. For Ross, for example, lying is always wrong, but it is wrong prima facie. It may be that in a particular situation my actual duty requires that I lie. Even though what I have done is prima facie wrong, it is the morally right thing to do if some other prima facie duty that requires lying in the case is more stringent than the prima facie duty to tell the truth. (Perhaps only by lying am I able to prevent a terrorist from blowing up an airplane.) I must be able to explain and justify my failure to tell the truth, and it is of course possible that I may not be able to do so. It may be that I was confused and misunderstood the situation or failed to consider other alternatives. I may have been wrong to believe that my actual duty required me to lie. However, even if I was correct in my belief, that I lied is still prima facie wrong. It is this fact (and for Ross it is a fact) that requires me to explain and justify my action.

We have considered only a few simple examples of prima facie duties, but Ross is more thorough and systematic than our examples might suggest. He offers a list of prima facie wrong. It is this fact (and for Ross it is a fact) that requires me to explain and justify my action.

1.   Duties of Fidelity: telling the truth, keeping actual and implicit promises, and not representing fiction as history.

2.   Duties of Reparation: righting the wrongs we have done to others.

3.   Duties of Gratitude: recognizing the services others have done for us.

4.   Duties of Justice: preventing a distribution of pleasure or happiness that is not in keeping with the merit of the people involved.

5.   Duties of Beneficence: helping to better the condition of other beings with respect to virtue, intelligence, or pleasure.

6.   Duties of Self-Improvement: bettering ourselves with respect to virtue or intelligence.

7.   Duties of Nonmaleficence: avoiding or preventing an injury to others.

Ross doesn't claim that this is a complete list of the prima facie duties that we recognize. However, he does believe that the duties on the list are all ones that we acknowledge and are willing to accept as legitimate and binding without argument. He believes that if we simply reflect on these prima facie duties we will see that they may be truly asserted. As he puts the matter:

> I . . . am claiming that we *know* them to be true. To me it seems as self-evident as anything could be, that to make a promise, for instance, is to create a moral claim on us in someone else. Many readers will perhaps say that they do *not* know this to be true. If so I certainly cannot prove it to them. I can only ask them to reflect again, in the hope that they will ultimately agree that they also know it to be true.

Notice that Ross explicitly rejects the possibility of providing us with reasons or arguments to convince us to accept his list of prima facie duties. We are merely invited to reflect on certain kinds of cases, like keeping promises, and Ross is convinced that this reflection will bring us to accept his claim that these are true duties. Ross, like other intuitionists, tries to get us to agree with his moral perceptions in much the same way as we might try to get people to agree with us about our color perceptions. We might, for example, show a paint sample to a friend and say, "Don't you think that looks blue? It does to me. Think about it for a minute."

We introduced the distinction between actual and prima facie duties to deal with those situations in which duties seem to conflict. The problem, as we can now state it, is this: What are we to do in a situation in which we recognize more than one prima facie duty and it is not possible for us to act in a way that will fulfill them all? We know, of course, that we should act in a way that satisfies our actual duty. But that is just our problem. What, after all, is our actual duty when our prima facie duties are in conflict?

Ross offers us two principles to deal with cases of conflicting duty. The first principle is designed to handle situations in which just two prima facie duties are in conflict: *That act is one's duty which is in accord with the more stringent prima facie obligation.*

The second principle is intended to deal with cases in which several prima facie duties are in conflict: *That act is one's duty which has the greatest balance of prima facie rightness over prima facie wrongness.*

Unfortunately, both these principles present problems in application. Ross does not tell us how we are to determine when an obligation is "more stringent" than another. Nor does he give us a rule for determining the "balance" of prima facie rightness over wrongness. Ultimately, according to Ross, we must simply rely upon our perceptions of the situation. There is no automatic or mechanical procedure that can be followed. If we learn the facts in the case, consider the consequences of our possible actions, and reflect on our prima facie duties, we should be able to arrive at a conclusion as to the best course of action—in Ross's view something that we as moral agents must and can do.

To return to specific cases, perhaps there is no direct way to answer the abstract question, Is the duty not to lie to a patient "more stringent" than the duty not to cause needless suffering? So much depends on the character and condition of the individual patient that an abstract determination of our duty based on "balance" or "stringency" is useless. However, knowing the patient, we should be able to perceive what the right course of action is.

Ross further believes that there are situations in which there are no particular difficulties about resolving the conflict between prima facie duties. For example, most of us would agree that, if we can save someone from serious injury by lying, then we have more of an obligation to save someone from injury than we do to tell the truth.

Ross's Ethics in the Medical Context

Ross's moral rules are not absolute in the sense that Kant's are; consequently, as with utilitarianism, it is not possible to say what someone's duty would be in an actual concrete situation. We can discuss in general, however, the advantages that Ross's theory brings to medical-moral issues. We shall mention only two for illustration.

First and most important is Ross's list of prima facie duties. The list of duties can serve an important function in the moral education of physicians, researchers, and other medical personnel. The list encourages each person responsible for patient care to reflect on the prima facie obligations that he or she has to-

ward those people and to set aside one of those obligations only when morally certain that another obligation takes precedence.

The specific duties imposed in a prima facie way are numerous and can be expressed in terms relevant to the medical context: do not injure patients; do not distribute scarce resources in a way that fails to recognize individual worth; do not lie to patients; show patients kindness and understanding; educate patients in ways useful to them; do not hold out false hopes to patients, and so on.

Second, like utilitarianism, Ross's ethics encourages us to show sensitivity to the unique features of situations before acting. Like Kant's ethics, however, Ross's also insists that we look at the world from a particular moral perspective. In arriving at decisions about what is right, we must learn the facts of the case and explore the possible consequences of our actions. Ultimately, however, we must guide our actions by what is right, rather than by what is useful, or by what will produce happiness, or anything of the kind.

Since for Ross actions are not always justified in terms of their results, we cannot say unequivocally "It's right to trick this person into becoming a research subject because the experiment may benefit thousands." Yet, we cannot say that it is always wrong for a researcher to trick a person into volunteering. An action is right or wrong regardless of what we think about it, but in a particular case circumstances might justify an experimenter in allowing some other duty to take precedence over the duty of fidelity.

Fundamentally, then, Ross's ethics offers us the possibility of gaining the advantages of utilitarianism without ignoring the fact that there seem to be duties with an undeniable moral force behind them that cannot be accounted for by utilitarianism. Ross's ethics accommodates not only our intuition that certain actions should be performed just because they are right but also our inclination to pay attention to the results of actions and not just the motives behind them.

Difficulties

The advantages Ross's ethics offers over both utilitarianism and Kantianism are offset by some serious difficulties. To begin with, it seems false that we all grasp the same principles. We are well aware that people's beliefs about what is right and about what their duties are result from the kind of education and experience that they have had. The ability to perceive what is good or right does not appear to be universally shared. Ross does say that the principles are the convictions of "the moral consciousness of the best people." In any ordinary sense of "best," there is reason to say that such people don't always agree on moral principles. If "best" means "morally best," then Ross is close to being circular: the best people are those who acknowledge the same prima facie obligations, and those who recognize the same prima facie obligations are the best people.

Some have objected that Ross's list of prima facie duties seems incomplete. For example, Ross does not explicitly say that we have a prima facie obligation not to steal, but most people would hold that if we have any prima facie duties at all, the duty not to steal must surely be counted among them. Of course, it is possible to say that stealing is covered by some other obligation—the duty of fidelity, perhaps, since stealing may violate a trust. Nevertheless, from a theory based on intuition, the omission of such duties leaves Ross's list peculiarly incomplete.

Further, some critics have claimed that it is not clear that there is always even a prima facie obligation to do some of the things Ross lists. Suppose that I promise to lie about a friend's physical condition so that he can continue to collect insurance payments. Some would say that I have no obligation at all to keep such an unwise promise. In such a case,

there would be no conflict of duties, because I don't have even a prima facie duty to keep such a promise.

Finally, Ross's theory, some have charged, seems to be false to the facts of moral disagreements. When we disagree with someone about an ethical matter, we consider reasons for and against some position. Sometimes the discussion results in agreement. But according to Ross's view this should not be possible. Although we may discuss circumstances and consequences and agree about the prima facie duties involved, ultimately I arrive at my judgment about the duty that is most stringent or has the greatest degree of prima facie rightness and you arrive at yours. At this point, it seems, there can be no further discussion, even though the two judgments are incompatible. Thus, a choice between the two judgments about what act should be performed becomes arbitrary.

Few contemporary philosophers would be willing to endorse Ross's ethical theory without serious qualifications. The need for a special kind of moral perception (or "intuition") marks the theory as unacceptable for most philosophers. Yet many would acknowledge that the theory has great value in illuminating such aspects of our moral experience as reaching decisions when we feel the pull of conflicting obligations. Furthermore, at least some would acknowledge Ross's prima facie duties as constituting an adequate set of moral principles.

RAWLS'S THEORY OF JUSTICE

In 1971 the Harvard philosopher John Rawls published a book called *A Theory of Justice*. The work continues to attract a considerable amount of attention and has been described by some as the most important book in moral and social philosophy of this century.

One commentator, R. P. Wolfe, points out that Rawls attempts to develop a theory that combines the strengths of utilitarianism with those of the deontological position of Kant and Ross, while avoiding the weaknesses of each view. Utilitarianism claims outright that happiness is fundamental and suggests a direct procedure for answering ethical-social questions. But it is flawed by its lack of a principle of justice. Kant and Ross make rightness a fundamental moral notion and stress the ultimate dignity of human beings. Yet neither provides a workable method for solving problems of social morality. Clearly, Rawls's theory promises much if it can succeed in uniting the two ethical traditions we have discussed.

The Original Position and the Principles of Justice

For Rawls the central task of government is to preserve and promote the liberty and welfare of individuals. Thus, principles of justice are needed to serve as standards for designing and evaluating social institutions and practices. They provide a way of resolving conflicts among the competing claims that individuals make and a means of protecting the legitimate interests of individuals. In a sense, the principles of justice constitute a blueprint for the development of a just society.

But how are we to formulate principles of justice? Rawls makes use of a hypothetical device he calls "the original position." Imagine a group of people like those who make up our society. These people display the ordinary range of intelligence, talents, ambitions, convictions, and social and economic advantages. They include both sexes and members of various racial and ethnic groups.

Furthermore, suppose that this group is placed behind what Rawls calls "a veil of ignorance." Assume that each person is made ignorant of his or her sex, race, natural endowments, social position, economic condition, and so on. Furthermore, assume that

these people are capable of cooperating with one another, that they follow the principles of rational decision making, and that they are capable of a sense of justice and will adhere to principles they agree to adopt. Finally, assume that they all desire what Rawls calls "primary goods": the rights, opportunities, powers, wealth, and such that are both worth possessing in themselves and are necessary to securing the more specific goods an individual may want.

Rawls argues that the principles of justice chosen by such a group will be just if the conditions under which they are selected and the procedures for agreeing on them are fair. The original position, with its veil of ignorance, characterizes a state in which alternative notions of justice can be discussed freely by all. Since the ignorance of the participants means that individuals cannot gain advantage for themselves by choosing principles that favor their own circumstances, the eventual choices of the participants will be fair. Since the participants are assumed to be rational, they will be persuaded by the same reasons and arguments. These features of the original position lead Rawls to characterize his view as "justice as fairness."

We might imagine at first that some people in the original position would gamble and argue for principles that would introduce gross inequalities in their society. For example, some might argue for slavery. If these people should turn out to be masters after the veil of ignorance is stripped away, they would gain immensely. But if they turn out to be slaves, then they would lose immensely. However, since the veil of ignorance keeps them from knowing their actual positions in society, it would not be rational for them to endorse a principle that might condemn them to the bottom of the social order.

Given the uncertainties of the original situation, there is a better strategy that these rational people would choose. In the economic discipline known as game theory, this strategy is called "maximin." When we choose in uncertain situations, this strategy directs us to select from the alternatives the one whose worst possible outcome is better than the worst possible outcome of the other alternatives. (If you don't know whether you're going to be a slave, you shouldn't approve a set of principles that permits slavery when you have other options.)

Acting in accordance with this strategy, Rawls argues that people in the original position would agree on the following two principles of justice:

> 1. Each person is to have an equal right to the most extensive total system of equal basic liberties compatible with a similar system of liberty for all.
> 2. Social and economic inequalities are to be arranged so that they are both: (a) to the greatest benefit of the least advantaged . . . , and (b) attached to offices and positions open to all under conditions of fair equality of opportunity.

For Rawls, these two principles are taken to govern the distribution of all social goods: liberty, property, wealth, and social privilege. The first principle has priority. It guarantees a system of equal liberty for all. Furthermore, because of its priority, it explicitly prohibits the bartering away of liberty for social or economic benefits. (For example, a society cannot withhold the right to vote from its members on the grounds that voting rights damage the economy.)

The second principle governs the distribution of social goods other than liberty. Although society could organize itself in a way that would eliminate differences in wealth and abolish the advantages that attach to different social positions, Rawls argues that those in the original position would not choose this form of egalitarianism. Instead, they would opt for the second principle of justice. This means that in a just society differences in wealth and social position can be tolerated only when they can be shown to benefit everyone and to benefit, in particular, those who have the fewest advantages. A just society is not one in which everyone is equal, but one in which inequalities must be demonstrated to be legitimate. Furthermore, there must be a genuine opportunity for acquiring membership in a group that enjoys special benefits. Those not qualified to enter medical schools because of past discrimination in education, for example, can claim a right for special preparation to qualify them. (Of course in a Rawlsian society there would be no discrimination to be compensated for.)

Rawls argues that these two principles are required to establish a just society. Furthermore, in distributing liberty and social goods, the principles guarantee the worth and self-respect of the individual. People are free to pursue their own conception of the good and fashion their own lives. Ultimately, the only constraints placed on them as members of society are those expressed in the principles of justice.

Yet Rawls also acknowledges that those in the original position would recognize that we have duties both to ourselves and to others. They would, for example, want to take measures to see that their interests are protected if they should meet with disabling accidents, become seriously mentally disturbed, and so on. Thus, Rawls approves a form of paternalism: others should act for us when we are unable to act for ourselves. When our preferences are known to them, those acting for us should attempt to follow what we would wish. Otherwise, they should act for us as they would act for themselves if they were viewing our situation from the standpoint of the original position. Paternalism is thus a duty to ourselves that would be recognized by those in the original position.

Rawls is also aware of the need for principles that bind and guide individuals as moral decision makers. He claims that those in the original position would reach agreement on principles for such notions as fairness in our dealings with others, fidelity, respect for persons, and beneficence. From these principles we gain some of our obligations to one another.

But, Rawls claims, there are also "natural duties" that would be recognized by those in the original position. Among those Rawls mentions are (1) the duty of justice—supporting and complying with just institutions, (2) the duty of helping others in need or jeopardy, (3) the duty not to harm or injure another, (4) the duty to keep our promises.

For the most part, these are duties that hold between or among people. They are only some of the duties that would be offered by those in the original position as unconditional duties. Thus, Rawls in effect endorses virtually the same duties as those that Ross presents as prima facie duties. Rawls realizes that the problem of conflicts of duty was left unsolved by Ross and so perceives the need for assigning priorities to duties—ranking them as higher and lower. Rawls believes that a full system of principles worked out from the original position would include rules for ranking duties. Rawls's primary concern, however, is with justice in social institutions, and he does not attempt to establish any rules for ranking.

Rawls's Theory of Justice in the Medical Context

Rawls's "natural duties" are virtually the same as Ross's prima facie duties. Consequently, most of what we said earlier about prima facie duties and moral decision making applies to Rawls.

Rawls endorses the legitimacy of paternalism, although he does not attempt to specify detailed principles to justify individual cases. He does tell us that we should consider the preferences of others when they are known to us and when we are in a situation in which we must act for them because they are unable to act for themselves. For example, suppose we know that a person approves of electro-convulsive therapy (shock treatments, or ECT) for the treatment of severe depression. If that person should become so depressed as to be unable to reach a decision about his own treatment, then we would be justified in seeing to it that he received ECT.

To take a similar case, suppose that you are a surgeon and have a patient who has expressed to you her wish to avoid numerous operations that may prolong her life six months or so but will be unable to restore her to health. If in operating you learned that she has a form of uterine cancer that had spread through her lower extremities and if in your best judgment nothing could be done to restore her to health, then it would be your duty to her to allow her to die as she chooses. Repeated operations would be contrary to her concept of her own good.

The most important question in exploring Rawls's theory is how the two principles of justice might apply to the social institutions and practices of medical care and research. Most obviously, Rawls's principles repair utilitarianism's flaw with respect to human experimentation. It would never be right, in Rawls's view, to exploit one group of people or even one person for the benefit of others. Thus, experiments in which people are forced to be subjects or are tricked into participating are ruled out. They involve a violation of basic liberties of individuals and of the absolute respect for persons that the principles of justice require.

A person has a right to decide what risks she is willing to take with her own life and health. Thus, voluntary consent is required before someone can legitimately become a research subject. However, society might decide to reward research volunteers with money, honors, or social privileges to encourage participation in research. Provided that the overall structure of society already conforms to the two principles of justice, this is a perfectly legitimate practice so long as it brings benefits (ideally) to everyone and the possibility of gaining the rewards of participation is open to all.

Regarding the allocation of social resources in the training of medical personnel (physicians, nurses, therapists, and so on), one may conclude that such investments are justified only if the withdrawal of the support would work to the disadvantage of those already most disadvantaged. Public money may be spent in the form of scholarships and institutional grants to educate personnel, who may then derive great social and economic benefits from their education. But for Rawls the inequality that is produced is not necessarily unjust. Society can invest its resources in this way if it brings benefits to those most in need of them.

The implication of this position seems to be that everyone is entitled to health care. First, it could be argued that health is among the "primary goods" that Rawls's principles are designed to protect and promote. After all, without health an individual is hardly in a position to pursue other more specific goods, and those in the original position might be imagined to be aware of this and to endorse only those principles of justice that would require providing at least basic health care to those in the society. Furthermore, it could be argued that the inequalities of the health-care system can be justified only if those in most need can benefit from them. Since this is not obviously the case with the present system, Rawls's principles seem to call for a reform that would provide health care to those who are unable to pay.

However, it is important to point out that it is not at all obvious that a demand to reform our health-care system follows from Rawls's position. For one thing, it is not clear that Rawls's principles are intended to be directly applied to our society as it is. Our society includes among its members people with serious disabilities and ones with both acute and chronic diseases. If Rawls's principles are intended to apply only to people with normal physical and psychological abilities and needs, as he sometimes suggests, then it is not clear that those who are ill can be regarded as appropriate candidates. If they are considered appropriate, then the results may be unacceptable. The principles of justice may require that we devote vast amounts of social resources to making only marginal improvements in the lives of those who are ill.

Furthermore, Rawls does not explicitly mention the promotion of health as one of the primary goods. It may seem reasonable to include it among them, given the significance of health as a condition for additional pursuits, but this is a point that requires support. (Norman Daniels is one who has argued for considering health a primary good.) This seems the most promising position to take if Rawls's principles are to be used as a basis for evaluating our current health policies and practices.

It seems reasonable to hold that Rawls's principles, particularly the second, can be used to restrict access to certain kinds of health care. In general, individuals may spend their money in any way they wish to seek their notions of what is good. Thus, if someone wants cosmetic surgery to change the shape of his chin and has the money to pay a surgeon, then he may have it done. But if medical facilities or personnel should become overburdened and unable to provide needed care for the more seriously afflicted, then the society would be obligated to forbid cosmetic surgery. By doing this it would then increase the net access to needed health care by all members of society. The rich who desired cosmetic surgery would not be permitted to exploit the poor who needed basic health care.

These are just a few of the possible implications that Rawls's theory has for medical research and practice. It seems likely that more and more applications of the theory will be worked out in detail in the future.

Difficulties

Rawls's theory is currently the subject of much discussion in philosophy. The debate is often highly technical, and a great number of objections have been raised. At present, however, there are no objections that would be acknowledged as legitimate by all critics. Rather than attempt to summarize the debate, we shall simply point to two aspects of Rawls's theory that have been acknowledged as difficulties.

One criticism concerns the original position and its veil of ignorance. Rawls does not permit those in the original position to know anything of their own purposes, plans, or interests—of their conception of the good. They do not know whether they prefer tennis to Tennyson, pleasures of mind over pleasures of the body. They are allowed to consider only those goods—self-respect, wealth, social position—that Rawls puts before them. Thus, critics have said, Rawls has excluded morally relevant knowledge. It is impossible to see how people could agree on principles to regulate their lives when they are so ignorant of their desires and purposes. Rawls seems to have biased the original position in his favor, and this calls into question his claim that the original position is a fair and reasonable way of arriving at principles of justice.

A second criticism focuses on whether Rawls's theory is really as different from utilitarianism as it appears to be. Rawls's theory may well permit inequalities of treatment under certain conditions in the same way that the principle of utility permits them. The principles of justice that were stated earlier apply, Rawls says, only when liberty can be effectively established and maintained. Rawls is very unclear about when a situation

may be regarded as one of this kind. When it is not, his principles of justice are ones of a "general conception." Under this conception, liberties of individuals can be restricted, provided that the restrictions are for the benefit of all. It is possible to imagine, then, circumstances in which we might force individuals to become experimental subjects both for their own benefit and for that of others. We might, for example, require that all cigarette smokers participate in experiments intended to acquire knowledge about lung and heart damage. Since everyone would benefit, directly or indirectly, from such knowledge, forcing their participation would be legitimate. Thus, under the general conception of justice, the difference between Rawls's principles and the principle of utility may, in practice, become vanishingly small.

NATURAL LAW ETHICS AND MORAL THEOLOGY

The general view that the rightness of actions is something determined by nature itself, rather than by the laws and customs of societies or the preferences of individuals, is called "natural law theory." Moral principles are thus regarded as objective truths that can be discovered in the nature of things by reason and reflection. The basic idea of the theory was expressed succinctly by the Roman philosopher Cicero (106–43 B.C.). "Law is the highest reason, implanted in Nature, which commands what ought to be done and forbids the opposite. This reason, when firmly fixed and fully developed in the human mind, is Law."

The natural law theory originated in classical Greek and Roman philosophy and has immensely influenced the development of moral and political theories. Indeed, all the ethical theories we have discussed are indebted to the natural law tradition. The reliance upon reason as a means of settling upon or establishing ethical principles and the emphasis on the need to reckon with the natural abilities and inclinations of human nature are just two of the threads that are woven into the theories that we have discussed.

Purposes, Reason, and the Moral Law as Interpreted by Roman Catholicism

The natural law theory of Roman Catholicism was given its most influential formulation in the thirteenth century by St. Thomas Aquinas (1225–1274). Contemporary versions of the theory are mostly elaborations and interpretations of Aquinas's basic statement. Thus, an understanding of Aquinas's views is important for grasping the philosophical principles that underlie the Roman Catholic position on such issues as abortion.

Aquinas was writing at a time in which a great number of the texts of Aristotle (384–322 B.C.) were becoming available in the West, and Aquinas's philosophical theories incorporated many of Aristotle's principles. A fundamental notion borrowed by Aquinas is the view that the universe is organized in a teleological way. That is, the universe is structured in such a way that each thing in it has a goal or purpose. Thus, when conditions are right, a tadpole will develop into a frog. In its growth and change, the tadpole is following "the law of its nature." It is achieving its goal.

Humans have a material nature, just as a tadpole does, and in their own growth and development they too follow a law of their material nature. But Aquinas also stresses that humans possess a trait that no other creature does—reason. Thus, the full development of human potentialities—the fulfillment of human purpose—requires that we follow the direction of the law of reason, as well as being subjected to the laws of material human nature.

The development of reason is one of our ends as human beings, but we also rely upon reason to determine what our ends are and how we can achieve them. It is this function of reason that leads Aquinas to identify reason as the source of the moral law. Reason is practical in its operation, for it directs our actions so that we can bring about certain results. In giving us directions, reason imposes an obligation on us, the obligation to bring about the results that it specifies. But Aquinas says that reason cannot arbitrarily set goals for us. Reason directs us toward our good as the goal of our action, and what that good is, is discoverable within our nature. Thus reason recognizes the basic principle "Good is to be done and evil avoided."

But this principle is purely formal, or empty of content. To make it a practical principle we must consider what the human good is. According to Aquinas, the human good is that which is suitable or proper to human nature. It is what is "built into" human nature in the way that, in a sense, a frog is already "built into" a tadpole. Thus, the good is that to which we are directed by our natural inclinations as both physical and rational creatures.

Like other creatures, we have a natural inclination to preserve our lives; consequently, reason imposes on us an obligation to care for our health, not to kill ourselves, and not to put ourselves in positions in which we might be killed. We realize through reason that others have a rational nature like ours, and we see that we are bound to treat them with the same dignity and respect that we accord ourselves. Furthermore, when we see that humans require a society to make their full development possible, we realize that we have an obligation to support laws and practices that make society possible.

Thus, for example, as we have a natural inclination to propagate our species (viewed as a "natural" good), reason places on us an obligation not to thwart or pervert this inclination. As a consequence, to fulfill this obligation within society, reason supports the institution of marriage.

Reason also finds in our nature grounds for procedural principles. For example, because everyone has an inclination to preserve his life and well-being, no one should be forced to testify against himself. Similarly, because all individuals are self-interested, no one should be permitted to be a judge in his own case.

Physical inclinations, under the direction of reason, point us toward our natural good. But, according to Aquinas, reason itself can also be a source of inclinations. For example, Aquinas says that reason is the source of our natural inclination to seek the truth, particularly the truth about the existence and nature of God.

Just from the few examples we have considered, it should be clear how Aquinas believed it was possible to discover in human nature natural goods. Relying upon these as goals or purposes to be achieved, reason would then work out the practical way of achieving them. Thus, through the subtle application of reason, it should be possible to establish a body of moral principles and rules. These are the doctrines of natural law.

Because natural law is founded on human nature, which is regarded as unchangeable, Aquinas regards natural law itself as unchangeable. Moreover, it is seen as the same for all people, at all times, and in all societies. Even those without knowledge of God can, through the operation of reason, recognize their natural obligations.

For Aquinas and for Roman Catholicism, this view of natural law is just one aspect of a broader theological framework. The teleological organization of the universe is attributed to the planning of a creator—goals or purposes are ordained by God. Furthermore, although natural law is discoverable in the universe, its ultimate source is divine wisdom and God's eternal law. Everyone who is rational is capable of grasping natural law. But because passions and irrational inclinations may corrupt human nature and because some people lack the abilities or time to work out the demands of natural law, God also chose to reveal our duties to us in explicit ways. The major source of revelation, of course, is taken to be the Biblical scriptures.

Natural law, scriptural revelation, the interpretation of the scriptures by the Church, Church tradition, and the teachings of the Church are regarded in Roman Catholicism as the sources of moral ideals and principles. By guiding one's life by them, one can develop the rational and moral part of one's nature and move towards the goal of achieving the sort of perfection that is suitable for humans.

This general moral-theological point of view is the source for particular Roman Catholic doctrines that have special relevance to medicine. We shall consider just two of the most important principles.

The Principle of Double Effect.   A particular kind of moral conflict arises when the performance of an action will produce both good and bad effects. On the basis of the good effect, it seems it is our duty to perform the action; but on the basis of the bad effect, it seems our duty not to perform it.

Let's assume that the death of a fetus is in itself a bad effect and consider a case like the following: A woman who is three months pregnant is found to have a cancerous uterus. If the woman's life is to be saved, the uterus must be removed at once. But if the uterus is removed, then the life of the unborn child will be lost. Should the operation be performed?

The principle of double effect is intended to help in the resolution of these kinds of conflicts. The principle holds that such an action should be performed only if the intention is to bring about the good effect and the bad effect will be an unintended or indirect consequence. More specifically, four conditions must be satisfied:

1. The action itself must be morally indifferent or morally good.

2. The bad effect must not be the means by which the good effect is achieved.

3. The motive must be the achievement of the good effect only.

4. The good effect must be at least equivalent in importance to the bad effect.

Are these conditions satisfied in the case that we mentioned? The operation itself, if this is considered to be the action, is at least morally indifferent. That is, in itself it is neither good nor bad. That takes care of the first condition. If the mother's life is to be saved, it will not be *by means of* killing the fetus. It will be by means of removing the cancerous uterus. Thus, the second condition is met. The motive of the surgeon, we may suppose, is not the death of the fetus but saving the life of the woman. If so, then the third condition is satisfied. Finally, since two lives are at stake, the good effect (saving the life of the woman) is at least equal to the bad effect (the death of the fetus). The fourth condition is thus met. Under ordinary conditions, then, these conditions would be considered satisfied and such an operation would be morally justified.

The principle of double effect is most often mentioned in a medical context in cases of abortion. But, in fact, it has a much wider range of application in medical ethics. It bears on cases of contraception, sterilization, organ transplants, and the use of extraordinary measures to maintain life.

The Principle of Totality.   The principle of totality can be expressed in this way: An individual has a right to dispose of his organs or to destroy their capacity to function only to the extent that the general well-being of the whole body demands it. Thus, it is clear that we have a natural obligation to preserve our lives, but, by the Roman Catholic view, we also have a duty to preserve the integrity of our bodies. This duty is based on the belief that each of our organs was designed by God to play a role in maintaining the functional integrity of our bodies, that each has a place in the divine plan. As we are the custodians of our bodies, not their owners, it is our duty to care for them as a trust.

The principle of totality has implications for a great number of medical procedures. Strictly speaking, even cosmetic surgery is morally right only when it is required to maintain or assure the normal functioning of the rest of the body. More important, procedures that are typically employed for contraceptive purposes—vasectomies and tubal ligations—are ruled out. After all, such procedures involve "mutilation" and the destruction of the capacity of the organs of reproduction to function properly. The principle of totality thus also forbids the sterilization of the mentally retarded.

As an ethical theory, natural law theory is sometimes described as teleological. In endorsing the principle "Good is to be done and evil avoided," the theory identifies a goal with respect to which the rightness of an action is to be judged. As the principle of double effect illustrates, the intention of the individual who acts is crucial to determining whether the goal is sought. In a sense, the intention of the action, what the individual wills, defines the action. Thus, "performing an abortion" and "saving a woman's life" are not necessarily the same action, even in those instances in which their external features are the same. Unlike utilitarianism, which is also a teleological theory, natural law theory is not consequentialist: the outcome of an action is not the sole feature to consider in determining the moral character of the action.

Applications of Roman Catholic Moral-Theological Viewpoints in the Medical Context

Roman Catholic ethicists and moral theologians have written numerous aspects of medical ethics and developed a body of widely accepted doctrine. We shall consider only four topics.

First, the application of the principle of double effect and the principle of totality have definite consequences in the area of medical experimentation. Since we hold our bodies in trust, we are responsible for assessing the degree of risk present in an experiment in which we are asked to be a subject. Thus, we need to be fully informed of the nature of the experiment and the risks that it holds for us. If after obtaining this knowledge we decide to give our consent, it must be given freely and not as the result of deception or coercion.

Because human experimentation carries with it the possibility of injury and death, the principle of double effect and its four strictures apply. If scientific evidence indicates that a sick person may benefit from participating in an experiment, then the experiment is morally justifiable. If, however, the evidence indicates that the chances of helping that person are slight and he or she may die or be gravely injured, then the experiment is not justified. In general, the likelihood of a person's benefitting from the experiment must exceed the danger of that person's suffering greater losses.

A person who is incurably ill may volunteer to be an experimental subject, even though she or he cannot reasonably expect personal gain in the form of improved health. The good that is hoped for is good for others, in the form of increased medical knowledge. Even here, however, there are constraints imposed by the principle of double effect. There must be no likelihood that the experiment will seriously injure, and the probable value of the knowledge expected to result must balance the risk run by the patient. Not even the incurably ill can be made subjects of trivial experiments.

The good sought by healthy volunteers is also the good of others. The same restrictions mentioned in connection with the incurably ill apply to experimenting on healthy people. Additionally, the principle of totality places constraints on what a person may volunteer to do with his or her body. No healthy person may submit to an experiment that involves the probability of serious injury, impaired health, mutilation, or death.

A second medical topic addressed by Roman Catholic theologians is whether "ordinary" or "extraordinary" measures are to be taken in the preservation of human life. While it is believed that natural law and divine law impose on us a moral obligation to preserve our lives, Catholic moralists have interpreted this obligation as requiring that we rely upon only ordinary means. In the medical profession, the phrase "ordinary means" is used to refer to medical procedures that are standard or orthodox, in contrast with those that are untried or experimental. But from the viewpoint of Catholic ethics, "ordinary" used in the medical context applies to "all medicines, treatments, and operations which offer a reasonable hope of benefit for the patient and which can be obtained and used without excessive expense, pain, or other inconvenience." Thus, by contrast, extraordinary means are those that offer the patient no reasonable hope or whose use causes serious hardship for the patient or others.

Medical measures that would save the life of a patient but subject her to years of pain or would produce in her severe physical or mental incapacities are considered extraordinary. A patient or her family are under no obligation to choose them, and physicians are under a positive obligation not to encourage their choice.

The third medical topic for consideration is euthanasia. In the Roman Catholic ethical view, euthanasia in any form is considered immoral. It is presumed to be a direct violation of God's dominion over creation and the human obligation to preserve life. The Ethical Directives for Catholic Hospitals is explicit on the matter of taking a life:

The direct killing of any innocent person, even at his own request, is always morally wrong. Any procedure whose sole immediate effect is the death of a human being is a direct killing. . . . Euthanasia ("mercy killing") in all its forms is forbidden. . . . The failure to supply the ordinary means of preserving life is equivalent to euthanasia.

According to this view, it is wrong to allow babies suffering from serious birth defects to die. If they can be saved by ordinary means, there is an obligation to do so. It is also wrong to act to terminate the lives of those hopelessly ill, either by taking steps to bring about their deaths or by failing to take steps to maintain their lives by ordinary means.

It is never permissible to hasten the death of a person as a direct intention. It is, however, permissible to administer drugs that alleviate pain. The principle of double effect suggests that giving such drugs is a morally justifiable action even though the drugs may indirectly hasten the death of a person.

Last, we may inquire how Roman Catholicism views abortion. According to the Roman Catholic view, from the moment of conception the conceptus (later, the fetus) is considered to be a person with all the rights of a person. For this reason, direct abortion at any stage of pregnancy is regarded as morally wrong. Abortion is "direct" when it results from a procedure "whose sole immediate effect is the termination of pregnancy." This means that what is generally referred to as therapeutic abortion, in which an abortion is performed to safeguard the life or health of the woman, is considered wrong. For example, a woman with serious heart disease who becomes pregnant cannot morally justify an abortion on the grounds that the pregnancy is a serious threat to her life. Even when the ultimate aim is to save the life of the woman, direct abortion is wrong.

We have already seen, however, that the principle of double effect permits the performance of an action that may result in the death of an unborn child if the action satisfies the four criteria for applying the principle. Thus, *indirect* abortion is considered to be morally permissible. That is, the abortion must be the outcome of some action (for example, removal of a cancerous uterus) that is performed for the direct and total purpose of treating a pathological condition affecting the woman. The end sought in direct abortion is the destruction of life, but the end sought in indirect abortion is the preservation of life.

Difficulties

Our discussion has centered on the natural law theory of ethics as it has been interpreted in Roman Catholic theology. Thus, there are two possible types of difficulties: those associated with natural law ethics in its own right and those associated with its incorporation into theology. The theological difficulties go beyond the scope of our aims and interests. We shall restrict ourselves to considering the basic difficulty that faces natural law theory as formulated by Aquinas. Since it is this formulation that has been used in Roman Catholic moral theology, we shall be raising a problem for it in an indirect way.

The fundamental difficulty with Aquinas's argument for natural law is caused by the assumption, borrowed from Aristotle, that the universe is organized in a teleological fashion. (This is the assumption that every kind of thing has a goal or purpose.) This assumption is essential to Aquinas's ethical theory, for he identifies the good of a thing with its natural mode of operation. Without the assumption, we are faced with the great diversity and moral indifference of nature. Inclinations, even when shared by all humans, are no more than inclinations. There are no grounds for considering them "goods," and they have no moral status. The universe is bereft of natural values.

Yet, there are many reasons to consider this assumption false. Physics surrendered the notion of a teleological organization in the world as long ago as the seventeenth century—the rejection of Aristotle's physics also entailed the rejection of Aristotle's teleological view of the world. This left biology as the major source of arguments in favor of teleology. But contemporary evolutionary theory shows that the apparent purposive character of evolutionary change can be accounted for by the operation of natural selection on random mutations. Also, the development and growth of organisms can be explained by the presence of genetic information that controls the processes. The tadpole develops into a frog because evolution has produced a genetic program that directs the sequence of complicated chemical changes. Thus, there seems to be no adequate grounds for asserting that the teleological organization of nature is anything more than apparent.

Science and "reason alone" do not support teleology. It can be endorsed only if one is willing to assume that any apparent teleological organization is the product of a divine plan. Yet, because all apparent teleology can be explained in nonteleological ways, this assumption seems neither necessary nor legitimate.

Without its foundation of teleology, Aquinas's theory of natural law ethics seems to collapse. This is not to say, of course, that some other natural law theory, one not requiring the assumption of teleology, might not be persuasively defended.

II. MAJOR MORAL PRINCIPLES

Making moral decisions is always a difficult and stressful task. Abstract discussions of issues never quite capture the feelings of uncertainty and self-doubt we characteristically experience when called upon to decide what ought to be done or to judge whether someone did the right thing. There are no mechanical processes or algorithms we can apply in a situation of moral doubt. There are no computer programs to supply us with the proper decision when given the relevant data.

In a very real sense, we are on our own when it comes to making ethical decisions. This does not mean that we are without resources and must decide blindly or even naively. When we have the luxury of time, when the need to make a decision is not pressing, then we may attempt to work out an answer to a moral question by relying upon a general ethical theory like those discussed earlier. However, in ordinary life we rarely have the opportunity or time to engage in an elaborate process of reasoning and analysis.

A more practical approach is to employ moral principles that have been derived from and justified by a moral theory. A principle such as "Avoid causing needless harm" can serve as a more direct guide to action and decision making than, say, Kant's categorical imperative. With such a principle in mind, we realize that, if we are acting as a physician, then we have a duty to use our knowledge and skills to protect our patients from injury. For example, we should not expose a patient to the needless risk of a diagnostic test that does not promise to yield useful information.

In this section, we will present and illustrate five moral principles. All are ones of special relevance to dealing with the ethical issues presented by decisions concerning medical care. The principles have their limitations. For one thing, they are in no sense complete. Moral issues arise, even in the context of medicine, for which they can supply no direct guidance. In other situations, the principles themselves may come into conflict and point toward incompatible solutions. (How can we both avoid causing harm and allow a terminally ill patient to die?) The principles themselves indicate no way such conflicts can be resolved, for, even taken together, they do not constitute a coherent moral theory. To resolve conflicts, it may be necessary to employ the more basic principles of such a theory.

It is fair to say that each of the five basic moral theories we have discussed endorses the legitimacy of these principles. Not all would formulate them in the same way, and not all would give them the same moral weight. Nevertheless, each theory would accept them as expressing appropriate guidelines for moral decision making.

Indeed, the best way to think about the principles is as guidelines. They are in no way rules that can be applied automatically. Rather, they express standards to be consulted in attempting to arrive at a justified decision. As such, they provide a basis for evaluating actions or policies as well as for making individual moral decisions. They help guarantee that our decisions are made in accordance with principles and not according to our whims or prejudices. By following them we are more likely to reach decisions that are reasoned, consistent, and applicable to similar cases.

THE PRINCIPLE OF NONMALEFICENCE

"Above all, do no harm" is perhaps the most famous and most quoted of all moral maxims in medicine. It captures in a succinct way what is universally considered to be an overriding duty of anyone who undertakes the care of a patient. We believe that in treating a patient a physician should not by carelessness, malice, inadvertence, or avoidable ignorance do anything that will cause injury to the patient.

The maxim is one expression of what is sometimes called in ethics the principle of nonmaleficence. The principle can be formu-

lated in various ways, but here is one relatively noncontroversial way of stating it: *We ought to act in ways that do not cause needless harm or injury to others.* Stated in a positive fashion, the principle tells us that we have a duty to avoid maleficence, that is to avoid harming or injuring other people.

In the most obvious case, we violate the principle of nonmaleficence when we intentionally do something we know will cause someone harm. For example, suppose that a surgeon during the course of an operation deliberately severs a muscle, knowing that by doing so he will cripple the patient. The surgeon is guilty of maleficence and is morally (as well as legally) blameworthy for his action.

The principle may also be violated when no malice or intention to do harm is involved. A nurse who carelessly gives a patient the wrong medication and causes the patient to suffer irreversible brain damage may have had no intention of causing the patient any injury. However, the nurse was negligent in his actions and failed to exercise due care in discharging his responsibilities. His actions resulted in an avoidable injury to his patient. Hence, he failed to meet his obligation of nonmaleficence.

The duty imposed by the principle of nonmaleficence is not a demand to accomplish the impossible. We realize that we cannot reasonably expect perfection in the practice of medicine. We know that the results of treatments are often uncertain and may cause more harm than good. We know that the knowledge we have of diseases is only partial and that decisions about diagnosis and therapy typically involve the exercise of judgment, with no guarantee of correctness. We know there is an uncertainty built into the very nature of things and that our power to control the outcome of natural processes is limited. Consequently, we realize that we cannot hold physicians and other health professionals accountable for every instance of death and injury involving patients under their care.

Nevertheless, we can demand that physicians and others live up to reasonable standards of performance. In the conduct of their professions, we can expect them to be cautious and diligent, patient and thoughtful. We can expect them to pay attention to what they are doing and to deliberate about whether a particular procedure should be done. In addition, we can expect them to possess the knowledge and skills relevant to the proper discharge of their duties.

These features and others like them make up the standards of performance that define what we have a right to expect from physicians and other health professionals. In the language of the law, these are the standards of "due care," and it is by reference to them that we evaluate the medical care given to patients. Failure to meet the standards opens practitioners (physicians, nurses, dentists, therapists) to the charge of moral or legal maleficence.

In our society, we have attempted to guarantee that at least some of the due-care standards are met by relying upon such measures as degree programs, licensing laws, certifying boards, and hospital credentials committees. Such an approach offers a way of seeing to it that physicians and others have acquired at least a minimum level of knowledge, skill, and experience before undertaking the responsibilities attached to their roles. The approach also encourages such values as diligence, prudence, and caution, but there is of course no way of guaranteeing that in a particular case a physician will exhibit those virtues. Haste, carelessness, and inattention are always possible, and the potential that a patient will suffer an injury from them is always present.

The standards of due care are connected in some respects with such factual matters as the current state of medical knowledge and training and the immediate circumstances in which a physician provides care. For example, in the 1920s and 1930s, it was not at all unusual for a general practitioner to perform relatively complicated surgery. This was particularly true of someone practicing in a rural area. In performing surgery, he would be acting in a reasonable and expected fashion and could not be legitimately charged with violating the principle of nonmaleficence.

However, the change in medicine from that earlier time to the present has also altered our beliefs about what is reasonable and expected. Today a general practitioner who has had no special training and is not board certified and yet performs surgery on his patients may be legitimately criticized for maleficence. The standards of due care in surgery are now higher and more exacting than they once were, and the general practitioner who undertakes to perform most forms of surgery causes his patients to undergo an unusual and unnecessary risk literally at his hands. Their interest would be better served if their surgery were performed by a trained and qualified surgeon.

Such a case also illustrates that no actual harm or injury must occur for someone to be acting in violation of the principle of nonmaleficence. The general practitioner performing surgery may not cause any injury to his patients, but he puts them in a position in which the possibility of harm to them is greater than it needs to be. It is in this respect that he is not exercising due care in his treatment and so can be charged with maleficence. He has subjected his patients to *unnecessary* risk, risk greater than they would be subject to in the hands of a trained surgeon.

It is important to stress that the principle of nonmaleficence does not require that a physician subject a patient to no risks at all. Virtually every form of diagnostic testing and medical treatment involves some degree of risk to the patient, and to provide medical care at all, a physician must often act in ways that involve a possible injury to the patient.

For example, a physician who takes a thorough medical history and performs a physical examination, then treats a patient with an antibiotic for bacterial infection cannot be held morally responsible if the patient suffers a severe drug reaction. That such a thing might happen is a possibility that cannot be foreseen in an individual case.

Similarly, a serious medical problem may justify subjecting the patient to a serious risk. (Gaining the consent of the patient is an obvious consideration, however.) A life-threatening condition, such as an occluded right coronary artery, may warrant coronary-bypass surgery, with all its attendant dangers.

In effect, the principle of nonmaleficence tells us to avoid needless risk and, when risk is an inevitable aspect of an appropriate diagnostic test or treatment, to minimize the risk as much as is reasonably possible. A physician who orders a lumbar puncture for a patient who complains of occasional headaches is acting inappropriately, given the nature of the complaint, and is subjecting his patient to needless risk. By contrast, a physician who orders such a test after examining a patient who has severe and recurring headaches, a fever, pain and stiffness in his neck, and additional key clinical signs is acting appropriately. The risk to the patient from the lumbar puncture is the same in both cases, but the risk is warranted in the second case and not in the first. A failure to act with due care violates the principle of nonmaleficence, even if no harm results, whereas acting with due care does not violate the principle, even if harm does result.

THE PRINCIPLE OF BENEFICENCE

"As to diseases, make a habit of two things—to help or at least to do no harm." This directive from the Hippocratic writings stresses that the physician has two duties. The second of them ("at least to do no harm") we dis-

cussed in connection with the principle of nonmaleficence. The first of them ("to help") we will consider here in connection with the principle of beneficence.

Like the previous principle, the principle of beneficence can be stated in various and different ways. Here is one formulation: *We should act in ways that promote the welfare of other people.* That is, we should help other people when we are able to do so.

Some philosophers have expressed doubt that we have an actual duty to help others. We certainly have a duty not to harm other people, but it has seemed to some that there are no grounds for saying that we have a duty to promote their welfare. We would deserve praise if we did, but we would not deserve blame if we did not. From this point of view, being beneficent is beyond the scope of duty.

We need not consider whether this view is correct in general. For our purposes, it is enough to realize that the nature of the relationship between a physician and a patient does impose the duty of acting in the patient's welfare. That is, the duty of beneficence is inherent in the role of physician. A physician who was not acting for the sake of the patient's good would, in a very real sense, not be acting as a physician.

That we recognize this as a duty appropriate to the physician's role is seen most clearly in cases in which the physician is also a researcher and his patient is also an experimental subject. In such instances, there is a possibility of a role conflict, for the researcher's aim of acquiring knowledge is not always compatible with the physician's aim of helping the patient. (See Chapter 5 for a discussion of this problem.)

The duty required by the principle of beneficence is inherent in the role not only of physicians but of all health professionals. Nurses, therapists, clinical psychologists, social workers, and others accept the duty of promoting the welfare of their patients or clients as an appropriate part of their responsibilities. We expect nurses and others to do good for us, and it is this expectation that leads us to designate them as belonging to what are often called "the helping professions."

The extent to which beneficence is required as a duty for physicians and others is not a matter easily resolved. In practice, we recognize that there are limits to what can be expected from even those who have chosen to make a career of helping others. We do not expect physicians to sacrifice completely their self-interest and welfare on behalf of their patients. We do not think their duty demands that they be totally selfless. If some do, we may praise them as secular saints or moral heroes, but that is because they go beyond the demands of duty. At the same time, we would have little good to say of a physician who always put her interest above that of her patients, who never made a personal sacrifice to serve their interests.

Just as there are standards of due care that explicitly and implicitly define what we consider to be right conduct in protecting patients from harm, so there seem to be implicit standards of beneficence. We obviously expect physicians to help patients by providing them with appropriate treatment. More than this, we expect physicians to be prepared to make *reasonable* sacrifices for the sake of their patients. Even in the age of "health-care teams," a single physician assumes responsibility for a particular patient when the patient is hospitalized or treated for a serious illness. It is this physician who is expected to make the crucial medical decisions, and we expect him or her to realize that discharging that responsibility may involve an interruption of private plans and activities. A surgeon who is informed that her postoperative patient has started to bleed can be expected to cancel her plan to attend a concert. Doing so is a reasonable duty imposed by the principle of beneficence. If she failed to discharge the duty, in

the absence of mitigating circumstances, she would become the object of disapproval by her patient and by her medical colleagues.

It would be very difficult to spell out exactly what duties are required by the principle of beneficence. Even if we limited ourselves to the medical context, there are so many ways of promoting someone's welfare and so many different circumstances to consider that it would be virtually impossible to provide anything like a catalogue of appropriate actions. However, such a catalogue is hardly necessary. Most people most often have a sense of what is reasonable and what is not, and it is this sense that we rely on in making judgments about whether physicians and others are fulfilling the duty of beneficence in their actions.

The principles of nonmaleficence and beneficence impose social duties also. In the most general terms, we look to society to take measures to promote the health and safety of its citizens. The great advances made in public health during the nineteenth century were made because the society recognized a responsibility to attempt to prevent the spread of disease. Water treatment plants, immunization programs, and quarantine restrictions were all in recognition of society's duty of nonmaleficence.

These and similar programs have been continued and augmented, and our society has also recognized a duty of beneficence in connection with health care. The Medicaid program for the poor and Medicare for the elderly are major efforts to see to at least some of the health needs of a large segment of the population. Prenatal programs for expectant mothers and public clinics are among the other social responses we have made to promote the health of citizens.

Less obvious than programs that provide direct medical care are ones that support medical research and basic science. Directly or indirectly, such programs contribute to meeting the health needs of our society.

Much basic research is relevant to acquiring an understanding of the processes involved in both health and disease, and much medical research is specifically aimed at the development of effective diagnostic and therapeutic measures.

In principle, social beneficence has no limits, but in practice it must. Social resources like tax revenues are in restricted supply, and the society must decide how they are to be spent. Housing and food for the poor, education, defense, the arts, and the humanities are just some of the areas demanding support in the name of social beneficence. Medical care is just one among many claimants, and we must decide as a society what proportion of our social resources we want to commit to medical care. Are we prepared to guarantee to all whatever medical care they need? Are we willing to endorse only a basic level of care? Do we want to say that what is available to some (the rich or well-insured) must be available to all (the poor and uninsured)? Just how beneficent we wish to be—and can afford to be—is a matter still under discussion (see Chapter 9).

THE PRINCIPLE OF UTILITY

The principle of utility can be formulated in this way: *We should act in such a way as to bring about the greatest benefit and the least harm.* As we discussed earlier, the principle is the very foundation of the moral theory of utilitarianism. However, the principle need not be regarded as unique to utilitarianism. It can be thought of as one moral principle among others that present us with a prima facie duty, and as such it need not be regarded as always taking precedence over others. In particular, we would never think it was justified to deprive someone of a right, even if by doing so we could bring benefit to many others.

We need not repeat the discussion of the principle of utility presented earlier, but it may be useful to consider here how the principle relates to the principles of nonmaleficence and beneficence. When we consider the problem of distributing social resources, it becomes clear that acting in accordance with the principles of nonmaleficence and beneficence usually involves tradeoffs. To use our earlier example, as a society we are concerned with providing for the health-care needs of our citizens. To accomplish this end, we support various programs—Medicare, Medicaid, hospital-building programs, medical research, and so on.

However, there are limits to what we can do. Medical care is not the only concern of our society. We are interested in protecting people from harm and in promoting their interests, but there are many forms of harm and many kinds of interest to be promoted. With finite resources at our disposal, the more money we spend on health care, the less we can spend on education, the arts, the humanities, and so on.

Even if we decided to spend more money on health care than we are currently spending, there would come a point at which we would receive only a marginal return for our money. General health would eventually reach such a level that it would be difficult to raise it still higher. To save even one additional life, we would have to spend a vast sum of money. By contrast, at the start of a health-care program, relatively little money can make a relatively big difference. Furthermore, money spent for marginal improvements would be directed away from other needs that had become even more crucial because of underfunding. Thus, we could not spend all our resources on health care without ignoring other social needs.

The aim of social planning is to balance the competing needs of the society. Taken alone, the principles of nonmaleficence and beneficence are of no help in resolving the conflicts among social needs. The principle of utility must come into play to establish and rank needs and to serve as a guide for determining to what extent it is possible to satisfy one social need in comparison with others. In effect, the principle imposes a social duty on us all to use our resources to do as much good as possible. That is, we must do the most good *overall*, even when this means we are not able to meet all needs in a particular area.

The application of the principle of utility is not limited to large-scale social issues, such as how to divide our resources among medical care, defense, education, and so on. We may also rely on the principle when we are deliberating about the choice of alternative means of accomplishing an aim. For example, we might decide to institute a mandatory screening program to detect infants with PKU but decide against a program to detect those with Tay-Sachs. PKU can often be treated successfully if discovered early enough, whereas early detection of Tay-Sachs makes little or no difference in the outcome of the disease. Furthermore, PKU is distributed in the general population, whereas Tay-Sachs occurs mostly in a special segment of the population. In general, then, the additional money spent on screening for Tay-Sachs would not be justified by the results. The money could do more good, produce more benefits, were it spent some other way.

The principle of utility is also relevant to making decisions about the diagnosis and treatment of individuals. For example, as we mentioned earlier, no diagnostic test can be justified if it causes the patient more risk than the information likely to be gained is worth. Invasive procedures are associated with a certain rate of injury and death (morbidity and mortality). It would make no sense to subject a patient to a kidney biopsy if the findings were not likely to affect the course of treatment or if the risk from the biopsy were greater than the risk of the suspected disease itself.

Attempts are well underway in medicine

to employ the formal theories of decision analysis to assist physicians in determining whether a particular mode of diagnosis, therapy, or surgery can be justified in individual cases. Underlying the details of formal analysis is the principle of utility, which directs us to act in a way that will bring about the greatest benefit and the least harm.

PRINCIPLES OF DISTRIBUTIVE JUSTICE

We expect (and can demand) to be treated justly in our dealings with other people and with institutions. If our insurance policy covers up to thirty days of hospitalization, then we expect a claim against the policy for that amount of time to be honored. If we arrive in an emergency room with a broken arm before the arrival of someone else with a broken arm, we expect to be attended to before that person.

We do not always expect that being treated justly will work to our direct advantage. Although we would prefer to keep all the money we earn, we realize that we must pay our share of taxes. If a profusely bleeding person arrives in the emergency room after we do, we recognize that he is in need of immediate treatment and should be attended to before we are.

Justice has at least two major aspects. Seeing to it that people receive that to which they are entitled, that their rights are recognized and protected, falls under the general heading of *noncomparative justice*. By contrast, *comparative justice* is concerned with the application of laws and rules and with the distribution of burdens and benefits.

The concern of comparative justice that is most significant to the medical context is *distributive justice*. As the name suggests, distributive justice concerns the distribution of such social benefits and burdens as medical services, welfare payments, public offices, taxes, and military service. In general, the distribution of income has been the focus of recent discussions of distributive justice. In medical ethics, the focus has been the distribution of health care. Is everyone in the society entitled to receive health-care benefits, whether or not she or he can pay for them? If so, then is everyone entitled to the same amount of health care? (See Chapter 9 for a discussion of this issue.)

Philosophical theories of justice attempt to resolve questions of distributive justice by providing a detailed account of the features of individuals and society that will justify our making distinctions in the ways we distribute benefits and burdens. If some people are to be rich and others poor, if some are to rule and others serve, then there must be some rational and moral basis for such distinctions. We look to theories of justice to provide us with such a basis. (See the earlier discussion of John Rawls's theory for an outstanding recent example.)

Theories of justice differ significantly, but at the core of all theories is the basic principle that "Similar cases ought to be treated in similar ways." The principle expresses the notion that justice involves fairness of treatment. For example, it is manifestly unfair to award two different grades to two people who score the same on a multiple-choice exam. If two cases are the same, then it is arbitrary or irrational to treat them differently. To justify different treatment, we would have to show that in some relevant respect the cases are also dissimilar.

This fairness principle is known as the *formal* principle of justice. It is called "formal" because, like a sentence with blanks, it must be filled in with information. Specifically, we must be told what factors or features are to be considered *relevant* in deciding whether or not two cases are similar. If two cases differ in *relevant* respects, we may be justified in treating them differently. We may do so without being either irrational or arbitrary.

Theories of distributive justice present us with *substantive* (or *material*) principles of justice. The theories present us with arguments to show why certain features or factors should be considered relevant in deciding whether cases are similar. The substantive principles can then be referred to in determining whether particular laws, practices, or public policies can be considered just. Further, the substantive principles can be employed as guidelines for framing laws and policies and for developing a just society.

Arguments in favor of particular theories of justice are too lengthy to present here. However, it is useful to consider briefly four substantive principles that have been offered by various theorists as ones worthy of acceptance. To a considerable extent, differences among these principles help explain present disagreements in our society about the ways in which such social "goods" as income, education, and health care should be distributed. Although the principles themselves direct the distribution of burdens (taxation, public service, and so on) as well as benefits, we will focus on benefits. The basic question answered by each principle is, "Who is entitled to what proportion of society's goods?"

The Principle of Equality

According to the principle of equality, all benefits and burdens are to be distributed equally. Everyone is entitled to the same size slice of the pie, and everyone must bear an equal part of the social load. The principle, strictly interpreted, requires a radical egalitarianism—everyone is to be treated the same in all respects.

The principle is most plausible for a society above the margin of production. When there is enough to go around but not much more, then it is manifestly unfair for some to have more than they need and for others to have less than they need. When a society is more affluent, the principle may lose some of its persuasiveness. When greater efforts by a few produce more goods than the efforts of the ordinary person, it may be unfair not to recognize the accomplishments of a few by greater rewards. Rawls's theory remains an egalitarian one, while providing a way to resolve this apparent conflict. According to Rawls, any departure from equality is arbitrary, unless it can be shown that the inequality will work out to *everyone's* advantage.

The Principle of Need

The principle of need is an extension of the egalitarian principle of equal distribution. If goods are parceled out according to individual need, those who have greater needs will receive a greater share. However, the outcome will be one of equality. Since the basic needs of everyone will be met, everyone will end up at the same level. The treatment of individuals will be equal, in this respect, even though the proportion of goods they receive will not be.

What is to count as a need is a significant question that cannot be answered by a principle of distribution alone. Obviously, basic biological needs (food, clothing, shelter) must be included, but what about psychological or intellectual needs? The difficulty of resolving the question of needs is seen in the fact that—even in our affluent society, the richest in the history of the world—we are still debating the question of whether health care should be available to all.

The Principle of Contribution

According to the principle of contribution, everyone should get back that proportion of social goods that is the result of his or her productive labor. If two people work to grow potatoes and the first works twice as long or twice as hard as the second, then the first should be entitled to twice as large a share of the harvest.

The difficulty with this principle in an in-dustrialized, capitalistic society is that contributions to production can take forms other than time and labor. Some people risk their money in investments needed to make production possible, and others contribute crucial ideas or inventions. How are comparisons to be made? Furthermore, in highly industrialized societies it is the functioning of the entire system, rather than the work of any particular individual, that creates the goods to be distributed. A single individual's claim on the outcome of the whole system may be very small.

Nonetheless, it is individuals who make the system work, so it does seem just that individuals should benefit from their contributions. If it is true that it is the system of social organization itself that is most responsible for creating the goods, then this is an argument for supporting the system through taxation and other means. If individual contributions count for relatively little (although for something), there may be no real grounds for attempting to distinguish among them in distributing social benefits.

The Principle of Effort

According to the principle of effort, the degree of effort made by the individual should determine the proportion of goods received by the individual. Thus, the file clerk who works just as hard as the president of a company should receive the same proportion of social goods as the president. Those who are lazy and refuse to exert themselves will receive proportionally less than those who work hard.

The advantage of the principle is that it captures our sense of what is fair—that those who do their best should be similarly rewarded, while those who do less than their best should be less well rewarded. The principle assumes that people have equal opportunities to do their best and that if they do not it is their own fault. One difficulty with this assumption is that, even if the society presents equal opportunities, nature does not. Some people are born with handicaps or meet with accidents, and their misfortunes may make it difficult for them to want to do their best, even when they are given the opportunity.

Each principle has its shortcomings, but this does not mean that adjustments cannot be made to correct their weaknesses. A complete theory of justice need not be limited in the number of principles that it accepts, and it is doubtful that any theory can be shown to be both fair and plausible if it restricts itself to only one principle. While all theories require adjustment, theories fall into types in accordance with the principles they emphasize. For example, Marxist theories select need as basic, while libertarian theories stress personal contribution as the grounds for distribution. Utilitarian theories employ that combination of principles that promises to maximize both private and public interests.

Joel Feinberg, to whom the preceding discussion is indebted, may be mentioned as an example of a careful theorist who recommends the adoption of a combination of principles. Feinberg sees the principle of equality based on needs as the basic determination of distributive justice. After basic needs have been satisfied, the principles of contribution and effort should be given the most weight.

According to Feinberg, when there is an economic abundance, then the claim to "minimally decent conditions" can reasonably be made for every person in the society. To have one's basic needs satisfied under such conditions amounts to a fundamental right. However, when everyone's basic needs are taken care of and society produces a surplus of goods, then considerations of contribution and effort become relevant. Those who contribute most to the increase of goods or those who work the hardest to produce it (or some combination) can legitimately lay claim to a greater share.

The principles of justice we have discussed may seem at first to be intolerably abstract and so irrelevant to the practical business of society. However, it is important to keep in mind that it is by referring to such principles that we criticize our society and its laws and practices. The claim that society is failing to meet some basic need of all of its citizens and that this is unfair or unjust is a powerful charge. It can be a call to action in the service of justice. If the claim can be demonstrated, it has more than rhetorical power. It imposes upon us all an obligation to eliminate the source of the injustice.

Similarly, in framing laws and formulating policies, we expect those who occupy the offices of power and influence to make their decisions in accordance with principles. Prominent among these must be principles of justice. It may be impossible in the conduct of daily business to apply any principle directly or exclusively, for we can hardly remake our society overnight. Yet if we are committed to a just society, then the principles of justice can at least serve as guidelines when policy decisions are made. They remind us that it is not always fair for the race to go to the swift.

THE PRINCIPLE OF AUTONOMY

The principle of autonomy can be stated this way: *Rational individuals should be permitted to be self-determining.* According to this formulation, we act autonomously when our actions are the result of our own choices and decisions. Thus, autonomy and self-determination are equivalent.

Autonomy is associated with the status we ascribe to rational beings as persons in the morally relevant sense. We are committed to the notion that persons are by their very nature uniquely qualified to decide what is in their own best interest. This is because, to use Kant's terms, they are ends in themselves, not means to some other end. As such, they have an inherent worth, and it is the duty of others to respect that worth and avoid treating them as though they were just ordinary parts of the world to be manipulated according to the will of someone else. A recognition of autonomy is a recognition of that inherent worth, and a violation of autonomy is a violation of our concept of what it is to be a person. To deny someone autonomy is to treat her or him as something less than a person.

This view of the nature of autonomy and its connection with our recognition of what is involved in being a person is shared by several significant moral theories. At the core of each theory is the concept of the rational individual as a moral agent who, along with other moral agents, possesses an unconditional worth. Moral responsibility itself is based on the assumption that such agents are free to determine their own actions and pursue their own aims.

Autonomy is significant not only because it is a condition for moral responsibility, but because it is through the exercise of autonomy that individuals shape their lives. We might not approve of what people do with their lives. It is sad to see talent wasted and opportunities for personal development rejected. Nevertheless, as we sometimes say, "It's *his* life." We recognize that people are entitled to attempt to make their lives what they want them to be and that it would be wrong for us to take control of their lives and dictate their actions, even if we could. We recognize that a person must walk to heaven or hell by his own freely chosen path.

Simply put, to act autonomously is to decide for one's self what to do. Of course, decisions are never made outside of a context, and the world and the people in it exert influence, impose constraints, and restrict opportunities. It is useful to call attention to three interrelated aspects of autonomy in order to get a better understanding of the ways in which autonomy can be exercised, denied, and restricted. We will look at autonomy in the contexts of actions, options, and decision making.

Autonomy and Actions

Consider the following situations:

A police officer shoves a demonstrator off the sidewalk during an abortion protest.

An attendant in a psychiatric ward warns a patient to stay in bed or be strapped down.

A corrections officer warns a prison inmate that if he does not donate blood he will not be allowed out of his cell to eat dinner.

A state law requires that anyone admitted to a hospital be screened for the AIDS antibody.

In each of these situations, either actual force, the threat of force, or potential penalties are employed to direct the actions of an individual toward some end. All involve some form of coercion, and the coercion is used to restrict the freedom of individuals to act as they might choose.

Under such circumstances, the individual ceases to be the agent who initiates the action as a result of his or her choice. The individual's initiative is set aside, wholly or partially, in favor of someone else's.

Autonomy is violated in such cases even if the individual intends to act in the way that is imposed or demanded. Perhaps the prison inmate would have donated blood anyway, and surely some people would have wanted to be screened for AIDS. However, the use of coercion makes the wishes or intentions of the individual partly or totally irrelevant to whether the act is performed.

Autonomy as the initiation of action through one's own intention and choice can clearly be restricted to a greater or lesser degree. Someone who is physically forced to become a subject in a medical experiment, as in a Nazi concentration camp, is totally deprived of autonomy. The same is true of someone tricked into becoming a subject without knowing it. In the infamous Tuskegee syphilis studies, some participants were led to believe they were receiving appropriate medical treatment, when in fact they were part of a control group in the experiment. The situation is somewhat different for someone who agrees to become a subject in order to receive needed medical care. Such a person is acting under strong coercion, but the loss of autonomy is not complete. It is at least possible to refuse to participate, even if the cost of doing so may be extremely high.

In situations more typical than those above, autonomy may be compromised, rather than denied. For example, someone who is by nature nonassertive or someone who is poor and uneducated may find it very difficult to preserve his power of self-determination when he becomes a patient in a hospital. Medical authority, represented by physicians and the hospital staff, may be so intimidating to such a person that he does not feel free to exercise his autonomy. In such a case, although no one may be deliberately attempting to infringe on the patient's autonomy, social and psychological factors may constitute a force so coercive that the patient feels he has no choice but to do what he is told.

Autonomy and Options

Autonomy involves more than freedom from duress in making decisions. There must be genuine possibilities to decide among. A forced option is no option at all, and anyone who is in the position of having to take what she can get can hardly be regarded as self-determining or as exercising free choice.

In our society, economic and social conditions frequently limit the options available in medical care. As a rule, the poor simply do not have the same choices available to them as the rich. Someone properly insured or financially well off who might be helped by a heart transplant can decide whether or not to undergo the risk of having one. That is an option not generally available to someone who is uninsured and poor.

Similarly, a woman who depends on Medicaid and lives in a state in which Medicaid funds cannot be used to pay for abortions may not have the option of having an abortion. Her choice is not a genuine one, for she lacks the means to implement it. The situation is quite different for a middle-class woman faced with the same question. She may decide against having an abortion, but whatever she decides, the choice is real. She is autonomous in a way that the poor woman is not.

Those who believe that one of the goals of our society is to promote and protect the autonomy of individuals have frequently argued that we must do more to offer all individuals the same range of health-care options. If we do not, they have suggested, then our society cannot be one in which everyone has an equal degree of autonomy. In a very real sense, those who are rich will have greater freedom of action than those who are poor.

Autonomy and Decision Making

More is involved in decision making than merely saying yes or no. In particular, relevant information is an essential condition for genuine decision making. We are exercising our autonomy in the fullest sense only when we are making *informed* decisions.

It is pointless to have options if we are not aware of them, and we can hardly be said to be directing the course of our lives if our decisions must be made in ignorance of information that is available and relevant to our choices. These are the reasons that lying and other forms of deception are so destructive of autonomy. If someone with a progressive and ordinarily fatal disease is not told about it by her physician, then she is in no position to decide how to shape what remains of her life. The lack of a crucial piece of information— that she is dying—is likely to lead her to make decisions different from the ones she would make were she in possession of the information.

Information is the key to protecting and preserving autonomy in most medical situations. A patient who is not informed of alternative forms of treatment and their associated risks is denied the opportunity to make his own wishes and values count for something in his own life. For example, someone with coronary artery disease who is not told of the relative merits of medical treatment with drugs but is told only that he is a candidate for coronary-artery bypass surgery, is in no position to decide what risks he wishes to take and what ordeals he is prepared to undergo. A physician who does not supply the patient with the information the patient needs is restricting the patient's autonomy. The principle of autonomy requires *informed* consent, for consent alone does not involve genuine self-determination.

Making decisions for "the good" of others (paternalism), without consulting their wishes, deprives them of their status as autonomous agents. For example, some people at the final stages of a terminal illness might prefer to be allowed to die without heroic intervention, while others might prefer to prolong their lives as long as medical skills and technological powers make possible. If a physician or family undertakes to make a decision in this matter on behalf of the patient, then no matter what their motive, they are denying to the patient the power of self-determination.

Because autonomy is so bound up with informed consent and decision making, special problems arise in the case of those unable to give consent and make decisions. Patients who are comatose, severely brain-damaged,

psychotic, or seriously mentally impaired are not capable of making decisions on their own behalf. The nature of their condition has already deprived them of their autonomy. Of course this does not mean that they have no status as moral persons or that they have no interests. It falls to others to see that their interests are served.

The situation is similar for those, such as infants and young children, who are incapable of understanding. Any consent that is given must be given by others. But what are the limits of consent that can be legitimately given for some other person? Consenting to needed medical care seems legitimate, but what about rejecting needed medical care? What about consenting to becoming a subject in a research program? These questions are as crucial as they are difficult to resolve.

Restrictions on Autonomy

Autonomy is not an absolute or unconditional value. We would regard it as absurd for someone to claim that he was justified in committing a murder because he was only exercising his power of self-determination. Such a defense would be morally ludicrous.

However, we do value autonomy and recognize a general duty to respect it and even to promote its exercise. We demand compelling reasons to justify restricting the power of individuals to make their own choices and direct their own lives.

We will briefly examine four principles that are frequently appealed to in justifying restrictions on autonomy. The principles have been discussed most in the context of social and legal theory, for it is through laws and penalties that a society most directly regulates the conduct of its citizens. However, the principles can also be appealed to to justify policies and practices of institutions (such as hospitals) and the actions of individuals that affect other people.

Appealing to a principle can provide, at best, only a prima facie justification. Even if a principle can be shown to apply to a particular case in which freedom of action is restricted, we may value the lost freedom more than what is gained by restricting it. Reasons suggested by the principle may not be adequately persuasive. Furthermore, the principles themselves are frequently the subjects of controversy, and, with the exception of the harm principle, it is doubtful that any of the principles would be universally endorsed by philosophers and legal theorists.

The Harm Principle.   According to the harm principle, we may restrict the freedom of people to act if the restriction is necessary to prevent harm to others. In the most obvious case, we may take action to prevent violence like rape, robbery, killing, or assault. We may act to protect someone who is in apparent risk of harm from the action of someone else. The risk of harm need not be the result of the intention to harm. Thus, we might take steps to see that a surgeon whose skills and judgment have been impaired through drug use is not permitted to operate. The risk that he poses to his patients warrants the effort to keep him from acting as he wishes.

The harm principle may also be used to justify laws that exert coercive force and so restrict freedom of action. Laws against homicide and assault are clear examples, but the principle extends also to the regulation of institutions and practices. People may be robbed at the point of a pen, as well as at the point of a knife, and the harm produced by fraud may be as great as that produced by outright theft. Careless or deceptive medical practitioners may cause direct harm to their patients, and laws that regulate the standards of medical practice restrict the freedom of practitioners for the protection of patients.

The Principle of Paternalism.   In its weak version, the principle of paternalism is no more than the harm principle applied to the individual himself. According to the prin-

ciple, we are justified in restricting someone's freedom to act if doing so is necessary to prevent him from harming himself. Thus, we might force an alcoholic into a treatment program and justify our action by claiming that we did so to prevent him from continuing to harm himself by his drinking.

In its strong version, the principle of paternalism justifies restricting someone's autonomy if by doing so we can benefit her. In such a case, our concern is not only with preventing the person from harming herself, but also with promoting her good in a positive way. The principle might be appealed to even in cases in which our actions go against the other's known wishes. For example, a physician might decide to treat a patient with a placebo (an inactive drug), even if she has asked to be told the truth about her medical condition and her therapy. He might attempt to justify his action by claiming that if the patient knew she was receiving a placebo, then the placebo would be less likely to be effective. Since taking the placebo while believing that it is an active drug makes her feel better, the physician may claim that by deceiving her he is doing something to help her.

Paternalism may be expressed in laws and public policies, as well as in private actions. Some have suggested the drug laws as a prime example of governmental paternalism. By making certain drugs illegal and inaccessible and by placing other drugs under the control of physicians, the laws aim to protect people from themselves. Self-medication is virtually eliminated, and the so-called recreational use of drugs is prohibited. The price for such laws is a restriction on individual autonomy. Some have argued that the price is too high and that the most the government should do is warn and educate the individual about the consequences of using certain drugs.

The Principle of Legal Moralism.   The principle of legal moralism holds that a legitimate function of the law is to enforce morality by turning the immoral into the illegal. Hence, the restrictions placed on actions by the law are justified by the presumed fact that the actions are immoral and so ought not to be performed.

To a considerable extent, laws express the values of a society and the society's judgments about what is morally right. In our society, homicide and theft are recognized as crimes, and those who commit them are guilty of legal, as well as moral, wrongdoing. Society attempts to prevent such crimes and to punish offenders.

The degree to which the law should embody moral judgments is a hard question. It is particularly difficult to answer in a pluralistic society like ours, in which there may be sharp differences of opinion about the moral legitimacy of some actions. Until quite recently, for example, materials considered obscene could not be freely purchased, birth-control literature could not be freely distributed nor contraceptives legally prescribed in some states, and the conditions of divorce were generally stringent and punitive. Even now many states outlaw homosexual solicitation and acts, and prostitution is generally illegal. The foundation for such laws is the belief by many that the practices proscribed are morally wrong.

The current heated debate over abortion reflects, in some of its aspects, the conflict between those who favor strong legal moralism and those who oppose it. Many who consider abortion morally wrong would also like to see it made illegal once more. Others, even though they may oppose abortion, believe that it is a private moral matter and that the attempt to regulate it by law is an unwarranted intrusion of state power.

The Welfare Principle. The welfare principle holds that it is justifiable to restrict individual autonomy if doing so will result in providing benefits to others. Those who endorse this principle are not inclined to think

that it demands a serious self-sacrifice for the welfare of others. Rather, in their view, an ideal application of the principle would be the case in which we give up just a little autonomy to bring about a great deal of benefit to others.

For example, transplant organs are in short supply at the moment because their availability depends mostly on their being freely donated. The situation could be dramatically changed by a law requiring that organs from the recently dead be salvaged and made available for use as transplants.

Such a law would end the present system of voluntary donation, and by doing so it would restrict our freedom to decide what is to be done with our bodies after death. However, it would be easy to argue that the tremendous value that others might gain from such a law easily outweighs the slight restriction on autonomy that it would involve.

These four principles are not the only ones that offer grounds for abridging the autonomy of individuals, but they are the most relevant to decision making and policy planning in medicine. It is important to keep in mind that merely appealing to a principle is not enough to warrant a limit on autonomy. A principle points in the direction of an argument, but it is no substitute for one. The high value we place on autonomy gives its preservation a high priority, and compelling considerations are required to justify compromising it. In the view of some philosophers, who endorse the position taken by Mill, only the harm principle can serve as grounds for legitimately restricting autonomy. Other theorists find persuasive reasons to do so in other principles.

III. RETROSPECT

The two major tasks of this chapter have been to provide information about several important ethical theories and to formulate and illustrate several generally accepted moral principles. One aim in performing these tasks was to make it easier to follow the arguments and discussions in the selections that make up the major part of this book.

Another and ultimately more serious aim has been to call attention to ethical theories and principles you may wish to consider adopting. From this standpoint, the problems and issues presented in the selections can be considered test cases for the theories and principles. You may find that some of the theories that we have discussed are inadequate to deal with certain moral issues in the medical context, although they may seem satisfactory in more common or simpler cases. Or you may discover that certain commonly accepted moral principles lead to contradictory results or to conclusions that you find difficult to accept. Other theories or principles may appear to give definite and persuasive answers to medical-moral problems, but you may find that they rest on assumptions that it does not appear reasonable to accept. Such a dialectical process of claims and criticism is slow and frustrating. Yet it offers the best hope of settling on theories and principles that we can accept with confidence and employ without misgivings.

During the last ten years, a great amount of effort has been expended addressing the moral problems of medical practice and research. Without question, progress has been made in developing a better understanding of a number of issues and securing agreement about how they are to be dealt with. Nevertheless, a large number of moral issues in medicine remain unsettled or even unexplored. Even in the absence of moral consensus on these issues, the demands of practical decision making generate a force that presses us for immediate solutions.

In such a situation, we cannot afford to try to settle all doubts about moral principles in an abstract way and only then apply them to problems in medicine. The dialectical process must be made practical. Formulating and testing theories and principles must go on at the same time as we are actually making moral decisions. We must do our best to discover the principles of aerodynamics while staying aloft.

To a considerable extent, that is what this book is about. Positions are taken and defended by the authors. But they, too, are aware that they are participating in a search for a satisfactory resolution to the problems they discuss, and few, if any, would regard their solutions as beyond criticism. Medical ethics is still an area in which there are more legitimate questions than there are satisfactory answers, but the answers that we do have are better supported and better reasoned than those available even ten years ago.

PART I

TERMINATION

CHAPTER 1

ABORTION

SOCIAL CONTEXT: THE ABORTION DISPUTE

Three women and two men parade the sidewalk in front of the red-brick building that houses Reproductive Health Services. They carry placards that read "Abortion = Murder," "Babies Are People," and "God Is Prolife." One of the men carries a glass jar containing the remains of a twenty-week-old fetus.

"They're killing babies in there!" one of the men yells at a woman going into the building. "What if your mother had had an abortion?" another picketer shouts. The woman glances at the group, then pointedly ignores them.

The demonstrators walk their posts three days a week, the days abortions are performed in the clinic. Those willing to stop to talk to them, they attempt to convince of the immorality of abortion. Women who admit to being pregnant and considering abortion are subjected to great verbal pressure. Sometimes tempers flare into open anger and fights break out. Patients of the clinic complain that they are being harassed. The protesters claim they are only exercising their freedom of speech and speaking out against a practice that is as wrong as any other form of murder.

The scene could be almost any place in the United States today. The tone of the abortion debate has become angry as some people, convinced of abortion's immorality, have adopted a more activist stance. Frustration at failing to make abortion illegal has encouraged some of its opponents to attempt to halt its practice by more direct means.

Although most antiabortion or prolife activists have limited themselves to peaceful demonstrations, a few have resorted to outright violence. During the last three years, there have been over thirty cases of bombing, firebombing, or arson at clinics where abortions are performed. In 1985 alone, 224 incidents of violence were reported at clinics throughout the country. Threatening letters and telephone calls to clinics have increased in frequency, and personal threats against physicians and their families are not unusual. In August of 1983, three men describing themselves as members of the Army of God abducted Dr. Hector Zevallos and his wife. Although the Zevalloses were released unharmed eight days later, the men reportedly threatened to kill them if President Reagan did not announce an end to legal abortions.

Physicians who regularly perform abortions and the personnel at clinics admit to feeling frightened by the possibility of violence. Some physicians have given up performing abortions, and some clinics have closed. Some physicians say that their patients have been intimidated, and that some have either avoided seeking abortions or obtained them at greater expense at hospitals.

Clearly, those who have chosen to employ violent means are only a small fraction of the total of abortion opponents. Established groups condemn the violence and continue to place emphasis on the traditional strategies of verbal persuasion, rational argument, and appeal to ethical or religious principles.

Quite apart from the violence, the conflict between opponents and supporters of abortion has become increasingly emotional. As each group attempts to win public support for its side, the techniques of persuasion have moved closer to the methods of propaganda and away from the standards of rational discussion. An insight into this shift of character in the public debate on abortion can be gained by considering some of the strategies and tactics adopted by organizations favoring abortion as an option, as well as by those opposed to it.

In 1985 the National Abortion Rights Action League (NARAL) adopted a campaign called "Abortion Rights: Silent No More." Its aim, according to the organization's leadership, is to take an approach towards abortion that is personal, appeals to the emotions, and directs attention to the woman, rather than to the fetus. On May 21, 1985, it held a "Speak Out" in Washington, D.C., to make public some of the reported thirty to forty thousand personal testimonials by women who reaffirmed the rightness of their decision to have an abortion and asserted the right of women to make such choices for themselves.

The campaign was initiated, in part, to counter the impact on public opinion of the release of a videotape called "The Silent Scream." The tape has been widely shown under the auspices of various groups opposed to abortion. It depicts a twelve-week-old fetus, which it describes in the narration as drawing back in pain and attempting to escape surgical instruments during the progress of an abortion. The narrator, Dr. Bernard Nathanson, was once the director of an abortion clinic but is now an outspoken abortion opponent.

At a meeting of the National Right to Life organization, held in Washington at the same time that the NARAL Speak Out, Dr. Nathanson stressed the propaganda value of the videotape. In his view the videotape will help turn opinion against abortion just as television coverage shifted public opinion from favoring the Vietnam war to opposing it. (Critics of the tape and of Dr. Nathanson have charged that a twelve-week fetus is not sufficiently developed neurologically to experience pain.)

A representative of the Moral Majority, commenting on the new tactics of the NARAL, is quoted as saying, "The campaign is just fine with us. We have combat-ready people to deal with emotional issues, legions of women who would testify about how they feel exploited by abortion." The founder of another group opposed to NARAL, Women Exploited by Abortion, described women who believed they made the right choice choosing an abortion as "emotionally ill."

In July 1985, the president of the National Organization for Women (NOW) announced that the group was initiating its own campaign. The aim of the "Campaign to Save Women's Lives: One Million Strong" was to collect one million signatures in support of maintaining abortion as a legal option.

The New Orleans meeting of NOW was picketed by some one hundred members of the Louisiana Right to Life Federation. They carried placards saying "Save the Baby" and "Abortion is Murder." The president of the federation said that she could not understand NOW's position, since "750,000 female babies are aborted every year . . . [and] that's an awful lot of women being denied their rights."

Despite the acrimonious character of much of current public controversy over abortion, it is important to keep in mind that the great majority of seriously concerned people neither employ nor endorse these extreme tactics. The abortion question raises substantial philosophical and moral issues that can and must be dealt with by rational discussion. Everyone who cares about living in a society guided by the principles of reason is obligated to attempt to raise the intellectual level of public and private discourse. Moral fervor and even outrage have their place in social and political life, but they can never substitute for rational inquiry.

Those who oppose abortion have continued to take legal measures to attempt to halt or slow its practice. One such effort was the subject of the 1983 Supreme Court decision in the case of *Akron* v. *Akron Center for Reproductive Health.* Since the ruling has been generally acknowledged as a reaffirmation of the position the Court took in *Roe* v. *Wade,* it is worthwhile to discuss briefly the issues involved.

In 1978 the City of Akron, Ohio, passed an ordinance intended by its sponsors to be a model for the regulation of abortion in all communities. The ordinance required that all abortions after the first trimester be performed in a hospital, that parental consent be obtained for minors, and that a twenty-four-hour waiting period be observed between the time of the patient's decision and the operation.

Further, the woman's physician was required to inform her personally that "the unborn child is a human life from the moment of conception" and to provide her with a description mentioning the physical characteristics of "the particular unborn child . . . including appearance, mobility, tactile sensitivity, including pain, perception, or re-

sponse." The physician was also required to warn the patient that "abortion is a major surgical procedure which can result in severe complications" and "severe emotional disturbances" and advise her that various agencies were available to assist her during and after pregnancy if she chose not to have an abortion.

Opponents of the Akron ordinance saw it as an attempt to discourage women from seeking abortions by placing a number of financial and psychological barriers in their way. The Supreme Court's six-to-three ruling affirmed this view. The Court held that the requirement that abortions after the first trimester be performed in a hospital could not be justified by considerations of the safety of the woman, because, up to the sixteenth week, the standard abortion procedures are safer than childbirth. Further, the Court held that the ordinance violated the discretion of the physician by requiring that the physician recite "a lengthy and inflexible list of information," rather than consult and advise the patient in making her decision. The requirement that the physician personally supply the information was rejected for lack of any demonstration that it would further the state's interest in the woman's health.

The Court did not deny the importance of informed consent in the case of abortion. It held, however, that the information provided to a woman should suit her particular needs and that her physician should assume the responsibility for supplying her with the appropriate information. The Court concluded that the reciting of information that the Akron ordinance required was apparently "designed not to inform the woman's consent but rather to persuade her to withhold it altogether." The "parade of horribles" required by the procedures seemed intended to deter women from exercising their constitutional right.

The Akron decision was a setback for those eager to see abortion restricted, if not wholly eliminated, by the law. However, the legal battles did not end. In 1985 the Supreme Court agreed to hear arguments on the Pennsylvania *Abortion Control Act,* essentially similar to the Akron ordinance. Ranking members of the Justice Department indicated that they would use the opportunity to urge the Court to reverse itself on the constitutional right to have an abortion that was established in *Row* v. *Wade* in 1973.

In June of 1986, the Supreme Court reaffirmed once more the doctrine of *Roe* v. *Wade.* However, the Court was deeply divided, and the five-to-four ruling has been interpreted by many as indicating that in the future the Court might reverse itself on the abortion issue.

The decision itself was hailed by advocates of abortion rights, but the division in the Court was seen as encouraging by those opposed to abortion.

CASE PRESENTATION
The Ordeal of Alice Wilson

Late in the afternoon on a September day, twelve-year-old Alice Wilson (as we will call her) was walking the eight blocks home from the public school she attended. She liked the walk, for the south St. Louis neighborhood she lived in was a generally pleasant place. Large, turn-of-the-century brick houses predominated, and the streets were lined with leafy sycamore trees.

But, like many urban areas, the neighborhood showed signs of decay. Several houses were abandoned, their windows boarded up with unpainted plywood. The streets were littered, and once well-tended front lawns were often hardly more than scraggly patches of weeds.

At the corner of Grand and Hervy, Alice left the well-traveled sidewalk through the business district and crossed the street to Shaw Park. By walking through the park, rather than around it, she could cut the distance to her house almost by half. She wouldn't dare go through the park after dark, but on that bright afternoon the park seemed beautiful and safe. She had walked through the park dozens of times, both alone and with her friends, and had never had any trouble.

That day was different. Alice stayed on the main asphalt path leading across the park and passed by the first picnic area. Then, just beyond that area, she was attacked by three teen-aged males. They were older and larger than Alice, and she had never seen them before. One grabbed her from behind and put his hand over her mouth so she couldn't scream. Another said they would kill her if she didn't keep quiet. They dragged her off the path and into a place surrounded by bushes. Then all three of them raped her.

Afterwards, the boys ran from the park, leaving Alice crying on the ground. She eventually recovered enough to dress herself and walk the rest of the way home. When her mother came home from work, Alice told her what had happened. Because Alice seemed to be basically unhurt, except for being frightened and distraught, Mrs. Wilson decided that Alice didn't need medical attention. Alice's father was dead so Mrs. Wilson was responsible for making decisions about her welfare.

Alice went back to school and resumed her normal life. But about a week later she developed a high fever and vaginal pains and discharges. Mrs. Wilson was sufficiently alarmed to take her daughter to the clinic of nearby South General Hospital.

After a physical examination and laboratory tests, Dr. Charles Kranski, a resident at South General working at the clinic, first talked with Alice, then presented the results to Mrs. Wilson. He explained that Alice was in generally good health, but the chances were quite high that she had been infected with gonorrhea as a result of the sexual assault. It would be necessary to wait for a culture to grow to be certain; meanwhile, Alice would be treated with a course of penicillin.

The most troubling news, however, was that Alice was pregnant from the rape. That would be an unfortunate thing to happen for any rape victim, but in Alice's case it was particularly terrible. Dr. Kranski explained that although Alice was old enough to conceive a child, she was not really old enough to have one. She was simply not sufficiently developed physiologically to undergo pregnancy. She might well have a spontaneous abortion, a miscarriage, but if she did not, the chances were very good that attempting to have the child might kill her.

Dr. Kranski told Mrs. Wilson that he had discussed Alice's case with two obstetricians and that they both agreed with him that the only reasonable course of action was for Alice to have an abortion as soon as possible. In fact, Dr. Kranski said, as soon as the venereal disease was controlled, he would like to schedule Alice for an abortion for therapeutic reasons. He had already explained the situation to Alice, he said, and she agreed to the abortion. But because she was still a minor, it was necessary to have Mrs. Wilson's consent before the operation could be performed.

To Dr. Kranski's surprise, Mrs. Wilson told him that she would not give her consent. "I belong to the Church of the Spiritual Life," she said. "We follow the commandment 'Thou shall not kill.' "

Thinking that she had not understood the implications of Alice's pregnancy, Dr. Kranski again explained that Alice would probably die unless she had an abortion. Because of Alice's youth and small size, he said, the developing fetus would severely compress her internal organs and perhaps rupture them. If that happened, she would probably bleed to death. Even if that did not happen, she might suffer irreversible liver or kidney damage.

Mrs. Wilson remained totally unmoved. "God will save my daughter's life, if He wants it saved," she said. "And God will abort the child she's carrying, if He wants it aborted."

Dr. Kranski gave up his attempt to secure Mrs. Wilson's approval for the abortion. Later, he explained the situation to the director of the clinic, Dr. Saul Mendlovitz. Dr. Mendlovitz took up the matter with the legal staff of South General Hospital, and it was decided to seek a court order permitting the abortion.

The appropriate legal steps were taken, and after a court hearing at which Mrs. Wilson was represented by a state-appointed attorney, South General Hospital was granted permission to take necessary medical steps to save the life of Alice Wilson. No appeal was filed.

Despite her mother's continued personal opposition, Alice Wilson underwent an abortion.

INTRODUCTION

Hardly more than a decade ago, most Americans considered abortion a crime so disgusting that it was rarely mentioned in public. Back-alley abortionists with dirty hands and unclean instruments were real enough, but they were also the villains of cautionary tales to warn women against being tempted into the crime. Abortion was the dramatic stuff of novels and movies portraying girls in trouble or women pushed to the brink. To choose to have an abortion was to choose to be degraded.

The Supreme Court decision in _Roe_ v. _Wade_ changed all that in 1973. The decision had the effect of legalizing abortion, and since then abortion has gained acceptance from a majority of the population. Yet controversy over the legitimacy of abortion continues to flare. Indeed, no other topic in medical ethics has attracted more attention or so polarized public opinion. The reason is understandable. In the abortion question, major moral, legal, and social issues are intertwined to form a problem of great subtlety and complexity.

Before focusing on some of the specific issues raised by abortion, we would do well to have in hand some of the relevant factual information about human developmental biology and the techniques of abortion.

Human Development and Abortion

Fertilization occurs when an ovum is penetrated by a sperm cell and the nuclei of the two unite to form a single cell containing forty-six chromosomes. This normally occurs in the Fallopian tube (or oviduct), a narrow tube leading from the ovary into the uterus (womb). The fertilized ovum—zygote, or conceptus—continues its passage down the Fallopian tube, and during its two to three day passage it undergoes a number of cell divisions that increase its size. (Rarely, the zygote does not descend but continues to develop in the Fallopian tube. Because the tube is so small, the pregnancy usually has to be terminated surgically.) After reaching the uterus, a pear-shaped organ, the zygote floats free in the intrauterine fluid. Here it develops into a blastocyst, a ball of cells surrounding a fluid-filled cavity.

By the end of the second week, the blastocyst becomes embedded in the wall of the uterus. At this point and until the end of the eighth week, it is known as an embryo. During the fourth and fifth weeks, organ systems begin to develop, and the external features take on a definitely human shape.

During the eighth week, brain activity usually becomes detectable. At this time, the embryo comes to be known as a fetus. Birth generally occurs about nine months after fertilization. It is customary to divide this time into three three-month periods, or trimesters. At present, pregnancy cannot be diagnosed with certainty by ordinary methods until ten to fourteen days after a woman has missed her menstrual period.

Abortion is the termination of pregnancy. It can occur because of internal biochemical factors or as a result of physical injury to the woman. Terminations from such causes are usually referred to as "spontaneous abortions," but they are also commonly called miscarriages.

Abortion can also be a deliberate process resulting from human intervention. The methods used in contemporary medicine depend to a great extent on the stage of the pregnancy. The earliest intervention involves the use of drugs (the morning-after pill) to prevent the embedding of the blastocyst in the uterine wall. Subsequent intervention during the first trimester (up to about twelve weeks) commonly employs one of two techniques. The first of the two is uterine or vacuum aspiration. The cervix, the narrow outer opening of the uterus, is dilated (widened) by instruments. Then a small tube is inserted into the uterus, and its contents are emptied by suction. The second commonly used procedure is dilation and curettage. The cervix is dilated and its contents are gently scraped out by the use of a curette, a spoon-shaped surgical instrument.

After sixteen weeks, when the fetus is too large to make the other methods practical, the most common abortion technique is saline injection. The fluid in the membrane sac (amnion) surrounding the fetus is withdrawn through a hollow needle and replaced by a solution of salt and water. This induces a miscarriage.

A second method, hysterotomy, is a surgical procedure in which the fetus is removed from the uterus through an incision. The procedure is the same as that known as Caesarean section and is rarely performed for the purpose of abortion.

These facts about pregnancy and abortion put us in a position to discuss some of the moral problems connected with them. We shall not be able to untangle the skein of issues wrapped around the abortion question. We shall only attempt to state a few of the more serious ones and to indicate the lines of argument that have been offered to support positions taken with respect to them. Afterwards, we will sketch out some possible responses that might be offered on the basis of the ethical theories we considered in the introductory chapter. Finally, we will present summary statements of the views taken by the authors of the selections that make up the bulk of this chapter.

The Status of the Fetus

It is absolutely crucial for the application of the principles of any moral theory that we have a settled opinion about the objects and subjects of morality. Although principles are generally stated with respect to rational individuals, every theory recognizes that there are people who in fact cannot be considered rational agents. For example, mental and physical incapacities may diminish or destroy rationality. But ethical theories generally recognize that we still have duties to people who are so incapacitated.

The basic problem that this raises is: Who or what is to be considered a person? Are there characteristics that we can point to and say that it is by virtue of possessing these characteristics that an individual must be considered a person and thus accorded moral treatment?

The abortion issue raises this question most particularly with regard to the fetus. (We will use the term "fetus," for the moment, to refer to the developing organism at any stage.) Just what is the status of the fetus in the world? We must find a satisfactory answer to this question, some writers have suggested, before we can resolve the general moral problem of abortion.

Let's consider the possible consequences of answering this question one way or the other. First, if a fetus is a person, then it has a serious claim to life. We must assert the claim on its behalf, for, like an unconscious person, the fetus is unable to do so. The claim of the fetus as a person must be given weight and respect in deliberating about any action that would terminate its life. Perhaps only circumstances as extreme as a threat to the life of the mother would justify abortion.

Assuming that the fetus is a person, then an abortion would be a case of killing and not something to be undertaken without reasons sufficient to override the fetus's claim to life.

In effect, only conditions of the same sort as would justify our killing an adult person (for example, self-defense) would justify our killing a fetus. Thus, the moral burden in every case would be to demonstrate that abortion is not a case of wrongful killing.

By contrast, if a fetus is *not* a person in a morally relevant sense, then abortion need not be considered a case of killing equivalent to the killing of an adult. In one view, it might be said that an abortion is not essentially different from an appendectomy. According to this way of thinking, a fetus is no more than a complicated clump of organic material, and its removal involves no serious moral difficulty.

In another view, it could be argued that even though the fetus is not a person, it is a *potential* person, and this is a significant and morally-relevant property. The fetus's very potentiality makes it unique and distinguishes it from a diseased appendix or a cyst or any other kind of organic material. Thus, because the fetus can become a person, abortion does present a moral problem. A fetus can be destroyed only for serious reasons. Thus, preventing a person from coming into existence must be justified to an extent comparable to the justification required for killing a person. (Some have suggested that the justification does not have to be identical because the fetus is only a potential person. The justifications we might present for killing a person would thus serve only as a guide for those that might justify abortion.)

So far we have used the word "fetus," and this usage tends to obscure the fact that human development is a process with many stages. Perhaps it is only in the later stages of development that the entity becomes a person. But exactly when might this happen?

The differences between a fertilized ovum and a fully-developed baby just a few minutes before birth are considerable. The ovum and the blastocyst seem just so much tissue. But the embryo and the fetus present more serious claims to being persons. Should abortion be allowed until the fetus becomes visibly human, or until the fetus shows heartbeat and brain waves, or until the fetus can live outside the uterus (becomes viable)?

The process of development is continuous, and so far it has proved impossible to find differences between stages that can be generally accepted as morally relevant. Some writers on abortion have suggested that it is useless to look for such differences, because any place where the line is drawn will be arbitrary. Others have claimed that it is possible to draw the line by relying on criteria that can be rationally defended. A few have even argued that a reasonable set of criteria for determining who shall be considered a person might even deny the status to infants.

Pregnancy, Abortion, and the Rights of Women

Pregnancy and fetal development are normal biological processes, and most women who choose to have a child carry it to term without unusual difficulties. However, it is important to keep in mind that even a normal pregnancy involves changes and stresses that are uniquely burdensome. Once the process of fetal growth is initiated, a woman's entire physiology is altered by the new demands placed on it and by the biochemical changes taking place within her body. For example, metabolic rate increases, the thyroid gland grows larger, the heart pumps more blood to meet fetal needs, and a great variety of hormonal changes take place. The growing fetus physically displaces the woman's internal organs and alters the size and shape of her body.

As a result of such changes, the pregnant woman may suffer a variety of ailments. More common ones include severe nausea and vomiting ("morning sickness"), muscle cramps, abdominal pain, anemia, tiredness, and headaches. For many women such complaints are relatively mild or infrequent, while for others they are severe or constant. Nausea and vomiting can lead to dehydration and malnutrition so serious as to be life-threatening. Women who suffer from diseases like diabetes are apt to face special health problems as a result of pregnancy.

Partly because of hormonal changes, women are also more likely to experience psychological difficulties when pregnant, such as emotional lability (mood swings), severe depression, and acute anxiety. Such conditions are often accompanied by quite realistic concerns about the loss of freedom associated with becoming a parent, compromised job status, loss of sexual attractiveness due to the change in body shape, and the pains and risks of childbirth.

The woman who intends to carry a child to term is also likely to have to alter her behavior in many ways. She may have to curtail the time she spends working, take a leave of absence, or even quit her job. Any career plans she has are likely to suffer. She may be unable to participate in social activities to the extent she previously did, and give up some entirely. In addition, if she recognizes an obligation to the developing fetus and is well informed, she may have to alter her diet, stop smoking, and strictly limit the amount of alcohol she consumes.

In summary, the physical and emotional price paid by a woman for a full-term pregnancy is high. Even a normal pregnancy, one that proceeds without any special difficulties, exacts a toll of discomfort, stress, restricted activity, and worry.

Women who wish to have a child are generally willing to undergo the rigors of pregnancy to satisfy this desire. But is it a woman's duty to nurture and carry to term an unwanted child? Pregnancies resulting from rape and incest are the kinds of dramatic cases frequently mentioned to emphasize the seriousness of the burden imposed on women. But the question is also important when the conditions surrounding the pregnancy are more ordinary.

Suppose that a woman becomes pregnant unintentionally and decides that having a child will be harmful to her career or her way of life. Or suppose that she simply does not wish to subject herself to the pains of pregnancy. Does a woman have a moral duty to see to it that the developing child comes to be born?

A number of writers have taken the position that women have an exclusive right to control their own reproductive function. In their view, such a right is based upon the generally recognized right to control what is done to our bodies. Since pregnancy is something that involves a woman's body, the woman concerned may legitimately decide whether to continue the pregnancy or terminate it. The decision is hers alone, and social or legal policies that restrict the free exercise of her right are unjustifiable.

Essentially the same point is sometimes phrased by saying that women own their bodies. Because their bodies are their own "property," women alone have the right to decide whether to become pregnant and, if pregnant unintentionally, whether to have an abortion.

Critics have pointed out that this general line of argument, taken alone, does not support the strong conclusion that women should be free from all constraints in making abortion decisions. Even granting that women's bodies are their own property, we nevertheless recognize restrictions on exercising property rights. We have no right to shoot trespassers, and we cannot endanger our neighbors by burning down our house. Similarly, if any legitimate moral claims can be made on behalf of the fetus, then the right of women to decide whether to have an abortion may not be unrestricted.

Some philosophers (Judith J. Thomson, for example) have taken the view that, although women are entitled to control their bodies and make abortion decisions, the decision to have an abortion must be supported by weighty reasons. They have suggested that even if we grant that a fetus is a person, its claim to life cannot be given unconditional precedence over the woman's claim to control her own life. She is entitled to autonomy and the right to arrange her life in accordance with her own concept of the good. It would be wrong for her to destroy the fetus for a trivial reason, but legitimate and adequate reasons for taking the life of the fetus might be offered.

Others, by contrast, have argued that when a woman becomes pregnant she assumes an obligation for the life of the fetus. It is, after all, completely dependent on her for its continued existence. She has no more right to take its life in order to seek her own best interest than she has to murder someone whose death may bring benefits to her.

Therapeutic Abortion

Abortion is sometimes required in order to save the life of the mother or in order to provide her with medical treatment that may correct some life-threatening condition. Abortion performed for such a purpose is ordinarily regarded as a case of self-defense. For this reason, it is almost universally considered to be morally unobjectionable. (Strictly speaking, the Roman Catholic view condemns abortion in all of its forms. It does approve of providing medical treatment for the mother, even if this results in the death of the fetus, but the death of the fetus must never be intended.)

If the principle of preserving the life and health of the mother justifies abortion, then what conditions fall under that principle? If a woman has cancer of the uterus and her life can be saved only by an operation that will result in the death of the fetus, then this clearly falls under the principle. But what about psychological conditions? Is a woman's mental health relevant to deciding whether an abortion is justified? What if a psychiatrist believes that a woman cannot face the physical rigors of pregnancy or bear the psychological stresses that go with it without developing severe psychiatric symptoms? Would such a judgment justify an abortion? Or is the matter of psychological health irrelevant to the abortion issue?

Consider, too, the welfare of the fetus. Suppose that prenatal tests or other reliable means indicate that the developing child suffers from serious abnormalities. (This was the case of the "thalidomide babies.") Is abortion for the purpose of preventing the birth of such children justifiable?

It might be argued that it is not, that an impaired fetus has as much right to its life as an impaired person. We do not, after all, consider it legitimate to kill people who become seriously injured or suffer from diseases that render them helpless. Rather, we care for them and work to improve their lives—at least we ought to.

Someone might argue, however, that abortion in such cases is not only justifiable, but a duty. (See, for example, the article by H. T. Engelhardt in Chapter 2.) It is our duty to kill the fetus to spare the person that it will become a life of unhappiness and suffering. We might even be said to be acknowledging the dignity of the fetus by doing what it might do for itself if it could, what any rational creature would do. Destroying such a fetus would spare future pain to the individual and his or her family and save society from an enormous expense. Thus we have not only the justification to kill such a fetus, but also the positive obligation to do so.

In this chapter, we will not deal explicitly with the issues that are raised by attempting to decide whether it is justifiable to terminate the life of an impaired fetus. Because such issues are directly connected with prenatal genetic diagnosis and treatment, we will dis-

cuss them more fully in Chapter 6. Nonetheless, in considering the general question of the legitimacy of abortion, it is important to keep such special considerations in mind.

Abortion and the Law

Abortion in our society has been a legal issue as well as a moral issue. Until the Supreme Court decision in *Roe* v. *Wade*, nontherapeutic abortion was illegal in virtually all states. And even now there are groups lobbying strongly for a Constitutional amendment that would protect a fetus's "right to life" and prohibit elective abortion.

The rightness or wrongness of abortion is a moral matter, one whose issues can be resolved only by appealing to a moral theory. Different theories may yield incompatible answers, and even individuals who accept the same theory may arrive at different conclusions.

Such a state of affairs raises the question of whether the moral convictions or conclusions of some people should be embodied in laws that govern the lives of all people in the society. The question can be put succinctly: Should the moral beliefs of some people serve as the basis for laws that will impose those beliefs on everyone?

There is no straightforward way of answering this general question. To some extent, which moral beliefs are at issue are a relevant consideration. So too are the political principles that we are willing to accept as basic to our society. Every ethical theory recognizes that there is a scope of action that must be left to individuals as moral agents acting freely on the basis of their own understanding and perceptions. Laws requiring the expression of benevolence or gratitude, for example, seem peculiarly inappropriate.

Yet, one of the major aims of a government is to protect the rights of its citizens. Consequently, a society must have just laws that recognize and enforce those rights. In a very real way, then, the moral theory that we hold and the conclusions arrived at on the basis of it will determine whether we believe that certain types of laws are justified. They are justified when they protect the rights recognized in our moral theories—when political rights reflect moral rights. (See the introduction to Chapter 9 for a fuller discussion of moral rights and their relation to political rights.)

An ethical theory that accords the status of a person to a fetus is likely to claim also that the laws of the society should recognize the rights of the fetus. A theory that does not grant the fetus this position is not likely to regard laws forbidding abortion as justifiable.

Ethical Theories and Abortion

Theories like those of Mill, Kant, Ross, and Rawls attribute to individuals autonomy or self-direction. An individual is entitled to control his or her own life, and it seems reasonable to extend this principle to apply to one's own body. If so, then a woman should have the right to determine whether or not she wishes to have a child. If she is pregnant with an unwanted child, then, no matter how she came to be pregnant, she might legitimately decide on an abortion. Utilitarianism also suggests this answer on consequential grounds. In the absence of other considerations, if it seems likely that having a child will produce more unhappiness than an abortion would, then an abortion would be justifiable.

If the fetus is considered to be a person, however, the situation is different for some theories. The Roman Catholic view holds that the fetus is an innocent person and that direct abortion is never justifiable. Even if the pregnancy is due to rape, the fetus cannot be held at fault and made to suffer through its death. Even though she may not wish to have the child, the mother has a duty to preserve the life of the fetus.

For deontological theories like those of Kant and Ross, the situation becomes more complicated. If the fetus is a person, then it has an inherent dignity and worth. It is an innocent life which cannot be destroyed except for the weightiest moral reasons. Those reasons may include the interests and wishes of the woman, but deontological theories provide no clear answer as to how those are to be weighed.

For utilitarianism, by contrast, even if the fetus is considered a person, the principle of utility may still justify an abortion. Killing a person is not, for utilitarianism, inherently wrong. (Yet, it is compatible with rule utilitarianism to argue that permitting elective abortion as a matter of policy would produce more unhappiness than forbidding abortion altogether. Thus, utilitarianism does not offer a definite answer to the abortion issue.)

As we have already seen, both utilitarianism and deontological theories can be used to justify therapeutic abortion. When the mother's life or health is at stake, then the situation may be construed as one of self-defense. Both Kant and Ross recognize that we each have a right to protect ourselves, even if it means taking the life of another person. For utilitarianism, preserving one's life is justifiable, for being alive is a necessary condition for all forms of happiness.

We have also indicated that abortion, "for the sake of the fetus" can be justified by both utilitarianism and deontological theories. If by killing the fetus we can spare it a life of suffering, minimize the sufferings of its family, and preserve the resources of the society, then abortion is legitimate on utilitarian grounds. In the terms of Kant and Ross, destroying the fetus might be a way of recognizing its dignity. If we assume that it is a person, then by sparing it a life of indignity and pain we are treating it in the way that a rational being would want to be treated.

The legitimacy of laws forbidding abortion is an issue that utilitarianism would resolve by considering their effects. If such laws promote the general happiness of the society, then they are justifiable. Otherwise, they are not. In general, Kant, Ross, Rawls, and natural law theory recognize intrinsic human worth and regard as legitimate laws protecting that worth, even if those holding this view are only a minority of the society. Thus, laws discriminating against blacks and women, for example, would be considered unjust on the basis of these theories. Laws enforcing equality, by contrast, would be considered just.

But what about fetuses? The Roman Catholic interpretation of natural law would regard the case as exactly the same. As full human persons, they are entitled to have their rights protected by law. Those who fail to recognize this are guilty of moral failure, and laws permitting abortion are the moral equivalent of laws permitting murder.

For Kant and other deontologists, the matter is less clear. So long as there is substantial doubt about the status of the fetus, it is not certain that it is legitimate to demand that the rights of fetuses be recognized and protected by law. It is clear that the issue of whether or not the fetus is considered a person is most often taken as the crucial one in the abortion controversy.

The Selections

All the issues we have discussed previously are dealt with in the selections in this chapter. Yet it is the last issue, the status of the fetus as a person, that dominates concern. In *Roe v. Wade* the U.S. Supreme Court declared unconstitutional a Texas statute that restricted legal abortions to cases in which the life of the mother was threatened. The decision implied that all such state laws regulating abortion were unconstitutional. In effect, then, the decision made abortion legal in the United States.

The decision rested, in part, on the rea-soning that a woman has a right to act for her own health and well-being as part of a more general right of privacy. The Court also considered the question of the legitimate limits of state interference to protect a woman's health and to protect the life of a fetus. The Court refused to recognize the fetus as a "person in the full sense" or to grant the right of the state to act on its behalf until the time (around the twenty-eighth week) that it can live outside the mother's body.

The ruling laid down three guidelines for regulating abortion: (1) until the end of the first trimester, the abortion decision is a medical one that must be left to the woman and her physician, (2) after the end of the first trimester, the state may regulate the abortion procedure in ways reasonably related to maternal health, (3) after the fetus is viable, the state may regulate or even prohibit abortion, except where it is necessary to preserve the life or health of the mother.

The Court faced the line-drawing problem and drew the line at viability. John T. Noonan, in our second reading, "An Almost Absolute Value in History," makes the moment of fertilization the stage at which the developing organism becomes a person. Noonan reviews the distinctions used by abortion proponents (viability, experience, quickening, attitudes of adults towards the fetus, social viability) and concludes that they are all illegitimate. By contrast, he argues that conception is the decisive moment of humanization—for it is then that the new being receives the genetic code of its parents.

The basic principle that should govern our attitude towards the fetus, Noonan claims, is a theological and humanistic one: Do not injure your fellow man without a reason. Thus, once the humanity of the fetus is perceived, abortion is never right except in "self-defense." With the exception of saving the mother's life then, abortion is immoral because it "violates the rational humanist tenet of the quality of human lives."

Judith Jarvis Thomson in her very influential "A Defense of Abortion" avoids the problem of determining when the fetus becomes a person. For the sake of argument only, she grants the conservative view that the fetus is a person from the moment of conception. She points out, however, that the conservative argument using this claim as a premise actually involves an additional unstated premise. The argument typically runs: The fetus is an innocent person; therefore, killing a fetus is always wrong. The argument requires that we assume that killing an innocent person is always wrong. But, Thomson claims, killing an innocent person is sometimes allowable. This is most clearly so when self-defense requires it.

Using several moral analogies, Thomson attempts to show that a fetus's right to life does not consist in the right not to be killed, but in the right not to be killed unjustly. The fetus's claim to life is not an absolute one which must always be granted unconditional precedence over the interests of its mother. Thus, abortion is not always permissible, but neither is it always impermissible. When the reasons for having an abortion are trivial, then abortion is not legitimate. When the reasons are serious and involve the health or welfare of the woman, then abortion is justifiable.

Mary Anne Warren in "On the Moral and Legal Status of Abortion" takes an even stronger position than Thomson, arguing that a woman's right to have an abortion is unrestricted. She attempts to show that there is no adequate basis for holding that the fetus has "a significant right to life" and that, whatever right can be appropriately granted to the fetus, it can never override a woman's right to protect her own interest and well-being. Accordingly, laws that restrict access to abortion are an unjustified violation of a woman's rights.

Warren is critical of both Noonan and Thomson. Noonan, she claims, fails to demonstrate that whatever is genetically human (the fetus) is also morally human (a person). Thomson, Warren argues, is mistaken in believing that it is possible both to grant that the fetus is a person and to produce a satisfactory defense of the right to obtain an abortion. Contrary to Thomson's aim, her central argument supports the right to abortion only in cases in which the woman is in no way responsible for her pregnancy.

Like Noonan, Warren conceives the basic issue in abortion to be the question of what properties something must possess to be a person in the moral sense. She offers five traits she believes anyone would accept as central and argues that the fetus, at all stages of development, possesses none of them. Since the fetus is not a person, it is not entitled to the full range of moral rights. That the fetus has the potential to become a person may give it a prima facie right to life, but the rights of an actual person always outweigh those of a potential person.

An apparent consequence of Warren's argument is that infanticide is justified as well as abortion. Warren argues in a postscript that it does not follow from her argument that infanticide is permissible under present social conditions, although under some other conditions it would be.

In the last selection in this chapter, "Responsible Women and Abortion Decisions," Martha Brandt Bolton takes on the difficult task of defining and defending a moderate position on abortion. She rejects both the conservative view that abortion is almost always a serious moral wrong and the radical view that abortion is always a morally neutral action.

Bolton argues that the conservative claim that the fetus is a person and so has the *same* rights as an "undisputed" person is mistaken. To respect the right of an undisputed person not to be killed, we need only refrain from killing him. However, not to kill a fetus requires nurturing, so a fetus has a right not to be killed only if it has the additional right to be nurtured. Thus, the fetus must be granted either a stronger right to support than we grant to undisputed persons or a weaker right not to be killed. Granting the fetus a stronger right, Bolton tries to show, leads to logical incoherence.

According to Bolton, the claim that abortion is morally neutral is also mistaken. That the fetus, if properly nurtured, will become a person entitles it to some consideration, and a pregnant woman has some obligation to nurture a fetus, although the obligation is not absolute. Furthermore, an abortion decision is not a purely personal matter, for it is made in a context of other interests and obligations. When such matters as the woman's ability to plan a "morally coherent life" and her responsibilities to her family and to the larger community are taken into account, then abortion may be morally permitted or even morally required.

Clearly, the Supreme Court decision did not resolve the philosophical difficulties posed by abortion. Making abortion legal did not necessarily make it moral. Making the end of the first trimester the beginning of legitimate state control is pragmatically useful, but it does not provide a satisfactory answer to the question of whether the fetus is a person.

Noonan's conservative view that the moment of conception is also the beginning of a person has a powerful simplicity, but because the differences between a fertilized ovum and an about-to-be-born baby are so great, it too seems arbitrary. It does violence to our perception that potentiality (the genetic code of DNA) is very different from actuality (a child), that a blueprint and a pile of building materials are very different from a house.

Thomson makes no effort to deal with criteria that would allow us to decide whether a fetus is a person. She does, however, call to our attention the important notion that we are sometimes justified in causing the death of an innocent person. This offers a means of considering the permissibility of abortion in a case-by-case way, without our having to secure agreement on the question of the status of the fetus.

Warren makes a strong case for the right of a woman to obtain an abortion, but her claim that this right can be asserted with equal force at all stages of fetal development, until the very moment of birth, does as much violence to our perception as Noonan's claim that the fetus is a person from the very moment of conception.

Most people are likely to feel the strongest sympathy for a moderate position like that taken by Bolton. Quite apart from the question of the soundness of her arguments, she calls attention to some of the realistic issues that are faced by women who must make a decision about abortion. In doing so, she makes it clear why the decision can involve great moral anguish.

The social problems of abortion show no signs of being resolved. At present, over a million abortions are performed every year in the United States. The 1985 Census Bureau statistics reported an average of 426 abortions per 1,000 live births nationwide, and in the District of Columbia there were more abortions than births—a ratio of 1,517 to 1,000. About one quarter of all abortions are paid for with tax money in the form of Medicaid payments.

In 1977 the Supreme Court ruled that states are under no obligation to fund elective abortions for the poor under the Medicaid program, and in 1980 the Court held that the federal government is not required to fund abortions of any kind. Medicaid is presently both a state and federally funded program. Some fourteen states, accounting for 75 percent of the women eligible for Medicaid, chose to continue to finance elective abortions with state funds. In those states, nearly 98 percent of the women seeking an abortion obtained one. In states providing no funding, about 20 percent of women wanting abortions were forced to continue their pregnancies. Those securing abortions either obtained money from private sources to pay for legal abortions or (in 4 percent of the cases) illegal ones.

Opponents of abortion have generally approved the Supreme Court decisions regarding abortion payments. By contrast, those who support elective abortion point out that the result of the decisions is to deny to some women an opportunity open to others.

Women with financial means will have no difficulty obtaining abortions, while those without money will have either to bear children they don't want or to take their chances with back-alley abortionists whose services they can afford.

Yet, should those who consider abortion a form of murder have to pay through taxes for an operation that commits it? This is just one of the moral dilemmas that must be worked out before the issue of the place of abortion in society can be resolved.

United States Supreme Court Decision in *Roe* v. *Wade*

Background Note: A pregnant single woman, Roe, brought a class-action suit against Wade, the District Attorney of Dallas County. Roe challenged the constitutionality of the Texas criminal abortion laws, which prohibited procuring or performing an abortion except on medical advice for the purpose of saving the mother's life. A three-judge District Court ruled that the abortion statutes were void, and Wade appealed directly to the Supreme Court. By seven to two the Court ruled in favor of Roe, and Justice Blackmun delivered the majority opinion. That opinion is abridged here and citations to other cases omitted. The decision was handed down on January 22, 1973.

Three reasons have been advanced to explain historically the enactment of criminal abortion laws in the 19th century and to justify their continued existence.

It has been argued occasionally that these laws were the product of a Victorian social concern to discourage illicit sexual conduct. Texas, however, does not advance this justification in the present case, and it appears that no court or commentator has taken the argument seriously. The appellants and *amici* contend, moreover, that this is not a proper state purpose at all and suggest that, if it were, the Texas statutes are overbroad in protecting it since the law fails to distinguish between married and unwed mothers.

A second reason is concerned with abortion as a medical procedure. When most criminal abortion laws were first enacted, the procedure was a hazardous one for the woman. This was particu-

larly true prior to the development of antisepsis. Antiseptic techniques, of course, were based on discoveries by Lister, Pasteur, and others first announced in 1867, but were not generally accepted and employed until about the turn of the century. Abortion mortality was high. Even after 1900, and perhaps until as late as the development of antibiotics in the 1940's, standard modern techniques such as dilation and curettage were not nearly so safe as they are today. Thus it has been argued that a State's real concern in enacting a criminal abortion law was to protect the pregnant woman, that is, to restrain her from submitting to a procedure that placed her life in serious jeopardy.

Modern medical techniques have altered this situation. Appellants and various *amici* refer to medical data indicating that abortion in early pregnancy, that is, prior to the end of first trimester, although not without its risk, is now relatively safe. Mortality rates for women undergoing early abortions, where the procedure is legal, appear to be as low as or lower than the rates for normal childbirth. Consequently, any interest of the State in protecting the woman from an inherently hazardous procedure, except when it would be equally dangerous for her to forego it, has largely disappeared. Of course, important state interests in the area of health and medical standards do remain. The state has a legitimate interest in seeing to it that abortion, like any other medical

United States Supreme Court, 410 U.S. 113, 93 S. Ct. 705. January 22, 1973.

procedure, is performed under circumstances that insure maximum safety for the patient. This interest obviously extends at least to the performing physician and his staff, to the facilities involved, to the availability of after-care, and to adequate provision for any complication or emergency that might arise. The prevalence of high mortality rates at illegal "abortion mills" strengthens, rather than weakens, the State's interest in regulating the conditions under which abortions are performed. Moreover, the risk to the woman increases as her pregnancy continues. Thus the State retains a definite interest in protecting the woman's own health and safety when an abortion is proposed at a late stage of pregnancy.

The third reason is the State's interest—some phrase it in terms of duty—in protecting prenatal life. Some of the argument for this justification rests on the theory that a new human life is present from the moment of conception. The State's interest and general obligation to protect life then extends, it is argued, to prenatal life. Only when the life of the pregnant mother herself is at stake, balanced against the life she carries within her, should the interest of the embryo or fetus not prevail. Logically, of course, a legitimate state interest in this area need not stand or fall on acceptance of the belief that life begins at conception or at some other point prior to live birth. In assessing the State's interest, recognition may be given to the less rigid claim that as long as at least *potential* life is involved, the State may assert interests beyond the protection of the pregnant woman alone.

Parties challenging state abortion laws have sharply disputed in some courts the contention that a purpose of these laws, when enacted, was to protect prenatal life. Pointing to the absence of legislative history to support the contention, they claim that most state laws were designed solely to protect the woman. Because medical advances have lessened this concern, at least with respect to abortion in early pregnancy, they argue that with respect to such abortions the laws can no longer be justified by any state interest. There is some scholarly support for this view of original purpose. The few state courts called upon to interpret their laws in the late 19th and early 20th centuries did focus on the State's interest in protecting the woman's health rather than in preserving the embryo and fetus. Proponents of this view point out that in

many States, including Texas, by statute or judicial interpretation, the pregnant woman herself could not be prosecuted for self-abortion or for cooperating in an abortion performed upon her by another. They claim that adoption of the "quickening" distinction through received common law and state statutes tacitly recognizes the greater health hazards inherent in late abortion and impliedly repudiates the theory that life begins at conception.

It is with these interests, and the weight to be attached to them, that this case is concerned.

The Constitution does not explicitly mention any right of privacy. In a line of decisions, however, going back perhaps as far as *Union Pacific R. Co.* v. *Botsford,* 141 U.S. 250, 251 (1891), the Court has recognized that a right of personal privacy, or a guarantee of certain areas or zones of privacy, does exist under the Constitution. In varying contexts the Court or individual Justices have indeed found at least the roots of that right in the First Amendment, in the Fourth and Fifth Amendments, in the penumbras of the Bill of Rights, in the Ninth Amendment, or in the concept of liberty guaranteed by the first section of the Fourteenth Amendment. These decisions make it clear that only personal rights that can be deemed "fundamental" or "implicit in the concept of ordered liberty" are included in this guarantee of personal privacy. They also make it clear that the right has some extension to activities relating to marriage, procreation, contraception, family relationships, and child rearing and education.

This right of privacy, whether it be founded in the Fourteenth Amendment's concept of personal liberty and restrictions upon state action, as we feel it is, or, as the District Court determined, in the Ninth Amendment's reservation of rights to the people, is broad enough to encompass a woman's decision whether or not to terminate her pregnancy. The detriment that the State would impose upon the pregnant woman by denying this choice altogether is apparent. Specific and direct harm medically diagnosable even in early pregnancy may be involved. Maternity, or additional offspring, may force upon the woman a distressful life and future. Psychological harm may be imminent. Mental and physical health may be taxed by child care. There is also the distress, for all concerned, associated with the unwanted child, and there is the problem of bringing a child into a family already unable, psychologically and otherwise, to care for it. In other cases, as in this one, the additional difficulties and continuing stigma of unwed motherhood may be involved. All these are factors the woman and her responsible physician necessarily will consider in consultation.

On the basis of elements such as these, appellants and some *amici* argue that the woman's right is absolute and that she is entitled to terminate her pregnancy at whatever time, in whatever way, and for whatever reason she alone chooses. With these we do not agree. Appellants' arguments that Texas either has no valid interest at all in regulating the abortion decision, or no interest strong enough to support any limitation upon the woman's sole determination, is unpersuasive. The Court's decisions recognizing a right of privacy also acknowledge that some state regulation in areas protected by that right is appropriate. As noted above, a state may properly assert important interests in safeguarding health, in maintaining medical standards, and in protecting potential life. At some point in pregnancy, these respective interests become sufficiently compelling to sustain regulation of the factors that govern the abortion decision. The privacy right involved, therefore, cannot be said to be absolute. In fact, it is not clear to us that the claim asserted by some *amici* that one has an unlimited right to do with one's body as one pleases bears a close relationship to the right of privacy previously articulated in the Court's decisions. The Court has refused to recognize an unlimited right of this kind in the past.

We therefore conclude that the right of personal privacy includes the abortion decision, but that this right is not unqualified and must be considered against important state interests in regulation.

We note that those federal and state courts that have recently considered abortion law challenges have reached the same conclusion. A majority, in addition to the District Court in the present case, have held state laws unconstitutional, at least in part, because of vagueness or because of overbreadth and abridgement of rights.

Although the results are divided, most of these courts have agreed that the right of privacy, however based, is broad enough to cover the abortion decision; that the right, nonetheless, is not absolute and is subject to some limitations; and that at some point the state interests as to protection of health, medical standards, and prenatal life, become dominant. We agree with this approach.

Where certain "fundamental rights" are involved, the Court has held that regulation limiting these rights may be justified only by a "compelling state interest" . . . and that legislative enactments must be narrowly drawn to express only the legitimate state interests at stake.

In the recent abortion cases courts have recognized these principles. Those striking down state laws have generally scrutinized the State's interest in protecting health and potential life and have concluded that neither interest justified broad limitations on the reasons for which a physician and his pregnant patient might decide that she should have an abortion in the early stages of pregnancy. Courts sustaining state laws have held that the State's determinations to protect health or prenatal life are dominant and constitutionally justifiable.

The District Court held that the appellee failed to meet his burden of demonstrating that the Texas statute's infringement upon Roe's rights was necessary to support a compelling state interest, and that, although the defendant presented "several compelling justifications for state presence in the area of abortions," the statutes outstripped these justifications and swept "far beyond any areas of compelling state interest." Appellant and appellee both contest that holding. Appellant, as has been indicated, claims an absolute right that bars any state imposition of criminal penalties in the area. Appellee argues that the State's determination to recognize and protect prenatal life from and after conception constitutes a compelling state interest. As noted above, we do not agree fully with either formulation.

A. The appellee and certain *amici* argue that the fetus is a "person" within the language and meaning of the Fourteenth Amendment. In support of this they outline at length and in detail the well-known facts of fetal development. If this suggestion of personhood is established, the appellant's case, of course, collapses, for the fetus' right to life is then guaranteed specifically by the Amendment. The appellant conceded as much on reargument. On the other hand, the appellee conceded on reargument that no case could be cited that holds that a fetus is a person within the meaning of the Fourteenth Amendment.

The Constitution does not define "person" in so many words. Section 1 of the Fourteenth Amendment contains three references to "person." . . . But in nearly all these instances, the use of the word is such that it has application only postnatally. None indicates, with any assurance, that it has any possible prenatal application.

All this, together with our observation, *supra,* that throughout the major portion of the 19th century prevailing legal abortion practices were far freer than they are today, persuades us that the word "person," as used in the Fourteenth Amendment, does not include the unborn. . . .

B. The pregnant woman cannot be isolated in her privacy. She carries an embryo and, later, a fetus, if one accepts the medical definitions of the developing young in the human uterus. See Dorland's Illustrated Medical Dictionary, 478–479, 547 (24th ed. 1965). The situation therefore is inherently different from marital intimacy, or bedroom possession of obscene material, or marriage, or procreation, or education, with which *Eisenstadt, Giswold, Stanley, Loving, Skinner, Pierce,* and *Meyer* were respectively concerned. As we have intimated above, it is reasonable and appropriate for a State to decide that at some point in time another interest, that of health of the mother or that of potential human life, becomes significantly involved. The woman's privacy is no longer sole and any right of privacy she possesses must be measured accordingly.

Texas urges that, apart from the Fourteenth Amendment, life begins at conception and is present throughout pregnancy, and that, therefore, the State has a compelling interest in protecting that life from and after conception. We need not resolve the difficult question of when life begins. When those trained in the respective disciplines of medicine, philosophy, and theology are unable to arrive at any consensus, the judiciary, at this point in the development of man's knowledge, is not in a position to speculate as to the answer.

It should be sufficient to note briefly the wide divergence of thinking on this most sensitive and difficult question. There has always been strong support for the view that life does not begin until live birth. This was the belief of the Stoics. It appears to be the predominant, though not the unanimous, attitude of the Jewish faith. It may be taken to represent also the position of a large segment of the Protestant community, insofar as that can be ascertained; organized groups that have taken a formal position on the abortion issue have generally regarded abortion as a matter for the conscience of the individual and her family. As we have noted, the common law found greater significance in quickening. Physicians and their scientific colleagues have regarded that event with less interest and have tended to focus either upon conception or upon live birth or upon the interim point at which the fetus becomes "viable," that is, potentially able to live outside the mother's womb, albeit with artificial aid. Viability is usually placed at about seven months (28 weeks) but may occur earlier, even at 24 weeks. The Aristotelian theory of "mediate animation," that held sway throughout the Middle Ages and the Renaissance in Europe, continued to be official Roman Catholic dogma until the 19th century, despite opposition to this "ensoulment" theory from those in the Church who would recognize the existence of life from the moment of conception. The latter is now, of course, the official belief of the Catholic Church. As one of the briefs *amicus* discloses, this is a view strongly held by many non-Catholics as well, and by many physicians. Substantial problems for precise definition of this view are posed, however, by new embryological data that purport to indicate that conception is a "process" over time, rather than an event, and by new medical techniques such as menstrual extraction, the "morning-after" pill, implantation of embryos, artificial insemination, and even artificial wombs.

In areas other than criminal abortion the law has been reluctant to endorse any theory that life, as we recognize it, begins before live birth or to accord legal rights to the unborn except in narrowly defined situations and except when the rights are contingent upon live birth. For example, the traditional rule of tort law had denied recovery for prenatal injuries even though the child was born alive. That rule has been changed in almost every jurisdiction. In most States recovery is said to be permitted only if the fetus was viable, or at least quick, when the injuries were sustained, though few courts have squarely so held. In a recent development, generally opposed by the commentators, some States permit the parents of a stillborn child to maintain an action for wrongful death because of prenatal injuries. Such an action, however, would appear to be one to vindicate the parents' interest and is thus consistent with the view that the fetus, at most, represents only the potentiality of life. Similarly, unborn children have been recognized as acquiring rights or interests by way of inheritance or other devolution of property, and have been represented by guardians *ad litem*. Perfection of the interests involved, again, has generally been contingent upon live birth. In short, the unborn have never been recognized in the law as persons in the whole sense.

In view of all this, we do not agree that, by adopting one theory of life, Texas may override the rights of the pregnant woman that are at stake. We repeat, however, that the State does have an important and legitimate interest in preserving and protecting the health of the pregnant woman, whether she be a resident of the State or a nonresident who seeks medical consultation and treatment there, and that it has still *another* important and legitimate interest in protecting the potentiality of human life. These interests are separate and distinct. Each grows in substantiality as the woman approaches term and, at a point during pregnancy, each becomes "compelling."

With respect to the State's important and legitimate interest in the health of the mother, the "compelling" point, in the light of present medical knowledge, is at approximately the end of the first trimester. This is so because of the now established medical fact . . . that until the end of the first trimester mortality in abortion is less than mortality in normal childbirth. It follows that, from and after this point, a State may regulate the abortion procedure to the extent that the regulation reasonably relates to the preservation and protection of maternal health. Examples of permissible state regulation in this area are requirements as to the qualifications of the person who is to perform the abortion; as to the licensure of that person; as to the facility in which the procedure is to be performed, that is, whether it must be a hospital or may be a clinic or some other place of less-than-hospital status; as to the licensing of the facility; and the like.

This means, on the other hand, that, for the period of pregnancy prior to this "compelling" point, the attending physician, in consultation with his patient, is free to determine, without regulation by the State, that in his medical judgment the patient's pregnancy should be terminated. If that decision is reached, the judgment may be effectuated by an abortion free of interference by the State.

With respect to the State's important and legitimate interest in potential life, the "compelling" point is at viability. This is so because the fetus then presumably has the capability of meaningful life outside the mother's womb. State regulation protective of fetal life after viability thus has both logical and biological justifications. If the State is interested in protecting fetal life after viability, it may go so far as to proscribe abortion during that period except when it is necessary to preserve the life or health of the mother.

Measured against these standards, Art. 1196 of the Texas Penal Code, in restricting legal abortions to those "procured or attempted by medical advice for the purpose of saving the life of the mother," sweeps too broadly. The statute makes no distinction between abortions performed early in pregnancy and those performed later, and it limits to a single reason, "saving" the mother's life, the legal justification for the procedure. The statute, therefore, cannot survive the constitutional attack made upon it here. . . .

To summarize and to repeat:

1. A state criminal abortion statute of the current Texas type, that excepts from criminality only a *life saving* procedure on behalf of the mother, without regard to pregnancy stage and without recognition of the other interests involved, is violative of the Due Process Clause of the Fourteenth Amendment.

   a. For the stage prior to approximately the end of the first trimester, the abortion decision and its effectuation must be left to the medical judgment of the pregnant woman's attending physician.

   b. For the stage subsequent to approximately the end of the first trimester, the State, in promoting its interest in the health of the mother, may, if it chooses, regulate the abortion procedure in ways that are reasonably related to maternal health.

c. For the stage subsequent to viability the State, in promoting its interest in the potentiality of human life, may, if it chooses, regulate, and even proscribe, abortion except where it is necessary, in appropriate medical judgment, for the preservation of the life or health of the mother.

2. The State may define the term "physician" . . . to mean only a physician currently licensed by the State, and may proscribe any abortion by a person who is not a physician as so defined. . . .

This holding, we feel, is consistent with the relative weights of the respective interests involved, with the lessons and example of medical and legal history, with the lenity of the common law, and with the demands of the profound problems of the present day. The decision leaves the State free to place increasing restrictions on abortion as the period of pregnancy lengthens, so long as those restrictions are tailored to the recognized state interests. The decision vindicates the right of the physician to administer medical treatment according to his professional judgment up to the points where important state interests provide compelling justifications for intervention. Up to those points the abortion decision in all its aspects is inherently, and primarily, a medical decision, and basic responsibility for it must rest with the physician. If an individual practitioner abuses the privilege of exercising proper medical judgment, the usual remedies, judicial and intra-professional, are available. . . .

An Almost Absolute Value in History

John T. Noonan, Jr.

The most fundamental question involved in the long history of thought on abortion is: How do you determine the humanity of a being? To phrase the question that way is to put in comprehensive humanistic terms what the theologians either dealt with as an explicitly theological question under the heading of "ensoulment" or dealt with implicitly in their treatment of abortion. The Christian position as it originated did not depend on a narrow theological or philosophical concept. It had no relation to theories of infant baptism.[1] It appealed to no special theory of instantaneous ensoulment. It took the world's view on ensoulment as that view changed from Aristotle to Zacchia. There was, indeed, theological influence affecting the theory of ensoulment finally adopted, and, of course, ensoulment itself was a theological concept, so that the position was always explained in theological terms. But the theological notion of ensoulment could easily be translated into humanistic language by substituting "human" for "rational soul"; the problem of knowing when a man is a man is common to theology and humanism.

If one steps outside the specific categories used by the theologians, the answer they gave can be analyzed as a refusal to discriminate among human beings on the basis of their varying potentialities. Once conceived, the being was recognized as man because he had man's potential. The criterion for humanity, thus, was simple and all-embracing: if you are conceived by human parents, you are human.

The strength of this position may be tested by a review of some of the other distinctions offered in the contemporary controversy over legalizing abortion. Perhaps the most popular distinction is in terms of viability. Before an age of so many months, the fetus is not viable, that is, it cannot be removed from the mother's womb and live apart from her. To that extent, the life of the fetus is absolutely dependent on the life of the mother. This dependence is made the basis of denying recognition to its humanity.

There are difficulties with this distinction. One is that the perfection of artificial incubation may make the fetus viable at any time: it may be removed and artificially sustained. Experiments with animals already show that such a procedure is possible. This hypothetical extreme case relates to an actual difficulty: there is considerable elasticity to the idea of viability. Mere length of life is not an exact measure. The viability of the fetus depends on the extent of its anatomical and functional development. The weight and length of the fetus are better guides to the state of its development than age, but weight and length vary. Moreover, different racial groups have different ages at which their fetuses are viable. Some evidence, for example, suggests that Negro fetuses mature more quickly than white fetuses. If viability is the norm, the standard would vary with race and with many individual circumstances.

The most important objection to this approach is that dependence is not ended by viability. The fetus is still absolutely dependent on someone's care in order to continue existence; indeed a child of one or three or even five years of age is absolutely dependent on another's care for existence; uncared for, the older fetus or the younger child will die as surely as the early fetus detached from the mother. The unsubstantial lessening in dependence at viability does not seem to signify any special acquisition of humanity.

A second distinction has been attempted in terms of experience. A being who has had experience, has lived and suffered, who possesses memories, is more human than one who has not. Humanity depends on formation by experience. The fetus is thus "unformed" in the most basic human sense.

This distinction is not serviceable for the embryo which is already experiencing and reacting. The embryo is responsive to touch after eight weeks and at least at that point is experiencing. At an earlier stage the zygote is certainly alive and responding to its environment. The distinction may also be challenged by the rare case where aphasia has erased adult memory: has it erased humanity? More fundamentally, this distinction leaves even the older fetus or the younger child to be treated as an unformed inhuman thing. Finally, it is not clear why experience as such confers humanity. It could be argued that certain central experiences such as loving or learning are necessary to make a man human. But then human beings who have failed to love or to learn might be excluded from the class called man.

A third distinction is made by appeal to the sentiments of adults. If a fetus dies, the grief of the parents is not the grief they would have for a living child. The fetus is an unnamed "it" till birth, and is not perceived as personality until at least the fourth month of existence when movements in the womb manifest a vigorous presence demanding joyful recognition by the parents.

Yet feeling is notoriously an unsure guide to the humanity of others. Many groups of humans have had difficulty in feeling that persons of another tongue, color, religion, sex, are as human as they. Apart from reactions to alien groups, we mourn the loss of a ten-year-old boy more than the loss of his one-day-old brother or his 90-year-old grandfather. The difference felt and the grief expressed vary with the potentialities extinguished, or the experience wiped out; they do not seem to point to any substantial difference in the humanity of baby, boy, or grandfather.

Distinctions are also made in terms of sensation by the parents. The embryo is felt within the womb only after about the fourth month. The embryo is seen only at birth. What can be neither seen nor felt is different from what is tangible. If the fetus cannot be seen or touched at all, it cannot be perceived as man.

Yet experience shows that sight is even more untrustworthy than feeling in determining humanity. By sight, color became an appropriate index for saying who was a man, and the evil of racial discrimination was given foundation. Nor can touch provide the test; a being confined by sickness, "out of touch" with others, does not thereby seem to lose his humanity. To the extent that touch still has appeal as a criterion, it appears to be a survival of the old English idea of "quickening"—a possible mistranslation of the Latin *animatus* used in the canon law. To that extent touch as a criterion seems to be dependent on the Aristotelian notion of ensoulment, and to fall when this notion is discarded.

Finally, a distinction is sought in social visibility. The fetus is not socially perceived as human. It cannot communicate with others. Thus, both subjectively and objectively, it is not a member of society. As moral rules are rules for the behavior of members of society to each other, they cannot be made for behavior toward what is not yet a member. Excluded from the society of men, the fetus is excluded from the humanity of men.[2]

By force of the argument from the consequences, this distinction is to be rejected. It is more subtle than that founded on an appeal to physical sensation, but it is equally dangerous in its implications. If humanity depends on social recognition, individuals or whole groups may be dehumanized by being denied any status in their society. Such a fate is fictionally portrayed in *1984* and has actually been the lot of many men in many societies. In the Roman empire, for example, condemnation to slavery meant the practical denial of most human rights; in the Chinese Communist world, landlords have been classified as enemies of the people and so treated as nonpersons by the state. Humanity does not depend on social recognition, though often the failure of society to recognize the prisoner, the alien, the heterodox as human has led to the destruction of human beings. Anyone conceived by a man and a woman is human. Recognition of this condition by society follows a real event in the objective order, however imperfect and halting the recognition. Any attempt to limit humanity to exclude some group runs the risk of furnishing authority and precedent for excluding other groups in the name of the consciousness or perception of the controlling group in the society.

A philosopher may reject the appeal to the humanity of the fetus because he views "humanity" as a secular view of the soul and because he doubts the existence of anything real and objective which can be identified as humanity. One answer to such a philosopher is to ask how he reasons about moral questions without supposing that there is a sense in which he and the others of whom he speaks are human. Whatever group is taken as the society which determines who may be killed is thereby taken as human. A second answer is to ask if he does not believe that there is a right and wrong way of deciding moral questions. If there is such a difference, experience may be appealed to: to decide who is human on the basis of

the sentiment of a given society has led to consequences which rational men would characterize as monstrous.

The rejection of the attempted distinctions based on viability and visibility, experience and feeling, may be buttressed by the following considerations: Moral judgments often rest on distinctions, but if the distinctions are not to appear arbitrary *fiat*, they should relate to some real difference in probabilities. There is a kind of continuity in all life, but the earlier stages of the elements of human life possess tiny probabilities of development. Consider for example, the spermatozoa in any normal ejaculate: There are about 200,000,000 in any single ejaculate, of which one has a chance of developing into a zygote. Consider the oocytes which may become ova: there are 100,000 to 1,000,000 oocytes in a female infant, of which a maximum of 390 are ovulated. But once spermatozoon and ovum meet and the conceptus is formed, such studies as have been made show that roughly in only 20 percent of the cases will spontaneous abortion occur. In other words, the chances are about 4 out of 5 that this new being will develop. At this stage in the life of the being there is a sharp shift in probabilities, an immense jump in potentialities. To make a distinction between the rights of spermatozoa and the rights of the fertilized ovum is to respond to an enormous shift in possibilities. For about twenty days after conception the egg may split to form twins or combine with another egg to form a chimera, but the probability of either event happening is very small.

It may be asked, What does a change in biological probabilities have to do with establishing humanity? The argument from probabilities is not aimed at establishing humanity but at establishing an objective discontinuity which may be taken into account in moral discourse. As life itself is a matter of probabilities, as most moral reasoning is an estimate of probabilities, so it seems in accord with the structure of reality and the nature of moral thought to found a moral judgment on the change in probabilities at conception. The appeal to probabilities is the most commonsensical of arguments, to a greater or smaller degree all of us base our actions on probabilities, and in morals, as in law, prudence and negligence are often measured by the account one has taken of the probabilities. If the chance is 200,000,000 to 1 that the movement in the bushes into which you shoot is a man's, I doubt if many persons would hold you careless in shooting; but if the chances are 4 out of 5 that the movement is a human being's, few would acquit you of blame. Would the argument be different if only one out of ten children conceived came to term? Of course this argument would be different. This argument is an appeal to probabilities that actually exist, not to any and all state of affairs which may be imagined.

The probabilities as they do exist do not show the humanity of the embryo in the sense of a demonstration in logic any more than the probabilities of the movement in the bush being a man demonstrate beyond all doubt that the being is a man. The appeal is a "buttressing" consideration, showing the plausibility of the standard adopted. The argument focuses on the decisional factor in any moral judgment and assumes that part of the business of a moralist is drawing lines. One evidence of the nonarbitrary character of the line drawn is the difference of probabilities on either side of it. If a spermatozoon is destroyed, one destroys a being which had a chance of far less than 1 in 200 million of developing into a reasoning being, possessed of the genetic code, a heart and other organs, and capable of pain. If a fetus is destroyed, one destroys a being already possessed of the genetic code, organs, and sensitivity to pain, and one which had an 80 percent chance of developing further into a baby outside the womb who, in time, would reason.

The positive argument for conception as the decisive moment of humanization is that at conception the new being receives the genetic code. It is this genetic information which determines his characteristics, which is the biological carrier of the possibility of human wisdom, which makes him a self-evolving being. A being with a human genetic code is man.

This review of current controversy over the humanity of the fetus emphasizes what a fundamental question the theologians resolved in asserting the inviolability of the fetus. To regard the fetus as possessed of equal rights with other humans was not, however, to decide every case where abortion might be employed. It did decide the case where the argument was that the fetus should be aborted for its own good. To say a being was human was to say it had a destiny to decide for itself which could not be taken from it by another man's decision. But human beings with equal rights often come in conflict with each other, and some decision must be made as whose claims are to prevail. Cases of conflict involving the fetus are different only in two respects: the total inability of the fetus to speak for itself and the fact that the right of the fetus regularly at stake is the right to life itself.

The approach taken by the theologians to these conflicts was articulated in terms of "direct" and "indirect." Again, to look at what they were doing from outside their categories, they may be said to have been drawing lines or "balancing values." "Direct" and "indirect" are spatial metaphors; "line-drawing" is another. "To weigh" or "to balance" values is a metaphor of a more complicated mathematical sort hinting at the process which goes on in moral judgments. All the metaphors suggest that, in the moral judgments made, comparisons were necessary, that no value completely controlled. The principle of double effect was no doctrine fallen from heaven, but a method of analysis appropriate where two relative values were being compared. In Catholic moral theology, as it developed, life even of the innocent was not taken as an absolute. Judgments on acts affecting life issued from a process of weighing. In the weighing, the fetus was always given a value greater than zero, always a value separate and independent from its parents. This valuation was crucial and fundamental in all Christian thought on the subject and marked it off from any approach which considered that only the parents' interests needed to be considered.

Even with the fetus weighed as human, one interest could be weighed as equal or superior: that of the mother in her own life. The casuists between 1450 and 1895 were willing to weigh this interest as superior. Since 1895, that interest was given decisive weight only in the two special cases of the cancerous uterus and the ectopic pregnancy. In both of these cases the fetus itself had little chance of survival even if the abortion were not performed. As the balance was once struck in favor of the mother whenever her life was endangered, it could be so struck again. The balance reached between 1895 and 1930 attempted prudentially and pastorally to forestall a multitude of exceptions for interests less than life.

The perception of the humanity of the fetus and the weighing of fetal rights against other human rights constituted the work of the moral analysts. But what spirit animated their abstract judgments? For the Christian community it was the injunction of Scripture to love your neighbor as yourself. The fetus as human was a neighbor; his life had parity with one's own. The commandment gave life to what otherwise would have been only rational calculation.

The commandment could be put in humanistic as well as theological terms: Do not injure your fellow man without reason. In these terms, once the humanity of the fetus is perceived, abortion is never right except in self-defense. When life must be taken to save life, reason alone cannot say that a mother must prefer a child's life to her own. With this exception, now of great rarity, abortion violates the rational humanist tenet of the equality of human lives.

For Christians the commandment to love had received a special imprint in that the exemplar proposed of love was the love of the Lord for his disciples. In the light given by this example, self-sacrifice carried to the point of death seemed in the extreme situations not without meaning. In the less extreme cases, preference for one's own interests to the life of another seemed to express cruelty or selfishness irreconcilable with the demands of love.

Notes

1. According to Glanville Williams (*The Sanctity of Human Life*, p. 193), "The historical reason for the Catholic objection to abortion is the same as for the Christian Church's historical opposition to infanticide: the horror of bringing about the death of an unbaptized child." This statement is made without any citation of evidence. [As previously argued], desire to administer baptism could, in the Middle Ages, even be urged as a reason for procuring an abortion. It is highly regrettable that the American Law Institute was apparently misled by Williams' account and repeated after him the same baseless statement. See American Law Institute, *Model Penal Code: Tentative Draft No. 9* (1959), p. 148, n. 12.

2. Thomas Aquinas gave an analogous reason against baptizing a fetus in the womb: "As long as it exists in the womb of the mother, it cannot be subject to the operation of the ministers of the Church as it is not known to men" (*In sententias Petri Lombardi* 4.6 1.1.2).

A Defense of Abortion[1]

Judith Jarvis Thomson

Most opposition to abortion relies on the premise that the fetus is a human being, a person, from the moment of conception. The premise is argued for, but, as I think, not well. Take, for example, the most common argument. We are asked to notice that the development of a human being from conception through birth into childhood is continuous; then it is said that to draw a line, to choose a point in this development and say "before this point the thing is not a person, after this point it is a person" is to make an arbitrary choice, a choice for which in the nature of things no good reason can be given. It is concluded that the fetus is, or anyway that we had better say it is, a person from the moment of conception. But this conclusion does not follow. Similar things might be said about the development of an acorn into an oak tree, and it does not follow that acorns are oak trees, or that we had better say they are. Arguments of this form are sometimes called "slippery slope arguments"—the phrase is perhaps self-explanatory—and it is dismaying that opponents of abortion rely on them so heavily and uncritically.

I am inclined to agree, however, that the prospects for "drawing a line" in the development of the fetus look dim. I am inclined to think also that we shall probably have to agree that the fetus has already become a human person well before birth. Indeed, it comes as a surprise when one first

Judith Jarvis Thomson, "A Defense of Abortion," Philosophy & Public Affairs, *Vol. 1, no. 1 (Fall 1971).*
Copyright © 1971 by Princeton University Press. Reprinted by permission of Princeton University Press.

learns how early in its life it begins to acquire human characteristics. By the tenth week, for example, it already has a face, arms and legs, fingers and toes; it has internal organs, and brain activity is detectable.[2] On the other hand, I think that the premise is false, that the fetus is not a person from the moment of conception. A newly fertilized ovum, a newly implanted clump of cells, is no more a person than an acorn is an oak tree. But I shall not discuss any of this. For it seems to me to be of great interest to ask what happens if, for the sake of argument, we allow the premise. How, precisely, are we supposed to get from there to the conclusion that abortion is morally impermissible? Opponents of abortion commonly spend most of their time establishing that the fetus is a person, and hardly any time explaining the step from there to the impermissibility of abortion. Perhaps they think the step too simple and obvious to require much comment. Or perhaps instead they are simply being economical in argument. Many of those who defend abortion rely on the premise that the fetus is not a person, but only a bit of tissue that will become a person at birth; and why pay out more arguments than you have to? Whatever the explanation, I suggest that the step they take is neither easy nor obvious, that it calls for closer examination than it is commonly given, and that when we do give it this closer examination we shall feel inclined to reject it.

I propose, then, that we grant that the fetus is a person from the moment of conception. How does the argument go from here? Something like this, I take it. Every person has a right to life. So the fetus has a right to life. No doubt the mother has a right to decide what shall happen in and to her body; everyone would grant that. But surely a person's right to life is stronger and more stringent than the mother's right to decide what happens in and to her body, and so outweighs it. So the fetus may not be killed; an abortion may not be performed.

It sounds plausible. But now let me ask you to imagine this. You wake up in the morning and find yourself back to back in bed with an unconscious violinist. A famous unconscious violinist. He has been found to have a fatal kidney ailment, and the Society of Music Lovers has canvassed all the available medical records and found that you alone have the right blood type to help. They have

therefore kidnapped you, and last night the violinist's circulatory system was plugged into yours, so that your kidneys can be used to extract poisons from his blood as well as your own. The director of the hospital now tells you, "Look, we're sorry the Society of Music Lovers did this to you—we would never have permitted it if we had known. But still, they did it, and the violinist now is plugged into you. To unplug you would be to kill him. But never mind, it's only for nine months. By then he will have recovered from his ailment, and can safely be unplugged from you." Is it morally incumbent on you to accede to this situation? No doubt it would be very nice of you if you did, a great kindness. But do you *have* to accede to it? What if it were not nine months, but nine years? Or longer still? What if the director of the hospital says, "Tough luck, I agree, but you've now got to stay in bed, with the violinist plugged into you, for the rest of your life. Because remember this. All persons have a right to life, and violinists are persons. Granted you have a right to decide what happens in and to your body, but a person's right to life outweighs your right to decide what happens in and to your body. So you cannot ever be unplugged from him." I imagine you would regard this as outrageous, which suggests that something really is wrong with that plausible-sounding argument I mentioned a moment ago.

In this case, of course, you were kidnapped; you didn't volunteer for the operation that plugged the violinist into your kidneys. Can those who oppose abortion on the ground I mentioned make an exception for a pregnancy due to rape? Certainly. They can say that persons have a right to life only if they didn't come into existence because of rape; or they can say that all persons have a right to life, but that some have less of a right to life than others, in particular, that those who came into existence because of rape have less. But these statements have a rather unpleasant sound. Surely the question of whether you have a right to life at all, or how much of it you have, shouldn't turn on the question of whether or not you are a product of a rape. And in fact the people who oppose abortion on the ground I mentioned do not make this distinction, and hence do not make an exception in case of rape.

Nor do they make an exception for a case in which the mother has to spend the nine months of her pregnancy in bed. They would agree that would be a great pity, and hard on the mother; but all the same, all persons have a right to life, the fetus is a person, and so on. I suspect, in fact, that they would not make an exception for a case in which, miraculously enough, the pregnancy went on for nine years, or even the rest of the mother's life.

Some won't even make an exception for a case in which continuation of the pregnancy is likely to shorten the mother's life; they regard abortion as impermissible even to save the mother's life. Such cases are nowadays very rare, and many opponents of abortion do not accept this extreme view. All the same, it is a good place to begin: a number of points of interest come out in respect to it.

1.

Let us call the view that abortion is impermissible even to save the mother's life "the extreme view." I want to suggest first that it does not issue from the argument I mentioned earlier without the addition of some fairly powerful premises. Suppose a woman has become pregnant, and now learns that she has a cardiac condition such that she will die if she carries the baby to term. What may be done for her? The fetus, being a person, has a right to life, but as the mother is a person too, so has she a right to life. Presumably they have an equal right to life. How is it supposed to come out that an abortion may not be performed? If mother and child have an equal right to life, shouldn't we perhaps flip a coin? Or should we add to the mother's right to life her right to decide what happens in and to her body. which everybody seems to be ready to grant—the sum of her rights now outweighing the fetus's right to life?

The most familiar argument here is the following. We are told that performing the abortion would be directly killing[3] the child, whereas doing nothing would not be killing the mother, but only letting her die. Moreover, in killing the child, one would be killing an innocent person, for the child has committed no crime, and is not aiming at his mother's death. And then there are a variety of ways in which this might be continued. (1) But as directly killing an innocent person is always and absolutely impermissible, an abortion may not be performed. Or, (2) as directly killing an innocent person is murder, and murder is always and absolutely impermissible, an abortion may not be performed.[4] Or, (3) as one's duty to refrain from directly killing an innocent person is more stringent than one's duty to keep a person from dying, an abortion may not be performed. Or, (4) if one's only options are directly killing an innocent person or letting a person die, one must prefer letting the person die, and thus an abortion may not be performed.[5]

Some people seem to have thought that these are not further premises which must be added if the conclusion is to be reached, but that they follow from the very fact that an innocent person has a right to life.[6] But this seems to me to be a mistake, and perhaps the simplest way to show this is to bring out that while we must certainly grant that innocent persons have a right to life, the theses in (1) through (4) are all false. Take (2), for example. If directly killing an innocent person is murder, and thus is impermissible, then the mother's directly killing the innocent person inside her is murder, and thus is impermissible. But it cannot seriously be thought to be murder if the mother performs an abortion on herself to save her life. It cannot seriously be said that she *must* refrain, that she *must* sit passively by and wait for her death. Let us look again at the case of you and the violinist. There you are, in bed with the violinist, and the director of the hospital says to you, "It's all most distressing, and I deeply sympathize, but you see this is putting an additional strain on your kidneys, and you'll be dead within the month. But you *have* to stay where you are all the same. Because unplugging you would be directly killing an innocent violinist, and that's murder, and that's impermissible." If anything in the world is true, it is that you do not commit murder, you do not do what is impermissible, if you reach around to your back and unplug yourself from that violinist to save your life.

The main focus of attention in writings on abortion has been on what a third party may or may not do in answer to a request from a woman for an abortion. This is in a way understandable. Things being as they are, there isn't much a woman can safely do to abort herself. So the question asked is what a third party may do, and what the mother may do, if it is mentioned at all, is deduced, almost as an afterthought, from what it is concluded that third parties may do. But it seems to me that to treat the matter in this way is to refuse to grant to the mother that very status of person which is so firmly insisted on for the fetus. For we cannot simply read off what a person may do from what a third party may do. Suppose you find yourself trapped in a tiny house with a growing child. I mean a very tiny house, and a rapidly growing child—you are already up against the wall of the house and in a few minutes you'll be crushed to death. The child on the other hand won't be crushed to death if nothing is done to stop him from growing he'll be hurt, but in the end he'll simply burst open the house and walk out a free man. Now I could well understand it if a bystander were to say, "There's nothing we can do for you. We cannot choose between your life and his, we cannot be the ones to decide who is to live, we cannot intervene." But it cannot be concluded that you too can do nothing, that you cannot attack it to save your life. However innocent the child may be, you do not have to wait passively while it crushes you to death. Perhaps a pregnant woman is vaguely felt to have the status of house, to which we don't allow the right of self-defense. But if the woman houses the child, it should be remembered that she is a person who houses it.

I should perhaps stop to say explicitly that I am not claiming that people have a right to do anything whatever to save their lives. I think, rather, that there are drastic limits to the right of self-defense. If someone threatens you with death unless you torture someone else to death, I think you have not the right, even to save your life, to do so. But the case under consideration here is very different. In our case there are only two people involved, one whose life is threatened, and one who threatens it. Both are innocent: the one who is threatened is not threatened because of any fault, the one who threatens does not threaten because of any fault. For this reason we may feel that we bystanders cannot intervene. But the person threatened can.

In sum, a woman surely can defend her life against the threat to it posed by the unborn child, even if doing so involves its death. And this shows not merely that the theses in (1) through (4) are

false; it shows also that the extreme view of abortion is false, and so we need not canvass any other possible ways of arriving at it from the argument I mentioned at the outset.

2.

The extreme view could of course be weakened to say that while abortion is permissible to save the mother's life, it may not be performed by a third party, but only by the mother herself. But this cannot be right either. For what we have to keep in mind is that the mother and the unborn child are not like two tenants in a small house which has, by an unfortunate mistake, been rented to both: the mother *owns* the house. The fact that she does adds to the offensiveness of deducing that the mother can do nothing from the supposition that third parties can do nothing. But it does more than this: it casts a bright light on the supposition that third parties can do nothing. Certainly it lets us see that a third party who says "I cannot choose between you" is fooling himself if he thinks this is impartiality. If Jones has found and fastened on a certain coat, which he needs to keep him from freezing, but which Smith also needs to keep him from freezing, then it is not impartiality that says "I cannot choose between you" when Smith owns the coat. Women have said again and again "This body is *my* body!" and they have reason to feel angry, reason to feel that it has been like shouting into the wind. Smith, after all, is hardly likely to bless us if we say to him, "Of course it's your coat, anybody would grant that it is. But no one may choose between you and Jones who is to have it."

We should really ask what it is that says "no one may choose" in the face of the fact that the body that houses the child is the mother's body. It may be simply a failure to appreciate this fact. But it may be something more interesting, namely the sense that one has a right to refuse to lay hands on people, even where it would be just and fair to do so, even where justice seems to require that somebody do so. Thus justice might call for somebody to get Smith's coat back from Jones, and yet you have a right to refuse to be the one to lay hands on Jones, a right to refuse to do physical violence to him. This, I think, must be granted. But then what should be said is not "no one may choose," but only "*I* cannot choose," and indeed not even this, but "*I* will not *act*," leaving it open that somebody else can or should, and in particular that anyone in a position of authority, with the job of securing people's rights, both can and should. So this is no difficulty. I have not been arguing that any given third party must accede to the mother's request that he perform an abortion to save her life, but only that he may.

I suppose that in some views of human life the mother's body is only on loan to her, the loan not being one which gives her any prior claim to it. One who held this view might well think it impartiality to say "I cannot choose." But I shall simply ignore this possibility. My own view is that if a human being has any just, prior claim to anything at all, he has a just, prior claim to his own body. And perhaps this needn't be argued for here anyway, since, as I mentioned, the arguments against abortion we are looking at do grant that the woman has a right to decide what happens in and to her body.

But although they do grant it, I have tried to show that they do not take seriously what is done in granting it. I suggest the same thing will reappear even more clearly when we turn away from cases in which the mother's life is at stake, and attend, as I propose we now do, to the vastly more common cases in which a woman wants an abortion for some less weighty reason than preserving her own life.

3.

Where the mother's life is not at stake, the argument I mentioned at the outset seems to have a much stronger pull. "Everyone has a right to life, so the unborn person has a right to life." And isn't the child's right to life weightier than anything other than the mother's own right to life, which she might put forward as ground for an abortion?

This argument treats the right to life as if it were unproblematic. It is not, and this seems to me to be precisely the source of the mistake.

For we should now, at long last, ask what it comes to, to have a right to life. In some views having a right to life includes having a right to be given at least the bare minimum one needs for continued life. But suppose that what in fact *is* the bare minimum a man needs for continued life is

something he has no right at all to be given? If I am sick unto death, and the only thing that will save my life is the touch of Henry Fonda's cool hand on my fevered brow, then all the same, I have no right to be given the touch of Henry Fonda's cool hand on my fevered brow. It would be frightfully nice of him to fly in from the West Coast to provide it. It would be less nice, though no doubt well meant, if my friends flew out to the West Coast and carried Henry Fonda back with them. But I have no right at all against anybody that he should do this for me. Or again, to return to the story I told earlier, the fact that for continued life that violinist needs the continued use of your kidneys does not establish that he has a right to be given the continued use of your kidneys. He certainly has no right against you that *you* should give him continued use of your kidneys. For nobody has any right to use your kidneys unless you give him this right—if you do allow him to go on using your kidneys, this is a kindness on your part, and not something he can claim from you as his due. Nor has he any right against anybody else that *they* should give him continued use of your kidneys. Certainly he had no right against the Society of Music Lovers that they should plug him into you in the first place. And if you now start to unplug yourself, having learned that you will otherwise have to spend nine years in bed with him, there is nobody in the world who must try to prevent you, in order to see to it that he is given something he has a right to be given.

Some people are rather stricter about the right to life. In their view, it does not include the right to be given anything, but amounts to, and only to, the right not to be killed by anybody. But here a related difficulty arises. If everybody is to refrain from killing that violinist, then everybody must refrain from doing a great many different sorts of things. Everybody must refrain from slitting his throat, everybody must refrain from shooting him—and everybody must refrain from unplugging you from him. But does he have a right against everybody that they shall refrain from unplugging you from him? To refrain from doing this is to allow him to continue to use your kidneys. It could be argued that he has a right against us that *we* should allow him to continue to use your kidneys. That is, while he had no right against us that we should give him the use of your kidneys, it might be argued that he anyway has a right against us that we shall not now intervene and deprive him of the use of your kidneys. I shall come back to third-party interventions later. But certainly the violinist has no right against you that *you* shall allow him to continue to use your kidneys. As I said, if you do allow him to use them, it is a kindness on your part, and not something you owe him.

The difficulty I point to here is not peculiar to the right of life. It reappears in connection with all the other natural rights, and it is something which an adequate account of rights must deal with. For present purposes it is enough just to draw attention to it. But I would stress that I am not arguing that people do not have a right to life—quite to the contrary, it seems to me that the primary control we must place on the acceptability of an account of rights is that it should turn out in that account to be a truth that all persons have a right to life. I am arguing only that having a right to life does not guarantee having either a right to be given the use of or a right to be allowed continued use of another person's body—even if one needs it for life itself. So the right to life will not serve the opponents of abortion in the very simple and clear way in which they seem to have thought it would.

4.

There is another way to bring out the difficulty. In the most ordinary sort of case, to deprive someone of what he has a right to is to treat him unjustly. Suppose a boy and his small brother are jointly given a box of chocolates for Christmas. If the older boy takes the box and refuses to give his brother any of the chocolates, he is unjust to him, for the brother has been given a right to half of them. But suppose that, having learned that otherwise it means nine years in bed with that violinist, you unplug yourself from him. You surely are not being unjust to him, for you gave him no right to use your kidneys, and no one else can have given him any such right. But we have to notice that in unplugging yourself, you are killing him; and violinists, like everybody else, have a right to life, and thus in the view we were considering just now, the right not to be killed. So here you do what he supposedly has a right you shall not do, but you do not act unjustly to him in doing it.

The emendation which may be made at this point is this: the right to life consists not in the right not to be killed, but rather in the right not to be killed unjustly. This runs a risk of circularity, but never mind: it would enable us to square the fact that the violinist has a right to life with the fact that you do not act unjustly toward him in unplugging yourself, thereby killing him. For if you do not kill him unjustly, you do not violate his right to life, and so it is no wonder you do him no injustice.

But if this emendation is accepted, the gap in the argument against abortion stares us plainly in the face: it is by no means enough to show that the fetus is a person, and to remind us that all persons have a right to life—we need to be shown also that killing the fetus violates its right to life, i.e., that abortion is unjust killing. And is it?

I suppose we may take it as a datum that in a case of pregnancy due to rape the mother has not given the unborn person a right to the use of her body for food and shelter. Indeed, in what pregnancy could it be supposed that the mother has given the unborn person such a right? It is not as if there were unborn persons drifting about the world, to whom a woman who wants a child says "I invite you in."

But it might be argued that there are other ways one can have acquired a right to the use of another person's body than by having been invited to use it by that person. Suppose a woman voluntarily indulges in intercourse, knowing of the chance it will issue in pregnancy, and then she does become pregnant; is she not in part responsible for the presence, in fact the very existence, of the unborn person inside? No doubt she did not invite it in. But doesn't her partial responsibility for its being there itself give it a right to the use of her body?[7] If so, then her aborting it would be more like the boys taking away the chocolates, and less like your unplugging yourself from the violinist—doing so would be depriving it of what it does have a right to, and thus would be doing it an injustice.

And then, too, it might be asked whether or not she can kill it even to save her own life: If she voluntarily called it into existence, how can she now kill it, even in self-defense?

The first thing to be said about this is that it is something new. Opponents of abortion have been so concerned to make out the independence of the fetus, in order to establish that it has a right to life, just as its mother does, that they have tended to overlook the possible support they might gain from making out that the fetus is *dependent* on the mother, in order to establish that she has a special kind·of responsibility for it, a responsibility that gives it rights against her which are not possessed by any independent person—such as an ailing violinist who is a stranger to her.

On the other hand, this argument would give the unborn person a right to its mother's body only if her pregnancy resulted from a voluntary act, undertaken in full knowledge of the chance a pregnancy might result from it. It would leave out entirely the unborn person whose existence is due to rape. Pending the availability of some further argument, then, we would be left with the conclusion that unborn persons whose existence is due to rape have no right to the use of their mothers' bodies, and thus that aborting them is not depriving them of anything they have a right to and hence is not unjust killing.

And we should also notice that it is not at all plain that this argument really does go even as far as it purports to. For there are cases and cases, and the details make a difference. If the room is stuffy, and I therefore open a window to air it, and a burglar climbs in, it would be absurd to say, "Ah, now he can stay, she's given him a right to the use of her house—for she is partially responsible for his presence there, having voluntarily done what enabled him to get in, in full knowledge that there are such things as burglars, and that burglars burgle." It would be still more absurd to say this if I had had bars installed outside my windows, precisely to prevent burglars from getting in, and a burglar got in only because of a defect in the bars. It remains equally absurd if we imagine it is not a burglar who climbs in, but an innocent person who blunders or falls in. Again, suppose it were like this: people-seeds drift about in the air like pollen, and if you open your windows, one may drift in and take root in your carpets or upholstery. You don't want children, so you fix up your windows with fine mesh screens, the very best you can buy. As can happen, however, and on very, very rare occasions does happen, one of the screens is defective; and a seed drifts in and takes root. Does the person-plant who now develops

have a right to the use of your house? Surely not—despite the fact that you voluntarily opened your windows, you knowingly kept carpets and upholstered furniture, and you knew that screens were sometimes defective. Someone may argue that you are responsible for its rooting, that it does have a right to your house, because after all you *could* have lived out your life with bare floors and furniture, or with sealed windows and doors. But this won't do—for by the same token anyone can avoid a pregnancy due to rape by having a hysterectomy, or anyway by never leaving home without a (reliable!) army.

It seems to me that the argument we are looking at can establish at most that there are *some* cases in which the unborn person has a right to the use of its mother's body, and therefore *some* cases in which abortion is unjust killing. There is room for much discussion and argument as to precisely which, if any. But I think we should sidestep this issue and leave it open, for at any rate the argument certainly does not establish that all abortion is unjust killing.

5.

There is room for yet another argument here, however. We surely must all grant that there may be cases in which it would be morally indecent to detach a person from your body at the cost of his life. Suppose you learn that what the violinist needs is not nine years of your life, but only one hour: all you need do to save his life is to spend one hour in that bed with him. Suppose also that letting him use your kidneys for that one hour would not affect your health in the slightest. Admittedly you were kidnapped. Admittedly you did not give anyone permission to plug him into you. Nevertheless it seems to me plain you *ought* to allow him to use your kidneys for that hour—it would be indecent to refuse.

Again, suppose pregnancy lasted only an hour, and constituted no threat to life or health. And suppose that a woman becomes pregnant as a result of rape. Admittedly she did not voluntarily do anything to bring about the existence of a child. Admittedly she did nothing at all which would give the unborn person a right to the use of her body. All the same it might well be said, as in the newly amended violinist story, that she *ought* to allow it to remain for that hour—that it would be indecent in her to refuse.

Now some people are inclined to use the term "right" in such a way that it follows from the fact that you ought to allow a person to use your body for the hour he needs, that he has a right to use your body for the hour he needs, even though he has not been given that right by any person or act. They may say that it follows also that if you refuse, you act unjustly toward him. This use of the term is perhaps so common that it cannot be called wrong; nevertheless it seems to me to be an unfortunate loosening of what we would do better to keep a tight rein on. Suppose that box of chocolates I mentioned earlier had not been given to both boys jointly, but was given only to the older boy. There he sits, stolidly eating his way through the box, his small brother watching enviously. Here we are likely to say, "You ought not to be so mean. You ought to give your brother some of those chocolates." My own view is that it just does not follow from the truth of this that the brother has any right to any of the chocolates. If the boy refuses to give his brother any, he is greedy, stingy, callous—but not unjust. I suppose that the people I have in mind will say it does follow that the brother has a right to some of the chocolates, and thus that the boy does act unjustly if he refuses to give his brother any. But the effect of saying this is to obscure what we should keep distinct, namely the difference between the boy's refusal in this case and the boy's refusal in the earlier case, in which the box was given to both boys jointly, and in which the small brother thus had what was from any point of view clear title to half.

A further objection to so using the term "right" that from the fact that A ought to do a thing for B, it follows that B has a right against A that A do it for him, is that it is going to make the question of whether or not a man has a right to a thing turn on how easy it is to provide him with it; and this seems not merely unfortunate, but morally unacceptable. Take the case of Henry Fonda again. I said earlier that I had no right to the touch of his cool hand on my fevered brow, even though I needed it to save my life. I said it would be frightfully nice of him to fly in from the West Coast to provide me with it, but that I had no right against him that he should do so. But suppose he isn't on the West Coast. Suppose he has only to walk across the room, place a hand briefly on my brow—and lo, my life is saved. Then surely he ought to do it, it would be indecent to refuse. Is it to be said, "Ah, well, it follows that in this case she has a right to the touch of his hand on her brow, and so it would be an injustice in him to refuse"? So that I have a right to it when it is easy for him to provide it, though no right when it's hard? It's rather a shocking idea that anyone's rights should fade away and disappear as it gets harder and harder to accord them to him.

So my own view is that even though you ought to let the violinist use your kidneys for the one hour he needs, we should not conclude that he has a right to do so—we should say that if you refuse, you are, like the boy who owns all the chocolates and will give none away, self-centered and callous, indecent in fact, but not unjust. And similarly, that even supposing a case in which a woman pregnant due to rape ought to allow the unborn person to use her body for the hour he needs, we should not conclude that he has a right to do so; we should conclude that she is self-centered, callous, indecent, but not unjust, if she refuses. The complaints are no less grave; they are just different. However, there is no need to insist on this point. If anyone does wish to deduce "he has a right" from "you ought," then all the same he must surely grant that there are cases in which it is not morally required of you that you allow that violinist to use your kidneys, and in which he does not have a right to use them, and in which you do not do him an injustice if you refuse. And so also for mother and unborn child. Except in such cases as the unborn person has a right to demand it—and we were leaving open the possibility that there may be such cases—nobody is morally *required* to make large sacrifices, of health, of all other interests and concerns, of all other duties and commitments, for nine years, or even for nine months, in order to keep another person alive.

6.

We have in fact to distinguish between two kinds of Samaritan: the Good Samaritan and what we might call the Minimally Decent Samaritan. The story of the Good Samaritan, you will remember, goes like this:

A certain man went down from Jerusalem to Jericho, and fell among thieves, which stripped him of his raiment, and wounded him, and departed, leaving him half dead.

And by chance there came down a certain priest that way: and when he saw him, he passed by on the other side.

And likewise a Levite, when he was at the place, came and looked on him, and passed by on the other side.

But a certain Samaritan, as he journeyed, came where he was; and when he saw him he had compassion on him.

And went to him, and bound up his wounds, pouring in oil and wine, and set him on his own beast, and brought him to an inn, and took care of him.

And on the morrow, when he departed, he took out two pence, and gave them to the host, and said unto him, "Take care of him; and whatsoever thou spendest more, when I come again, I will repay thee." (Luke 10:30–35)

The Good Samaritan went out of his way, at some cost to himself, to help one in need of it. We are not told what the options were, that is, whether or not the priest and the Levite could have helped by doing less than the Good Samaritan did, but assuming they could have, then the fact they did nothing at all shows they were not even Minimally Decent Samaritans, not because they were not Samaritans, but because they were not even minimally decent.

These things are a matter of degree, of course, but there is a difference, and it comes out perhaps most clearly in the story of Kitty Genovese, who, as you will remember, was murdered while thirty-eight people watched or listened, and did nothing at all to help her. A Good Samaritan would have rushed out to give direct assistance against the murderer. Or perhaps we had better allow that it would have been a Splendid Samaritan who did this, on the ground that it would have involved a risk of death for himself. But the thirty-eight not only did not do this, they did not even trouble to pick up a phone to call the police. Minimally Decent Samaritanism would call for doing at least that, and their not having done it was monstrous.

After telling the story of the Good Samaritan, Jesus said, "Go, and do thou likewise." Perhaps he meant that we are morally required to act as the Good Samaritan did. Perhaps he was urging peo-ple to do more than is morally required of them. At all events it seems plain that it was not morally required of any of the thirty-eight that he rush out to give direct assistance at the risk of his own life, and that it is not morally required of anyone that he give long stretches of his life—nine years or nine months—to sustaining the life of a person who has no special right (we were leaving open the possibility of this) to demand it.

Indeed, with one rather striking class of exceptions, no one in any country in the world is *legally* required to do anywhere near as much as this for anyone else. The class of exceptions is obvious. My main concern here is not the state of the law in respect to abortion, but it is worth drawing attention to the fact that in no state in this country is any man compelled by law to be even a Minimally Decent Samaritan to any person; there is no law under which charges could be brought against the thirty-eight who stood by while Kitty Genovese died. By contrast, in most states in this country women are compelled by law to be not merely Minimally Decent Samaritans, but Good Samaritans to unborn persons inside them. This doesn't by itself settle anything one way or the other, because it may well be argued that there should be laws in this country—as there are in many European countries—compelling at least Minimally Decent Samaritanism.[8] But it does show that there is a gross injustice in the existing state of the law. And it shows also that the groups currently working against liberalization of abortion laws, in fact working toward having it declared unconstitutional for a state to permit abortion, had better start working for the adoption of Good Samaritan laws generally, or earn the charge that they are acting in bad faith.

I should think, myself, that Minimally Decent Samaritan laws would be one thing, Good Samaritan laws quite another, and in fact highly improper. But we are not here concerned with the law. What we should ask is not whether anybody should be compelled by law to be a Good Samaritan, but whether we must accede to a situation in which somebody is being compelled—by nature, perhaps—to be a Good Samaritan. We have, in other words, to look now at third-party interventions. I have been arguing that no person is morally required to make large sacrifices to sustain the life of another who has no right to demand them, and this even where the sacrifices do not include life itself; we are not morally required to be Good Samaritans or anyway Very Good Samaritans to one another. But what if a man cannot extricate himself from such a situation? What if he appeals to us to extricate him? It seems to me plain that there are cases in which we can, cases in which a good Samaritan would extricate him. There you are, you were kidnapped, and nine years in bed with that violinist lie ahead of you. You have your own life to lead. You are sorry, but you simply cannot see giving up so much of your life to the sustaining of his. You cannot extricate yourself, and ask us to do so. I should have thought that—in light of his having no right to the use of your body—it was obvious that we do not have to accede to your being forced to give up so much. We can do what you ask. There is no injustice to the violinist in our doing so.

7.

Following the lead of the opponents of abortion, I have throughout been speaking of the fetus merely as a person, and what I have been asking is whether or not the argument we began with, which proceeds only from the fetus's being a person, really does establish its conclusion. I have argued that it does not.

But of course there are arguments and arguments, and it may be said that I have simply fastened on the wrong one. It may be said that what is important is not merely the fact that the fetus is a person, but that it is a person for whom the woman has a special kind of responsibility issuing from the fact that she is its mother. And it might be argued that all my analogies are therefore irrelevant—for you do not have that special kind of responsibility for that violinist, Henry Fonda does not have that special kind of responsibility for me. And our attention might be drawn to the fact that men and women both *are* compelled by law to provide support for their children.

I have in effect dealt (briefly) with this argument in section 4 above; but a (still briefer) recapitulation now may be in order. Surely we do not have any such "special responsibility" for a person unless we have assumed it, explicitly or implicitly. If a set of parents do not try to prevent pregnancy, do not obtain an abortion, but rather take it home

with them, then they have assumed responsibility for it, they have given it rights, and they cannot *now* withdraw support from it at the cost of its life because they now find it difficult to go on providing for it. But if they have taken all reasonable precautions against having a child, they do not simply by virtue of their biological relationship to the child who comes into existence have a special responsibility for it. They may wish to assume responsibility for it, or they may not wish to. And I am suggesting that if assuming responsibility for it would require large sacrifices, then they may refuse. A Good Samaritan would not refuse—or anyway, a Splendid Samaritan, if the sacrifices that had to be made were enormous. But then so would a Good Samaritan assume responsibility for that violinist; so would Henry Fonda, if he is a Good Samaritan, fly in from the West Coast and assume responsibility for me.

8.

My argument will be found unsatisfactory on two counts by many of those who want to regard abortion as morally permissible. First, while I do argue that abortion is not impermissible, I do not argue that it is always permissible. There may well be cases in which carrying the child to term requires only Minimally Decent Samaritanism of the mother, and this is a standard we must not fall below. I am inclined to think it a merit of my account precisely that it does *not* give a general yes or a general no. It allows for and supports our sense that, for example, a sick and desperately frightened fourteen-year-old schoolgirl, pregnant due to rape, may of *course* choose abortion, and that any law which rules this out is an insane law. And it also allows for and supports our sense that in other cases resort to abortion is even positively indecent. It would be indecent in the woman to request an abortion, and indecent in a doctor to perform it, if she is in her seventh month, and wants the abortion just to avoid the nuisance of postponing a trip abroad. The very fact that the arguments I have been drawing attention to treat all cases of abortion, or even all cases of abortion in which the mother's life is not at stake, as morally on a par ought to have made them suspect at the outset.

Second, while I am arguing for the permissibility of abortion in some cases, I am not arguing for the right to secure the death of the unborn child. It is easy to confuse these two things in that up to a certain point in the life of the fetus it is not able to survive outside the mother's body; hence removing it from her body guarantees its death. But they are importantly different. I have argued that you are not morally required to spend nine months in bed, sustaining the life of that violinist; but to say this is by no means to say that if, when you unplug yourself, there is a miracle and he survives, you then have a right to turn round and slit his throat. You may detach yourself even if this costs him his life; you have no right to be guaranteed his death, by some other means, if unplugging yourself does not kill him. There are some people who will feel dissatisfied by this feature of my argument. A woman may be utterly devastated by the thought of a child, a bit of herself, put out for adoption and never seen or heard of again. She may therefore want not merely that the child be detached from her, but more, that it die. Some opponents of abortion are inclined to regard this as beneath contempt—thereby showing insensitivity to what is surely a powerful source of despair. All the same, I agree that the desire for the child's death is not one which anybody may gratify, should it turn out to be possible to detach the child alive.

At this place, however, it should be remembered that we have only been pretending throughout that the fetus is a human being from the moment of conception. A very early abortion is surely not the killing of a person, and so is not dealt with by anything I have said here.

Notes

1. I am very much indebted to James Thomson for discussion, criticism, and many helpful suggestions.

2. Daniel Callahan, *Abortion: Law, Choice and Morality* (New York, 1970), p. 373. This book gives a fascinating survey of the available information on abortion. The Jewish tradition is surveyed in David M. Feldman, *Birth Control in Jewish Law* (New York, 1968). part 5, the Catholic tradition in John T. Noonan, Jr., "An Almost Absolute Value in History," in *The Morality of Abortion*, ed. John T. Noonan, Jr. (Cambridge, Mass., 1970).

3. The term "direct" in the arguments I refer to is a technical one. Roughly, what is meant by "direct killing" is either killing as an end in itself, or killing as a means to some end, for example, the end of saving someone else's life. See note 6, below, for an example of its use.

4. Cf. *Encyclical Letter of Pope Pius XI on Christian Marriage*, St. Paul Editions (Boston, n.d.), p. 32: "However much we may pity the mother whose health and even life is gravely imperiled in the performance of the duty allotted to her by nature, nevertheless what could ever be a sufficient reason for excusing in any way the direct murder of the innocent? This is precisely what we are dealing with here." Noonan (*The Morality of Abortion*, p. 43) reads this as follows: "What cause can ever avail to excuse in any way the direct killing of the innocent? For it is a question of that."

5. The thesis in (4) is in an interesting way weaker than those in (1), (2), and (3): they rule out abortion even in cases in which both mother *and* child will die if the abortion is not performed. By contrast, one who held the view expressed in (4) could consistently say that one needn't prefer letting two persons die to killing one.

6. Cf. the following passage from Pius XII, *Address to the Italian Catholic Society of Midwives*: "The baby in the maternal breast has the right to life immediately from God.—Hence there is no man, no human authority, no science, no medical, eugenic, social, economic or moral 'indication' which can establish or grant a valid juridical ground for a direct deliberate disposition of an innocent human life, that is a disposition which looks to its destruction either as an end or as a means to another end perhaps in itself not illicit.—The baby, still not born, is a man in the same degree and for the same reason as the mother" (quoted in Noonan, *The Morality of Abortion*, p. 45).

7. The need for a discussion of this argument was brought home to me by members of the Society for Ethical and Legal Philosophy, to whom this paper was originally presented.

8. For a discussion of the difficulties involved, and a survey of the European experience with such laws, see *The Good Samaritan and the Law*, ed. James M. Ratcliffe (New York, 1966).

On the Moral and Legal Status of Abortion ⸻

Mary Anne Warren

We will be concerned with both the moral status of abortion, which for our purposes we may define as the act which a woman performs in voluntarily terminating, or allowing another person to terminate, her pregnancy, and the legal status which is appropriate for this act. I will argue that, while it is not possible to produce a satisfactory defense of a woman's right to obtain an abortion without showing that a fetus is not a human being, in the morally relevant sense of that term, we ought not to conclude that the difficulties involved in determining whether or not a fetus is human make it impossible to produce any satisfactory solution to the problem of the moral status of abortion. For it is possible to show that, on the basis of intuitions which we may expect even the opponents of abortion to share, a fetus is not a person, and hence not the sort of entity to which it is proper to ascribe full moral rights.

Of course, while some philosophers would deny the possibility of any such proof,[1] others will deny that there is any need for it, since the moral permissibility of abortion appears to them to be too obvious to require proof. But the inadequacy of this attitude should be evident from the fact that both the friends and the foes of abortion consider their position to be morally self-evident. Because proabortionists have never adequately come to grips with the conceptual issues surrounding abortion, most if not all, of the arguments which they advance in opposition to laws restricting access to abortion fail to refute or even weaken the traditional antiabortion argument, i.e., that a fetus is a human being, and therefore abortion is murder.

These arguments are typically of one of two sorts. Either they point to the terrible side effects of the restrictive laws, e.g., the deaths due to illegal abortions, and the fact that it is poor women who suffer the most as a result of these laws, or else they state that to deny a woman access to abortion is to deprive her of her right to control her own body. Unfortunately, however, the fact that restricting access to abortion has tragic side effects does not, in itself, show that the restrictions are unjustified, since murder is wrong regardless of the consequences of prohibiting it; and the appeal to the right to control one's body, which is generally construed as a property right, is at best a rather feeble argument for the permissibility of abortion. Mere ownership does not give me the right to kill innocent people whom I find on my property, and indeed I am apt to be held responsible if such people injure themselves while on my property. It is equally unclear that I have any moral right to expel an innocent person from my property when I know that doing so will result in his death.

Furthermore, it is probably inappropriate to describe a woman's body as her property, since it seems natural to hold that a person is something distinct from her property, but not from her body. Even those who would object to the identification of a person with his body, or with the conjunction of his body and his mind, must admit that it would be very odd to describe, say, breaking a leg, as damaging one's property, and much more appropriate to describe it as injuring one*self*. Thus it is probably a mistake to argue that the right to obtain an abortion is in any way derived from the right to own and regulate property.

But however we wish to construe the right to abortion, we cannot hope to convince those who consider abortion a form of murder of the existence of any such right unless we are able to produce a clear and convincing refutation of the traditional antiabortion argument, and this has not, to my knowledge, been done. With respect to the two most vital issues which that argument involves, i.e., the humanity of the fetus and its implication for the moral status of abortion, confusion has prevailed on both sides of the dispute.

Thus, both proabortionists and antiabortionists have tended to abstract the question of

Reprinted from The Monist, LaSalle, Illinois 61301, Vol. 57, no. 1, with permission of the author and the publisher. "Postscript on Infanticide" reprinted from The Problem of Abortion, Second Edition, edited by Joel Feinberg (Belmont, Calif.: Wadsworth, 1984).

whether abortion is wrong to that of whether it is wrong to destroy a fetus, just as though the rights of another person were not necessarily involved. This mistaken abstraction has led to the almost universal assumption that if a fetus is a human being, with a right to life, then it follows immediately that abortion is wrong (except perhaps when necessary to save the woman's life), and that it ought to be prohibited. It has also been generally assumed that unless the question about the status of the fetus is answered, the moral status of abortion cannot possibly be determined.

Two recent papers, one by B. A. Brody,[2] and one by Judith Thomson,[3] have attempted to settle the question of whether abortion ought to be prohibited apart from the question of whether or not the fetus is human. Brody examines the possibility that the following two statements are compatible: (1) that abortion is the taking of innocent human life, and therefore wrong; and (2) that nevertheless it ought not to be prohibited by law, at least under the present circumstances.[4] Not surprisingly, Brody finds it impossible to reconcile these two statements, since, as he rightly argues, none of the unfortunate side effects of the prohibition of abortion is bad enough to justify legalizing the *wrongful* taking of human life. He is mistaken, however, in concluding that the incompatibility of (1) and (2), in itself, shows that "the legal problem about abortion cannot be resolved independently of the status of the fetus problem" (p. 369).

What Brody fails to realize is that (1) embodies the questionable assumption that if a fetus is a human being, then of course abortion is morally wrong, and that an attack on *this* assumption is more promising, as a way of reconciling the humanity of the fetus with the claim that laws prohibiting abortion are unjustified, than is an attack on the assumption that if abortion is the wrongful killing of innocent human beings then it ought to be prohibited. He thus overlooks the possibility that a fetus may have a right to life and abortion still be morally permissible, in that the right of a woman to terminate an unwanted pregnancy might override the right of the fetus to be kept alive. This immorality of abortion is no more demonstrated by the humanity of the fetus, in itself, than the immorality of killing in self-defense is demonstrated by the fact that the assailant is a human being. Neither is it demonstrated by the

innocence of the fetus, since there may be situations in which the killing of innocent human beings is justified.

It is perhaps not surprising that Brody fails to spot this assumption, since it has been accepted with little or no argument by nearly everyone who has written on the morality of abortion. John Noonan is correct in saying that "the fundamental question in the long history of abortion is, How do you determine the humanity of a being?"[5] He summarizes his own antiabortion argument, which is a version of the official position of the Catholic Church, as follows:

> . . . it is wrong to kill humans, however poor, weak, defenseless, and lacking in opportunity to develop their potential they may be. It is therefore morally wrong to kill Biafrans. Similarly, it is morally wrong to kill embryos.[6]

Noonan bases his claim that fetuses are human upon what he calls the theologians' criterion of humanity: that whoever is conceived of human beings is human. But although he argues at length for the appropriateness of this criterion, he never questions the assumption that if a fetus is human then abortion is wrong for exactly the same reason that murder is wrong.

Judith Thomson is, in fact, the only writer I am aware of who has seriously questioned this assumption; she has argued that, even if we grant the antiabortionist his claim that a fetus is a human being, with the same right to life as any other human being, we can still demonstrate that, in at least some and perhaps most cases, a woman is under no moral obligation to complete an unwanted pregnancy.[7] Her argument is worth examining, since if it holds up it may enable us to establish the moral permissibility of abortion without becoming involved in problems about what entitles an entity to be considered human, and accorded full moral rights. To be able to do this would be a great gain in the power and simplicity of the proabortion position, since, although I will argue that these problems can be solved at least as decisively as can any other moral problem, we should certainly be pleased to be able to avoid having to solve them as part of the justification of abortion.

On the other hand, even if Thomson's argument does not hold up, her insight, i.e., that it prone to the sort of illness the only cure for which is the use of someone else's bloodstream for nine months, and that because of this there has been formed a society of music lovers who agree that whenever a violinist is stricken they will draw lots and the loser will, by some means, be made the one and only person capable of saving him. Now then, would you be obligated to cooperate in curing the violinist if you had voluntarily joined this society, knowing the possible consequences, and then your name had been drawn and you had been kidnapped? Admittedly, you did not promise ahead of time that you would, but you did deliberately place yourself in a position in which it might happen that a human life would be lost if you did not. Surely this is at least a prima facie reason for supposing that you have an obligation to stay in bed with the violinist. Suppose that you had gotten your name drawn deliberately; surely *that* would be quite a strong reason for thinking that you had such an obligation.

It might be suggested that there is one important disanalogy between the modified violinist case and the case of an unwanted pregnancy, which makes the woman's responsibility significantly less, namely, the fact that the fetus *comes into existence* as the result of the result of the woman's actions. This fact might give her a right to refuse to keep it alive, whereas she would not have had this right had it existed previously, independently, and then as a result of her actions become dependent upon her for its survival.

My own intuition, however, is that x has no more right to bring into existence, either deliberately or as a foreseeable result of actions he could have avoided, a being with full moral rights (y), and then refuse to do what he knew beforehand would be required to keep that being alive, than he has to enter into an agreement with an existing person, whereby he may be called upon to save that person's life, and then refuse to do so when so called upon. Thus x's responsibility for y's existence does not seem to lessen his obligation to keep y alive, if he is also responsible for y's being in a situation in which only he can save him.

Whether or not this intuition is entirely correct, it brings us back once again to the conclusion that once we allow the assumption that a fetus has full moral rights it becomes an extremely complex

and difficult question whether and when abortion is justifiable. Thus the Thomson analogy cannot help us produce a clear and persuasive proof of the moral permissibility of abortion. Nor will the opponents of the restrictive laws thank us for anything less; for their conviction (for the most part) is that abortion is obviously *not* a morally serious and extremely unfortunate, even though sometimes justified act, comparable to killing in self-defense or to letting the violinist die, but rather is closer to being a morally neutral act, like cutting one's hair.

The basis of this conviction, I believe, is the realization that a fetus is not a person, and thus does not have a full-fledged right to life. Perhaps the reason why this claim has been so inadequately defended is that it seems self-evident to those who accept it. And so it is, insofar as it follows from what I take to be perfectly obvious claims about the nature of personhood, and about the proper grounds for ascribing moral rights, claims which ought, indeed, to be obvious to both the friends and foes of abortion. Nevertheless, it is worth examining these claims, and showing how they demonstrate the moral innocuousness of abortion, since this apparently has not been adequately done before.

II

The question which we must answer in order to produce a satisfactory solution to the problem of the moral status of abortion is this: How are we to define the moral community, the set of beings with full and equal moral rights, such that we can decide whether a human fetus is a member of this community or not? What sort of entity, exactly, has the inalienable rights to life, liberty, and the pursuit of happiness? Jefferson attributed these rights to all *men*, and it may or may not be fair to suggest that he intended to attribute them *only* to men. Perhaps he ought have attributed them to all human beings. If so, then we arrive, first, at Noonan's problem of defining what makes a being human, and, second, at the equally vital question which Noonan does not consider, namely, What reason is there for identifying the moral community with the set of all human beings, in whatever way we have chosen to define that term?

1. On the Definition of 'Human'

One reason why this vital second question is so frequently overlooked in the debate over the moral status of abortion is that the term 'human' has two distinct, but not often distinguished, senses. This fact results in a slide of meaning, which serves to conceal the fallaciousness of the traditional argument that since (1) it is wrong to kill innocent human beings, and (2) fetuses are innocent human beings, then (3) it is wrong to kill fetuses. For if 'human' is used in the same sense in both (1) and (2) then, whichever of the two senses is meant, one of these premises is question-begging. And if it is used in two different senses then of course the conclusion doesn't follow.

Thus, (1) is a self-evident moral truth,[9] and avoids begging the question about abortion, only if 'human being' is used to mean something like 'a full-fledged member of the moral community.' (It may or may not also be meant to refer exclusively to members of the species *Homo sapiens*.) We may call this the *moral* sense of 'human.' It is not to be confused with what we will call the *genetic* sense; i.e., the sense in which *any* member of the species is a human being, and no member of any other species could be. If (1) is acceptable only if the moral sense is intended, (2) is non-question-begging only if what is intended is the genetic sense.

In "Deciding Who is Human," Noonan argues for the classification of fetuses with human beings by pointing to the presence of the full genetic code, and the potential capacity for rational thought (p. 135). It is clear that what he needs to show, for his version of the traditional argument to be valid, is that fetuses are human in the moral sense, the sense in which it is analytically true that all human beings have full moral rights. But, in the absence of any argument showing that whatever is genetically human is also morally human, and he gives none, nothing more than genetic humanity can be demonstrated by the presence of the human genetic code. And, as we will see, the *potential* capacity for rational thought can at most show that an entity has the potential for *becoming* human in the moral sense.

2. Defining the Moral Community

Can it be established that genetic humanity is sufficient for moral humanity? I think that there are very good reasons for not defining the moral community in this way. I would like to suggest an alternative way of defining the moral community, which I will argue for only to the extent of explaining why it is, or should be, self-evident. The suggestion is simply that the moral community consists of all and only *people*, rather than all and only human beings;[10] and probably the best way of demonstrating its self-evidence is by considering the concept of personhood, to see what sorts of entity are and are not persons, and what the decision that a being is or is not a person implies about its moral rights.

What characteristics entitle an entity to be considered a person? This is obviously not the place to attempt a complete analysis of the concept of personhood, but we do not need such a fully adequate analysis just to determine whether and why a fetus is or isn't a person. All we need is a rough and approximate list of the most basic criteria of personhood, and some idea of which, or how many, of these an entity must satisfy in order to properly be considered a person.

In searching for such criteria, it is useful to look beyond the set of people with whom we are acquainted, and ask how we would decide whether a totally alien being was a person or not. (For we have no right to assume that genetic humanity is necessary for personhood.) Imagine a space traveler who lands on an unknown planet and encounters a race of beings utterly unlike any he has ever seen or heard of. If he wants to be sure of behaving morally toward these beings, he has to somehow decide whether they are people, and hence have full moral rights, or whether they are the sort of thing which he need not feel guilty about treating as, for example, a source of food.

How should he go about making this decision? If he has some anthropological background, he might look for such things as religion, art, and the manufacturing of tools, weapons, or shelters, since these factors have been used to distinguish our human from our prehuman ancestors, in what seems to be closer to the moral than the genetic sense of 'human.' And no doubt he would be right to consider the presence of such factors as good evidence that the alien beings were people, and morally human. It would, however, be overly anthropocentric of him to take the absence of these things as adequate evidence that they were not, since we can imagine people who have progressed beyond, or evolved without ever developing, these cultural characteristics.

I suggest that the traits which are most central to the concept of personhood, or humanity in the moral sense, are, very roughly, the following:

1. consciousness (of objects and events external and/or internal to the being), and in particular the capacity to feel pain;

2. reasoning (the *developed* capacity to solve new and relatively complex problems);

3. self-motivated activity (activity which is relatively independent of either genetic or direct external control);

4. the capacity to communicate, by whatever means, messages of an indefinite variety of types, that is, not just with an indefinite number of possible contents, but on indefinitely many possible topics;

5. the presence of self-concepts, and self-awareness, either individual or racial, or both.

Admittedly, there are apt to be a great many problems involved in formulating precise definitions of these criteria, let alone in developing universally valid behavioral criteria for deciding when they apply. But I will assume that both we and our explorer know approximately what (1)–(5) mean, and that he is also able to determine whether or not they apply. How, then, should he use his findings to decide whether or not the alien beings are people? We needn't suppose that an entity must have *all* of these attributes to be properly considered a person; (1) and (2) alone may well be sufficient for personhood, and quite probably (1)–(3) are sufficient. Neither do we need to insist that any one of these criteria is *necessary* for personhood, although once again (1) and (2) look like fairly good candidates for necessary conditions, as does (3), if 'activity' is construed so as to include the activity of reasoning.

All we need to claim, to demonstrate that a fetus is not a person, is that any being which satisfies *none* of (1)–(5) is certainly not a person. I consider this claim to be so obvious that I think anyone who denied it, and claimed that a being which satisfied none of (1)–(5) was a person all the same, would thereby demonstrate that he had no notion at all of what a person is—perhaps because he had

confused the concept of a person with that of genetic humanity. If the opponents of abortion were to deny the appropriateness of these five criteria. I do not know what further arguments would convince them. We would probably have to admit that our conceptual schemes were indeed irreconcilably different, and that our dispute could not be settled objectively.

I do not expect this to happen, however, since I think that the concept of a person is one which is very nearly universal (to people), and that it is common to both proabortionists and antiabortionists, even though neither group has fully realized the relevance of this concept to the resolution of their dispute. Furthermore, I think that on reflection even the antiabortionists ought to agree not only that (1)–(5) are central to the concept of personhood, but also that it is a part of this concept that all and only people have full moral rights. The concept of a person is in part a moral concept; once we have admitted that *x* is a person we have recognized, even if we have not agreed to respect, *x*'s right to be treated as a member of the moral community. It is true that the claim that *x* is a *human being* is more commonly voiced as part of an appeal to treat *x* decently than is the claim that *x* is a person, but this is either because 'human being' is here used in the sense which implies personhood, or because the genetic and moral senses of 'human' have been confused.

Now if (1)–(5) are indeed the primary criteria of personhood, then it is clear that genetic humanity is neither necessary nor sufficient for establishing that an entity is a person. Some human beings are not people, and there may well be people who are not human beings. A man or woman whose consciousness has been permanently obliterated but who remains alive is a human being which is no longer a person; defective human beings, with no appreciable mental capacity, are not and presumably never will be people; and a fetus is a human being which is not yet a person, and which therefore cannot coherently be said to have full moral rights. Citizens of the next century should be prepared to recognize highly advanced, self-aware robots or computers, should such be developed, and intelligent inhabitants of other worlds, should such be found, as people in the fullest sense, and to respect their moral rights. But to ascribe full moral rights to an entity which is not a person is as absurd as to ascribe moral obligations and responsibilities to such an entity.

3. Fetal Development and the Right to Life

Two problems arise in the application of these suggestions for the definition of the moral community to the determination of the precise moral status of a human fetus. Given that the paradigm example of a person is a normal adult being, then (1) How like this paradigm, in particular how far advanced since conception, does a human being need to be before it begins to have a right to life by virtue, not of being fully a person as of yet, but of being *like* a person? and (2) To what extent, if any, does the fact that a fetus has the *potential* for becoming a person endow it with some of the same rights? Each of these questions requires some comment.

In answering the first question, we need not attempt a detailed consideration of the moral rights of organisms which are not developed enough, aware enough, intelligent enough, etc., to be considered people, but which resemble people in some respects. It does seem reasonable to suggest that the more like a person, in the relevant respects, a being is, the stronger is the case for regarding it as having a right to life, and indeed the stronger its right to life is. Thus we ought to take seriously the suggestion that, insofar as "the human individual develops biologically in a continuous fashion . . . the rights of a human person might develop in the same way."[11] But we must keep in mind that the attributes which are relevant in determining whether or not an entity is enough like a person to be regarded as having some of the same moral rights are no different from those which are relevant to determining whether or not it is fully a person—i.e., are no different from (1)–(5)—and that being genetically human, or having recognizably human facial and other physical features, or detectable brain activity, or the capacity to survive outside the uterus, are simply not among these relevant attributes.

Thus it is clear that even though a seven- or eight-month fetus has features which make it apt to arouse in us almost the same powerful protective instinct as is commonly aroused by a small infant, nevertheless it is not significantly more

personlike than is a very small embryo. It is *somewhat* more personlike; it can apparently feel and respond to pain, and it may even have a rudimentary form of consciousness, insofar as its brain is quite active. Nevertheless, it seems safe to say that it is not fully conscious, in the way that an infant of a few months is, and that it cannot reason, or communicate messages of indefinitely many sorts, does not engage in self-motivated activity, and has no self-awareness. Thus, in the *relevant* respects, a fetus, even a fully developed one, is considerably less personlike than is the average mature mammal, indeed the average fish. And I think that a rational person must conclude that if the right to life of a fetus is to be based upon its resemblance to a person, then it cannot be said to have any more right to life than, let us say, a newborn guppy (which also seems to be capable of feeling pain), and that a right of that magnitude could never override a woman's right to obtain an abortion, at any stage of her pregnancy.

There may, of course, be other arguments in favor of placing legal limits upon the stage of pregnancy in which an abortion may be performed. Given the relative safety of the new techniques of artificially inducing labor during the third trimester, the danger to the woman's life or health is no longer such an argument. Neither is the fact that people tend to respond to the thought of abortion in the later stages of pregnancy with emotional repulsion, since mere emotional responses cannot take the place of moral reasoning in determining what ought to be permitted. Nor, finally, is the frequently heard argument that legalizing abortion, especially late in the pregnancy, may erode the level of respect for human life, leading, perhaps, to an increase in unjustified euthanasia and other crimes. For this threat, if it is a threat, can be better met by educating people to the kinds of moral distinctions which we are making here than by limiting access to abortion (which limitation may, in its disregard for the rights of women, be just as damaging to the level of respect for human rights).

Thus, since the fact that even a fully developed fetus is not personlike enough to have any significant right to life on the basis of its personlikeness shows that no legal restrictions upon the stage of pregnancy in which an abortion may be performed can be justified on the grounds that we should protect the rights of the older fetus; and since there is no other apparent justification for such restrictions, we may conclude that they are entirely unjustified. Whether or not it would be *indecent* (whatever that means) for a woman in her seventh month to obtain an abortion just to avoid having to postpone a trip to Europe, it would not, in itself, be *immoral*, and therefore it ought to be permitted.

4. Potential Personhood and the Right to Life

We have seen that a fetus does not resemble a person in any way which can support the claim that it has even some of the same rights. But what about its *potential*, the fact that if nurtured and allowed to develop naturally it will very probably become a person? Doesn't that alone give it at least some right to life? It is hard to deny that the fact that an entity is a potential person is a strong prima facie reason for not destroying it; but we need not conclude from this that a potential person has a right to life, by virtue of that potential. It may be that our feeling that it is better, other things being equal, not to destroy a potential person is better explained by the fact that potential people are still (felt to be) an invaluable resource, not to be lightly squandered. Surely, if every speck of dust were a potential person, we would be much less apt to conclude that every potential person has a right to become actual.

Still, we do not need to insist that a potential person has no right to life whatever. There may well be something immoral, and not just imprudent, about wantonly destroying potential people, when doing so isn't necessary to protect anyone's rights. But even if a potential person does have some prima facie right to life, such a right could not possibly outweigh the right of a woman to obtain an abortion, since the rights of any actual person invariably outweigh those of any potential person, whenever the two conflict. Since this may not be immediately obvious in the case of a human fetus, let us look at another case.

Suppose that our space explorer falls into the hands of an alien culture, whose scientists decide to create a few hundred thousand or more human beings, by breaking his body into its component cells, and using these to create fully developed human beings, with, of course, his genetic code. We may imagine that each of these newly created men will have all of the original man's abilities, skills, knowledge, and so on, and also have an individual self-concept, in short that each of them will be a bona fide (though hardly unique) person. Imagine that the whole project will take only seconds, and that its chances of success are extremely high, and that our explorer knows all of this, and also knows that these people will be treated fairly. I maintain that in such a situation he would have every right to escape if he could, and thus to deprive all of these potential people of their potential lives; for his right to life outweighs all of theirs together, in spite of the fact that they are all genetically human, all innocent, and all have a very high probability of becoming people very soon, if only he refrains from acting.

Indeed, I think he would have a right to escape even if it were not his life which the alien scientists planned to take, but only a year of his freedom, or, indeed, only a day. Nor would he be obligated to stay if he had gotten captured (thus bringing all these people-potentials into existence) because of his own carelessness, or even if he had done so deliberately, knowing the consequences. Regardless of how he got captured, he is not morally obligated to remain in captivity for *any* period of time for the sake of permitting any number of potential people to come into actuality, so great is the margin by which one actual person's right to liberty outweighs whatever right to life even a hundred thousand potential people have. And it seems reasonable to conclude that the rights of a woman will outweigh by a similar margin whatever right to life a fetus may have by virtue of its potential personhood.

Thus, neither a fetus's resemblance to a person, nor its potential for becoming a person provides any basis whatever for the claim that it has any significant right to life. Consequently, a woman's right to protect her health, happiness, freedom, and even her life,[12] by terminating an unwanted pregnancy, will always override whatever right to life it may be appropriate to ascribe to a fetus, even a fully developed one. And thus, in the absence of any overwhelming social need for every possible child, the laws which restrict the right to obtain an abortion, or limit the period of pregnancy during which an abortion may be performed, are a wholly unjustified violation of a woman's most basic moral and constitutional rights.[13]

Postscript on Infanticide, February 26, 1982

One of the most troubling objections to the argument presented in this article is that it may appear to justify not only abortion but infanticide as well. A newborn infant is not a great deal more personlike than a nine-month fetus, and thus it might seem that if late-term abortion is sometimes justified, then infanticide must also be sometimes justified. Yet most people consider that infanticide is a form of murder, and thus never justified.

While it is important to appreciate the emotional force of this objection, its logical force is far less than it may seem at first glance. There are many reasons why infanticide is much more difficult to justify than abortion, even though if my argument is correct neither constitutes the killing of a person. In this country, and in this period of history, the deliberate killing of viable newborns is virtually never justified. This is in part because neonates are so very *close* to being persons that to kill them requires a very strong moral justification—as does the killing of dolphins, whales, chimpanzees, and other highly personlike creatures. It is certainly wrong to kill such beings just for the sake of convenience, or financial profit, or "sport."

Another reason why infanticide is usually wrong, in our society, is that if the newborn's parents do not want it, or are unable to care for it, there are (in most cases) people who are able and eager to adopt it and to provide a good home for it. Many people wait years for the opportunity to adopt a child, and some are unable to do so even though there is every reason to believe that they would be good parents. The needless destruction of a viable infant inevitably deprives some person or persons of a source of great pleasure and satisfaction, perhaps severely impoverishing their lives. Furthermore, even if an infant is considered to be unadoptable (e.g., because of some extremely severe mental or physical handicap) it is still wrong in most cases to kill it. For most of us

value the lives of infants, and would prefer to pay taxes to support orphanages and state institutions for the handicapped rather than to allow unwanted infants to be killed. So long as most people feel this way, and so long as our society can afford to provide care for infants which are unwanted or which have special needs that preclude home care, it is wrong to destroy any infant which has a chance of living a reasonably satisfactory life.

If these arguments show that infanticide is wrong, at least in this society, then why don't they also show that late-term abortion is wrong? After all, third trimester fetuses are also highly personlike, and many people value them and would much prefer that they be preserved, even at some cost to themselves. As a potential source of pleasure to some family, a viable fetus is just as valuable as a viable infant. But there is an obvious and crucial difference between the two cases: once the infant is born, its continued life cannot (except, perhaps, in very exceptional cases) pose any serious threat to the woman's life or health, since she is free to put it up for adoption, or, where this is impossible, to place it in a state-supported institution. While she might prefer that it die, rather than being raised by others, it is not clear that such a preference would constitute a right on her part. True, she may suffer greatly from the knowledge that her child will be thrown into the lottery of the adoption system, and that she will be unable to ensure its well-being, or even to know whether it is healthy, happy, doing well in school, etc.; for the law generally does not permit natural parents to remain in contact with their children, once they are adopted by another family. But there are surely better ways of dealing with these problems than by permitting infanticide in such cases. (It might help, for instance, if the natural parents of adopted children could at least receive some information about their progress, without necessarily being informed of the identity of the adopting family.)

In contrast, a pregnant woman's right to protect her own life and health clearly outweighs other people's desire that the fetus be preserved—just as, when a person's life or limb is threatened by some wild animal, and when the threat cannot be removed without killing the animal, the person's right to self-protection outweighs the desires of those who would prefer that the animal not be harmed. Thus, while the moment of birth may not mark any sharp discontinuity in the degree to which an infant possesses a right to life, it does mark the end of the mother's absolute right to determine its fate. Indeed, if and when a late-term abortion could be safely performed without killing the fetus, she would have no absolute right to insist on its death (e.g., if others wish to adopt it or to pay for its care), for the same reason that she does not have a right to insist that a viable infant be killed.

It remains true that according to my argument neither abortion nor the killing of neonates is properly considered a form of murder. Perhaps it is understandable that the law should classify infanticide as murder or homicide, since there is no other existing legal category which adequately or conveniently expresses the force of our society's disapproval of this action. But the moral distinction remains, and it has several important consequences.

In the first place, it implies that when an infant is born into a society which—unlike ours—is so impoverished that it simply cannot care for it adequately without endangering the survival of existing persons, killing it or allowing it to die is not necessarily wrong—provided that there is no *other* society which is willing and able to provide such care. Most human societies, from those at the hunting and gathering stage of economic development to the highly civilized Greeks and Romans, have permitted the practice of infanticide under such unfortunate circumstances, and I would argue that it shows a serious lack of understanding to condemn them as morally backward for this reason alone.

In the second place, the argument implies that when an infant is born with such severe physical anomalies that its life would predictably be a very short and/or very miserable one, even with the most heroic of medical treatment, and where its parents do not choose to bear the often crushing emotional, financial and other burdens attendant upon the artificial prolongation of such a tragic life, it is not morally wrong to cease or withhold treatment, thus allowing the infant a painless death. It is wrong (and sometimes a form of murder) to practice involuntary euthanasia on persons, since they have the right to decide for themselves whether or not they wish to continue to live. But terminally ill neonates cannot make this decision for themselves, and thus it is incumbent upon responsible persons to make the decision for them, as best they can. The mistaken belief that infanticide is always tantamount to murder is responsible for a great deal of unnecessary suffering, not just on the part of infants which are made to endure needlessly prolonged and painful deaths, but also on the part of parents, nurses, and other involved persons, who must watch infants suffering needlessly, helpless to end that suffering in the most humane way.

I am well aware that these conclusions, however modest and reasonable they may seem to some people, strike other people as morally monstrous, and that some people might even prefer to abandon their previous support for women's right to abortion rather than accept a theory which leads to such conclusions about infanticide. But all that these facts show is that abortion is not an isolated moral issue; to fully understand the moral status of abortion we may have to reconsider other moral issues as well, issues not just about infanticide and euthanasia, but also about the moral rights of women and of nonhuman animals. It is a philosopher's task to criticize mistaken beliefs which stand in the way of moral understanding, even when—perhaps especially when—those beliefs are popular and widespread. The belief that moral strictures against killing should apply equally to *all* genetically human entities, and *only* to genetically human entities, is such an error. The overcoming of this error will undoubtedly require long and often painful struggle; but it must be done.

Notes

1. For example, Roger Wertheimer, who in "Understanding the Abortion Argument" (*Philosophy and Public Affairs*, 1, No. 1 [Fall, 1971], 67–95), argues that the problem of the moral status of abortion is insoluble, in that the dispute over the status of the fetus is not a question of fact at all, but only a question of how one responds to the facts.
2. B. A. Brody, "Abortion and the Law," *The Journal of Philosophy*, 68, No. 12 (June 17, 1971), 357–69.
3. Judith Thomson, "A Defense of Abortion," *Philosophy and Public Affairs*, 1, No. 1 (Fall, 1971), 47–66.
4. I have abbreviated these statements somewhat, but not in a way which affects the argument.
5. John Noonan, "Abortion and the Catholic

Church: A Summary History," *Natural Law Forum,* 12 (1967), 125.

6. John Noonan, "Deciding Who Is Human," *Natural Law Forum,* 13 (1968), 134.

7. "A Defense of Abortion."

8. We may safely ignore the fact that she might have avoided getting raped, e.g., by carrying a gun, since by similar means you might likewise have avoided getting kidnapped, and in neither case does the victim's failure to take all possible precautions against a highly unlikely event (as opposed to reasonable precautions against a rather likely event) mean that he is morally responsible for what happens.

9. Of course, the principle that it is (always) wrong to kill innocent human beings is in need of many other modifications, e.g., that it may be permissible to do so to save a greater number of other innocent human beings, but we may safely ignore these complications here.

10. From here on, we will use 'human' to mean genetically human, since the moral sense seems closely connected to, and perhaps derived from, the assumption that genetic humanity is sufficient for membership in the moral community.

11. Thomas L. Hayes, "A Biological View," *Commonweal,* 85 (March 17, 1967), 677–78; quoted by Daniel Callahan, in *Abortion, Law, Choice, and Morality* (London: Macmillan & Co., 1970).

12. That is, insofar as the death rate, for the woman, is higher for childbirth than for early abortion.

13. My thanks to the following people, who were kind enough to read and criticize an earlier version of this paper: Herbert Gold, Gene Glass, Anne Lauterbach, Judith Thomson, Mary Mothersill, and Timothy Binkley.

Responsible Women and Abortion Decisions

Martha Brandt Bolton

I

When a pregnant woman considers whether or not to seek an abortion, is she facing a choice between doing what is morally wrong and doing what is morally right, or is her choice without moral significance? There are two answers to this question which have become familiar to all of us, and I want to argue that both of them are wrong.

One answer comes from those who hold that the fetus is already a living human being and a person; they hold that a fetus, like every other person, has a right not to be deliberately killed. Some who hold this view allow that circumstances may permit the killing of the fetus—for example, when it is necessary to save the life of the pregnant woman. Generally speaking, however, according to those who advocate the fetus' "right to life," the decision to have an abortion is comparable to the decision to murder. Thus, they hold that in general, abortions are morally wrong.

The second familiar answer to our question is that, in general, an abortion has no moral significance; it is not morally wrong, but neither is it morally permissible or right. It is a personal and private decision comparable to the decision to have an abscessed tooth pulled or a bothersome tumor removed. According to this view, neither the fetus nor anyone else has rights which are violated by abortion. A woman is free to have, or not to have, an abortion as she chooses. I should clarify at once a point about this position that abortion is morally insignificant. It must be distinguished from that taken by a majority of the Supreme Court in the 1973 decision that laws prohibiting abortion during the first three months of pregnancy are unconstitutional. The Court found that abortion does not violate anyone's *constitutional* rights, and it is not the sort of action which the *state* has an interest in prohibiting. The position with which I am concerned has it that abortion violates no one's *moral* rights and cannot be prohibited, or required, on *moral* grounds.

As I have said, I think that both of these familiar views about the morality of abortion are wrong. Let me begin with the anti-abortionists,

Reprinted with permission from Having Children, *Onora O'Neill and William Ruddick, eds. (New York: Oxford University Press, 1979).*

who claim that a fetus has a right not to be killed comparable to that of any person. Anti-abortionists make this claim, in part, because they hold that a fetus is already a person.[1] The thought that a newly conceived fetus is a person seems absurd to some, but it seems credible to others. The reason is that there is no readily available or widely accepted view about exactly what a person is.

One distinctive characteristic of persons is that they are entitled to special consideration. We are obligated to treat the lives, needs, and desires of other *persons* with consideration equal to that we think should be given to our own. For instance, conflicts between my needs and wants and those of other persons cannot automatically be decided in favor of me; the others have rights against my actions, and I am morally obligated to respect them. It is true that I may have moral obligations to animals, which are clearly not persons. But the point about persons is that I have *special* obligations to them, and they have *particular* rights that limit what it is morally permissible for me to do. The category of persons is in part a moral one; having certain rights and participating in a certain network of obligations is at least part of what it is to be a person.

The problem is that we do not know how to describe, in a general way, what creatures entitled to this special consideration must be like. We all agree about most cases we confront (although historically there has been debate about black people and women, in general). But even the most sensitive and honest of us can conceive of cases in which we would not know what to think.

One sort of puzzling case concerns creatures that are clearly not biological humans or *homo sapiens*. Imagine the moral questions that might arise if we encountered highly developed forms of life on other planets, or if we discovered creatures who are the "missing link" in the evolution of humans from apes. Should we force such creatures to work for us? Should we eat them? What about cross-breeding? Non-fictional cases may actually be at hand. Does the gorilla from the San Francisco Zoo, who is able to use language, have any of the rights of a person? The biological facts do not provide answers to these questions. Creatures that are indisputably not *homo sapiens* may nevertheless be entitled to the special consideration we owe to *persons*. By the same token, the

fact that a creature *is* a biological human being does not settle such questions either. Consider cases of extreme criminal insanity or humans deep in coma with no hope of regaining consciousness. No doubt, we do have certain obligations to these humans, but we probably do not have the full range of obligations that we have to others in our community. If so, then a human being may be a person at one stage of his/her biological life and a non-person at other stages. Whether or not this is the case, and which stages of development are person-stages, will not be settled by biological facts about us.

II

Anti-abortionists begin the discussion of the morality of abortion with the claim that a fetus is a person. Most base this claim on biological facts, but as I have said, such facts do not settle the question. Others, recognizing that there is legitimate doubt that a fetus is a person, reason that the fetus should be given the benefit of the doubt. From there, anti-abortionists argue that it is a fundamental right of a person not to be deliberately killed.[2] This right is forfeited in certain circumstances where killing is justified, most notably in self-defense.[3] But the fact is that these circumstances rarely arise in pregnancy; they are confined to cases in which the life or health of the pregnant woman is seriously threatened by the presence of the fetus. Thus, a fetus cannot be killed (or can only very rarely be killed) if the fetus has the rights of a person.

I have already said that the assumption that a fetus is a person is unfounded, but I think that the anti-abortionist has a more serious problem. I think the claim that the fetus has the *same* rights as an undisputed person does can be shown to be clearly wrong.[4] If I am correct in thinking that a fetus cannot have the same right not to be killed as an undisputed person has, then the anti-abortionists are wrong when they prohibit abortion on grounds that persons as such have a right not to be killed.

To see the incoherence in the anti-abortionists' argument, we need to look at the gaps in their account of what is at stake in an abortion. They emphasize the fetus' alleged "right to life." They do not emphasize a matter which is equally important. This is that if a pregnant woman is obligated not to kill a fetus, then she is obligated to do a great deal more than that. She can meet the alleged obligation not to kill only if she takes on the various obligations involved in bearing and having a child. At the least, she must nurture the fetus, carry it to term, and give it birth; she must then care for the infant or make alternative arrangements for its care. Of course, there may be others willing to adopt the infant and raise the child; but we should not lose sight of the fact that for some babies there are not likely to be adoptive parents. For pregnant women whose potential babies will not be accepted for adoption, the responsibilities involved in caring for the fetus loom very large. For any pregnant woman, the only way to avoid killing a fetus is to take responsibility for nurturing and giving birth to it; for some, the alternative is undertaking to care for and raise a child. Anti-abortionists insist on the fetus' right not to be killed; they discount the fact that a fetus has the right *only if* it also has a right to be nurtured by the pregnant woman and raised by her or someone else.

It is important to describe the fetus' alleged right in this way, rather than in the way in which anti-abortionists typically do. Respecting the right of another person not to be killed is relatively simple. It is a matter of refraining from doing something. But respecting a fetus' right to be nurtured and developed involves a complex pattern of activities which form a prominent, demanding, and (in some cases) permanent part of one's life. It is relatively easy to live without deliberately killing someone; but it may require an indefinitely large commitment of time, energy, emotion, and physical resources to nurture and care for a child. Furthermore, the obligation not to kill is conceptually simple; it extends to *all* other persons, and the situations in which it is forfeited are familiar (for instance, self-defense). In contrast, the obligation to nurture and develop others is conceptually complex. It is not entirely clear how much of one's resources such obligations demand, nor is it clear how far they extend. Surely they do not extend to *all* other persons, for anyone's personal resources are too slight to meet such massive demands. By the same token, the limitations on any one person's resources make it inevitable that obligations to help different persons will conflict; some will

have to be chosen over others. When anti-abortionists emphasize the obligation not to kill a fetus, they make it seem as if our obligations to fetuses were as simple as our obligations not to kill other persons. But this is seriously misleading. Fetuses differ from persons in that a pregnant woman cannot avoid killing a fetus unless she undertakes to nurture and develop it. Her obligations to a fetus cannot be any more simple than her obligations to help in the growth and development of others who may need it; and I have suggested that these obligations are complex and limited.

Let me illustrate what I mean when I say that obligations to aid the development and growth of others are limited and complex. Consider a mother with several children, one of whom has a disability which retards normal development. Suppose that with expensive treatment and patient training, the retarded child will slowly develop many capacities that other children acquire rapidly and without special help. The woman's resources are limited; her money, time, physical strength, and emotional capacity are not inexhaustible. Developing a certain capacity in the retarded child—say, the ability to make short unaccompanied trips outside the house—may put a severe strain on her resources. Her time and energy are needed to support the family, and she hasn't the money to engage someone else to work with the special child. There is a point beyond which she is not morally required to devote resources to the growth and development of the special child. Because her resources are limited, she must choose how they will be used. Her obligations to aid the special child are limited not only by her own strength and resources but also by her obligations to the other children. The mere fact that a child needs help in order to develop does not always establish an overriding obligation for the mother to meet the need.

So far, I have been considering limitations on the mother's obligation to supply what is needed for the child to develop a specific skill. This affects the child's prospects for a satisfying life, but not the child's life itself. But clearly, similar considerations bear on the resources required to sustain the child's basic care. If resources are severely strained, the mother may have to relinquish all care of the child. Usually, she can make satisfactory alternative arrangements, and there is surely nothing morally wrong about her doing so. Even if alternative arrangements are not available, she may be forced to stop caring for the child if her resources are sufficiently strained. The point is that her obligations to support the development of a particular child are limited by her situation, and they are complex. Both her resources and her other obligations determine their extent.

I have been saying that a mother does not have *limitless* obligations to aid in the development of a child, or even to sustain a child's life. The same holds for any one person's obligations to support the growth, or even the life, of any other person. The basic fact that any one person's time, energy, and other resources have limits makes it absurd to suggest otherwise.

There are, then, *two* features of a person's rights and obligations which are relevant to the issue of abortion, and the anti-abortionists' insistence on one of them obscures the other. The features are: first, that a person has a right not to be killed which extends to virtually all circumstances except those of self-defense; and second, that any one person's obligations to aid another's growth or sustain another's life must, in the nature of the case, have limits.

Where the rights and obligations of undisputed persons are concerned, these fundamental features are fully compatible. One person's obligation to sustain the life of another stops at a certain point; at that point, the other's requirements may not be fully met and he/she may die. In refusing further aid, a person does not violate the other's right not to be killed; he/she may only be acting responsibly given his/her other commitments and in any case, there are limits to the extent to which anyone is obligated to sustain the life of another. Let us see how this works in a couple of cases. Consider a family supporting an elderly member who needs expensive medical care; suppose the medical situation worsens, and care becomes prohibitively expensive for the family. To reserve enough money to supply other basic needs, they must withdraw financial support for the medical care and, as a result, the elderly person dies. The withdrawal of support is regrettable, but not morally wrong; surely the elderly person's right not to be killed has not been violated. The elderly person is simply left to his/her own resources; when they

do not suffice, the person is allowed to die. Or, consider a situation in which one person rescues another from nearly drowning and administers artificial respiration. For a while, the artificially provided oxygen sustains the victim's life, but the life-sustaining activity of the rescuer cannot be continued indefinitely. At some point, the person must be returned to his/her own means of sustaining life and, if they are inadequate, the person must be allowed to die. The death is by drowning; no one would suggest that the person was killed by the one who attempted to save his/her life. No one would think that the victim's right not to be killed had been violated. In cases like these, where one person's life is sustained by the activities or resources of another, we can distinguish between two sorts of actions: (i) the one person's ceasing the activity which sustains the other's life and (ii) the one person's deliberately killing the other. Actions of the first sort do not violate a person's right not to be the victim of actions of the second sort.

I suggest that what enables us to make this important distinction is that persons typically have resources of *their own* for sustaining their lives. At some time in their lives, undisputed persons have carried on their own life functions without direct dependence upon others. When such a person's life functions are later sustained by someone else, we suppose the person has (currently inadequate) resources to which he/she can be returned.

However, a fetus is importantly different from an undisputed person. We cannot distinguish between the pregnant woman's withdrawing her support for its life functions and her killing it.[5] I suggest that the reason is that a fetus, or at least one not yet viable, has no resources of its *own* for carrying on life functions.[6] A fetus cannot be returned to its own resources and allowed to die. If the woman ceases her support for its life, we seem forced to say that the fetus has been killed. So, whereas we can reconcile the limits on our obligations to sustain the life of an undisputed person with our obligation not to kill such a person, we *cannot* do so in the case of a (previable) fetus. It is this that convinces me that a fetus cannot have the *same* right not to be killed that an undisputed person has.

Let me summarize. An undisputed person

has a right not to be deliberately killed and (at best) a right to limited aid in growth and sustaining his/her life from a particular other person. Now consider a fetus. If a fetus has a right not to be deliberately killed (except in self-defense), then it has a right to be nurtured by the pregnant woman, and this is *not* a limited claim on her resources. Thus, a fetus has a right to demand more than an undisputed person does, and so its rights are not *the same* as such a person's are. On the other hand, if a fetus has only the same right to help from the pregnant woman that an undisputed person has, then there are limits to her obligations to it. Then, there will be a point at which the woman's obligations cease and the fetus can be killed, even though the killing is not done in self-defense. It follows, again, that a fetus does not have *the same* rights that an undisputed person does. A fetus cannot be accorded one of the relevant rights which undisputed persons have without also being given either a stronger right to help or a weaker right not to be killed than we accord to such persons.[7] Thus, a fetus cannot have the same right not to be killed that undisputed persons have.

III

If my view so far is correct, anti-abortionists cannot coherently support a general prohibition against abortion by appeal to the claim that a fetus has the rights of a person. Their response may be that, in fact, a pregnant woman's obligations to a fetus are *stronger* than her obligations to a person.[8] Anti-abortionists may claim she has a special duty to care for the fetus, so that her obligations to it are not limited in the ways obligations to other persons are. Accordingly, an anti-abortionist might persist in maintaining that aborting a fetus is generally morally wrong.

I think that this anti-abortionist position also is untenable. In particular, it distorts the situation of a woman as a morally responsible agent. It appeals, on the one hand, to the pregnant woman's ability to choose to do what is morally right (concerning abortion); on the other, it implies that she cannot be a responsible participant in a full moral life. Let me explain why I think that this is so.

The important fact about a pregnant woman's moral situation is the one I have been emphasizing: if she does not have an abortion, she must shoulder the more or less extensive and demanding responsibility of caring for the fetus. Now, many women have the various resources required to nurture the fetus and care for the potential child, or at least to make arrangements for its care. But many other women *do not*, and we need to be particularly concerned about their situation. Suppose that a pregnant woman knows that she cannot properly care for the fetus, or that the needs of the potential child will not be met. To undertake to nurture the fetus and give birth to a child, given her situation, would be morally irresponsible; it would be to accept obligations which she *knows* she cannot meet. No coherent moral rule requires a person to accept obligations which he/she knows cannot be fulfilled. Yet this is precisely what the anti-abortionists' moral stance requires of a pregnant woman in this situation. It requires that she refrain from abortion, and she cannot do so without incurring obligations to care for the fetus; in the sorts of circumstances with which I am concerned, she knows she must fail to meet them.[9]

Situations of the sort in question are, unfortunately, not merely hypothetical. Consider a case in which there is extreme emotional trauma connected with the woman's pregnancy, so that she is deeply ambivalent about the fetus. Such emotional ambivalence could be the result of her having been the victim of rape, or it could result from the unexpected death of the father of the fetus, or from the extreme youth and immaturity of the mother. The woman may recognize that her emotional ambivalence will keep her from providing adequate care for the fetus. It is important to realize that her inability to care for the fetus may be a genuine one which would be impossible to overcome. In another sort of case, she may know that she will be unable to provide adequate care for the fetus, either because she is addicted to alcohol or other harmful drugs or because she does not have access to the proper food or medical care. Or, she may know that she will be unable to care for the potential child and, further, that no one else in her community will be willing or able to do so.[10] Of course, pregnant women who face grave difficulties of these sorts are sometimes able to overcome them, especially if help from others in the community is available. But there will inevitably be cases in which it would be unreasonable, even irresponsible, to think that the difficulties could be overcome. Sometimes the resources required to nurture a fetus and care for a child are simply not available to a particular pregnant woman. For a woman in such a situation, the anti-abortionists' position has absurd implications. It implies that she is morally obligated to undertake responsibilities which she knows she must fail to meet. In brief, it places on her a moral responsibility to do what is morally irresponsible.

In less dire circumstances, a pregnant woman is still placed in an anomalous moral situation by the anti-abortionists' position. That position gives her an overriding obligation to care for the fetus. Now, what if the woman has already made important commitments which conflict with her developing the fetus? What if others are depending upon her? She has a responsibility to take reasonable precautions against conception, but responsible action of this sort is not a guarantee against pregnancy. If her obligation to the fetus takes precedence, she must fail to follow through on her commitments. But then, she should never have taken them on. Knowing that she might become pregnant, she should have recognized that she might be unable to fulfill her commitments. Accepting them was irresponsible. She should have avoided projects of helping others in which they could come to depend upon her, because she was liable to incur overriding obligations to a fetus. Thus, throughout child-bearing years, a woman can act responsibly only by truncating her participation in activities in which others come to depend upon her. But I think this is untenable, for it is central to the life of a morally responsible person to aspire to projects of this sort.

I think it is also central to the life of a morally responsible person that he/she develop abilities which make him/ her a useful, productive, contributing member of the community.[11] Doing so often requires large commitments of a person's time, thought, and other personal resources; such commitments are liable to conflict with the activity of nurturing a fetus and raising a child. So, while moral responsibility generally involves a more or less demanding program of developing one's contribution to the community, the anti-abortionists' view requires that a woman refrain from that sort of program. I think that this account of the moral situation of a woman is untenable.

IV

I have argued that the anti-abortionist position that abortion is virtually always wrong is untenable, but I think the other extreme position—that abortion is morally neutral—is equally mistaken. As I have said, I do not think that a fetus can usefully be regarded as a person in discussions of abortion. But it seems to me that the mere fact that it will become a human being, if properly nurtured, indicates that it is entitled to some sort of consideration.[12] I am inclined to think that a pregnant woman has some obligation to nurture a fetus although her obligation is far from absolute.

Further, it is clear that the decision to have, or *not* to have, an abortion does not affect the pregnant woman, alone. It determines whether or not a new member will be brought into the woman's family, her living situation, and her community. Its outcome stands to affect a wide range of others, favorably or unfavorably; their welfare and interests are at stake. Moreover, decisions concerning abortions often occur in situations where there are conflicting commitments and obligations. So, the decision to have an abortion, or not to have one, is not a purely personal matter without moral significance.[13]

I now want to say something about what sorts of considerations generally seem to bear upon the problem of the moral value of a particular abortion.[14] There seem to me to be (at least) three sorts of considerations relevant to the decision. The first is that as a potential human being, a fetus has some claim to be nurtured; like other claims on her aid, this one can be overridden by other factors in a particular woman's situation. The second relevant consideration is the way in which bearing a child, and possibly raising it, fits into the life of the pregnant woman; she must be able to plan a morally coherent life. Will nurturing the fetus prevent her from fulfilling important obligations to others? Will it prevent her from pursuing her plans for becoming a productive and useful member of her community? Is she in a situation in which she can successfully meet her responsibility to the fetus, if she undertakes to nurture it? It seems to me that the answers to these questions are critical. They may indicate that abortion is morally permissible, and they may even indicate that it is morally required. The third relevant consideration is the way in which having a child will affect others in the woman's family, living situation, and the larger community with which she identifies. If their welfare would be severely diminished by her child-raising activity, then I think she ought not to engage in it. On the other hand, if the welfare of others in her community would be enhanced by her having the child, then I think this is relevant. She then has some obligation to have the child, just as she has some obligation to undertake other projects which contribute to the well-being of others. As a morally sensitive person, she ought to pursue some projects of this sort, but there are limits to her obligations to pursue any one in particular. Let me fill in some of the details.

I believe the most important consideration is how bearing and raising a child would fit into the pregnant woman's life. As I have said, nurturing and developing a child requires a major commitment of one's mental and physical resources. A fetus has some claim on these resources, but it does not take precedence over the claims of others to whom the woman has conflicting obligations. She must choose those projects for helping others and strengthening her productive capability which she will pursue. Projects which interest her, engage her particular skills and talents, and those she will find especially rewarding may be given preference over others. If these factors suggest that she is better suited to other projects, then I think she is not morally obligated to nurture the fetus instead; in such cases, abortion is permissible. I am not suggesting that it is morally permissible to ignore all projects of helping others or contributing to their welfare. It is just that it must be permissible to exercise some control over the projects one undertakes; otherwise, it would be impossible to lead a coherent, morally responsible life.[15]

Consider a couple of examples. Take a young woman in college studying to go to medical school and looking forward to the practice of medicine. If she decides to give birth to a child, and especially if she decides to raise it, she is unlikely to complete her studies.[16] She must choose between nurturing the fetus and preparing herself to help her community in other ways. I see no reason why she should be obligated to choose one project rather than the other. It is a question of which she is more interested in, which she considers more important, which she finds herself better suited to pursue. What about a teen-aged woman who is emotionally immature and, in addition, has no means of supporting herself? If she cannot successfully meet the obligations involved in nurturing the fetus—say, because of her immaturity or the ridicule to which she is subject in her community—then I think it is absurd to suggest that she is morally required to do so. In another sort of case, a pregnant woman may already have begun projects which make large demands on her resources. They may be projects of raising other children, working with the elderly in her community, or employment in which others are counting on her continued participation. She may face a choice between failing to meet her obligations to others (in case she bears the child) and seeking an abortion. I think she is permitted to choose abortion. In extreme cases of dependence of others on her, she may even be required to seek abortion.

The final consideration relevant to the decision to have an abortion is the welfare of the pregnant woman's family, living companions, and the members of the larger community with which she identifies. Situations in which the welfare of these persons is endangered by her having a child are rare; but suppose, for example, that the family or community does not have resources to feed or care for an additional member, or that the fetus will have a tendency to infection or to socially destructive acts which the community is unable to control. In such cases, the interest of others in preserving their lives or health is violated by admitting the child into their community, and it seems to me that the woman ought not to bear the child (at least in that community). In most such cases, I think the woman would not want to bear the child, since she identifies with the community. Even if she does want to bear the child, I think she ought not to endanger others by doing so.

There are also cases in which others stand to benefit from the pregnant woman's bearing a child. Suppose, for example, that her family needs additional members to help with the production of food, to protect itself, or to carry on some other activity of value to them. Or, there may be those in the woman's community anxious to adopt the child. Another case is found among certain American Indian tribes; they have so few members that there is danger that the gene pool will become too small to sustain a healthy population. Now, the pregnant woman is in a position to benefit these others by having the child, and I think she ought to choose some projects which benefit others. The relevant factors are by now familiar: does she have conflicting prior obligations? Is the strain on her resources excessive? Does she strongly prefer alternative projects for contributing to the welfare of others?[17] If so, her obligation to have the child is overridden. If not, then she ought to have it. The (possible) benefit to others functions like the background claim of the fetus to be nurtured. Both provide reasons why a pregnant woman should decide against abortion and choose to nurture the fetus. But other facts about her situation are also relevant, and the reasons against nurturing the child may outweigh these reasons for it. In a wide variety of situations, abortion may be morally permitted, and in some it is morally required.[18]

Notes

1. For an account of the anti-abortionist position, see Roger Wertheimer, "Understanding the Abortion Argument," *Philosophy and Public Affairs*, 1, 1971. The official Roman Catholic stance on abortion is more complex, and elusive, than the ones discussed here; see Susan T. Nicholson, "The Roman Catholic Doctrine of Therapeutic Abortion," in *Feminism and Philosophy*, ed. by Mary Vetterling-Braggin, Frederick A. Elliston, and Jane English (Totowa, N.J.: Littlefield, Adams, 1977).

2. This argument has most fully and forcefully been made by Baruch Brody in *Abortion and the Sanctity of Human Life* (Cambridge, Mass.: M.I.T. Press, 1975); also see John Finnis, "The Rights and Wrongs of Abortion," *Philosophy and Public Affairs*, 2, 1973.

3. It is difficult to say whether there are other circumstances in which killing is justified—e.g., in cases of capital punishment, or where many lives may be saved by killing a few. It is also difficult to say precisely what sorts of self-defense justify killing—e.g., how immediate and violent the threat must be, how severe the threatened bodily harm must be. Some of these issues are discussed in Brody, op. cit.

4. Of course, no one claims that a fetus has all the rights of a mature person. The fetus is claimed to have the same right as an undisputed person not to be killed, and it is this claim that I want to dispute.

5. Some defenses of the morality of abortion in a fairly wide range of cases depend upon a distinction between removing the fetus and killing it. The general argument is that the pregnant woman may have a right to have the fetus removed, even though she has no right to have killed. See Judith Jarvis Thomson, "A Defense of Abortion," *Philosophy and Public Affairs*, 1, 1971, and Nicholson, op. cit. My view is that where a previable fetus is concerned, the distinction will not bear this weight.

6. Strictly speaking, this is true only of a fetus prior to the time at which it becomes viable (sometime after the twenty-fourth week, as things now stand). My claim is that as long as no distinction can be made between withdrawing support of the fetus and killing it, the fetus cannot have the same rights that undisputed persons do. In cases where this distinction can be made, I offer no reason to think that fetuses cannot be treated as undisputed persons.

7. In some of the most interesting discussions of abortion, this point is ignored. Having decided to treat a fetus as a person, the discussants must proceed to make dubious claims about the rights undisputed persons would have in situations comparable to those of fetuses. Thus, Thomson, op. cit., maintains that you are not morally obligated to refrain from killing another person by refusing him/her "the use of your body" when granting it is excessively burdensome. But Brody, op. cit., counters that a person has a right not to be killed, no matter what burdens this restraint places on others (including use of their bodies). Thomson begins with (something like) the point that a person's obligations to aid another are limited and ends by distorting the other's right not to be killed. Brody begins with a person's right not to be killed and ends by distorting another's obligations to aid the person. There appears to be no way to resolve this dispute. The problem, I think, is that the conflict concerns the rights persons are supposed to have in a sort of situation in which undisputed persons are *never found*; and the fact that they are never found in such situations is an indispensable condition of their having the rights they do. In the crucial case, undisputed persons are simply *dis*analogous to fetuses.

8. This would seem to be a better strategy, in any case. For our paradigms of persons are mature, capable, and relatively autonomous adults. Fetuses are much more like very young children than paradigmatic persons. Moreover, it would

generally be conceded that a parent's obligations to care for his/her children are much stronger than his/her obligations to help other persons in general.

9. At the same time, a woman who recognizes that she would be unable to fulfill obligations to a fetus or child should take reasonable measures to prevent conception. A pregnant woman in this situation may, or may not, have accepted the responsibility to use whatever safe, effective, and humane means of contraception are available to her. However, in either case, I think that she cannot be morally required to bear responsibilities she knows she cannot meet.

10. The extent to which a woman's activities must be curtailed to meet the obligations involved in nurturing a fetus obviously depends upon the degree to which her community supports her activity. Thus, the absurdity of the anti-abortionists' position, whether it makes reasonable development of a full moral life more or less compatible with meeting one's obligations to fetuses, depends upon the arrangements in any particular community. This, in itself, is reason to be suspicious of the view that abortion, in itself and regardless of the circumstances of the pregnant woman, is morally wrong.

11. There is not space here to argue for the connection between development of one's capacities and a fully moral life; for one interesting treatment, see Larry Blum et al., "Altruism and Women's Oppression," *Philosophical Forum*, 5, 1973–74.

12. This consideration does not seem to me to extend to human eggs or sperms, or other substances which could be developed into human beings. The ovum and sperm are "ingredients" that yield a human being, whereas it is the fetus that be-

comes a human being. Further, the fact that the genetic makeup of the fetus is determined, whereas that of an egg or sperm is not, seems to be relevant.

13. Different arguments for a similar view are given by Jane English, "Abortion and the Concept of a Person," *Canadian Journal of Philosophy*, 5, 1975.

14. I will consider only women who did not choose to become pregnant. It is important to remember that a woman may well have accepted the responsibility to use reasonable contraception techniques and still have become pregnant.

15. For a discussion of the role of abortion in exercising responsible control over one's life, see Howard Cohen, "Abortion and the Quality of Life," in *Philosophy and Feminism*, op. cit.

16. If her community provides far-reaching support for child-bearing and rearing-activity, the conflict between having a child and other sorts of useful activity can be greatly diminished. The support provided by public institutions, or other agencies, bears on the decision to have an abortion in almost every case. It is an unfortunate consequence that those who receive least support from their society (the poor and disadvantaged) will be morally required to seek abortion more frequently than those who receive more support. This injustice results from injustice elsewhere in the society.

17. For discussion of the obligations a black woman has to contribute to her community by bearing children, see Toni Cade, "On the Issue of Roles," in *The Black Woman*, ed. by Toni Cade (New York: New American Library, 1970).

18. Thanks are due to Amèlie Rorty, Martin Bunzl, and Onora O'Neill for useful comments on various versions of this paper which began as a talk to undergraduates.

CASE RETROSPECTIVE
Mrs. Sherri Finkbine and the Thalidomide Tragedy

Background Note: The following case concerns an event that took place before the U.S. Supreme Court decision in Roe v. Wade *was handed down in 1973. That decision had the effect of legalizing abortion in the United States. Before the decision, most state laws permitted abortion only for the purpose of saving the life of the mother. The case presented here illustrates the kinds of problems faced by many women who sought an abortion for other reasons.*

In 1962 Mrs. Sherri Finkbine was the mother of four normal children and was pregnant. Her health was good, but she was having some trouble sleeping. Rather than talking with her doctor, she simply took some of the tranquilizers that her husband had brought back from a trip to Europe. The tranquilizers were widely used there, and, like aspirin, they could simply be bought over the counter.

Subsequently, Mrs. Finkbine read an article that told of the great increase in the number of deformed children being born in Europe. Some of the children's arms and legs failed to develop or developed only in malformed ways; other children were blind and deaf or had seriously defective internal organs. The birth defects had been traced to the use in pregnancy of a supposedly harmless and widely-used tranquilizer. Its active ingredient was thalidomide.

Mrs. Finkbine was worried enough to ask her doctor to find out if the pills she had been taking contained thalidomide. They did. When he learned this, her doctor told her, "The odds are so against you that I am recommending termination of pregnancy." He explained that getting approval for an abortion should not be difficult. She had good medical reasons and all she had to do was to explain them to the three-member medical board of Phoenix.

Mrs. Finkbine agreed with her doctor's advice. But then she began to think that maybe it was her duty to inform other women who may have been taking thalidomide about its disastrous consequences. She called a local newspaper and told her story to the editor. He agreed not to use her name, but on a front page, bordered in black, he used the headline "BABY-DEFORMING DRUG MAY COST WOMAN HER CHILD HERE."

The story was picked up by the wire services, and it was not long before Mrs. Finkbine's identity became known. The medical board had already approved her request for an abortion, but because of the great publicity her case received, they canceled their approval. The State of Arizona abortion statute legally sanctioned abortion only when it was required to save the life of the mother. The board was afraid that their decision might be challenged in court and that the decision could not stand up to the challenge.

Mrs. Finkbine became the object of a great outpouring of antiabortion feelings. *Il Osservatore Romano*, the official Vatican newspaper, condemned Mrs. Finkbine and her husband as murderers. Although she received some letters of support, others were abusive. One writer said: "I hope someone takes the other four children and strangles them, because it is all the same thing." Another wrote from the perspective of the fetus: "Mommy, please dear Mommy, let me live. Please, please, I want to live. Let me love you, let me see the light of day, let me smell a rose, let me sing a song, let me look into your face, let me say Mommy."

Although Mrs. Finkbine tried to obtain a legal abortion outside her own state, she was unable to do so. Eventually, she went to Sweden. After a rigorous investigation by a medical board, Mrs. Finkbine was given an abortion in a Swedish hospital.

Mrs. Finkbine saw her own problem as solved at last. But she continued to have sympathy with those thousands of potential parents of thalidomide children who lacked the money to follow the course of action she had been forced to take by abortion laws she considered to be restrictive and inhumane.

Decision Scenario 1 ···

Ruth Perkins is twenty-four years old, and her husband Carl Freedon is four years older. Both are employed, Ruth as a junior executive for Laporte Gas Transmission and Carl as a librarian at the San Antonio Free Library. Their combined income is over forty thousand dollars a year.

Perkins and Freedon live up to their income. They have an eleven-room house with a tennis court in a high-priced San Antonio suburb, they both dress well, and Carl is a modest collector of sports cars (three MG-TDs). Both like to travel, and they try to get out of the country at least twice a year—Europe for a month in the summer and Mexico or the Caribbean for a couple of weeks during the winter.

Perkins and Freedon have no children. They agreed when they were married that children would not be a part of their plan for life together. They were distressed when Ruth became pregnant and at first refused to face the problem. They worried about it for several months, considering arguments for and against abortion. At last they decided that Ruth should have an abortion.

"I don't see why I have to go through with

this interview," Ruth said to the woman at the Morton Hospital Counseling Center.

"It's required of all who request an abortion," the counselor explained. "We think it's better for a person to be sure what she is doing so she won't regret it later."

"My husband and I are certain," Ruth said. "A child doesn't fit in at all with our life style. We go out a lot and we like to do things. A child would just get in the way."

"A child can offer many pleasures," the woman said.

"I don't doubt it. If some want them, that's fine with me. We don't. Besides, we both have careers that we're devoted to. I'm not about to quit my job to take care of a child, and the same is true of my husband."

"How long have you been pregnant?"

Ruth looked embarrassed. "Almost six months," she said. "Carl and I weren't sure what we wanted to do at first. It took a while for us to get used to the idea."

"You don't think you waited too long?"

"That's stupid," Ruth said. She could hardly keep her voice under control. "I didn't mean that personally. But Carl and I have a right to live our lives the way we want. So far as we are concerned a six-month fetus is not a person. If we want to get rid of it, that's our business."

"Would you feel the same if it were a child already born?"

"I might," Ruth said. "I mean, a baby doesn't have much personality or anything does it?"

"I take it you're certain you want the abortion."

"Absolutely. My husband and I think it's the right thing for us. If others think we're wrong . . . well, it's their right to think what they please."

How might Warren's arguments be used to support Perkins's position?

Could someone who accepts Thomson's arguments consider abortion justified in this case?

Would Bolton consider the harm to Perkins and Freedon a relevant consideration?

Do you believe Perkins is right about a six-month fetus's not being a person? If not, why not?

If a person believes abortion is a kind of murder, can she legitimately endorse the tolerant position taken by Perkins?

Decision Scenario 2 ....

It happened after a concert. Sixteen-year-old Mary Pluski had gone with three of her friends to hear Bruce Springsteen at Chicago's new Blanton Auditorium. After the concert, in a crowd estimated at eleven thousand, Mary became separated from the other three girls. She decided that the best thing to do was to meet them at the car.

But when she got to the eight-story parking building, Mary realized she wasn't sure what level they had parked on. She thought it might be somewhere in the middle so she started looking on the fourth floor. While she was walking down the aisles of cars, two men in their early twenties, one white and the other black, stopped her and asked if she was having some kind of trouble.

Mary explained the situation to them, and one of the men suggested that they get his car and drive around inside the parking building. Mary hesitated, but both seemed so polite and genu-inely concerned to help that she decided to go with them.

Once they were in the car, however, the situation changed. They drove out of the building and toward the South Side. Mary pleaded with them to let her out of the car, but they refused. They threatened her with violence if she called for help or tried to escape from the car. Then, some seven miles from the auditorium, the driver stopped the car in a dark area behind a vacant building. Mary was then raped by both men.

Mary was treated at Allenworth Hospital and released into the custody of her parents. She filed a complaint with the police, but her troubles were not yet over. Two weeks after she missed her menstrual period, tests showed that Mary was pregnant.

"How do you feel about having this child?" asked Sarah Ruben, the Pluski family physician.

"I hate the idea," Mary said. "I feel guilty about it, though. I mean, it's not the child's fault."

"Let me ask a delicate question," said Dr. Ruben. "I know from what you've told me before that you and your boyfriend have been having sex. Can you be sure this pregnancy is not really the result of that?"

Mary shook her head. "Not really. I use my diaphragm, but I know it doesn't give a hundred percent guarantee."

"That's right. Now, does it make any difference to you who the father might be, so far as a decision about terminating the pregnancy is concerned?"

"If I were sure that it was Bob, I guess the problem would be even harder," Mary said.

"There are some tests we can use to give us that information," Dr. Ruben said. "But that would mean waiting for the embryo to develop into a fetus. It would be easier and safer to terminate the pregnancy now."

Mary started crying. "I don't want a child," she said. "I don't want any child. I don't care who's the father, it was forced on me and I want to get rid of it."

"I'll make the arrangements," said Dr. Ruben.

Would Thomson's position recognize abortion here as a form of self-defense?

Would Noonan consider abortion immoral in this case?

Suppose the fetus is a person; would the maxim in this case satisfy the categorical imperative?

Does Mary's uncertainty about the father add any special moral difficulties?

Why would Bolton consider Mary's age relevant?

Decision Scenario 3 ···

"I don't want no more children," Mrs. Hinson said. "I've already got five, and I can't look after them the way they should be looked after. My husband's been gone three years. I don't know where he is but I know he ain't coming back."

After two years as a psychiatric social worker, David Rossum found Mrs. Hinson's situation familiar. He looked around the small living room. It was clean but crowded with broken second-hand furniture. Cheap dime-store metal frames lined the top of the television set. Children smiled in the blurry color snapshots.

"You're sure you're pregnant?" Rossum asked.

"The doctor at the clinic told me so," Mrs. Hinson said. "He gave me a paper to prove it. But I'm already on the welfare and the ADC. I can't do right by my children if I have another one to take care of."

"And you can't count on the father of this child to help you?"

"I can't count on him for nothing," said Mrs. Hinson. "I don't even see him anymore."

"So what do you want to do?" Rossum asked. He knew the answer, but the main part of his job was just listening.

"I want an abortion. That's what I want. But the people at the clinic, they told me I'd have to talk to you people first. If you won't say it's okay they won't do it, because there won't be nobody to pay for it."

"That's right," Rossum said. "You've got to have an authorization from our agency for any kind of special medical procedure of a non-emergency kind."

Suppose that you are David Rossum. On what grounds would you authorize (or refuse to authorize) Mrs. Hinson's request? If you were opposed to all abortions on moral grounds, ought you to allow this to influence your decision?

Does the reasoning in the Supreme Court decision (Roe v. Wade) apply in this case?

Do Rawls's principles of justice suggest a legitimate social policy to cover such cases?

Does the principle of utility?

If the fetus is a person, are there sufficient reasons for considering abortion here a case of justified killing?

Decision Scenario 4 ··

Clare Macwurter was twenty-two years old chronologically, but mentally she remained a child. As a result of her mother's prolonged and difficult labor, Clare had been deprived of an adequate blood-oxygen supply during her birth. The consequence was that she suffered irreversible brain damage.

Clare enjoyed life and was generally a happy person. She couldn't read, but she liked listening to music and watching television, although she could rarely understand the stories. She was physically attractive and, with the help of her parents, she could care for herself.

Clare was also interested in sex. When she was seventeen, she and a fellow student at the special school they attended had been caught having intercourse. Clare's parents had been told about the incident, but after Clare left the school the following year, they took no special precautions to ensure that Clare would not become sexually involved with anyone. After all, she stayed at home with her mother every day, and, besides, it was a matter they didn't much like to think about.

The Macwurters were both surprised and upset when Clare became pregnant. At first they couldn't imagine how it could have happened. Then they recalled that on several occasions Clare had been sent to stay at the house of Mr. Macwurter's brother and his wife while Mrs. Macwurter went shopping.

John Macwurter at first denied that he had anything to do with Clare's pregnancy. But during the course of a long and painful conversation with his brother, he admitted that he had sexual relations with Clare.

"I wasn't wholly to blame," John Macwurter said. "I mean, I know I shouldn't have done it. But still, she was interested in it, too. I didn't really rape her. Nothing like that."

The Macwurters were at a loss about what they should do. The physician they consulted told them that Clare would probably have a perfectly normal baby. But of course Clare couldn't really take care of herself, much less a baby. She was simply unfit to be a mother. Mrs. Macwurter, for her part, was not eager to assume the additional responsibilities of caring for another child. Mr. Macwurter would be eligible to retire in four more years, and the couple had been looking forward to selling their house and moving back to the small town in Oklahoma where they had first met and then married. The money they had managed to save, plus insurance and a sale of their property, would permit them to place Clare in a long-term care facility after their deaths. Being responsible for another child would both ruin their plans and jeopardize Clare's future well-being.

"I never thought I would say such a thing," Mrs. Macwurter told her husband, "but I think we should arrange for Clare to have an abortion."

"That's killing," Mr. Macwurter said.

"I'm not so sure it is. I don't really know. But even if it is, I think it's the best thing to do."

Mrs. Macwurter made the arrangements with Clare's physician for an abortion to be performed. When Mr. Macwurter asked his brother to pay for the operation, John Macwurter refused. He explained that he was opposed to abortion and so it would not be right for him to provide money to be used in that way.

Can the reasoning in Roe v. Wade *be applied in this case? After all, the person involved is not mentally competent and cannot be expected to exercise any right of privacy.*

Could Thomson's defense of abortion be employed here to show that the proposed abortion is permissible?

Why would Noonan oppose abortion here? What alternatives might he recommend? What if it were likely that the baby would be defective? Would this alter the situation for Noonan?

Do the traits Warren lists as central to the concept of personhood require that we think Clare Macwurter as not being a person in a morally relevant sense?

Decision Scenario 5 ···

Daniel Bocker was worried. The message his secretary had taken merely said, "Go to see Dr. Tai at 3:30 today." He hadn't been asked if 3:30 was convenient for him, and he hadn't been given a reason for coming in.

Mr. Bocker knew it would have to do with his wife Mary. She had been suffering a lot of pain during her pregnancy, and the preceding week she had been examined by a specialist that Dr. Tai, her gynecologist, had sent her to see. The specialist had performed a thorough examination and taken blood, tissue, and urine samples, but he had told Mary nothing.

"Thank you for coming in," Dr. Tai said. "I want to talk to you before I talk to your wife, because I need your help."

"The tests showed something bad, didn't they?" Mr. Bocker said. "Something is wrong with the baby."

"The baby is fine, but there is something wrong with your wife, something very seriously wrong. She has what we call uterine neoplasia."

"Is that cancer?"

"Yes it is," said Dr. Tai. "But I don't want either of you to panic about it. It's not at a very advanced stage, and at the moment it's localized. If an operation is performed very soon, then she has a good chance to make a full recovery. The standard figures show about 80 percent success."

"But what about the baby?"

"The pregnancy will have to be terminated," Dr. Tai said. "And I should tell you that your wife will not be able to have children after the operation."

Mr. Bocker sat quietly for a moment. He had always wanted children; for him a family without children was not a family at all. He and Mary had talked about having at least three, and the one she was pregnant with now was the first.

"Is it possible to save the baby?" he asked Dr. Tai.

"Mrs. Bocker is only in her fourth month; there is no chance the child could survive outside her body."

"But what if she didn't have the operation? Would the baby be normal?"

"Probably so, but the longer we wait to perform the operation, the worse your wife's chances become. I don't want to seem to tell you what to do, but my advice is for your wife to have an abortion and to undergo the operation as soon as it is reasonably possible."

"But she might recover, even if she had the child and then had the operation, mightn't she?"

"It's possible, but her chances of recovery are much less. I don't know what the exact figures would be, but she would be running a terrible risk."

Mr. Bocker understood what Dr. Tai was saying, but he also understood what he wanted.

"I'm not going to encourage Mary to have an abortion," he said. "I want her to have a child, and I think she wants that, too."

"What if she wants to have a better chance to live? I think the decision is really hers. After all, it's her life that is at stake."

"But it's not just her decision," Mr. Bocker said. "It's a family decision, hers and mine. I'm not going to agree to an abortion, even if she does want one. I'm going to try to get her to take the extra risk and have the child before she has the operation."

"I think that's the cruelest, most immoral thing I've ever heard," Dr. Tai said.

Would the doctrine of double effect justify taking steps to treat Mrs. Bocker's illness, even at the cost of terminating her pregnancy?

Would both Noonan and Thomson see the situation as one in which considerations of self-defense are relevant?

It is sometimes said that the father of a child also has a right to decide whether an abortion is to be performed. Would Daniel Bocker be justified in urging his wife to take the risk of having the child?

Does the categorical imperative have any relevance in determining whether an abortion is morally right in this case?

Decision Scenario 6 ··

Mrs. Lois Bishop (as we will call her) learned that she was carrying twins at the same time that she learned one of the twins had Down's syndrome.

"There's no question in my mind," she said. "I want to have an abortion. I had the tests done in the first place to do what I could to guarantee that I would have a normal, healthy child. I knew from the first that there was a possibility that I would have to have an abortion, so I'm prepared for it."

Her obstetrician, Dr. George Savano, nodded. "I understand that," he said. "You are certainly within your rights to ask for an abortion, and I can arrange for you to have one. But there is another possibility, an experimental one, that you might want to consider as an option."

The possibility consisted of the destruction of the abnormally developing fetus. In the end, it was the possibility that Mrs. Bishop chose. A long, thin needle was inserted through Mrs. Bishop's abdomen and guided into the heart of the fetus. A solution was then injected directly into the fetal heart.

Although there was a risk that Mrs. Bishop would have a miscarriage, she did not. The surviving twin continued to develop normally, and Mrs. Bishop had an uneventful delivery. The child, a boy, is now over five years old.

Dr. Savano was criticized by some physicians as "misusing medicine," but he rejects such charges. Mrs. Bishop also has no regrets, for if the procedure had not been performed, she would have been forced to abort both twins.

What sort of utilitarian argument might be offered to justify Dr. Savano's experimental procedure in this case?

Can the doctrine of double effect justify the procedure that terminates the life of the Down's syndrome twin? After all, Mrs. Bishop is concerned with preserving the life of the twin that is developing normally. She chooses the experimental procedure in order to avoid an abortion.

The procedure leads to the death of a developing fetus so one might say that it is morally equivalent to abortion. Are there any morally relevant features that distinguish this case from more ordinary cases involving abortion?

Decision Scenario 7 ··

Helen and John Kent waited nervously in the small consulting room while Laurie Stent, their Genetic Counselor, went to tell Dr. Charles Blatz they had arrived to talk to him.

"I regret that I have some bad news for you," Dr. Blatz told them. "The karyotyping that we do after the amniocentesis shows a chromosomal abnormality."

He looked at them, and Helen felt she could hardly breathe. "What is it?" she asked.

"It's a condition known as Trisomy-21, and it produces a birth defect we call Down's syndrome. You may have heard of it under the old name of mongolism."

"Oh, God," John said. "How bad is it?"

"Such children are always mentally retarded," Dr. Blatz said. "Some are severely retarded and others just twenty or so points below average. They have some minor physical deformities, and they sometimes have heart damage.

They typically don't live beyond their thirties, but by and large, they seem happy and have good dispositions."

Helen and John looked at each other with great sadness. "What do you think we should do?" Helen asked. "Should I have an abortion, and then we could try again?"

"I don't know," John said. "I really don't know. You've had a hard time being pregnant these last five months, and you'd have to go through that again. Besides, there's no guarantee this wouldn't happen again."

"But this won't be the normal baby we wanted," Helen said. "Maybe in the long run we'll be even unhappier than we are now."

According to the doctrine in Roe v. Wade, *who is to decide whether Helen Kent has an abortion? Are there any restrictions on the decision?*

Explain the nature of the conflict between the positions taken by Noonan and Warren that arises in this case.

If one accepts Thomson's view, what factors are relevant to deciding whether an abortion is justifiable in this instance?

If one accepts Bolton's position, how might one argue that abortion is justifiable here? How might one argue that abortion is not justifiable?

CHAPTER 2

TREATING OR TERMINATING: THE PROBLEM OF IMPAIRED INFANTS

SOCIAL CONTEXT: THE BABY DOE CASES

In Bloomington, Indiana, in 1982, a child was born with Down's syndrome and esophageal atresia. The parents and the physicians of the infant, who became known as Baby Doe, decided against the surgery that was needed to open the esophagus and allow the baby to be fed. The decision was upheld by the courts, and six days after birth, Baby Doe died of starvation and dehydration.

A month later, in May of 1982, the Secretary of Health and Human Services (HHS) notified hospitals that any institution receiving federal funds could not lawfully "withhold from a handicapped infant nutritional sustenance or medical or surgical treatment required to correct a life-threatening condition if (1) the withholding is based on the fact that the infant is handicapped and (2) the handicap does not render treatment or nutritional sustenance contraindicated."

Ten months later, acting under instructions from President Reagan, an additional and more detailed regulation was issued. Hospitals were required to display a poster in neonatal intensive care units and pediatric wards indicating that "discrimination" against handicapped infants was a violation of federal law. The poster also listed a toll-free, twenty-four-hour "hotline" number for reporting suspected violations. In addition, the regulations authorized representatives of HHS to take "immediate remedial action" to protect infants. Further, hospitals were required to permit HHS investigators access to the hospital and to relevant patient records.

A group of associations, including the American Academy of Pediatrics, brought suit against HHS in an attempt to stop the regulations from becoming legally effective. Judge Gerhard Gesell of the U.S. District Court ruled in April 1983, that HHS had not followed the proper procedures in putting the regulations into effect and so they were invalid. In particular, the regulations were issued without notifying and consulting with those affected by them, a procedure that is legally required to avoid arbitrary bureaucratic actions. The judge held that while HHS had considered relevant factors in identifying a problem, it had failed to consider the effects of the use of the hotline number. An "anonymous tipster" could cause "the sudden descent of Baby Doe squads" on hospitals, and "monopolizing physician and nurse time and making hospital charts and records unavailable during treatment, can hardly be presumed to produce quality care for the infant."

Furthermore, Judge Gesell held, the main purpose of the regulations was apparently to "require physicians treating newborns to take into account wholly medical risk-benefit considerations and to prevent parents from having any influence upon decisions as to whether further medical treatment is desirable." The regulations explored no other ways to prevent "discriminatory medical care." In his conclusion, Judge Gesell held that federal regulations dealing with imperiled newborns should "reflect caution and sensitivity" and that "wide public comment prior to rule-making is essential."

The Department of Health and Human Services responded to the court decision by drafting another regulation (July 5, 1983) that attempted to resolve the procedural objection that invalidated the first. Sixty days were allowed for the filing of written comments. Since the substance of the regulation was virtually the same, the proposal was widely contested, and on January 12, 1984, another set of regulations was published. Although changing some of the more controversial requirements of the original regulations and providing for infant-care advisory committees, the regulations were still the object of controversy and criticism.

Meanwhile, a second Baby Doe case had become the focus of public attention and legal action. On October 11, 1983, an infant who became known as Baby Jane Doe was born in Port Jefferson (Long Island), New York. Baby Jane Doe suffered from meningomyelocele, anencephaly, and hydrocephaly. (See the introduction to this chapter for an explanation of these conditions.) Her parents were told that without surgery the child might be expected to live from two weeks to two years, while with surgery she might survive twenty years. However, she would be severely retarded, epileptic, paralyzed, and likely to have constant urinary and bladder infections.

The parents consulted with neurologists, a Roman Catholic priest, nurses, and social workers. In the end, they decided that surgery was not in the best interest of the child and opted, instead, for the use of antibiotics to prevent infection of the exposed spinal nerves. "We love her very much," her mother said, "and that's why we made the decision we did."

Lawrence Washburn, Jr., a lawyer who for a number of years had initiated lawsuits on behalf of the unborn and handicapped, somehow learned that Baby Jane Doe was being denied life-prolonging surgery and entered a petition on her behalf before the New York State Supreme Court. Because Mr. Washburn was not related to the infant and had no personal knowledge of her condition or of her parents' decision, his legal standing in the case was questionable, and the court appointed William E. Weber to represent the interest of Baby Jane Doe. After a hearing, the judge ruled that the infant was in need of surgery to preserve her life and authorized Mr. Weber to consent.

This decision was reversed on appeal. The court held that the parents' decision was in the best interest of the infant. Hence, the state had no basis to intervene. The ruling was then appealed to the New York Court of Appeals and upheld. The court held that the parents' right to privacy was invaded when a person totally unrelated and with no knowledge of the infant's condition and treatment entered into litigation in an attempt to challenge the discharge of parental responsibility. However, the main grounds for allowing the ruling to stand were procedural, for the suit had not followed New York law requiring that the state intervene in the treatment of children only through the family court.

In the cases of both Baby Doe and Baby Jane Doe, the federal government went to court to demand the medical records of the infants. In both cases, the government charged that decisions against treatment represented discrimination against the handicapped. However, the courts consistently rejected the government's demands. In June of 1985, the Supreme Court agreed to hear arguments to decide whether the federal laws that protect the handicapped against discrimination also apply to the treatment of imperiled newborns who are denied life-prolonging treatment.

On May 15, 1985, the third anniversary of

the death of Baby Doe, the Department of Health and Human Services' final "Baby Doe" regulation went into effect. The regulation was an implementation of an amendment to the Child Abuse Prevention and Treatment Act that was passed into law in October 1985. The amendment was the result of negotiations between some nineteen groups representing right-to-life advocates, the disabled, the medical professions, and members of Congress.

The regulation extended the term "medical neglect" to cover cases of "withholding of medically indicated treatment from a disabled infant with a life-threatening condition." Such treatment was defined as

> the failure to respond to the infant's life-threatening conditions by providing treatment (including appropriate nutrition, hydration, and medication) which, in the treating physician's (or physicians') reasonable medical judgement, will be most likely to be effective in ameliorating or correcting all such conditions . . .

Withholding treatment, but not food and water, was not "medical neglect" in three kinds of cases:

1. The infant is chronically and irreversibly comatose.

2. The provision of such treatment would merely prolong dying, not be effective in ameliorating or correcting all of the infant's life-threatening conditions, or otherwise be futile in terms of the survival of the infant.

3. The provision of such treatment would be virtually futile in terms of the survival of the infant, and the treatment itself under such circumstances would be inhumane.

The regulation defined "reasonable medical judgment" as "a medical judgment that would be made by a reasonably prudent physician knowledgeable about the case and the treatment possibilities with respect to the medical conditions involved." State child protection service agencies were designated as the proper organizations to see to it that infants were not suffering "medical neglect," and, in order to receive any federal funds, such agencies were required to develop a set of procedures to carry out this function.

On June 9, 1986, the Supreme Court, in a five-to-three ruling with one abstention, struck down the Baby Doe regulations. The Court held that there was no evidence that hospitals had discriminated against impaired infants or had refused treatments sought by parents. Accordingly, there was no basis for federal intervention.

Justice John Paul Stevens, in the majority opinion, stressed the absence of any law that might serve as a basis for federal intervention. According to Justice Stevens, no federal law requires hospitals to treat impaired infants without parental consent. Nor does the government have the right "to give unsolicited advice either to parents, to hospitals, or to state officials who are faced with difficult treatment decisions concerning handicapped children." Furthermore, state child-protection agencies "may not be conscripted against their will as the foot soldiers in a Federal crusade."

Representatives of hospitals and those directly involved in neonatal care were generally relieved by the Supreme Court decision. In their arguments before the Court, they had claimed that federal "Baby Doe squads arriving within hours after birth" had second-guessed the agonizing decisions made by parents and physicians and that this had "a devastating impact on the parents."

The Court decision once again places the major responsibility for making decisions about withholding life-sustaining treatment from imperiled newborns on families and physicians acting in consultation.

One recommendation made in the Baby

Doe regulations may continue to have influence. The regulations encouraged hospitals to establish Infant Care Review Committees, and similar recommendations have been made by the President's Commission for the Study of Ethical Problems in Medicine and by the American Academy of Pediatrics. Exactly how such committees might operate, how they would be composed, and what powers they should have continues to be a matter of discussion and disagreement.

The proper role of government, the power of committees, and the responsibilities of parents are merely some of the problems that form the complex of moral issues associated with imperiled and impaired infants.

CASE PRESENTATION
Baby Owens: Down's Syndrome and Duodenal Atresia

On a chill December evening in 1976 Dr. Joan Owens pushed through the plateglass doors of Midwestern Medical Center and walked over to the admitting desk. Dr. Owens was a physician in private practice and regularly visited Midwestern to attend to her patients.

But this night was different. Dr. Owens was coming to the hospital to be admitted as a patient. She was pregnant, and shortly after nine o'clock she began having periodic uterine contractions. Dr. Owens recognized them as the beginnings of labor pains. She was sure of this not only because of her medical knowledge but also because the pains followed the same pattern they had before her other three children were born.

While her husband, Phillip, parked the car, Dr. Owens went through the formalities of admission. She was not particularly worried, for the birth of her other children had been quite normal and uneventful. But the pains were coming more frequently now, and she was relieved when she completed the admission process and was taken to her room. Phillip came with her, bringing her small blue suitcase of personal belongings.

At eleven-thirty that evening, Dr. Owens gave birth to a four-and-a-half pound baby girl. The plastic bracelet fastened around her wrist identified her as Baby Owens and listed her patient number as 23-764-2509.

Dr. Owens was groggy from exhaustion and from the medication she had received. But when the baby was shown to her, she saw at once that it was not normal. The baby's head was misshapen and the skin around her eyes strangely formed. Dr. Owens recognized that her daughter had Down's syndrome.

"Clarence," she called to her obstetrician. "Is the baby mongoloid?"

"We'll talk about it after your recovery," Dr. Clarence Ziner said.

"Tell me now," said Dr. Owens. "Examine it!"

Dr. Ziner made a hasty examination of the child. He had already seen that Dr. Owens was right and was doing no more than making doubly certain. A more careful examination would have to be made later.

When Dr. Ziner confirmed Joan Owens's suspicion, she did not hesitate to say what she was thinking. "Get rid of it," she told Dr. Ziner. "I don't want a mongoloid child."

Dr. Ziner tried to be soothing. "Just sleep for a while now," he told her. "We'll talk about it later."

Four hours later, a little after five in the morning and before it was fully light, Joan Owens woke up. Phillip was with her, and he had more bad news to tell. A more detailed examination had shown that the child's small intestine had failed to develop properly and was closed off in one place—the condition known as duodenal atresia. It could be corrected by a relatively simple surgical procedure, but until surgery was performed, the child could not be fed. Phillip had refused to consent to the operation until he had talked to his wife.

Joan Owens had not changed her mind: she did not want the child. "It wouldn't be fair to the other children to raise them with a mongoloid," she told Phillip. "It would take all of our time, and we wouldn't be able to give David, Sean, and Melinda the love and attention they need."

"I'm willing to do whatever you think best," Phillip said. "But what can we do?"

"Let the child die," Joan said. "If we don't consent to the surgery, the baby will die soon. And that's what we have to let happen."

Phillip put in a call for Dr. Ziner, and when he arrived in Joan's room, they told him of their decision. He was not pleased with it.

"The surgery has very low risk," he said. "The baby's life can almost certainly be saved. We can't tell how retarded she'll be, but most DS children get along quite well with help from their families. The whole family will grow to love her."

"I know," Joan said. "And I don't want that to happen. I don't want us to center our lives around a defective child. Phillip and I and our other children will be forced to lose out on many of life's pleasures and possibilities."

"We've made up our minds," Phillip said. "We don't want the surgery."

"I'm not sure the matter is as simple as that," Dr. Ziner said. "I'm not sure we can legally just let the baby die. I'll have to talk to the Director and the hospital attorney."

At six in the morning, Dr. Ziner called Dr. Felix Entraglo, the Director of Midwestern Medical Center, and Isaac Putnam, the head of the center's legal staff. They agreed to meet at nine o'clock to talk over the problem presented to them by the Owenses.

They met for two hours. It was Putnam's opinion that the hospital would not be legally liable if Baby Owens were allowed to die because her parents refused to give consent for necessary surgery.

"What about getting a court order requiring surgery?" Dr. Entraglo asked. "That's the sort of thing we do when an infant requires a blood transfusion or immunization and his parents' religious beliefs make them refuse consent."

"This case is not exactly parallel," said Mr. Putnam. "Here we're talking about getting a court to force parents to allow surgery to save the life of a defective infant. The infant will still be defective after the surgery, and I think a court would be reluctant to make a family undergo significant emotional and financial hardships when the parents have seriously deliberated about the matter and decided against surgery."

"But doesn't the child have some claim in this situation?" Dr. Ziner asked.

"That's not clear," said Mr. Putnam: "In general we assume that parents will act for the sake of their child's welfare, and when they are reluctant to do so, we look to the courts to act for the child's welfare. But in a situation like this . . . who can say? Is the Owens baby really a person in any legal or moral sense?"

"I think I can understand why a court would hesitate to order surgery," said Dr. Entraglo. "What sort of life would it be for a family when they had been pressured into accepting a child they didn't want. It would turn a family into a cauldron of guilt and resentment mixed in with love and concern. In this case, the lives of five normal people would be profoundly altered for the worse."

"So we just stand by and let the baby die?" asked Dr. Ziner.

"I'm afraid so," Dr. Entraglo said.

It took twelve days for Baby Owens to die. Her lips and throat were moistened with water to lessen her suffering, and in a small disused room set apart from the rooms of patients, she was allowed to starve to death.

Many nurses and physicians thought it was wrong that Baby Owens was forced to die such a lingering death. Some thought it was wrong for her to have to die at all, but such a protracted death seemed needlessly cruel. Yet they were cautioned by Dr. Entraglo that anything done to shorten the baby's life would probably constitute a criminal action. Thus, fear of being charged with a crime kept the staff from administering any medication to Baby Owens.

The burden of caring for the dying baby fell on the nurses in the obstetrics ward. The physicians avoided the child entirely, and it was the nurses who had to see to it that she received her water and was turned in her bed. This was the source of much resentment among the nursing staff, and a few nurses refused to have anything to do with the dying child. Most kept their ministrations to an absolute minimum.

But one nurse, Sara Ann Moberly, was determined to make Baby Owens's last days as comfortable as possible. She held the baby, rocked her, and talked soothingly to her when she cried. Doing all for the baby that she could do soothed Sara Ann as well.

But even Sara Ann was glad when Baby Owens died. "It was a relief to me," she said. "I almost couldn't bear the frustration of just sitting there day after day and doing nothing that could really help her."

INTRODUCTION

If we could speak of nature in human terms, we would often say that it is cruel and pitiless. Nowhere does it seem more heartless than in the case of babies born into the world with severe physical impairments and deformities. The birth of such a child transforms an occasion of expected joy into one of immense sadness. It forces the child's parents to make a momentous decision at a time they are least prepared to reason clearly: Shall they insist that everything be done to save the child's life? Or shall they request that the child be allowed an easeful death?

Nor can physicians and nurses escape the burden that the birth of such a child delivers. Committed to saving lives, can they condone the death of that child? What shall the physician say to the parents when they turn to him for advice? No one involved in the situation can escape the moral agonies that it brings.

To see more clearly what the precise moral issues are in such cases, we need to consider some of the factual details that may be involved in them. We need also to mention other kinds of moral considerations that may be relevant to deciding how an impaired newborn child is to be dealt with by those who have the responsibility to decide.

GENETIC AND CONGENITAL IMPAIRMENTS

The development of a child to the point of birth is an unimaginably complicated process, and there are many ways in which it can go wrong. Two kinds of errors are most frequently responsible for producing impaired children.

1. *Genetic errors.* The program of information that is coded into DNA (the genetic material) may be in some way abnormal because of the occurrence of a mutation. Consequently, when the DNA blueprint is "read" and its instructions followed, the child that develops will be impaired. The defective gene may have been inherited or it may be due to a new mutation.

2. *Congenital errors.* "Congenital" means only "present at birth," and, since genetic defects have results that are present at birth, the term is misleading. Ordinarily, however, the phrase is used to designate errors that result during the developmental process. The impairment, then, is not in the original blueprint (genes) but either results from genetic damage or from the reading of the blueprint. The manufacture and assembly of the materials that constitute the child's development are affected.

We know that many factors can influence fetal development. Radiation (such as x rays), drugs (such as thalidomide), chemicals (such as mercury), and nutritional deficiencies can all cause changes in an otherwise normal process. Also, biological disease agents, such as certain viruses or spirochetes, may intervene in development. They may alter the machinery of the cells, interfere with the formation of tissues, and defeat the carefully programmed process that leads to a normal child.

Genetic impairments are inherited; they are the outcome of the genetic endowment of the child. A carrier of defective genes who has children can pass on the genes. Congenital impairments are not inherited and cannot be passed on. This point is of great theoretical and practical importance. With proper genetic counseling, individuals belonging to families in which certain diseases "run" can assess the risk that their children might be impaired. Also, some genetic diseases can be diagnosed before birth. A blood test for the presence of the substance alphafetoprotein can indicate the likelihood of neural tube defects characteristic of spina bifida. Ultrasound can be used to confirm or detect these or other developmental anomalies. In a procedure known as amniocentesis, fluid is drawn from the uterus, and cells from the developing embryo are examined for genetic abnormalities. (The newer procedure of chorion sampling takes the cells directly from the fetal membrane.) If abnormalities are present, the woman may decide to have an abortion rather than give birth to an impaired child. A recognition of some kinds of developmental errors can lead to efforts to eliminate the impairments by controlling the factors responsible for them. (For additional information on genetic errors, screening, and attempts to correct their results, see the introduction to Chapter 7.)

Once the impaired child is born, the medical and moral problems are immediate. Let us consider now some of the defects commonly found in newborn children. Our focus will be on what they are rather than on what caused them, for so far as the moral issue is concerned in a particular case, how the child came to be impaired is of no importance.

Down's Syndrome

This is a genetic disease first identified in 1866 by the English physician J. L. H. Down. Normally, humans have twenty-three pairs of chromosomes, but Down's syndrome results from the presence of an extra chromosome. The condition is called Trisomy-21, for

instead of a twenty-first pair of chromosomes, the affected person has a twenty-first *triple*. (Less often, the syndrome is produced when the string of chromosomes gets twisted and chromosome pair number 21 sticks to number 15.)

In ways not wholly understood, the normal process of development is altered by this extra chromosome. The child is born with retardation and various physical abnormalities. Typically, these are relatively minor and include such features as a broad skull, a large tongue, and an upward slant of the eyelids. It is this last feature that led to the name "mongolism" for the condition.

Down's syndrome occurs in about one of every thousand births. It occurs most frequently in women over the age of thirty-five, although it is not known why this should be so. In 1984 researchers discovered that certain chromosomes sometimes contain an extra copy of a segment known as the "nucleolar organizing region." This abnormality seems linked to Down's syndrome, and families in which either parent has the abnormality are twenty times more likely to have an afflicted child. Researchers hope to use this information to develop a reliable screening test.

There is no cure for Down's syndrome—no way to compensate for the abnormality of the development process. Those with the defect generally have an IQ of about 50–80 and usually require the care and help of others. They can be taught easy tasks, and despite their impairment those with Down's syndrome usually seem to be quite happy people.

Spina Bifida

Spina bifida is a general name for birth defects that involve an opening in the spine. In development, the spine of the child fails to fuse properly, and often the open vertebrae permit the membrane covering the spinal cord to protrude to the outside. The membrane sometimes forms a bulging, thin sac that contains spinal fluid and nerve tissue. When nerve tissue is present, the condition is called myelomeningocele. This form of spina bifida is a very severe one.

Complications arising from spina bifida must often be treated surgically. The initial condition, the opening in the spine, must be closed up. In severe cases, the sac is removed and the nerve tissue inside is placed within the spinal canal. Normal skin is then grafted over the area. The danger of an infection of the meninges (meningitis) is great; thus, treatment with antibiotic drugs is also necessary.

Furthermore, a child with spina bifida is also likely to require orthopedic operations to attempt to correct the deformities of the legs and feet that occur because of muscle weakness and lack of muscular control due to nerve damage. The bones of such children are thin and brittle, and fractures are frequent.

A child born with spina bifida is virtually always paralyzed to some extent. Generally, the paralysis is below the waist. Because of the nerve damage, the child will have limited sensation in the lower part of the body. This means that he will have no control over his bladder or bowels. The lack of bladder control may result in infection of the bladder, urinary tract, and kidneys, because the undischarged urine may serve as a breeding place for microorganisms. Surgery may help with the problem of lack of control of the bladder and bowels.

Spina bifida occurs in between one and ten per 1,000 births. For reasons not understood, the rate in white families of low socioeconomic status is three times higher than that in families of higher socioeconomic status. The rate in the black population is less than half of that in the white population.

Spina bifida is almost always accompanied by hydrocephaly.

Hydrocephaly

This term literally means "water on the brain." When, for whatever reasons, the flow of fluid through the spinal canal is blocked, the cerebrospinal fluid produced within the brain cannot escape. Pressure build-up from the fluid can cause brain damage, and if it is not released the child will die. Although hydrocephaly is frequently the result of spina bifida, it can have several causes and can develop late in a child's life.

Treatment requires surgically inserting a thin tube, or shunt, to drain the fluid from the skull to the heart or abdomen where it can be absorbed. The operation can save the baby's life, but physical and mental damage is frequent. Placing the shunt and getting it to work properly are difficult tasks that may require many operations. If hydrocephaly accompanies spina bifida (and it almost always does), it is treated first.

Anencephaly

This term means literally "without brain." In this condition, the brain is partially or almost totally absent. The defect is related to spina bifida, for in some forms the bones of the skull are not completely formed and leave an opening through which brain material bulges to the outside.

In some cases, death is a virtual certainty. Other cases can be dealt with in much the same way as is spina bifida. Ordinarily, the individual is so severely retarded that he has minimum control over bodily movements and functions. There is never hope for improvement by any known means.

Esophageal Atresia

In medical terms, an atresia is the closing of a normal opening or canal. The esophagus is the muscular tube that extends from the back of the throat to the stomach. Sometimes the tube forms without an opening, or it does not completely develop so that it does not extend to the stomach. The condition must be corrected by surgery in order that the child may get food into its stomach. The chances of success in such surgery are very high.

Duodenal Atresia

The duodenum is the upper part of the small intestine. Food from the stomach empties into it. When the duodenum is closed off, food cannot pass through and be digested. Surgery can repair this condition and is successful in most cases.

An estimated six percent of all live births, some 200,000 infants a year, require intensive neonatal care. The afflictions that we have singled out for special mention are those that are most often the source of major moral problems. Those correctable by standard surgical procedures present no special moral difficulties. But even they are often involved with other impairments, such as Down's syndrome, that make them important factors in moral deliberations.

ETHICAL THEORIES AND THE PROBLEM OF BIRTH IMPAIRMENTS

A great number of serious moral issues are raised by impaired newborns. Should they be given only ordinary care or should special efforts be made to save their lives? Should they be given no care and allowed to die? Should they be killed in a merciful manner? Who should decide what is in the interest of the child? Might acting in the interest of the child require not acting to save the child's life?

A more basic question that cuts even deeper than these concerns the status of the newborn. It is virtually the same as the question raised in Chapter 1 about the fetus. Namely, are severely impaired newborns persons? It might be argued that some infants are so severely impaired that they should not be considered persons in a relevant moral sense. Not only do they lack the capacity to function, but they lack even the potentiality for ordinary psychological and social development. In this respect, they are worse off than most maturing fetuses.

If this view is accepted, then the principles of our moral theories do not require that we act to preserve the lives of impaired newborns. We might, considering their origin, be disposed to show them some consideration and treat them benevolently—perhaps in the same way we might deal with animals that are in a similarly hopeless condition. We might kill them or allow them to die as a demonstration of our compassion.

One major difficulty with this view is that it is not at all clear which impaired infants could legitimately be considered nonpersons. Birth defects vary widely in severity, and, unless one is prepared to endorse infanticide generally, it is necessary to have defensible criteria for distinguishing among newborns. Also, one must defend a general concept of person that would make it reasonable to regard human offspring as occupying a different status.

By contrast, it might be claimed that the fact that a newborn is a human progeny is sufficient to consider it a person. Assuming that this is so, the question becomes, "How ought we to treat a severely impaired infant person?" Just because they are infants, impaired newborns cannot express wishes, make claims, or enter into deliberations. All that is done concerning them must be done by others.

A utilitarian might decide that the social and personal cost (the suffering of the infant, the anguish of the parents and family, the monetary cost to society) of saving the life of such an infant is greater than the social and personal benefits that can be expected. Accordingly, such a child should not be allowed to live, and it should be killed as painlessly as possible to minimize its suffering. Yet a rule utilitarian might claim, on the contrary, that the rule "Save every child where possible" would, in the long run, produce more utility than disutility.

The natural-law position of Roman Catholicism is that even the most defective newborn is a human person. Yet this view does not require that extraordinary means be used to save the life of such a child. The suffering of the family, great expense, and the need for multiple operations would be reasons for providing only ordinary care. Ordinary care does not mean that every standard medical procedure that might help should be followed. It means only that the defective newborn should receive care of the same type provided for a normal infant. It would be immoral to kill the child or to cause its death by withholding all care.

If the infant is a person, then Kant would regard it as possessing an inherent dignity and value. But the infant in its condition lacks the capacity to reason and to express its will. How, then, should we, acting as its agents, treat it? Kant's principles provide no clear-cut answer. The infant does not threaten our own existence, and we have no grounds for killing it. But, it could be argued, we should allow the child to die. We can imaginatively put ourselves in the place of the infant. Although it would be morally wrong to will our own death (which, Kant claimed, would involve a self-defeating maxim), we might express our autonomy and rationality by choosing to refuse treatment that would prolong a painful and hopeless life. If this is so, then we might act in this way on behalf of the defective child. We might allow the child to die. Indeed, it may be our duty to do so. A similar line of argument from Ross's viewpoint might lead us to decide that, although we have a prima facie duty to preserve the child's life, our actual duty is to allow it to die.

Another basic question remains: Who is to make the decision about how an impaired newborn is to be treated? Traditionally, the assumption has been that this is a decision best left to the infant's parents and physicians. Because they can be assumed to have the highest concern for his welfare and the most knowledge about its condition and prospects, they are the ones who should have the primary responsibility for deciding his fate. If there is reason to believe that they are not acting in a responsible manner, then it becomes the responsibility of the courts to guarantee that the interests of the infant are served.

Hardly any responsible person advocates heroic efforts to save the lives of infants who are most severely impaired, and hardly anyone advocates not treating infants with relatively simple and correctable impairments. The difficult cases are those that fall somewhere along the continuum. Advances in medical management and technology can now save the lives of many infants who earlier would have died relatively quickly, and yet we still lack the power to provide those infants with a life that we might judge to be worthwhile. Yet a failure to treat such infants does not invariably result in their deaths, and a failure to provide them with early treatment may mean that they are even more impaired than they would be otherwise.

No one believes that we currently have a satisfactory solution to this dilemma. It is important to keep in mind that it is not a purely intellectual problem. The context in which particular decisions are made is one of doubt and confusion and genuine anguish.

THE SELECTIONS

John A. Robertson in his essay, "Examination of Arguments in Favor of Withholding Ordinary Medical Care from Defective Infants," defends a conservative natural-law position in criticizing two arguments in favor of withholding "necessary but ordinary" medical care from impaired infants. He rejects the claim made by Michael Tooley that infants are not persons and argues that, on the contrary, there is no nonarbitrary consideration that requires us to protect the past realization of conceptual capability but not its potential realization.

The second argument that Robertson considers is one to the effect that we have no obligation to treat defective newborns when the cost of doing so greatly outweighs the benefits (a utilitarian argument). In criticism, Robertson claims that we have no way of judging this. Life itself may be of sufficient worth to an impaired person to offset his or her suffering, and the suffering and cost to society are not sufficient to justify withholding care.

Contrary to Robertson, H. T. Engelhardt in "Ethical Issues in Aiding the Death of Young Children" contends that children are not persons in the full sense. They must exist in and through their families. Thus parents, in conference with a physician who provides information, are the appropriate ones to decide whether to treat an impaired newborn when (1) there is not only little likelihood of a full human life, but also there is the likelihood of suffering if the life is prolonged, or (2) the cost of prolonging the life is very great.

Engelhardt further argues that it is reasonable to speak of a *duty* not to treat an impaired infant when this will only prolong a painful life or would only lead to a painful death. He bases his claim on the legal notion of a "wrongful life." This notion suggests that there are cases in which nonexistence would be better than existence under the conditions in which a person must live. Life can thus be seen as an injury, rather than as a gift.

John Arras, in the last selection, raises the question of whether there are differences between normal and gravely impaired infants that justify withholding life-sustaining treat-

ment from the impaired. The "best interest" of the child standard seems to point to morally relevant distinctions. It is clearly in the best interest of the normal child to live, but is this always the case with the impaired child? The standard has the advantage of focusing on the child's interest, rather than (as with utilitarianism) on the interest of the parents or society. However, Arras points to a number of serious problems in interpreting and applying the standard in individual cases. Furthermore, Arras claims, in the final analysis the best-interest standard makes the absence of pain the only real moral consideration.

Arras argues that this is an unacceptable result and that other features, such as the ability to communicate and to give and receive love, are also morally relevant. Without acknowledging their relevance, we cannot even attribute any human interests to the child. Thus, according to Arras, we need a supplementary standard that is "geared to the presence or absence of distinctly human capacities." Such a "relational potential standard" rests on the ethical principle that biological human life is only a relative good. This means that in applying the standard we must face up to the difficult task of assessing the factors that make human life valuable to its possessors. In effect, we must attempt to determine a "threshold of meaningful human life."

In 1973 R. S. Duff and A. G. M. Campbell shocked the public by reporting that during a thirty-month period forty-three infants at the Yale–New Haven Hospital had been permitted to die. Each of the children suffered from one or more severe birth defects. Although the staff of the hospital took no steps to end the lives of the infants, treatment was withheld from them.

Such decisions had been made for years in hospitals throughout the world. Sometimes they were made by physicians acting alone and sometimes by physicians in consultation with families. But almost never had the situation been discussed openly and publicly.

Now there is more openness about the whole complex of moral and human problems presented by impaired newborns. There is a greater willingness to consider the possibility that saving the life of a child might not be the right act to perform, that it may even be our duty to assist the child's dying. In any case, the time of covert decisions and half-guilty conferences has passed. The issues are there, they are known to be there, and they must be faced.

Examination of Arguments in Favor of Withholding Ordinary Medical Care from Defective Infants

John A. Robertson

This [selection] considers two arguments in favor of withholding necessary but ordinary medical care from defective infants, and concludes that neither is persuasive. . . .

1. Defective Infants Are Not Persons

Children born with congenital malformations may lack human form and the possibility of ordinary, psychosocial development. In many cases mental retardation is or will be so profound, and physical incapacity so great, that the term "persons" or "humanly alive"[1] have odd or questionable meaning when applied to them. In these cases the infant's physical and mental defects are so severe that they will never know anything but a vegetative existence, with no discernible personality, sense of self, or capacity to interact with others. Withholding ordinary medical care in such cases, one may argue, is justified on the ground that these infants are not persons or human beings in the ordinary or legal sense of the term, and therefore do not possess the right of care that persons possess.

Central to this argument is the idea that living products of the human uterus can be classified into offspring that are persons, and those that are not. Conception and birth by human parents does not automatically endow one with personhood and its accompanying rights. Some other characteristic or feature must be present in the organism for personhood to vest,[3] and this the defective infant arguably lacks. Lacking that property, an organism is not a person or deserving to be treated as such.

Before considering what "morally significant features" might distinguish persons from nonpersons, and examining the relevance of such features to the case of the defective infant, we must face an initial objection to this line of inquiry. The objection questions the need for any distinction among human offspring because of

the monumental misuse of the concept of 'humanity' in so many practices of discrimination and atrocity throughout history. Slavery, witchhunts and wars have all been justified by their perpetrators on the grounds that they held their victims to be less than fully human. The insane and the criminal have for long periods been deprived of the most basic necessities for similar reasons, and been excluded from society. . . .

. . . Even when entered upon with the best of intentions, and in the most guarded manner, the enterprise of basing the protection of human life upon such criteria and definitions is dangerous. To question someone's humanity or personhood is a first step to mistreatment and killing.[4]

Hence, according to this view, human parentage is a necessary and sufficient condition for personhood, whatever the characteristics of the offspring, because qualifying criteria inevitably lead to abuse and untold suffering to beings who are

Reprinted by permission of the publisher from "Involuntary Euthanasia of Defective Newborns: A Legal Analysis," Stanford Law Review 27 (1975): 246–261. Copyright 1975 by the Board of Trustees of the Leland Stanford Junior University. Editor's Note: The footnotes in this essay have been renumbered.

unquestionably human. Moreover, the human species is sufficiently different from other sentient species that assigning its members greater rights on birth alone is not arbitrary.

This objection is indeed powerful. The treatment accorded slaves in the United States, the Nazi denial of personal status to non-Aryans, and countless other incidents, testify that man's inhumanity to man is indeed greatest when a putative nonperson is involved.[5] Arguably, however, a distinction based on gross physical form, profound mental incapacity, and the very existence of personality or selfhood, besides having an empirical basis in the monstrosities and mutations known to have been born to women[6] is a basic and fundamental one. Rather than distinguishing among the particular characteristics that persons might attain through the contingencies of race, culture, and class, it merely separates out those who lack the potential for assuming any personal characteristics beyond breathing and consciousness.

This reply narrows the issue: should such creatures be cared for, protected, or regarded as "ordinary" humans? If such treatment is not warranted, they may be treated as nonpersons. The arguments supporting care in all circumstances are based on the view that all living creatures are sacred, contain a spark of the divine, and should be so regarded. Moreover, indentifying those human offspring unworthy of care is a difficult task and will inevitably take a toll on those whose humanity cannot seriously be questioned. At this point the argument becomes metaphysical or religious and immune to resolution by empirical evidence, not unlike the controversy over whether a fetus is a person.[7] It should be noted, however, that recognizing all human offspring as persons, like recognizing the fetus to be a person,[8] does not conclude the treatment issue.[9]

Although this debate can be resolved only by reference to religious or moral beliefs, a procedural solution may reasonably be considered. Since reasonable people can agree that we ordinarily regard human offspring as persons, and further, that defining categories of exclusion is likely to pose special dangers of abuse, a reasonable solution is to presume that all living human offspring are persons. This rule would be subject to exception only if it can be shown beyond a reasonable doubt that certain offspring will never possess the minimal properties that reasonable persons ordinarily associate with human personality. If this burden cannot be satisfied, then the presumption of personhood obtains.

For this purpose I will address only one of the many properties proposed as a necessary condition of personhood—the capacity for having a sense of self—and consider whether its advocates present a cogent account of the nonhuman. Since other accounts may be more convincingly articulated, this discussion will neither exhaust nor conclude the issue. But it will illuminate the strengths and weaknesses of the personhood argument and enable us to evaluate its application to defective infants.

Michael Tooley has recently argued that a human offspring lacking the capacity for a sense of self lacks the rights to life or equal treatment possessed by other persons.[10] In considering the morality of abortion and infanticide, Tooley considers "what properties a thing must possess in order to have a serious right to life,"[11] and he concludes that:

> [h]aving a right to life presupposes that one is capable of desiring to continue existing as a subject of experiences and other mental states. This in turn presupposes both that one has the concept of such a continuing entity and that one believes that one is oneself such an entity. So an entity that lacks such a consciousness of itself as a continuing subject of mental states does not have a right to life.[12]

However, this account is at first glance too narrow, for it appears to exclude all those who do not presently have a desire "to continue existing as a subject of experiences and other mental states." The sleeping or unconscious individual, the deranged, the conditioned, and the suicidal do not have such desires, though they might have had them or could have them in the future. Accordingly, Tooley emphasizes the capability of entertaining such desires, rather than their actual existence.[13] But it is difficult to distinguish the capability for such desires in an unconscious, conditioned, or emotionally disturbed person from the capability existing in a fetus or infant. In all cases the capability is a future one; it will arise only if certain events occur, such as normal growth and development in the case of the infant, and removal of the disability in the other cases. The infant, in fact, might realize its capability[14] long before disabled adults recover emotional balance or consciousness.

To meet this objection, Tooley argues that the significance of the capability in question is not solely its future realization (for fetuses and infants will ordinarily realize it), but also its previous existence and exercise.[15] He seems to say that once the conceptual capability has been realized, one's right to desire continued existence permanently vests, even though the present capability for desiring does not exist, and may be lost for substantial periods or permanently. Yet, what nonarbitrary reasons require that we protect the past realization of conceptual capability but not its potential realization in the future? As a reward for its past realization? To mark our reverence and honor for someone who has realized that state? Tooley is silent on this point.

Another difficulty is Tooley's ambiguity concerning the permanently deranged, comatose, or conditioned. Often he phrases his argument in terms of a temporary suspension of the capability of conceptual thought.[16] One wonders what he would say of someone permanently deranged, or with massive brain damage, or in a prolonged coma. If he seriously means that the past existence of a desire for life vests these cases with the right to life, then it is indeed difficult to distinguish the comatose or deranged from the infant profoundly retarded at birth. Neither will ever possess the conceptual capability to desire to be a continuing subject of experiences. A distinction based on reward or desert seems arbitrary, and protection of life applies equally well in both cases. Would Tooley avoid this problem by holding that the permanently comatose and deranged lose their rights after a certain point because conceptual capacity will never be regained? This would permit killing (or at least withholding of care) from the insane and comatose—doubtless an unappealing prospect.[17] Moreover, we do not ordinarily think of the insane, and possibly the comatose, as losing personhood before their death. Although their personality or identity may be said to change, presumably for the worse, or become fragmented or minimal, we still regard them as specific persons. If a "self" in some minimal sense exists here then the profoundly retarded, who at least is conscious, also may be considered a self, albeit a minimal one. Thus, one may argue that Tooley fails to provide a convincing account of criteria distinguishing persons and nonpersons. He both excludes beings we ordinarily think of as persons—infants, deranged, conditioned, possibly the comatose—and fails to articulate criteria that convincingly distinguish the nonhuman.[18] But, even if we were to accept Tooley's distinction that beings lacking the potential for desire and a sense of self are not persons who are owed the duty to be treated by ordinary medical means, this would not appear to be very helpful in deciding whether to treat the newborn with physical or mental defects. Few infants, it would seem, would fall into this class.[19] First, those suffering from malformations, however gross, that do not affect mental capabilities would not fit the class of nonpersons. Second, frequently even the most severe cases of mental retardation cannot be reliably determined until a much later period;[20] care thus could not justifiably be withheld in the neonatal period, although this principle would permit nontreatment at the time when nonpersonality is clearly established.[21] Finally, the only group of defective newborns who would clearly qualify as nonpersons is anencephalics, who altogether lack a brain, or those so severely brain-damaged that it is immediately clear that a sense of self or personality can never develop. Mongols, myelomeningoceles, and other defective infants from whom ordinary care is now routinely withheld would not qualify as nonpersons. Thus, even the most coherent and cogent criteria of humanity are only marginally helpful in the situation of the defective infant. We must therefore consider whether treatment can be withheld on grounds other than the claim that such infants are not persons.

2. No Obligation to Treat Exists When the Costs of Maintaining Life Greatly Outweigh the Benefits

If we reject the argument that defective newborns are not persons, the question remains whether circumstances exist in which the consequences of treatment as compared with nontreatment are so undesirable that the omission of care is justified. As we have seen, the doctrine of necessity permits one to violate the criminal law when essential to prevent the occurrence of a greater evil.[22] The circumstances, however, when the death of a nonconsenting person is a lesser evil than his continuing life are narrowly circumscribed, and do not include withholding care from defective infants.[23] Yet many parents and physicians deeply committed to the loving care of the newborn think that treating severely defective infants causes more harm than good, thereby justifying the withholding of ordinary care.[24] In their view the suffering and diminished quality of the child's life do not justify the social and economic costs of treatment. This claim has a growing commonsense appeal, but it assumes that the utility or quality of one's life can be measured and compared with other lives, and that health resources may legitimately be allocated to produce the greatest personal utility. This argument will now be analyzed from the perspective of the defective patient and others affected by his care.

a. The Quality of the Defective Infant's Life

Comparisons of relative worth among persons, or between persons and other interests, raise moral and methodological issues that make any argument that relies on such comparisons extremely vulnerable. Thus the strongest claim for not treating the defective newborn is that treatment seriously harms the infant's own interests, whatever may be the effects on others. When maintaining his life involves great physical and psychosocial suffering for the patient, a reasonable person might conclude that such a life is not worth living. Presumably the patient, if fully informed and able to communicate, would agree. One then would be morally justified in withholding lifesaving treatment if such action served to advance the best interests of the patient.[25]

Congenital malformations impair development in several ways that lead to the judgment that deformed retarded infants are "a burden to themselves."[26] One is the severe physical pain, much of it resulting from repeated surgery that defective infants will suffer.[27] Defective children also are likely to develop other pathological features, leading to repeated fractures, dislocations, surgery, malfunctions, and other sources of pain. The shunt, for example, inserted to relieve hydrocephalus, a common problem in defective children, often becomes clogged, necessitating frequent surgical interventions.[28]

Pain, however, may be intermittent and manageable with analgesics. Since many infants and adults experience great pain, and many defective infants do not, pain alone, if not totally unmanageable, does not sufficiently show that a life is so worthless that death is preferable. More important are the psychosocial deficits resulting from the child's handicaps. Many defective children never can walk even with prosthesis, never interact with normal children, never appreciate growth, adolescence, or the fulfillment of education and employment, and seldom are even able to care for themselves. In cases of severe retardation, they may be left with a vegetative existence in a crib, incapable of choice or the most minimal response to stimuli. Parents or others may reject them, and much of their time will be spent in hospitals, in surgery, or fighting the many illnesses that beset them. Can it be said that such a life is worth living?

There are two possible responses to the quality-of-life argument. One is to accept its premises but to question the degree of suffering in particular cases, and thus restrict the justification for death to the most extreme cases. The absence of opportunities for schooling, career, and interaction may be the fault of social attitudes and the failings of healthy persons, rather than a necessary result of congenital malformations. Psychosocial suffering occurs because healthy, normal persons reject or refuse to relate to the defective, or hurry them to poorly funded institutions. Most nonambulatory, mentally retarded persons can be trained for satisfying roles. One cannot assume that a nonproductive existence is necessarily unhappy; even social rejection and nonacceptance can be mitigated.[29] Moreover, the psychosocial ills of the handicapped often do not differ in kind from those experienced by many persons. With training and care, growth, development, and a full range of experiences are possible for most people with physical and mental handicaps. Thus, the claim that death is a far better fate than life cannot in most cases be sustained.

This response, however, avoids meeting the quality-of-life argument on its strongest grounds. Even if many defective infants can experience growth, interaction, and most human satisfactions if nurtured, treated, and trained, some infants are so severely retarded or grossly deformed that their response to love and care, in fact their capacity to be conscious, is always minimal. Although mongoloid and nonambulatory spina bifida children may experience an existence we would hesitate to adjudge worse than death, the profoundly retarded, nonambulatory, blind, deaf infant who will spend his few years in the back-ward cribs of a state institution is clearly a different matter.

To repudiate the quality-of-life argument, therefore, requires a defense of treatment in even these extreme cases. Such a defense would question the validity of any surrogate or proxy judgments of the worth or quality of life when the wishes of the person in question cannot be ascertained. The essence of the quality-of-life argument is a proxy's judgment that no reasonable person can prefer the pain, suffering, and loneliness of, for example, life in a crib at an IQ level of 20, to an immediate, painless death.

But in what sense can the proxy validly conclude that a person with different wants, needs, and interests, if able to speak, would agree that such a life were worse than death? At the start one must be skeptical of the proxy's claim to objective disinterestedness. If the proxy is also the parent or physician, as has been the case in pediatric euthanasia, the impact of treatment on the proxy's interests, rather than solely on those of the child, may influence his assessment. But even if the proxy were truly neutral and committed only to caring for the child, the problem of egocentricity and knowing another's mind remains. Compared with the situation and life prospects of a "reasonable man," the child's potential quality of life indeed appears dim. Yet a standard based on healthy, ordinary development may be entirely inappropriate to this situation. One who has never known the pleasures of mental operation, ambulation, and social interaction surely does not suffer from their loss as much as one who has. While one who has known these capacities may prefer death to a life without them, we have no assurance that the handicapped person, with no point of comparison, would agree. Life, and life alone, whatever its limitations, might be of sufficient worth to him.[30]

One should also be hesitant to accept proxy assessments of quality-of-life because the margin of error in such predictions may be very great. For instance, while one expert argues that by a purely clinical assessment he can accurately forecast the minimum degree of future handicap an individual will experience,[31] such forecasting is not infallible,[32] and risks denying care to infants whose disability might otherwise permit a reasonably acceptable quality-of-life. Thus given the problems in ascertaining another's wishes, the proxy's bias to personal or culturally relative interests, and the unreliability of predictive criteria, the quality-of-life argument is open to serious question. Its strongest appeal arises in the case of a grossly deformed, retarded, institutionalized child, or one with incessant unmanageable pain, where continued life is itself torture. But these cases are few, and cast doubt on the utility of any such judgment. Even if the judgment occasionally may be defensible, the potential danger of quality-of-life assessments may be a compelling reason for rejecting this rationale for withholding treatment.[33]

b. The Suffering of Others

In addition to the infant's own suffering, one who argues that the harm of treatment justifies violation of the defective infant's right to life usually relies on the psychological, social, and economic costs of maintaining his existence to family and society. In their view the minimal benefit of treatment to persons incapable of full social and physical development does not justify the burdens that care of the defective infant imposes on parents, siblings, health professionals, and other patients. Matson, a noted pediatric neurosurgeon, states:

> [I]t is the doctor's and the community's responsibility to provide [custodial] care and to minimize suffering; but, at the same time, it is also their responsibility not to prolong such individual, familial, and community suffering unnecessarily, and not to carry out multiple procedures and prolonged, expensive, acute hospitalization in an infant whose chance for acceptable growth and development is negligible.[34]

Such a frankly utilitarian argument raises problems. It assumes that because of the greatly curtailed orbit of his existence, the costs or suffering of others is greater than the benefit of life to the child. This judgment, however, requires a coherent way of measuring and comparing interpersonal utilities, a logical-practical problem that utilitarianism has never surmounted.[35] But even if such comparisons could reliably show a net loss from treatment, the fact remains that the child must sacrifice his life to benefit others. If the life of one individual, however useless, may be sacrificed for the benefit of any person, however useful, or for the benefit of any number of persons, then we have acknowledged the principle that rational utility may justify any outcome.[36] As many philosophers have demonstrated, utilitarianism can always permit the sacrifice of one life for other interests, given the appropriate arrangement of utilities on the balance sheet.[37] In the absence of principled grounds for such a decision, the social equation involved in mandating direct, involuntary euthanasia[38] becomes a difference of degree, not kind, and we reach the point where protection of life depends solely on social judgments of utility.

These objections may well be determinative.[39] But if we temporarily bracket them and examine the extent to which care of the defective infant subjects others to suffering, the claim that inordinate suffering outweighs the infant's interest in life is rarely plausible. In this regard we must examine the impact of caring for defective infants on the family, health professions, and society-at-large.

The Family. The psychological impact and crisis created by birth of a defective infant is devastating.[40] Not only is the mother denied the normal tension release from the stresses of pregnancy,[41] but both parents feel a crushing blow to their dignity, self-esteem and self-confidence.[42] In a very short time, they feel grief for the loss of the normal expected child, anger at fate, numbness, disgust, waves of helplessness, and disbelief.[43] Most feel personal blame for the defect, or blame their spouse. Adding to the shock is fear that social position and mobility are permanently endangered.[44] The transformation of a "joyously awaited experience into one of catastrophe and profound psychological threat[45] often will reactivate unresolved maturational conflicts. The chances for social pathology—divorce, somatic complaints, nervous and mental disorders—increase and hard-won adjustment patterns may be permanently damaged.[46]

The initial reactions of guilt, grief, anger, and loss, however, cannot be the true measure of family suffering caused by care of a defective infant, because these costs are present whether or not the parents choose treatment. Rather, the question is to what degree treatment imposes psychic and other costs greater than would occur if the child were not treated. The claim that care is more costly rests largely on the view that parents and family suffer inordinately from nurturing such a child.

Indeed, if the child is treated and accepted at home, difficult and demanding adjustments must be made. Parents must learn how to care for a disabled child, confront financial and psychological uncertainty, meet the needs of other siblings, and work through their own conflicting feelings. Mothering demands are greater than with a normal child, particularly if medical care and hospitalization are frequently required.[47] Counseling or professional support may be nonexistent or difficult to obtain.[48] Younger siblings may react with hostility and guilt, older with shame and anger.[49] Often the normal feedback of child growth that renders the turmoil of childrearing worthwhile develops more slowly or not at all. Family resources can be depleted (especially if medical care is needed), consumption patterns altered, or standards of living modified.[50] Housing may have to be found closer to a hospital, and plans for further children changed.[51] Finally, the anxieties, guilt, and grief present at birth may threaten to recur or become chronic.[52]

Yet, although we must recognize the burdens and frustrations of raising a defective infant, it does not necessarily follow that these costs require nontreatment, or even institutionalization. Individual and group counseling can substantially alleviate anxiety, guilt, and frustration, and enable parents to cope with underlying conflicts triggered by the birth and the adaptations required.[53] Counseling also can reduce psychological pressures on siblings, who can be taught to recognize and accept their own possibly hostile feelings and the difficult position of their parents. They may even be taught to help their parents care for the child.[54]

The impact of increased financial costs also may vary.[55] In families with high income or adequate health insurance, the financial costs are manageable. In others, state assistance may be available.[56] If severe financial problems arise or pathological adjustments are likely, institutionalization, although undesirable for the child, remains an option.[57] Finally, in many cases, the experience of living through a crisis is a deepening and enriching one, accelerating personality maturation, and giving one a new sensitivity to the needs of spouse, siblings, and others. As one parent of a defective child states: "In the last months I have come closer to people and can understand them more. I have met them more deeply. I did not know there were so many people with troubles in the world."[58]

Thus, while social attitudes regard the handicapped child as an unmitigated disaster, in reality the problem may not be insurmountable, and often may not differ from life's other vicissitudes. Suffering there is, but seldom is it so overwhelming or so imminent that the only alternative is death of the child.[59]

Health professionals. Physicians and nurses also suffer when parents give birth to a defective child, although, of course, not to the degree of the parents. To the obstetrician or general practitioner the defective birth may be a blow to his professional identity. He has the difficult task of informing the parents of the defects, explaining their causes, and dealing with the parents' resulting emotional shock. Often he feels guilty for failing to produce a normal baby.[60] In addition, the parents may project anger or hostility on the physician, questioning his professional competence or seeking the services of other doctors.[61] The physician also may feel that his expertise and training are misused when employed to maintain the life of an infant whose chances for a productive existence are so diminished. By neglecting other patients, he may feel that he is prolonging rather than alleviating suffering.

Nurses, too, suffer role strain from care of the defective newborn. Intensive-care-unit nurses may work with only one or two babies at a time. They face the daily ordeals of care—the progress and relapses—and often must deal with anxious parents who are themselves grieving or ambivalent toward the child. The situation may trigger a nurse's own ambivalence about death and mothering, in a context in which she is actively working to keep alive a child whose life prospects seem minimal.[62]

Thus, the effects of care on physicians and nurses are not trivial, and must be intelligently confronted in medical education or in management of a pediatric unit. Yet to state them is to make clear that they can but weigh lightly in the decision of whether to treat a defective newborn. Compared with the situation of the parents, these burdens seem insignificant, are short term, and most likely do not evoke such profound emotions. In any case, these difficulties are hazards of the profession—caring for the sick and dying will always produce strain. Hence, on these grounds alone it is difficult to argue that a defective person may be denied the right to life.

Society. Care of the defective newborn also imposes societal costs, the utility of which is questioned when the infant's expected quality-of-life is so poor. Medical resources that can be used by infants with a better prognosis, or throughout the health-care system generally, are consumed in providing expensive surgical and intensive-care services to infants who may be severely retarded, never lead active lives, and die in a few months or years. Institutionalization imposes costs on taxpayers and reduces the resources available for those who might better benefit from it,[63] while reducing further the quality of life experienced by the institutionalized defective.

One answer to these concerns is to question the impact of the costs of caring for defective newborns. Precise data showing the costs to taxpayers or the trade-offs with health and other expenditures do not exist. Nor would ceasing to care for the defective necessarily lead to a reallocation within the health budget that would produce net savings in suffering or life;[64] in fact, the released resources might not be reallocated for health at all.[65] In any case, the trade-offs within the health budget may well be small. With advances in prenatal diagnosis of genetic disorders, many deformed infants who would formerly require care will be aborted beforehand.[66] Then, too, it is not clear that the most technical and expensive procedures always constitute the best treatment for certain malformations.[67] When compared with the almost seven percent of the GNP now spent on health,[68] the money in the defense budget, or tax revenues generally, the public resources required to keep defective newborns alive seem marginal, and arguably worth the commitment to life that such expenditures reinforce. Moreover, as the Supreme Court recently recognized,[69] conservation of the taxpayer's purse does not justify serious infringement of fundamental rights. Given legal and ethical norms against sacrificing the lives of nonconsenting others, and the imprecisions in diagnosis and prediction concerning the eventual outcomes of medical care,[70] the social-cost argument does not compel nontreatment of defective newborns.[71]

Notes

1. Commentary, *The Ethics of Surgery in Newborn Infants*, 8 CLINICAL PEDIATRICS 251 (1969); *cf.* Grunberg, *Who Lives and Dies?*, N.Y. Times, Apr. 22, 1974, at 35, col. 2.

2. *Id.* While the proposition appears to draw some support from Bracton's statement in a noncriminal context that a monster is not a human being, "Quia partus monstruosus est cum non nascatur ut homo," *cited* in G. WILLIAMS, THE SANCTITY OF LIFE AND THE CRIMINAL LAW 20–21 (1957), no case has ever held that a live human offspring is not a human being because of certain physical or mental deficits, and therefore may be killed. *See* G. WILLIAMS, *supra*, at 20–24. The state, in the exercise of its *parens patriae* power to protect persons incapacitated by infancy, neglect, or mental incompetence, recognizes that many "persons" incapable of leading an ordinary or normal life are nevertheless persons with rights and interests to be protected. *See, e.g.,* Herr, *Retarded Children and the Law: Enforcing the Constitutional Rights of the Mentally Retarded*, 23 SYR. L. REV. 995 (1972). Even a slave was protected by the law of homicide even though incapable of full social interaction. *See, e.g.,* Fields v. State, 1 Yager's Rep. 156 (Tenn. 1829). Thus, a judge in Maine recently had little difficulty in concluding that a deformed child with multiple anomalies and brain damage was "at the moment of live birth . . . a human being entitled to the fullest protection of the law." Maine Medical Center v. Houle, No. 74–145, at 4 (Super. Ct., Cumberland Cty., Feb. 14, 1974).

3. *See* Tooley, *Abortion and Infanticide*, 2 PHIL. & PUB. AFFAIRS 37, 51 (1972).

4. Bok, *Ethical Problems of Abortion*, 2 HASTINGS CENTER STUDIES, Jan. 1974, at 33, 41.

5. *See* Alexander, *Medical Science under Dictatorship*, 241 NEW ENG. J. MED. 39 (1949).

6. T. BECK & J. BECK, ELEMENTS OF MEDICAL JURISPRUDENCE 422 (11th ed. 1960).

7. *See* Tribe, *Foreword—Toward a Model of Roles in the Due Process of Life and Law*, HARV. L. REV. 1, 18–20 (1973).

8. *See* Thomson, *A Defense of Abortion*, 1 PHIL. AND PUB. AFFAIRS 47 (1971).

9. *See* notes [22–71] *infra* and accompanying text.

10. Tooley, *supra* note [3] at 49.

11. *Id.* at 37.

12. *Id.* at 49.

13. *Id.* at 50.

14. Tooley concedes that the infant attains this capacity in the first year of life, though further research is necessary to identify the exact time. *Id.* at 64.

15. *Correspondence*, 2 PHIL. & PUB. AFFAIRS 419 (1973).

16. *Id.* at 421–23.

17. A somewhat similar approach to the definition of personhood by Richard McCormick also fails to cogently distinguish the case of the deranged. McCormick argues that if the potential for human relationships "is simply nonexistent or would be utterly submerged and undeveloped in the mere struggle to survive, that life has achieved its potential" and ordinary care need not be provided. McCormick, *To Save or Let Die—The Dilemma of Modern Medicine*, 229 J.A.M.A. 172, 175 (1974). But would we sanction withholding antibiotics from an insane person suffering a serious infection simply because his capacity to enter into human relationships had become minimal?

18. John Rawls makes a similar argument for the proposition that not all human offspring are entitled to "equal basic rights" of liberty or "the guarantees of justice," *see* J. RAWLS, A THEORY OF JUSTICE 504–10 (1971), and is equally unsuccessful in articulating convincing criteria. His argument arises in the course of a discussion of the features of human beings which entitle them, as opposed to plants, animals, and machines, to be treated in accordance with the principles of justice. To be owed or entitled to equal justice one must possess a certain capacity not present in all human organisms. The capacity is moral personality: "Moral persons are distinguished by two features: First, they are capable of having (and are assumed to have) a conception of their good (as expressed by a rational plan of life); and second they are capable of having (and are assumed to acquire) a sense of justice, a normally effective desire to apply and to act upon the principles of justice, at least to a certain minimum degree." *Id.* at 505. Moral personality qualifies one to be treated with justice, because the principles of justice are derived from the choices which moral persons in the original position desiring to maximize their own (but unknown) good would make; "We use the characterization of

the person in the original position to single out the kinds of beings to whom the principles chosen apply. After all, the parties are thought of as adopting those criteria to regulate their common institutions and their conduct toward one another: and the description of their nature enters into the reasoning by which these principles are selected. Thus equal justice is owed to those who have the capacity to take part in and to act in accordance with the public understanding of the initial situation." *Id.*

Rawls, unlike Tooley, accepts the potential rather than present or soon-to-be-assumed capability for moral personality, which includes infants and those "who could take part in the initial agreement, were it not for fortuitous circumstances. . . ." *Id.* at 504. Although he is hesitant in describing moral personality as both a necessary and sufficient condition for justice, he does distinguish those "who have lost their realized capacity temporarily through misfortune, accident, or mental stress" from those "more or less permanently deprived of moral personality," who "may present a difficulty." *Id.* at 510. However, even if creatures lacking this capacity are not entitled to strict justice, "it does not follow that there are no requirements at all in regard to them, [n]or in our relations with the natural order. Certainly it is wrong to be cruel to animals and the destruction of a whole species can be a great evil. The capacity for feelings of pleasure and pain and for the forms of life of which animals are capable clearly imposes duties of compassion and humanity in their case." *Id.* at 512.

Rawls' position, however, is not strictly necessary for the "natural completion of justice as fairness." While Rawls needs to distinguish human claims from those of machines, plants, and animals, such a distinction can stand without dividing human organisms into two classes—the privileged and nonprivileged to enjoy justice. The need for persons in the original position to have certain capacities does not necessarily entail that the principles chosen apply only to those blessed in the natural lottery with the capacity to choose in the original position. Surely those whose capacity for justice or a life plan has been ended by accident or mental disturbance do not lose equal liberty. Why then should incapacity at birth disqualify one? If I understand Rawls correctly those in the original position would protect themselves against such a contingency by deriving principles which apply to all human offspring, whatever their capacity for a sense of justice or a life plan at any stage of life. Thus Rawls' statement that "[t]hose who can give justice are owed justice," *id.* at 510, need not

exclude those who by accident or natural infirmity are incapable of giving justice.

19. Warkany, for example, reports the incidence of anencephaly, the absence of all or most of an infant's brain, as approximately 1 in 1,000 for children born in hospital wards, but notes that "remarkable variations have been reported from different areas." J. WARKANY, [*Congenital Malformations*, (1971)], at 189.

20. *Id.* at 39.

21. But other factors might lead to treatment at this later point in time. For example, if care and nurturing occur immediately after birth, a strong mother-child bond is built, which might prevent mothers from deciding to withhold care when a serious defect is discovered weeks later. Barnett, Leiderman, Globstein & Klaus, *Neonatal Separation: The Maternal Side of Interactional Deprivation*, 45 PEDIATRICS 197, 197–99 (1970); Kennel & Klaus, *Care of the Mother of the High Risk Infant*, 14 CLIN. OBSTET. & GYNECOL. 926, 930–36 (1971).

22. *See* notes 157–64 and accompanying text [in the original].

23. *See* notes 169–80 and accompanying text [in the original].

24. See Duff and Campbell, *Moral and Ethical Dilemmas in the Special-Care Nursery*, 289 NEW ENG. J. MED. 890 (1973).

25. The perspective that the mere saving of life is not enough unless the lives are "worth saving" is well represented in the medical literature. Lorber, in discussing the process of selecting spina bifida infants for treatment, states: "Severe degree of paralysis is the most generally adopted reason for withholding treatment, but incontinence, severe hydrocephalus, gross deformities and social conditions are also taken into account. . . . There is no doubt that the future quality of life of many patients with myelomeningocele depends at least partly on the speed, efficiency and comprehensiveness of treatment from birth onwards—and often throughout their lives. Nevertheless, there are large numbers who are so severely handicapped at birth that those who survive are bound to suffer from a combination of major physical defects. In addition, many will be retarded in spite of everything that can be done for them. It is not necessary to enumerate all that this means to the patient, the family and the community in terms of suffering, deprivation, anxiety, frustration, family stress and financial cost. The large majority surviving at present have yet to reach the most

difficult period of adolescence and young adult life and the problems of love, marriage and employment." Lorber, [*Results of Treatment of Myelomeningocele,* DEVELOP. MED. & CHILD NEURO. 13 (1971): 279–303], at 279, *citing* Rickham & Mawdsley, "The Effect of Early Operation on the Survival of Spina Bifida Cystica," *Develop. Med. & Child Neurol.* 20 (Supp. 11, 1966) at 20. He summarizes the results of treating 524 cases of myelomeningocele on an unselected basis: "In summary, at the most 7 per cent of those admitted have less than grossly crippling disabilities and may be considered to have a quality of life not inconsistent with self-respect, earning capacity, happiness and even marriage. The next 20 per cent are also of normal intelligence and some may be able to earn their living in sheltered employment, but their lives are full of illness and operations. They are severely handicapped and are unlikely to live a full life-span. They are at a risk of sudden death from shunt complications or are likely to die of renal failure at an early age. The next 14 per cent are even more severely handicapped because they are retarded. They are unlikely to earn their living and their opportunities in life will be severely restricted. They will always be totally dependent on others." *Id.* at 286. He concludes that "[i]t is unlikely that many would wish to save a life which will consist of a long succession of operations, hospital admissions and other deprivations, or if the end result will be a combination of gross physical defects with retarded intellectual development." *Id.* at 300.

26. Smith & Smith, *Selection for Treatment in Spina Bifida Cystica,* 4 BRIT. MED. J. 189, 195 (1973).

27. *See* Lorber, *supra* note [25], at 284.

28. Ames & Schut, *Results of Treatment of 171 Consecutive Myelomeningoceles—1963 to 1968,* 52 PEDIATRICS 466, 469 (1972); Shurtleff & Foltz, *A Comparative Study of Meningomyelocele Repair or Cerebrospinal Fluid Shunt As Primary Treatment in Ninety Children,* DEVELOP. MED. & CHILD NEURO. 57 (Supp. 13, 1967).

29. *See* E. GOFFMAN, STIGMA: NOTES ON THE MANAGEMENT OF SPOILED IDENTITY 57–129 (1963).

30. *Cf.* Gleitman v. Cosgrove, 49 N.J. 22, 227 A.2d 689 (1967). The court denied plaintiff's right to collect damages for being born with deformities when a defendant physician was allegedly negligent in informing the plaintiff's mother of rubella, which would have led her to seek an abortion. The court stated: "It is basic to the human condition to seek life and hold on to it however heavily burdened. If Jeffrey could have been asked as to whether his life should be snuffed out before his full term of gestation could run its course, our felt intuition of human nature tells us he would almost surely choose life with defects as against no life at all." *Id.* at 30, 227 A.2d at 693.

Similarly, in the case of *In re* Hudson, 13 Wash. 2d. 673, 126 P.2d 765 (1942), a child was held not to be neglected when her parent refused to consent to life-endangering surgery to correct a gross deformity that made normal development and interaction impossible: "As we read the evidence, it is admitted by all concerned that . . . the child may not survive the ordeal of amputation; nevertheless, every one except the child's mother is willing, desirous, that the child be required to undergo the operation. Implicit in their position is their opinion that it would be preferable that the child die instead of going through life handicapped by the enlarged, deformed left arm. That may be to some today the humane, and in the future it may be the generally accepted, view. However, we have not advanced or retrograded to the stage where, in the name of mercy, we may lawfully decide that one shall be deprived of life rather than continue to exist crippled or burdened with some abnormality. That right of decision is a prerogative of the Creator." *Id.* at 684, 126 P.2d at 771. *See also* Cooke, [*Whose Suffering?* J. OF PEDIATRICS 80 (1971)], at 906–08.

31. *See* Lorber, *supra* note [25], at 299.

32. In Lorber's series, 20% of 110 infants "with major adverse criteria at birth were of normal intellectual development at 2–4 years of age, though all [had] severe physical handicaps and their life expectation [was] short." *Id.* at 300. Moreover, other researchers question the adequacy of Lorber's selection criteria. Ames and Schut, for example, in a report on unselected treatment cases of myelomeningocele find "it is not always possible to determine potential at birth," and report success with infants that Lorber would not have selected. *See* Ames & Schut, *supra* note [28], at 469–70.

33. If this judgment is to be made, it is essential that the circumstances in which nontreatment may be said to be in a patient's best interests be specified beforehand by an authoritative body, and that procedures which assure that a particular case falls within such criteria be followed. *See* notes 272–77 and accompanying text [in the original].

34. Matson, *Surgical Treatment of Myelomeningocele,* 42 PEDIATRICS 225, 226 (1968).

35. J. RAWLS, *supra* note [18], at 90–91.

36. *Cf.* Silving, *Euthanasia: A Study in Comparative Criminal Law,* 103, U. PA. L. REV. 350, 356 (1954).

37. *See, e.g.,* J. RAWLS, *supra* note [18], at 22–27.

38. Alexander, *supra* note [5], at 39.

39. The New Jersey Supreme Court, for example, would clearly reject a balancing test in such situations. *See* Gleitman v. Cosgrove, 49 N.J. 22, 227 A.2d 689 (1967).

40. "The experience of learning that your child is defective immediately after birth can still be categorized among the most painful and stigmatizing experiences of modern people. It is as if the parents' raison d'etre were called into question before an imagined parental bar of justice and an ontological blow dealt to their hopes of continuing their identities." Fletcher, [*Attitudes Towards Defective Newborns*, Hastings Center Studies 2 (1974)], at 34.

41. *See* Goodman, [*Continuing Treatment of Parents with Congenitally Defective Infants*, Social Work 9, no. 1, at 92]. *See generally* Kennel & Klaus, *supra* note [21].

42. Bentovim, *Emotional Disturbances of Handicapped Pre-School Children and Their Families—Attitudes to the Child*, 3 Brit. Med. J. 579, 580 (1972); Giannini & Goodman, *Counseling Families During the Crisis Reaction to Mongolism*, 67 Am. J. Mental Deficiency 740, 740–741 (1962); Goodman, *supra* note [41]; Mandelbaum & Wheeler, *The Meaning of A Defective Child to Parents*, 41 Social Casework 360 (1960); Schild, *Counselling with Parents of Retarded Children Living at Home*, 9 Social Work 86 (1964); Zachary, *Ethical and Social Aspects of Treatment of Spina Bifida*, The Lancet, Aug. 3, 1968, at 274–75.

43. *See* note [42], *supra*.

44. *See* Giannini & Goodman, *supra* note [42], at 743.

45. Goodman, *supra* note [41], at 92.

46. *Id.* at 93.

47. *See* Hunt, *Implications of the Treatment of Myelomeningocele for the Child and his Family*, The Lancet, Dec. 8, 1973, at 1308, 1309–10; Zachary, *supra* note [42], at 275.

48. Hunt, *supra* note [47], at 1310.

49. *Id.* at 1309; Bentovim, *supra* note [42], at 581.

50. Zachary, *supra* note [42], at 275.

51. Hunt, *supra* note [47], at 1310.

52. "At each stage there may be a fresh feeling of loss: the precarious balance is once more shattered, rage, depression, rejecting feelings, fear of battering, strain, somatic aches and pains, may be the result. Problems such as financial difficulties, poor housing, marital strain, pressure from siblings can compound such problems. Social life can be severely restricted and the handicapped child then has to cope with the additional handicap of a withdrawn, preoccupied, depressed, angry and hopeless parent, as well as the effect of the handicap itself." Bentovim, *supra* note [42], at 581.

53. *See, e.g.,* Cohen [*The Impact of the Handicapped Child on the Family*, Social Casework 43 (1962): 137]; Giannini & Goodman, *supra* note [42]; Schild, *supra* note [42], at 86.

54. *See* citations in note [53] *supra*.

55. The financial impact of caring for the defective child is difficult to estimate and varies with the seriousness of the defect, the resultant medical costs, health insurance coverage, and state assistance programs. For example, it may cost the parents of a child born with spina bifida from $5,000 to more than $40,000 to pay for the necessary operations, hospital care, medication, doctor's checkups, and braces. Interview with Peggy Miezio, Wis. Spina Bifida Ass'n, Aug. 24, 1974.

Since almost 180 million Americans in 1971 were covered by some form of health insurance, Health Insurance Institute, 1972–73 Source Book of Health Insurance Data 19 (1972), many parents find that insurance covers at least some of the costs. Until recently many policies excluded coverage for disorders commencing before the age of 15 days, and thus did not cover such congenital disorders as spina bifida, Down's syndrome, or cystic fibrosis. *See, e.g.,* Kissil v. Beneficial Nat'l Life Ins., 64 N.J. 555, 319 A.2d 67 (1974). Recently, several states have passed legislation requiring health insurance policies to cover newborn children from the day of birth. *See, e.g.,* Cal. Ins. Code § 10119 (West 1972). In addition, even if the policy lawfully excludes coverage of deformed newborns, indications are that in many cases, because of "social pressures," insurance companies cover newborn infants from the day of birth. Interview with Roy Anderson, Office of Comm'r of Ins. Madison, Wis., Aug. 22, 1974.

In addition to the availability of coverage, two other problems face parents of defective newborns. One is the limits of such coverage. If the medical expenses of the child are high, and the coverage limits of the policy low, parents may have to resort to use of savings or income, or seek state aid. Second, even if a parent were covered by a group policy, the coverage does not transfer if the primary insured leaves the business from which he obtained his policy. Availability of insurance coverage depends on "insurability," and as it is virtually impossible for a family to obtain new coverage for a handicapped child after birth, the families are, in effect, "locked into" their group policy, with a resulting decrease in mobility.

For families with inadequate or no insurance

coverage and who lack the means to absorb high expenditures for care of a deformed newborn, the availability of state assistance becomes crucial. In general, fairly adequate state aid is available to parents who do not wish to institutionalize their child. In California, for example, the state Crippled Children Services offers extensive aid for families with deformed children. When a deformed child requires medical attention that the parents are unable to afford, the parents, hospital, or family doctor may contact the local health department, which will then determine if the child is "medically eligible" for the services of the Crippled Children Department. A diagnostic evaluation of the child's condition is performed and an estimate is made of the cost of care. The Crippled Children Services then determines if the family is financially eligible for aid. An allowable income level is set according to several factors, and below a certain level (presently $6,300 for a family of four), all expenses are paid by the state. Above this level, the families pay an amount not greater than one-half of the difference between their income and the cost-of-living allowance level. Hospital expenses, medication, braces, nursing care–all the needs of the deformed child–are provided, and the only limit on aid is the agency's budget. Telephone interview with Darleen Gibben, State Crippled Children Services, Sacramento, Cal., Aug. 22, 1974.

For retarded children without serious physical defects, state aid, whether the child is institutionalized or not, is available depending on parental income. Telephone interview with Robert Baldo, Regional Center for Developmentally Disabled, Sacramento, Cal., Aug. 22, 1974.

Similar systems of aid for both physical and mental handicaps, and special education needs, are available in Illinois, Telephone interview with Dr. Graham Blanton, Director of Developmental Disabilities, Dep't of Mental Health and Developmental Disabilities, Springfield, Ill., Aug. 22, 1974; and in Wisconsin, Telephone interview with Elie Asleson, Bureau of Handicapped Children, Dep't of Health and Social Services, Madison, Wis., Aug. 27, 1974; and presumably in other states, since much of the state budget for these services is federally funded.

Although the data is too incomplete to conclude that care of a defective newborn will never severely drain a family's financial resources, it seems clear that the impact can be cushioned or minimized by institutionalization of the child, health insurance, or state aid. Obviously, if legislative policy remains committed to the value of life, a strong argument may be made that the taxpayers as a whole rather than individual families or insurance holders should bear the cost of care.

I am indebted to Marsha Peckham for clarification of the financial issues involved in the care of the defective newborn.

56. *See* note [55] *supra.*

57. Moreover, parental rights and obligations can be terminated. *See* note 37 [in the original].

58. *Quoted in* Johns, *Family Reactions to the Birth of a Child with a Congenital Abnormality,* 26 Obstet. & Gynecol. Survey 635, 637 (1971).

59. Since parents and physicians now view treatment and acceptance of a defective child as discretionary with the parents, acceptance may be viewed as a gift on the part of the parents to the child. Because of the child's defects, however, the debt or obligation owed to the donor by the recipient of a gift cannot be repaid, and few substitutions for that debt seem available. Given the frequency with which families donate organs to ailing members, it may be that the defective infant situation is not structured to maximize the chance of parental giftgiving. *See* R. Fox & J. Swayze, The Courage To Fail: A Social View of Organ Transplants and Dialysis 20–27 (1974).

60. Kennel & Klaus, *supra* note [21], at 946. This is particularly true if a physician identifies with the family and its values. "The physician may feel a sense of having failed the family with whom he has a relationship—and his own emotions and feelings come into play—seemingly to a greater extent than with lower class families. His recommendations may be influenced unconsciously by his discomfort with the situation and his strong desire to 'save' the family." Giannini & Goodman, *supra* note [42], at 744.

61. Cohen, *supra* note [53], at 138.

62. Author's observations at conference concerning treatment of a defective newborn at St. Mary's Hospital, Madison, Wis., Apr. 15, 1974.

63. "It may be true that further advances should improve the outlook for many, but unfortunately the basic defect is usually so severe that the children will always be severely handicapped in spite of any advances which can be foreseen today. Meanwhile it may be best to concentrate our therapeutic efforts on those who can truly benefit from treatment. If all the most severe cases are treated, the pressure of work will be such that adequate time cannot be devoted to the less severely affected who would benefit most." Lorber, *supra* note [25], at 300.

64. For example, the resources instead might be used to

increase physicians' salaries or the profits of drug or medical supply industries.

65. Resources presently consumed in the care of the defective may have been appropriated for that purpose only, and if not so utilized, will be withdrawn.

66. For instance, amniocentesis carried out on pregnant women over 35—the most risky age for Down's syndrome—should reduce the incidence of mongolism and the attendant problems of care. *Cf.* Smith, *On Letting Some Babies Die,* HASTINGS CENTER STUDIES, Vol. 2, No. 2, at 37, 45 (1974).

67. *See* Ames & Schut, *supra* note [28], at 467–70, which emphasizes the counseling and shunting of spina bifida babies rather than more elaborate and expensive intervention. *See also* C. FRIED, [AN ANATOMY OF VALUES (1970)], at 200–06.

68. Mechanic, *Problems in the Future Organization of Medical Practice*, 35 LAW & CONTEMP. PROB. 233, 234 (1970).

69. Memorial Hosp. v. Maricopa County, 415 U.S. 250 (1974).

70. *See* note [32] *supra* and accompanying text.

71. Moreover, although the case is unlikely to arise in medically developed nations, imagine, for example, that two myelomeningocele infants both need a shunt, orthopedic surgery, and other services, but resources are so limited that either complete care can be given to one and custodial care to the other, or both can be given only minimal care. Complete care for Baby *A* would lead to ambulation and normal intelligence, while complete care for Baby *B* would still leave him severely retarded and nonambulatory. Minimal care for both would leave both nonambulatory and retarded. Or suppose that resources would permit only one surgical procedure to correct duodenal atresia, but both a Down's syndrome and a normal baby need the operation. In either situation one may argue that physicians should be able to allocate scarce medical resources on the basis of their perception of which allocation will produce the most "good." Presumably, an outcome where the normal infant survives would be chosen. However, one may question whether, in situations of scarcity, distributive justice is satisfied by anything but a random or a first-come-first-served allocation, or an allocation system indifferent to the personal characteristics of each infant. To allocate health resources on the basis of prospective quality of life or social utility would raise in all but a few extreme cases the difficult task of (1) determining and measuring quality, and (2) specifying criteria for a nonarbitrary conclusion that quality X is better than quality Y. As David Smith observes: "Such an approach leads one to think that the ideal result is either a 'perfect' baby or a dead baby. And the root problems of this way of looking at the issue are that both the human rights of defectives and the imperfection of all babies are glossed over." Smith, *supra* note [66], at 46 (footnote omitted).

Thus, one may argue that even here qualitative or utilitarian judgments are out of place, for these depend on nonobjective, culturally relative standards of quality. The lot of some is improved by making others worse off, yet the reasons for preferring one group are not compelling on nonarbitrary grounds. Unless one were willing to accept the principle that medical decisionmakers may opt to maximize social utility when limited resources require a selection among patients, then the defective newborn could not be denied treatment because of his defects alone. Fortunately, this dilemma, which arose frequently when hemodialysis resources were in short supply, does not yet seem to have arisen in the case of defective newborns. *See* C. FRIED, *supra* note [67], at 200–06; Katz, *Process Design for Selection of Hemodialysis and Organ Transplant Recipients*, 22 BUFF. L. REV. 373 (1973).

Ethical Issues in Aiding the Death of Young Children

H. Tristram Engelhardt, Jr.

Euthanasia in the pediatric age group involves a constellation of issues that are materially different from those of adult euthanasia.[1] The difference lies in the somewhat obvious fact that infants and young children are not able to decide about their own futures and thus are not persons in the same sense that normal adults are. While adults usually decide their own fate, others decide on behalf of young children. Although one can argue that euthanasia is or should be a personal right, the sense of such an argument is obscure with respect to children. Young children do not have any personal rights, at least none that they can exercise on their own behalf with regard to the manner of their life and death. As a result, euthanasia of young children raises special questions concerning the standing of the rights of children, the status of parental rights, the obligations of adults to prevent the suffering of children, and the possible effects on society of allowing or expediting the death of seriously defective infants.

What I will refer to as the euthanasia of infants and young children might be termed by others infanticide, while some cases might be termed the withholding of extraordinary life-prolonging treatment.[2] One needs a term that will encompass both death that results from active intervention and death that ensues when one simply ceases further therapy.[3] In using such a term, one must recognize that death is often not directly but only obliquely intended. That is, one often intends only to treat no further, not actually to have death follow, even though one knows death will follow.[4]

Finally, one must realize that deaths as the result of withholding treatment constitute a significant proportion of neonatal deaths. For example, as high as 14 percent of children in one hospital have been identified as dying after a decision was made not to treat further, the presumption being that the children would have lived longer had treatment been offered.[5]

Even popular magazines have presented accounts of parental decisions not to pursue treatment.[6] These decisions often involve a choice between expensive treatment with little chance of achieving a full, normal life for the child and "letting nature take its course,"[7] with the child dying as a result of its defects. As this suggests, many of these problems are products of medical progress. Such children in the past would have died. The quandaries are in a sense an embarrassment of riches; now that one *can* treat such defective children, *must* one treat them? And, if one need not treat such defective children, may one expedite their death?

I will here briefly examine some of these issues. First, I will review differences that contrast the euthanasia of adults to euthanasia of children. Second, I will review the issue of the rights of parents and the status of children. Third, I will suggest a new notion, the concept of the "injury of continued existence," and draw out some of its implications with respect to a duty to prevent suffering. Finally, I will outline some important questions that remain unanswered even if the foregoing issues can be settled. In all, I hope more to display the issues involved in a difficult question than to advance a particular set of answers to particular dilemmas.

For the purpose of this paper, I will presume that adult euthanasia can be justified by an appeal to freedom. In the face of imminent death, one is usually choosing between a more painful and more protracted dying and a less painful or less protracted dying, in circumstances where either choice makes little difference with regard to the discharge of social duties and responsibilities. In the case of suicide, we might argue that, in general, social duties (for example, the duty to support one's family) restrain one from taking one's own life. But in the face of imminent death and in the presence of the pain and deterioration

This article first appeared in the book Beneficient Euthanasia, *edited by Marvin Kohl, published by* Prometheus Books, Buffalo, N.Y., 1975, and is reprinted by permission.

of a fatal disease, such duties are usually impossible to discharge and are thus rendered moot. One can, for example, picture an extreme case of an adult with a widely disseminated carcinoma, including metastases to the brain, who because of severe pain and debilitation is no longer capable of discharging any social duties. In these and similar circumstances, euthanasia becomes the issue of the right to control one's own body, even to the point of seeking assistance in suicide. Euthanasia is, as such, the issue of assisted suicide, the universalization of a maxim that all persons should be free, *in extremis*, to decide with regard to the circumstances of their death.

Further, the choice of positive euthanasia could be defended as the more rational choice: the choice of a less painful death and the affirmation of the value of a rational life. In so choosing, one would be acting to set limits to one's life in order not to live when pain and physical and mental deterioration make further rational life impossible. The choice to end one's life can be understood as a noncontradictory willing of a smaller set of states of existence for oneself, a set that would not include a painful death. As such, it would not involve a desire to destroy oneself. That is, adult euthanasia can be construed as an affirmation of the rationality and autonomy of the self.[7]

The remarks above focus on the active or positive euthanasia of adults. But they hold as well concerning what is often called passive or negative euthanasia, the refusal of life-prolonging therapy. In such cases, the patient's refusal of life-prolonging therapy is seen to be a right that derives from personal freedom, or at least from a zone of privacy into which there are no good grounds for social intervention.[8]

Again, none of these considerations apply directly to the euthanasia of young children, because they cannot participate in such decisions. Whatever else pediatric, in particular neonatal, euthanasia involves, it surely involves issues different from those of adult euthanasia. Since infants and small children cannot commit suicide, their right to assisted suicide is difficult to pose. The difference between the euthanasia of young children and that of adults resides in the difference between children and adults. The difference, in fact, raises the troublesome question of whether young children are persons, or at least whether

they are persons in the sense in which adults are. Answering that question will resolve in part at least the right of others to decide whether a young child should live or die and whether he should receive life-prolonging treatment.

The Status of Children

Adults belong to themselves in the sense that they are rational and free and therefore responsible for their actions. Adults are *sui juris*. Young children, though, are neither self-possessed nor responsible. While adults exist in and for themselves, as self-directive and self-conscious beings, young children, especially newborn infants, exist for their families and those who love them. They are not, nor can they in any sense be, responsible for themselves. If being a person is to be a responsible agent, a bearer of rights and duties, children are not persons in a strict sense. They are, rather, persons in a social sense: others must act on their behalf and bear responsibility for them. They are, as it were, entities defined by their place in social roles (for example, mother-child, family-child) rather than beings that define themselves as persons, that is, in and through themselves. Young children live as persons in and through the care of those who are responsible for them, and those responsible for them exercise the children's rights on their behalf. In this sense children belong to families in ways that most adults do not. They exist in and through their family and society.

Treating young children with respect has, then, a sense different from treating adults with respect. One can respect neither a newborn infant's or very young child's wishes nor its freedom. In fact, a newborn infant or young child is more an entity that is valued highly because it will grow to be a person and because it plays a social role as if it were a person.[9] That is, a small child is treated as if it were a person in social roles such as mother-child and family-child relationships, though strictly speaking the child is in no way capable of claiming or being responsible for the rights imputed to it. All the rights and duties of the child are exercised and "held in trust" by others for a future time and for a person yet to develop.

Medical decisions to treat or not to treat a

neonate or small child often turn on the probability and cost of achieving that future status—a developed personal life. The usual practice of letting anencephalic children (who congenitally lack all or most of the brain) die can be understood as a decision based on the absence of the possibility of achieving a personal life. The practice of refusing treatment to at least some children born with meningomyelocele can be justified through a similar, but more utilitarian, calculus. In the case of anencephalic children one might argue that care for them as persons is futile since they will never be persons. In the case of a child with meningomyelocele, one might argue that when the cost of cure would likely be very high and the probable lifestyle open to attainment very truncated, there is not a positive duty to make a large investment of money and suffering. One should note that the cost here must include not only financial costs but also the anxiety and suffering that prolonged and uncertain treatment of the child would cause the parents.

This further raises the issue of the scope of positive duties not only when there is no person present in a strict sense, but when the likelihood of a full human life is also very uncertain. Clinical and parental judgment may and should be guided by the expected lifestyle and the cost (in parental and societal pain and money) of its attainment. The decision about treatment, however, belongs properly to the parents because the child belongs to them in a sense that it does not belong to anyone else, even to itself. The care and raising of the child falls to the parents, and when considerable cost and little prospect of reasonable success are present, the parents may properly decide against life-prolonging treatment.

The physician's role is to present sufficient information in a usable form to the parents to aid them in making a decision. The accent is on the absence of a positive duty to treat in the presence of severe inconvenience (costs) to the parents; treatment that is very costly is not obligatory. What is suggested here is a general notion that there is never a duty to engage in extraordinary treatment and that "extraordinary" can be defined in terms of costs. This argument concerns children (1) whose future quality of life is likely to be seriously compromised and (2) whose present treatment would be very costly. The issue is that of

the circumstances under which parents would not be obliged to take on severe burdens on behalf of their children or those circumstances under which society would not be so obliged. The argument should hold as well for those cases where the expected future life would surely be of normal quality, though its attainment would be extremely costly. The fact of little likelihood of success in attaining a normal life for the child makes decisions to do without treatment more plausible because the hope of success is even more remote and therefore the burden borne by parents or society becomes in that sense more extraordinary. But very high costs themselves could be a sufficient criterion, though in actual cases judgments in that regard would be very difficult when a normal life could be expected.[10]

The decisions in these matters correctly lie in the hands of the parents, because it is primarily in terms of the family that children exist and develop—until children become persons strictly, they are persons in virtue of their social roles. As long as parents do not unjustifiably neglect the humans in those roles so that the value and purpose of that role (that is, child) stands to be eroded (thus endangering other children), society need not intervene. In short, parents may decide for or against the treatment of their severely deformed children.

However, society has a right to intervene and protect children for whom parents refuse care (including treatment) when such care does not constitute a severe burden and when it is likely that the child could be brought to a good quality of life. Obviously, "severe burden" and "good quality of life" will be difficult to define and their meanings will vary, just as it is always difficult to say when grains of sand dropped on a table constitute a heap. At most, though, society need only intervene when the grains clearly do not constitute a heap, that is, when it is clear that the burden is light and the chance of a good quality of life for the child is high. A small child's dependence on his parents is so essential that society need intervene only when the absence of intervention would lead to the role "child" being undermined. Society must value mother-child and family-child relationships and should intervene only in cases where (1) neglect is unreasonable and therefore would undermine respect and care for children, or (2) where societal intervention would prevent children from suffering unnecessary pain.[11]

The Injury of Continued Existence

But there is another viewpoint that must be considered: that of the child or even the person that the child might become. It might be argued that the child has a right not to have its life prolonged. The idea that forcing existence on a child could be wrong is a difficult notion, which, if true, would serve to amplify the foregoing argument. Such an argument would allow the construal of the issue in terms of the perspective of the child, that is, in terms of a duty not to treat in circumstances where treatment would only prolong suffering. In particular, it would at least give a framework for a decision to stop treatment in cases where, though the costs of treatment are not high, the child's existence would be characterized by severe pain and deprivation.

A basis for speaking of continuing existence as an injury to the child is suggested by the proposed legal concept of "wrongful life." A number of suits have been initiated in the United States and in other countries on the grounds that life or existence itself is, under certain circumstances, a tort or injury to the living person.[12] Although thus far all such suits have ultimately failed, some have succeeded in their initial stages. Two examples may be instructive. In each case the ability to receive recompense for the injury (the tort) presupposed the existence of the individual, whose existence was itself the injury. In one case a suit was initiated on behalf of a child against his father alleging that his father's siring him out of wedlock was an injury to the child.[13] In another case a suit on behalf of a child born of an inmate of a state mental hospital impregnated by rape in that institution was brought against the state of New York.[14] The suit was brought on the grounds that being born with such historical antecedents was itself an injury for which recovery was due. Both cases presupposed that nonexistence would have been preferable to the conditions under which the person born was forced to live.

The suits for tort for wrongful life raise the issue not only of when it would be preferable not to have been born but also of when it would be *wrong* to cause a person to be born. This implies that someone should have judged that it would have been preferable for the child never to have had existence, never to have been in the position to judge that the particular circumstances of life were intolerable.[15] Further, it implies that the person's existence under those circumstances should have been prevented and that, not having been prevented, life was not a gift but an injury. The concept of tort for wrongful life raises an issue concerning the responsibility for giving another person existence, namely, the notion that giving life is not always necessarily a good and justifiable action. Instead, in certain circumstances, so it has been argued, one may have a duty *not* to give existence to another person. This concept involves the claim that certain qualities of life have a negative value, making life an injury, not a gift; it involves, in short, a concept of human accountability and responsibility for human life. It contrasts with the notion that life is a gift of God and thus similar to other "acts of God" (that is, events for which no man is accountable). The concept thus signals the fact that humans can now control reproduction and that where rational control is possible humans are accountable. That is, the expansion of human capabilities has resulted in an expansion of human responsibilities such that one must now decide when and under what circumstances persons will come into existence.

The concept of tort for wrongful life is transferable in part to the painfully compromised existence of children who can only have their life prolonged for a short, painful, and marginal existence. The concept suggests that allowing life to be prolonged under such circumstances would itself be an injury of the person whose painful and severely compromised existence would be made to continue. In fact, it suggests that there is a duty not to prolong life if it can be determined to have a substantial negative value for the person involved.[16] Such issues are moot in the case of adults, who can and should decide for themselves. But small children cannot make such a choice. For them it is an issue of justifying prolonging life under circumstances of painful and compromised existence. Or, put differently, such cases indicate the need to develop social canons to allow a decent death for children for whom the only possibility is protracted, painful suffering.

I do not mean to imply that one should develop a new basis for civil damages. In the field of medicine, the need is to recognize an ethical category, a concept of wrongful continuance of existence, not a new legal right. The concept of injury for continuance of existence, the proposed analogue of the concept of tort for wrongful life, presupposes that life can be of a negative value such that the medical maxim *primum non nocere* ("first do no harm") would require not sustaining life.[17]

The idea of responsibility for acts that sustain or prolong life is cardinal to the notion that one should not under certain circumstances further prolong the life of a child. Unlike adults, children cannot decide with regard to euthanasia (positive or negative), and if more than a utilitarian justification is sought, it must be sought in a duty not to inflict life on another person in circumstances where that life would be painful and futile. This position must rest on the facts that (1) medicine now can cause the prolongation of the life of seriously deformed children who in the past would have died young and that (2) it is not clear that life so prolonged is a good for the child. Further, the choice is made not on the basis of costs to the parents or to society but on the basis of the child's suffering and compromised existence.

The difficulty lies in determining what makes life not worth living for a child. Answers could never be clear. It seems reasonable, however, that the life of children with diseases that involve pain and no hope of survival should not be prolonged. In the case of Tay-Sachs disease (a disease marked by a progressive increase in spasticity and dementia usually leading to death at age three or four), one can hardly imagine that the terminal stages of spastic reaction to stimuli and great difficulty in swallowing are at all pleasant to the child (even insofar as it can only minimally perceive its circumstances). If such a child develops aspiration pneumonia and is treated, it can reasonably be said that to prolong its life is to inflict suffering. Other diseases give fairly clear portraits of lives not worth living: for example, Lesch-Nyhan disease, which is marked by mental retardation and compulsive self-mutilation.

The issue is more difficult in the case of children with diseases for whom the prospects for normal intelligence and a fair lifestyle do exist, but where these chances are remote and their realization expensive. Children born with meningomyelocele present this dilemma. Imagine, for example, a child that falls within Lorber's fifth category (an IQ of sixty or less, sometimes blind, subject to fits, and always incontinent). Such a child has little prospect of anything approaching a normal life, and there is a good chance of its dying even with treatment.[18] But such judgments are statistical. And if one does not treat such children, some will still survive and, as John Freeman indicates, be worse off if not treated.[19] In such cases one is in a dilemma. If one always treats, one must justify extending the life of those who will ultimately die anyway and in the process subjecting them to the morbidity of multiple surgical procedures. How remote does the prospect of a good life have to be in order not to be worth great pain and expense?[20] It is probably best to decide, in the absence of a positive duty to treat, on the basis of the cost and suffering to parents and society. But, as Freeman argues, the prospect of prolonged or even increased suffering raises the issue of active euthanasia.[21]

If the child is not a person strictly, and if death is inevitable and expediting it would diminish the child's pain prior to death, then it would seem to follow that, all else being equal, a decision for active euthanasia would be permissible, even obligatory.[22] The difficulty lies with "all else being equal," for it is doubtful that active euthanasia could be established as a practice without eroding and endangering children generally, since, as John Lorber has pointed out, children cannot speak in their own behalf.[23] Thus, although there is no argument in principle against the active euthanasia of small children, there could be an argument against such practices based on questions of prudence. To put it another way, even though one might have a duty to hasten the death of a particular child, one's duty to protect children in general could override that first duty. The issue of active euthanasia turns in the end on whether it would have social consequences that refraining would not, on whether (1) it is possible to establish procedural safeguards for limited active euthanasia and (2) whether such practices would have a significant adverse effect on the treatment of small children in general. But since these are procedural issues dependent on sociological facts, they are not open to an answer within the confines of this article. In any event, the concept of the injury of continued existence provides a basis for the justification of the passive euthanasia of small children—a practice already widespread and somewhat established in our society—beyond the mere absence of a positive duty to treat.[24]

Conclusion

Though the lack of certainty concerning questions such as the prognosis of particular patients and the social consequence of active euthanasia of children prevents a clear answer to all the issues raised by the euthanasia of infants, it would seem that this much can be maintained: (1) Since children are not persons strictly but exist in and through their families, parents are the appropriate ones to decide whether or not to treat a deformed child when (a) there is not only little likelihood of full human life but also great likelihood of suffering if the life is prolonged, or (b) when the cost of prolonging life is very great. Such decisions must be made in consort with a physician who can accurately give estimates of cost and prognosis and who will be able to help the parents with the consequences of their decision. (2) It is reasonable to speak of a duty not to treat a small child when such treatment will only prolong a painful life or would in any event lead to a painful death. Though this does not by any means answer all the questions, it does point out an important fact—that medicine's duty is not always to prolong life doggedly but sometimes is quite the contrary.

Notes

1. I am grateful to Laurence B. McCullough and James P. Morris for their critical discussion of this paper. They may be responsible for its virtues, but not for its shortcomings.

2. The concept of extraordinary treatment as it has been developed in Catholic moral theology is useful: treatment is extraordinary and therefore not obligatory if it involves great costs, pain, or inconvenience, and is a grave burden to oneself or others without a reasonable expectation that such treatment would be successful. See Gerald Kelly, S. J., *Medico-Moral Problems* (St. Louis: The Catholic Hospital Association Press, 1958), pp. 128–141. Difficulties are hidden in terms such as "great costs" and "reasonable expectation," as well as in terms such as "successful." Such ambiguity reflects the fact that precise operational definitions are not available. That is, the precise meaning of "great," "reasonable," and "successful" are inextricably bound to particular circumstances, especially particular societies.

3. I will use the term euthanasia in a broad sense to indicate a deliberately chosen course of action or inaction that is known at the time of decision to be such as will expedite death. This use of euthanasia will encompass not only positive or active euthanasia (acting in order to expedite death) and negative or passive euthanasia (refraining from action in order to expedite death), but acting and refraining in the absence of a direct intention that death occur more quickly (that is, those cases that fall under the concept of double effect). See note 4.

4. But both active and passive euthanasia can be appreciated in terms of the Catholic moral notion of double effect. When the doctrine of double effect is invoked, one is strictly not intending euthanasia, but rather one intends something else. That concept allows actions or omissions that lead to death (1) because it is licit not to prolong life *in extremis* (allowing death is not an intrinsic evil), (2) if death is not actually willed or actively sought (that is, the evil is not directly willed), (3) if that which is willed is a major good (for example, avoiding useless major expenditure of resources or serious pain), and (4) if the good is not achieved by means of the evil (for example, one does not will to save resources or diminish pain *by* the death). With regard to euthanasia the doctrine of double effect means that one need not expend major resources in an endeavor that will not bring health but only prolong dying and that one may use drugs that decrease pain but hasten death. See Richard McCormick, *Ambiguity in Moral Choice* (Milwaukee: Marquette University Press, 1973). I exclude the issue of double effect from my discussion because I am interested in those cases in which the good may follow directly from the evil—the death of the child. In part, though, the second section of this paper is concerned with the concept of proportionate good.

5. Raymond S. Duff and A. G. M. Campbell, "Moral and Ethical Dilemmas in the Special-Care Nursery," *The New England Journal of Medicine,* 289 (Oct. 25, 1973), pp. 890–894.

6. Roger Pell, "The Agonizing Decision of Joanne and Roger Pell," *Good Housekeeping* (January 1972), pp. 76–77, 131–135.

7. This somewhat Kantian argument is obviously made in opposition to Kant's position that suicide involves a default of one's duty to oneself ". . . to preserve his life simply because he is a person and must therefore recognize a duty to himself (and a strict one at that)," as well as a contradictory volition: "that man ought to have the authorization to withdraw himself from all obligation, that is, to be free to act as if no authorization at all were required for this withdrawal, involves a contradiction. To destroy the subject of morality in his own person is tantamount to obliterating from the world . . ." Immanuel Kant, *The Metaphysical Principles of Virtue: Part II of the Metaphysics of Morals*, trans. James Ellington (Indianapolis: Bobbs-Merrill, 1964), p. 83; Akademie Edition, VI, 422–423.

8. Norman L. Cantor, "A Patient's Decision to Decline Life-Saving Medical Treatment: Bodily Integrity Versus the Preservation of Life," *Rutgers Law Review*, 26 (Winter 1972), p. 239.

9. By "young child" I mean either an infant or child so young as not yet to be able to participate, in any sense, in a decision. A precise operational definition of "young child" would clearly be difficult to develop. It is also not clear how one would bring older children into such decisions. See, for example, Milton Viederman, "Saying 'No' to Hemodialysis: Exploring Adaptation," and Daniel Burke, "Saying 'No' to Hemodialysis: An Acceptable Decision," both in *The Hastings Center Report*, 4 (September 1974), pp. 8–10, and John E. Schowalter, Julian B. Ferholt, and Nancy M. Mann, "The Adolescent Patient's Decision To Die," *Pediatrics*, 51 (January 1973), pp. 97–103.

10. An appeal to high costs alone is probably hidden in judgments based on statistics: even though there is a chance for a normal life for certain children with apparently severe cases of meningomyelocele, one is not obliged to treat since that chance is small, and the pursuit of that chance is very expensive. Cases of the costs being low but the expected suffering of the child being high will be discussed under the concept of the injury of continued existence. It should be noted that none of the arguments in this paper bear on cases where neither the cost nor the suffering of the child is considerable. Cases in this last category probably include, for example, children born with mongolism complicated only by duodenal atresia.

11. I have in mind here the issue of physicians, hospital administrators, or others being morally compelled to seek an injunction to force treatment of the child in the absence of parental consent. In these circumstances, the physician, who is usually best acquainted with the facts of the case, is the natural advocate of the child.

12. G. Tedeschi, "On Tort Liability for 'Wrongful Life,' " *Israel Law Review*, 1 (1966), p. 513.

13. Zepeda v. Zepeda: 41 Ill. App. 2d 240, 190 N.E. 2d 849 (1963).

14. Williams v. State of New York: 46 Misc. 2d 824, 260 N.Y.S. 2d 953 (Ct. Cl., 1965).

15. Torts: "Illegitimate Child Denied Recovery Against Father for 'Wrongful Life,' " *Iowa Law Review*, 49 (1969), p. 1009.

16. It is one thing to have a conceptual definition of the injury of continued existence (for example, causing a person to continue to live under circumstances of severe pain and deprivation when there are no alternatives but death) and another to have an operational definition of that concept (that is, deciding what counts as such severe pain and deprivation). This article has focused on the first, not the second, issue.

17. H. Tristram Engelhardt, Jr., "Euthanasia and Children: The Injury of Continued Existence," *The Journal of Pediatrics*, 83 (July 1973), pp. 170–171.

18. John Lorber, "Results of Treatment of Myelomeningocele," *Developmental Medicine and Child Neurology*, 13 (1971), p. 286.

19. John M. Freeman, "The Shortsighted Treatment of Myelomeningocele: A Long-Term Case Report," *Pediatrics*, 53 (March 1974), pp. 311–313.

20. John M. Freeman, "To Treat or Not To Treat," *Practical Management of Meningomyelocele*, ed. John Freeman (Baltimore: University Park Press, 1974), p. 21.

21. John Lorber, "Selective Treatment of Myelomeningocele: To Treat or Not To Treat," *Pediatrics*, 53 (March 1974), pp. 307–308.

22. I am presupposing that no intrinsic moral distinctions exist in cases such as these, between acting and refraining, between omitting care in the hope that death will ensue (that is, rather than the child living to be even more defective) and acting to ensure that death will ensue rather than having the child live under painful and seriously compromised circumstances. For a good discussion of the distinction between acting and refraining, see Jonathan Bennett, "Whatever the Consequences," *Analysis*, 26 (January 1966), pp. 83–102; P. J. Fitzgerald, "Acting and Refraining," *Analysis*, 27 (March 1967), pp. 133–139; Daniel Dinello, "On Killing and Letting Die," *Analysis*, 31 (April 1971), pp. 83–86.

23. Lorber, "Selective Treatment of Myelomeningocele," p. 308.

24. Positive duties involve a greater constraint than negative duties. Hence it is often easier to establish a duty not to do something (not to treat further) than a duty to do something (to actively hasten death). Even allowing a new practice to be permitted (for example, active euthanasia) requires a greater attention to consequences than does establishing the absence of a positive duty. For example, at common law there is no basis for action against a person who watches another drown without giving aid; this reflects the difficulty of establishing a positive duty.

Toward an Ethic of Ambiguity

John D. Arras

The Best Interests of the Child

How are we to show equal concern and respect for gravely impaired newborns? Are there any differences between otherwise normal children and certain gravely impaired babies that might justify allowing the latter to die through the intentional withholding of medical treatments?

One important and plausible candidate for a morally relevant distinction between normal and certain anomalous newborns resides in the notion of their respective "best interests."[1] Continued life is obviously in the interests of the normal child, but what of the child impaired by profound brain damage, whose days will be measured by operations and whose pain will be unrelieved by the communication of human sympathy? Would it not be in this child's best interests to die, rather than endure a life of meaningless suffering? And if so, would that not provide us with a morally relevant distinction?

The case for allowing the deaths of anomalous newborns on the ground of their "best interests" is by far the most compelling argument for infant euthanasia. By focusing on *the child's* interests, this standard avoids morally dubious utilitarian justifications based on the well-being of other interested parties, such as parents, siblings, or even of society at large. And by giving *full weight* to the child's interests, this approach can justify nontreatment in certain cases without having to make the (usually pernicious) assumption that the child is a nonperson with no standing in the human community. Despite these advantages, however, the best-interest standard presents staggering problems of interpretation and application.

A Preliminary Objection

Before coming to these problems, we must confront a direct challenge to the legitimacy of the best-interest standard itself. Certain theologians and jurists who oppose any resort to "quality-of-life" judgments on behalf of voiceless patients have argued that the best-interest standard forces us to make an impossible comparison. Although we can and should compare better life against worse life, they argue, we cannot compare the advantages of life, even with severe disabilities, against the state of nonbeing initiated by death. Since all our everyday evaluations take place against the backdrop of the assumed value of life, it is said, we cannot make the comparison of life against nonlife demanded by the best-interest standard without foundering on conceptual incoherence.[2]

While this is not the occasion to launch a lengthy metaphysical explanation of how a state of nonexistence might be "preferable" to certain states of existence—how can someone be better off dead?—two points can be made in response to those who claim that death can *never* be in the best interests of a nondying child. First, we can concede that a belief in the desirability of life grounds our everyday judgments of "better" and "worse," while still maintaining that the moral choices posed by the plight of the impaired newborn are

Reproduced by permission. © The Hastings Center. Hastings Center Report, 14 (April 1984): 25–33.
Editor's Note: This is a shortened version of the original article, and the footnotes have been renumbered.

anything but ordinary. Although we usually profess an implicit faith in the conceptual connection between our notions of "life" and "good," the profoundly anomalous and severely brain-damaged child shatters this everyday faith and severs the assumed connection.

In such cases, it is not at all obvious that mere life remains a good to the afflicted person; rather, it seems as though the child's illness has eclipsed the possibility of enjoying those normal human goods that ordinarily predispose us to say that life is good.[3] Moreover, while the existence of severe disabilities threatens to sever our everyday connection between "life" and "good," another item of everyday faith remains unshaken: We continue to believe that pain and suffering are evil, and that beneficence largely consists in abolishing, or at least ameliorating, these twin scourges of humankind. If an act of mercy killing were to deliver a child from a life of unmitigated pain—if only to a state of nonexistence rather than beatitude—it would take a profoundly dogmatic temperament to deny that death was in the child's best interest. Opponents of infant euthanasia could perhaps find other reasons to oppose such an act—for example, the belief that humans have no right to dispose of their own or anyone else's life—but merely on the grounds of individual well-being, there is no denying that death would be better than a life of intense and constant pain.

Second, if it were impossible for us to detach ourselves from our everyday grounding in the belief that life is good, if we could not wish someone else dead for his or her own sake, then the same difficulty would attach to first-person judgments as well. If it were in principle impossible to say that death would serve the best interests of any child, then it would be equally impossible for any rational adult to conclude that, given a bleak prognosis and the prospect of burdensome treatments, he or she would be better off dead. I doubt that the more thoughtful opponents of euthanasia would wish to embrace such a result. Even conservative theologians such as Paul Ramsey restrict their rejection of quality-of-life reasoning—and hence their rejection of "excessive burdensomeness" as a test of extraordinary means—to the class of voiceless patients who have not developed a value system that would allow them to assess the quality of future life for themselves.[4]

Ramsey explicitly grants to the competent adult the right to refuse treatments that would render continued life a burden. In order to assume this stance, he must admit the possibility that death would be in the best interest of certain persons, but this admission pulls the rug out from under the claim that, in principle, we cannot judge death to be in a child's best interest. The most that can be said is that no one has the right to make such judgments, or that allowing adults to make them for children will result in mistaken choices or downright abuse. We cannot say that, in principle, life (even with crushing impairments and constant pain) cannot even be compared with death. At best, such a denial is an unfortunate overstatement; at worst, it could be placed in the service of an overbearing medical paternalism. Indeed, what better way to thwart the choices of mature adults than to deny them the very capacity rationally to choose between an earlier death without treatment and a life of suffering with treatment?

In sum, we can say that death is not always and everywhere the greatest evil that could befall a person. Afflictions of the body and mind might conspire to render continued life a burden for certain individuals, for whom death might be viewed as a benefit—or at least as the lesser of two evils. As the President's Commission recently concluded, the best interests of the child—rather than a spurious nondiscrimination principle—should be our guide. Normally, of course, treatment will clearly be in a child's best interest. But the Commission granted the possibility that some permanent handicaps might be "so severe that continued existence would not be a net benefit to the infant."[5] Our next problem, then, is to determine with more precision how a best-interest standard might be applied and to discuss some weighty problems of interpretation.

Prognostic Uncertainty

One problem will plague efforts to implement any proposed criterion of nontreatment: medical and prognostic uncertainty.[6] Decisions must often be made regarding life or death in the absence of reliable data regarding a particular child's future life prospects. No matter where we draw the line separating "meaningful" from "excessively burdensome" life, we will often have to decide under conditions of great uncertainty. The spectrum of neonatal disabilities is very wide, as is the spectrum of disability *within* particular disease categories. The mere presence of Down's syndrome or of spina bifida does not by itself indicate how disabled a child will be. Some Down's children are profoundly retarded, while others turn out to be sufficiently intelligent to live at home with their families or in group homes and eventually to work productively in a sheltered setting. The problem is that, except for a few classes of disease, physicians cannot accurately predict the degree of a child's eventual impairment. This problem is compounded by our ability to diminish a child's eventual degree of disability by some means of vigorous medical and educational interventions. In the absence of reliable prognostic indicators of future quality of life, the rationality of nontreatment decisions for defective neonates is bound to be diminished. Any medical ethic that places a great value on human life must look with suspicion upon nontreatment decisions taken in the absence of reliable medical information.

While medical uncertainty threatens to undermine the application of *any* set of criteria for nontreatment based on quality of life, the best-interest standard is subject to further difficulties of interpretation. It may well turn out that, all things considered, death may serve the best interests of a severely afflicted infant; but before we can reach this conclusion, two important questions must be resolved. First, we must know what burdens to the child are admissible in our moral calculations of benefit and burden. Do any and all burdens to the child count, or only certain kinds? Second, we must have a clearer idea of the point of view from which these burdens will be assessed. Shall it be the viewpoint of the gravely impaired child or of the normal adult?

Which Burdens Shall Count?

So far, we have listed physical ailments that might befall a child and render excessively burdensome a prolongation of his or her life. Now we must consider whether burdens attributable to the child's socioeconomic status can be counted alongside strictly medical burdens as contributing to an excessively burdensome life and, if so, whether such burdens morally *ought* to be so counted.

In addition to suffering from the retardation associated with Down's syndrome, the repeated surgeries associated with spina bifida, or the iatrogenic toll of respirator therapy for premature infants, a child may suffer from a host of nonmedical problems. She may, if allowed to live, suffer from parental rejection. Plagued by frustration, guilt, and disappointment, parents can and do neglect their impaired children—or, worse yet, abuse them. Or the parents may love and wish to care for their child, yet be too ill-equipped to care for her at home and too poor to place her in an acceptable institution. Such parents face the dilemma of keeping their child at home, where the demands of caring for her disabilities are likely to drain their economic and emotional resources, or handing her over to an institution that is likely to be underfinanced and understaffed. At such an institution, the severely impaired child is likely to be relegated to some back ward where she will suffer from lack of love, human contact, and even basic care.[7]

"Clearly," it might be argued, "subjecting the anomalous child to this sort of institutionalized deprivation amounts to a harm of considerable proportion. In the absence of better alternatives to institutionalization, such as it is today in many economically deprived areas, these children should be relieved of potentially crushing burdens by means of an early, merciful death."

This is a plausible argument. Unquestionably the abuse and neglect attributable to a family's inability to cope or to pay for humane care can amount to substantial burdens for the child. And so long as burdensomeness to the child remains the crucial criterion involved in the best-interest standard, why shouldn't social as well as purely medical burdens count in our overall calculations? Indeed, if socially induced burdens can make continued life excessively burdensome for a severely retarded child relegated to some back ward, logic would seem to compel us to weigh them as heavily as any other kind of burden. The important thing, it might be said, is not the source of the burden, but its effect on the child. If parental neglect, social ostracism, and degrading conditions can make life unbearable, why shouldn't they be a part of our moral deliberations?

In spite of its initial plausibility, this line of reasoning runs afoul of the nondiscrimination principle. If it would be in a wealthy child's best interest to receive life-sustaining therapies, justice demands that a poor child with a similar medical condition and prognosis also receive the same treatment. Like cases should be treated alike. (The same can be said on behalf of children born to parents rich and poor alike who are unable or unwilling to nurture them. The parents' inadequacies are not the fault of their children.)

True, in our previous discussion of medically induced burdens we suggested that certain disabilities could be so severe as to render an anomalous child significantly different from a normal child for purposes of moral analysis. We said then that such disabilities could prompt us to deny the premise that the severely impaired child was still "like" the normal child in all relevant respects, and thus to deny the conclusion that such children must receive "like" treatment. We argued, finally, that the severely impaired child was unlike the normal child precisely in the sense that her best interests would not be served by further treatment or continued existence. Why not repeat the same argument here with regard, this time, to socially related burdens?

The answer to this eminently sensible question is that, whereas an extremely poor medical prognosis and quality of life can make for a significant moral difference between two babies, the same cannot be said of differences in wealth. Degree of wealth is never a morally significant difference between two potential recipients of basic health care. If a certain medical procedure is deemed to be truly beneficial and offered to a wealthy child with severe disabilities, it must also be offered to the similarly situated poor child. The latter is not responsible for the lack of concern of her parents, or for their inability to afford dignified and humane follow-up care. To say that the wealthy child should live (because her anomalies are not so severe as to make life too burdensome) but that the poor child with similar prognosis should die (because of further burdens imposed by her poverty) is to indulge in the rankest kind of discrimination. For purposes of moral analysis, these two patients are identical, and they should therefore receive similar treatment. That is the demand of simple justice—unless we hold that being rich in itself makes the wealthy impaired child more deserving of health care than the poor child, an unlikely concession for us to make.

A policy that allowed us to consider socially induced burdens would not only be profoundly unjust; it would also most likely impede efforts to improve the plight of the institutionalized, poor, imperiled child. Historically, one of the most potent arguments in favor of social reform has rested on the existence of human suffering and deprivation. Could we expect vigorous efforts to reform public institutions housing severely impaired children once the suffering and neglect that characterize such institutions have become publicly recognized as good reasons for killing these newborns? My sympathies lie entirely with Paul Ramsey's response to the suggestion that a child's poverty ought to count in her constellation of publicly recognized burdens. "That's one way," says Ramsey, "to remove every evening the human debris that has accumulated since morning." For the great majority of these handicapped infants, radical social reform—not "beneficent" euthanasia—is the answer.

The procedural implication of this argument about justice is that we should attempt to distinguish clearly between "treatment decisions" and decisions regarding the child's ultimate placement.[8] In other words, worries about the child's future life with a potentially abusive parent or in a hopelessly inadequate state institution should not be allowed to influence treatment decisions. Even though socially induced burdens can join forces with strictly physical disabilities to make a life excessively burdensome to its bearer, we must base our treatment decisions solely on the extent of medical disabilities. To take social factors into account is to act unjustly toward the child.

At this point in the argument, we have clearly entered a "moral blind alley"—that is, a situation so structured that whatever course we take, we end up doing something morally unacceptable.[9] Ordinarily this structure takes the form of a conflict between two disparate moral concerns—namely, doing good and doing justice. Morality, through the principle of beneficence, requires us to increase people's happiness and mitigate their unhappiness. But another moral principle enjoins us to respect persons' rights and to do justice. When these conflicting demands meet head-on in a concrete situation, the stage is set for an ethical dilemma. How can they be reconciled?

As Ronald Dworkin has contended, a concern

for rights and justice can function as a "trump card" in moral and political argument with regard to competing utilitarian considerations.[10] When there is a conflict between the demands of utility and the requirements of justice, we usually say that the former must simply yield to the latter. Pointing to the good or bad consequences said to flow from the performance or omission of an act is usually said to be an insufficient (or even irrelevant) justification if that act or omission happens to be unjust. For example, we say that a citizen's right to speak freely must be respected, even though rather serious consequences (such as public disturbances) may ensue from the exercise of that right. In this sort of case, the right course is clear—we should let the individual speak—and there is no serious moral dilemma. One moral concern has simply eclipsed another.

Sometimes circumstances may be so extreme and the consequences so dreadful that the priority of justice can no longer be maintained. When this happens, an agent enters a moral blind alley. He must choose, but all of his alternatives are morally unacceptable. If he does the "right" thing, the act required by strict justice, then catastrophic results will follow: if he violates the demands of justice, he avoids terrible consequences at the cost of doing a deed that should never be done. In such cases, one may prudently decide to violate rights and justice in order to avoid catastrophe, but this does not always count as a complete justification. "Moral traces" of the demands of justice remain, even when circumstances make it plain that justice must be violated. Simply put, it does not become *all right:* we are left with dirty hands.[11]

Winston Churchill faced such a moral dilemma in World War II—should he launch rocket attacks on German civilian populations, thereby killing hundreds of innocent persons, or risk losing the war? I suspect that we face a similar dilemma in the case of the impoverished impaired newborn. If we take the child's socially caused burdens into account—such as the likelihood of being neglected in a state institution—we may rightly decide that death would be better than such a fate. Allowing such a child to die would be a merciful act, averting an unbearable life for the child; but it would also be unjust. As we have seen, it is profoundly unjust to afford differential treatment to impaired newborns on the basis of socioeconomic factors. However, if we avert our eyes from the child's subsequent fate in a barren state institution, we act justly but possibly consign the child to a miserable life in a warehouse for discarded humans—a catastrophic result, to be sure.

It would appear, then, that we are confronted by a genuine moral dilemma occasioned by social conditions of poverty and inequity. Here, as elsewhere in the field of biomedical ethics, straightforward appeals to notions of right and justice—abstracted from a social context of profound injustice—can lead to morally disastrous results.[12] So long as these unjust social conditions persist, so long as the rich gravely impaired child enjoys a bearable quality of life denied to a poor counterpart, the door of the neonatal nursery will continue to open onto a moral blind alley. Rather than serve as an invitation to resignation, however, this conclusion underscores the necessity of increased social (governmental) support of the handicapped. Surely, any society that insists upon a controversial strict standard of justice concerning nontreatment decisions—a standard that will weigh heaviest upon those parents most in need of psychological and financial support—surely, such a society thereby incurs a corresponding duty to support those who must bear the burden it imposes.

What Standard Will Measure the Burden?

There are essentially two possibilities: we can adopt either the point of view of the rational adult or that of the anomalous child. According to some philosophers, we ought to adopt the viewpoint of the mature adult or the so-called "reasonable person."[13] "Since incompetent creatures are incompetent," writes Joseph Margolis, "we judge as rational adults of normal sensibilities would. It is in this sense that the decision to bring to an end the lives of selected fetuses and infants . . . is *conceptually parasitic* on the decision of the competent to end their own lives. . . ."

Although this approach is flawed, it has a certain appealing modesty. It does not require us to plumb the depths of the incompetent person's psyche to discern there what the incompetent patient "really wants." Such modesty is becoming when the patient for whom we are to decide has not left us any evidence of how he or she would decide: it is especially becoming when the patient lacks the very capacity to develop a value system in the first place. Although courts have recently ascribed to themselves or to guardians the right to make so-called "substituted judgments" for voiceless patients, and although the proxy decision makers have been legally charged with the (impossible?) task of deciding as the patient would decide, were he or she miraculously to become competent for an instant, I suspect that they end up attempting to judge as any rational adult of normal sensitivities would. And for good reason.

In the absence of explicit or implicit value judgments from the incompetent patient, what else do we have to go on? How do we know whether or not the permanently incompetent patient would judge life under present circumstances to be worth the candle? Far from being endowed with the Herculean powers of discernment required by such a task, we can only ask what the "vast majority" of adults would want, should such a fate befall them. This sort of judgment might still be very difficult to render, but at least we would be familiar with the grounds of our decision. Presumably, we all have some rough idea of when life would no longer be meaningful or worth living *for us*.

Despite its commonsensical appeal, two different objections have been lodged against invoking a "reasonable person" standard in the case of impaired newborns. The first merely points to the probability of abuse: a reasonable-person standard, based on what the vast majority of people would want, leaves the child unprotected against the whims and vagaries of normal adults. This prospect leads some critics to reject out of hand any consideration of quality of life in the treatment of newborns.

This objection is itself somewhat ambiguous. It could be taken to mean that a reasonable-person standard is theoretically acceptable, but would tend to be too easily abused in practice. This objection may or may not be sound. Empirical studies would have to be adduced showing that the likelihood of abuse is so great that any and all quality-of-life judgments based on adult sensibilities should be banished. In the absence of such evidence, an abrupt dismissal of a best-interest standard would appear to be unsupported.

Another objection goes to the heart of the matter. According to this version, put forth by John Robertson and others, the problem lies in the reasonable-person standard itself, not in our penchant for misusing it. Any standard of judgment based on the sensibilities of normal adults, it is claimed, will necessarily be prejudicial to the best interests of impaired children. In contrast to the point about the inevitability of abuse, this objection assumes the appropriateness of a best-interest standard but insists that any criterion based on the values of normal adults is bound systematically to distort our judgments of what is truly in a child's best interests. This version of the objection thus poses a direct challenge to Margolis's assumption that decisions on behalf of incompetent children must be conceptually parasitic on the standards appealed to by normal adults in deciding to end their own lives.

Come to think of it, why should the sentiments of normal adults be used as the touchstone of meaningful life for imperiled newborns? Although most normal adults are no doubt well-meaning and genuinely concerned not to abuse their standard of judgment, they are undoubtedly biased in favor of normalcy. Being normal themselves, competent adults have naturally pitched their value systems on the solid ground of normalcy. But it is precisely through the mediation of these values that adults are supposed to evaluate the disabilities of the child and assess their implications for the value of continued life. It is only natural to expect that, were the question put to them, many normal adults, having grown accustomed to the social and intellectual satisfactions that normalcy makes possible, would rather die than live without these basic human capacities. But as John Robertson pointed out in a classic article:

> Yet a standard based on healthy, ordinary development may be entirely inappropriate to this situation. One who has never known the pleasures of mental operation, ambulation, and social interaction surely does not suffer from their loss as much as one who has. While one who has known these capacities may prefer death to a life without them, we have no assurance that the handicapped person, with no point of comparison, would agree. Life, and life alone, whatever its

limitations, might be of sufficient worth to him.[14]

Echoing Robertson's point, the President's Commission recently warned against adopting the viewpoint of normal adults in assessing the best interests of anomalous children. While conceding that responsible parties must try to ground their judgments on considerations that would move a competent decision maker to forego treatment—thereby barring the consideration of idiosyncratic value judgments—the President's Commission strongly recommended that benefits and burdens be weighed from the incompetent infant's own perspective. We must ask not whether a normal adult would rather die than suffer from severe mental and physical impairments, but rather whether this child, who has never known the satisfactions and aspirations of the normal world, would prefer nothing to what he or she has.

If the best interests of the child is to be our standard of judgment, the viewpoint of the child is clearly the most appropriate measure of benefits and burdens. The standard of the reasonable adult, based as it is on the capacities and expectations of normalcy, would introduce a systematic bias into our considerations. Everywhere, it would have us see dashed hopes and frustration, rather than opportunities for growth and strategies of meaningful accommodation. Adopting the child's viewpoint would be difficult in practice, but it would conform more closely to the spirit of the best-interest standard. The issue, after all, is the welfare of this child, not the hopes and fears of adults that might be projected onto the child.

As the Commission rightly points out, this interpretation of the best-interest standard yields a very strict policy. For one thing, it stresses the child's well-being, to the exclusion of any and all considerations of the child's negative impact on others. Nontreatment of a nondying impaired child could not be justified on the ground that ongoing care would drain the family (or the state) of its financial resources or deprive siblings of the love and attention that they deserve.[15] In addition, this gloss of the best-interest standard would clearly have mandated life-saving treatments in most of the cases that have generated public controversy in recent years. While normal adults might prefer, for themselves, death to mental retardation, it cannot plausibly be argued that the average Down's syndrome child would see death as being in his or her best interest. To the contrary, persons with Down's syndrome derive great satisfaction from their lives. From their point of view, life is good and worth living, no matter how limited others might think their lives to be. The main difference separating them from us lies not in our capacity for enjoying life and for sharing love, but rather, it has been plausibly suggested, in their "congenital inability to hate."[16]

The Limits of the Best-Interest Standard

This standard, interpreted from the impaired child's viewpoint, is indeed strict—and rightly so. When human lives are at stake, we do not want to substitute, no matter how unconsciously, the fears of normal adults for the genuine best interests of impaired children. It has not been generally appreciated, however—not even by the President's Commission—just how strict this child-relative standard can become when pushed to the extreme limits of human disability.

The first hint of a problem with the application of this standard can be found in Robertson's initial article championing the viewpoint of the impaired child. Immediately following his convincing refutation of the claim that death would be a better fate than life for most "mongoloid" and nonambulatory spina bifida children, Robertson reached the same conclusion in the "worse case"—that is, "the profoundly retarded, nonambulatory, blind, deaf infant who will spend his few years in the back-ward cribs of a state institution. . . ."[17] Even in such an extreme case, where the Commission would no doubt be most likely to concede that "continued existence would not be a net benefit to the infant," Robertson refuses to sanction nontreatment and death. How do we know, he asks, that such a child with wants, needs, and interests so different from our own would prefer the abyss to his back-ward existence? How can we be sure that, for such a child, life and life alone would not be of sufficient worth?

Assuming that the infant is not in pain and has no conscious experience of suffering, Robertson's doubts appear to be well founded. Of course, if this child were also suffering inordinately from the side effects of invasive therapies or from the underlying condition itself—in addition to other multiple handicaps—that would be a different story. As we have already seen, unremitting and unrelievable pain can transform a person's continued existence from an unquestioned benefit into a harsh burden. But suppose the child suffers no pain. He lies there in his crib, blind, deaf, and uncomprehending. Never having experienced the satisfactions of normalcy, the infant is neither horrified by his plight, nor depressed by his neglect in the state institution or by the thought of his impending doom. He just lies there. Can we say with moral certitude that it is in the child's best interest to die?

I think not. We can say that, for such a severely impaired child, life cannot have much significance or value. Indeed, it is difficult to understand in what sense such a child can have any interests to which a best-interest standard might apply. Nevertheless, strictly from this infant's point of view, it is far from clear that death would be preferable to such a life. As Robertson implies, the mere act of subsisting on the back ward—vegetating, if you will—might well be deemed "worth the candle" by this child if, miraculously, he could survey his situation with the clarity of a competent person. "It's certainly not much," he might ruefully admit to himself, "but it's better than nothing. They feed me, change me, occasionally cuddle me. And I'm not in any pain to speak of. So why not just play out the meager hand that I've been dealt?"

This eerie soliloquy, spoken by a child who will never speak, will play to mixed reviews. For some, it will furnish convincing evidence that the best-interest standard, interpreted from the child's point of view, mandates treatment even in the worst cases (provided that the child is not in pain). Others, while (correctly) agreeing with this conclusion, will see in it evidence, not that such children should be kept alive, but rather that, in such extreme cases, the best-interest standard has been pushed beyond the pale of its capabilities. They will contend, rightly I think, that when pushed this far the best-interest standard generates results that conflict with moral common sense.

Consider, for example, the plight of the child born with Trisomy 13, a chromosomal disorder associated with severe mental retardation and severe physical impairments. The child's brain is so malformed that she will never possess the capacity to think or to communicate with others. And, as if these deficits were not sufficient, she is doomed to an early death. If treated aggressively and vigilantly, however, she might well live for months, or perhaps even for a year. Although she is probably not properly classified as a "dying patient" according to Surgeon General Koop's taxonomy,[18] this child will soon die never having had an intelligible thought, never having given or acknowledged love, never having experienced anything beyond simply "being there."

The fact that the child-based best-interest standard would mandate treatment even in the face of a prognosis bereft of any distinctly human potentiality reveals a feature of that standard that has so far gone unnoticed. In such extreme cases, the best-interest standard tends to view the absence of pain as the only morally relevant consideration. No matter that the infant is doomed to a life of very short duration, and lacks the capacity for any distinctively human development or activity; so long as the child does not experience any severe burdens, interpreted from her point of view, the fact that she can anticipate no distinctly human benefits is of no moral consequence.

But this seems wrong. The presence or absence of such characteristics as the ability to think, to communicate, to give and receive love, seems to be highly relevant from a moral point of view. Indeed, in the absence of these capacities, how can we attribute any human interests to the child on which a best-interest standard might operate? By narrowing the range of meaningful data to the presence or absence of unrelievable pain, the best-interest standard consigns itself in extreme cases to operating in a moral vacuum. The result is an indiscriminate mandate to treat, to keep alive, that flies in the face of common sense. When confronted with such cases, one wants to ask, not whether treatment will further the infant's best interests, but rather whether the child's impoverished level of existence is worth sustaining.

Beyond the Best-Interest Standard

Far from advancing the conclusion that even the worst case ought to receive life-sustaining treatments, our hypothetical soliloquy reveals the limits of the best-interest standard; in so doing, it underscores our need for a supplementary standard geared to the presence or absence of distinctly human capacities.[19] The ethical principle that justifies this standard is the proposition that biological human life is only a relative good. In the absence of certain distinctly human capacities—for self-consciousness and relating to other people—the usual connection between biological life and our notion of the good is effectively severed. Just as the presence of unrelievable pain can preclude the attainment of those basic human goods that make life worth living, so the absence of fundamental human capacities can render a life valueless, both to its possessor and to others. (This is not to deny that families can derive great satisfactions from caring for such severely impaired children and may well desire to keep them alive. But this particular reason for sustaining their lives has nothing to do with the child's best interests.) Without these qualities, no distinctly human good can be achieved. When this point is reached, the duty to sustain life loses its hold on caregivers.

Since such grievously afflicted children have no distinctly human capacities, and thus no human interests, the activity of keeping them alive is pointless from the moral point of view. Indeed, in these worst cases, it is a mistake to inquire about the best interests of such children or to insist that decisions to terminate treatment be made solely in terms of the child's good. As the previous discussion of the best-interest standard revealed, the only interest that can intelligibly be attributed to children lacking self-consciousness or relational potential is an interest in avoiding pain and suffering. Since, for them, continued existence does not offer the prospect of achieving any human good, we cannot sensibly attribute to such children an interest in sustaining their lives. Consequently, those who bear the responsibility for them are under no ethical obligation to prolong their lives by means of medical treatments.

In contrast to the misapplied best-interest standard, which sought to fasten onto the subjective preferences of the severely impaired child, this "relational potential standard" must issue from a social, intersubjective inquiry into the conditions of a valuable human life. Although any attempt to define the parameters of "meaningful human life" will doubtless meet with suspicion—or even with extreme hostility—this sort of inquiry makes a great deal more sense than the convoluted speculations required by a best-interest standard pushed beyond its limits. The search for a threshold of meaningful human life might well be difficult and fraught with the danger of abuse—how many pogroms and genocidal campaigns have been justified by their victims' alleged lack of "basic humanity"?—but the search for the secret preferences of patients lacking the capacity for self-knowledge and human relations is, I would argue, an essentially misguided venture.

The futility of this search is illustrated by the paradoxical subjective tests the courts have applied in extreme cases. In the famous *Saikewicz* case, for example, the judge bids us to reach a decision that "would be made by the incompetent person, if that person were competent, but taking into account the present and future incompetency of the individual as one of the factors which would necessarily enter into the decision-making process of the competent person."[20] Although the language of the President's Commission avoids the transparent absurdity of the *Saikewicz* formula, its recommendation amounts to the same thing: we are to base our judgments on grounds that "would lead a *competent* decisionmaker . . . to forego treatment" while, at the same time, "adopting the viewpoint of the *incompetent* patient" (emphasis added). Given the impossibility of this charge in the case of children lacking any relational potential or capacity for choosing a system of values, we are faced with two alternatives. We can either attempt to sustain the lives of such patients in spite of their empty prognoses, or we can engage in the risky business of designating a threshold of meaningful human life. The latter alternative might well be dangerous, but the former is pointless and burdensome to parents and society.

The Beginning of Wisdom

Two distinctions between normal infants and certain severely anomalous children are morally relevant. Just as a child might be excessively burdened by his treatments or underlying disease, so a child may lack certain basic human capacities. Such pain and lack of capacities mark significant moral differences between these anomalous children and their normal counterparts. Just as we ought to extend similar treatment to similar cases, we should also be prepared to extend dissimilar treatment to dissimilar cases. Since the nondiscrimination principle forbids differential treatment only in the absence of morally relevant distinctions between people, and since excessive burdens or the lack of relational potential constitute relevant distinctions, the nondiscrimination principle does not forbid nontreatment in the sorts of cases we have been discussing.

We are confronted here with an enormously difficult and complex moral issue. Contrary to the opinion of those who would simplify this problem beyond all recognition—either by mandating treatment for all children, or by allowing parents or health professionals unbridled discretion—I have tried, following Kierkegaard's example, " . . . to create [or at least acknowledge] difficulties everywhere. . . ."[21]

Ethical ambiguity pervades the issue. Most seriously impaired children should be treated, some should be allowed to die. Substantive principles are available, but their application is fraught with difficulty and danger. Although this pervasive ambiguity is difficult to live with, we can be sure that attempts to ignore it, to reduce the problem to a simple formula, will lead to an illusory and counterproductive quest for moral certainty.

Notes

1. President's Commission, *Deciding to Forego Life-Sustaining Treatments,* pp. 134–36, 217–23.

2. Versions of this argument appear in Paul Ramsey, *Ethics at the Edges of Life* (New Haven: Yale University Press, 1978), pp. 206–07, 240 n. 11; and in Paul Camenisch, "Abortion for the Sake of the Fetus." *Hastings Center Report* 6 (April 1976), 38–41. See also *Gleitman v. Cosgrove,* 49 N.J. 22, 227 A.2d 689 (1967): "It is basic to the human condition to seek life and hold on to it however heavily burdened."

3. Philippa Foot, "Euthanasia." *Philosophy and Public Affairs* 6 (1977), 94–96.

4. Ramsey, *Ethics at the Edges of Life,* pp. 154–59, 225.

5. President's Commission, *Deciding to Forego Life-Sustaining Treatment,* p. 218. On closer inspection, this particular gloss of the best-interest standard turns out to be dangerously overinclusive. Continued existence is not a "net benefit" for many people who would nevertheless opt for life over death. Here we should be talking about handicaps so severe that continued existence would be marked by constant pain and suffering. This lapse in the Commission report was called to my attention by Alan Fleischman.

6. See, e.g., Norman Fost, "How Decisions are Made: A Physician's View," in C. A. Swinyard, ed., *Decision Making and the Defective Newborn* (Springfield, Ill.: Charles C. Thomas, 1978), pp. 220–30.

7. For a vivid description of how bad the conditions can get in such institutions, see *New York State Association of Retarded Children* v. *Rockefeller* 357 Fed. Supp. 752 (Eastern Division, NY 1973).

8. Ramsey, *Ethics at the Edges of Life,* pp. 202–03.

9. Thomas Nagel, "War and Massacre," in Marshall Cohen, et al., eds., *War and Moral Responsibility* (Princeton, NJ: Princeton University Press, 1974), p. 23.

10. Dworkin, *Taking Rights Seriously,* pp. xi, 171–72.

11. Nagel, "War and Massacre," 16–17. See also Robert Nozick. "Moral Complications and Moral Structures," *Natural Law Forum* 13 (1968), 1–50.

12. This theme is developed at length in my essay, "The Right to Die on the Slippery Slope," *Social Theory and Practice* 8 (Fall 1982), 285–328. See also Nancy Rhoden, "The Limits of Liberty: Deinstitutionalization, Homelessness, and Libertarian Theory," *Emory Law Journal* 32 (Spring 1982), 375–440.

13. See Robert Veatch, *Death, Dying, and the Biological Revolution* (New Haven, CT: Yale University Press, 1976), pp. 124–36; and Joseph Margolis, "Human Life: Its Worth and Bringing It to an End," in Marvin Kohl, ed., *Infanticide and the Value of Life* (Buffalo, NY: Prometheus, 1978), pp. 180–91.

14. John Robertson, "Involuntary Euthanasia of Defective Newborns," *Stanford Law Review* 27 (1975), 254.

15. For an opposing view, see Carson Strong, "Defective Infants and Their Impact on Families: Ethical and Legal Considerations," *Law, Medicine and Health Care* (September 1983), pp. 168–81.

16. Louis Lasagna, "Murder Most Foul," *The Sciences* 22 (August-September 1982). Dr. Lasagna is the father of a twenty-year-old with Down's syndrome.

17. Robertson, "Involuntary Euthanasia of Defective Newborns," p. 254.

18. According to Dr. Koop, "For such [dying] infants, neither medicine nor law can be of any help. And neither medicine nor law should prolong these infants' process of dying." Statement before Hearing on Handicapped Newborns, Subcommittee on Select Education Committee on Education and Labor, U.S. House of Representatives (September

16, 1982). Quoted in President's Commission, *Deciding to Forego Life-Sustaining Treatment*, pp. 219–20, n. 81.

19. Such a standard is worked out by Richard McCormick, S. J., in "To Save or Let Die: The Dilemma of Modern Medicine," *Journal of the American*

Medical Association 229, No. 2 (July 8, 1974), 172–76.

20. *Superintendent of Belchertown State School* v. *Saikewicz*, 370 NE 2d 417 (1977).

21. Robert Bretall, ed., *A Kierkegaard Anthology* (New York, NY: Modern Library, 1936), p. 194.

Decision Scenario 1 ....

I had been working as a bioethics advisor at University Hospital for three months before I was called in to consult on a pediatrics case. Dr. Savano, the attending obstetrician, asked me to meet with him and Dr. Hinds, one of the staff surgeons, to talk with the father of a newborn girl.

I went to the consulting room with Dr. Savano, and he introduced me and Dr. Hinds to Joel Blake. From what Dr. Savano had already told me, I knew that Mr. Blake was in his early twenties and worked as a clerk at a discount store called the Bargain Barn. The baby's mother was Hilda Godgeburn, and she and Mr. Blake were not married.

Mr. Blake was very nervous. He knew that the baby had been born just three hours or so before and that Ms. Godgeburn was in very good condition. But Dr. Savano had not told him anything about the baby.

"I'm sorry to have to tell you this," Dr. Savano said. "But the baby was born with severe defects."

"My God," Blake said. "What's the matter?"

"It's a condition called spina bifida," Dr. Savano said. "There's a hole in the baby's back just below the shoulder blades, and some of the nerves from the spine are protruding through it. The baby will have little or no control over her legs, and she won't be able to control her bladder or bowels." Dr. Savano paused to see if Mr. Blake was understanding him. "The legs and feet are also deformed to some extent because of the defective spinal nerves."

Mr. Blake was shaking his head, paying close attention but hardly able to accept what he was being told.

"There's one more thing," Dr. Savano said. "The spinal defect is making the head fill up with liquid from the spinal canal. That's putting pressure on the brain. We can be sure that the brain is already damaged, but if the pressure continues, the child will die."

"Is there anything that can be done?" Blake asked. "Anything at all?"

Dr. Savano nodded to Dr. Hinds. "We can do a lot," Dr. Hinds said. "We can drain the fluid from the head, repair the opening in the spine, and later we can operate on the feet and legs."

"Then why aren't you doing it?" Mr. Blake asked. "Do I have to agree to it? If I do, then I agree. Please go ahead."

"It's not that simple," Dr. Hinds said. "You see, we can perform surgery, but that won't turn your baby into a normal child. She will always be paralyzed and mentally retarded. To what extent, we can't say now. Her bodily wastes will have to be drained to the outside by the means of artificial devices that we'll have to connect surgically. There will have to be several operations, probably, to get the drain from her head to work properly. A number of operations on her feet will be necessary."

"Oh, God," Mr. Blake said. "Hilda and I can't take it. We don't have enough money for the operations. And even if we did, we would have to spend the rest of our lives taking care of the child."

"The child could be put into a state institution," Dr. Hinds said.

"That's even worse," Mr. Blake said. "Just handing our problem to somebody else. And what kind of life would she have? A pitiful, miserable life."

None of the rest of us said anything. "You said she would die without the operation to drain her head," Mr. Blake said. "How long would that take?"

"A few hours perhaps," Dr. Savano said. "But we can't be sure. It may take several days, and conceivably she might not die at all."

"Oh, God," Mr. Blake said again. "I don't want her to suffer. Can she just be put to sleep painlessly?"

Dr. Savano didn't answer the question. He seemed not even to hear it. "We'll have to talk to Ms. Godgeburn also," he said. "And before you make up your mind for good, I want you to talk with the bioethics advisor. You two discuss the matter, and the advisor will perhaps bring out some things you haven't thought about. Dr. Hinds will leave you both together now. Let me know when you've reached your final decision and we'll talk again."

Assume that you are the bioethics advisor in this case. Would you attempt to persuade Mr. Blake

that attempts should be made to save the child's life?

Do you think he is right in asking that the child be painlessly killed? If such killing is not legally permissible, is this relevant to deciding whether the child should be saved if possible? What considerations for and against such an attempt might you mention to help Mr. Blake in reaching a decision?

Are there any arguments in what you have read that seem to you entirely persuasive in such a case?

What factual considerations (if any) do you consider relevant to resolving the moral issues here?

Decision Scenario 2 ....

Brookhaven, as we will call it, is a long-term health care institution in the Washington metropolitan area. Most of Brookhaven's patients are in residence there for only a few months: either they succumb to their ailments and die or they recover sufficiently to return to their homes.

But for some patients death has no immediate likelihood, nor is recovery a possibility. They linger on at Brookhaven, day after day and year after year. Juli Meyers is such a patient, although that is not really her name.

Juli is seventeen and has been in Brookhaven for six years. But before Brookhaven there were other institutions. In fact, Juli has spent most of her life in hospitals and special care facilities. But Juli does not seem to be aware of any of this.

At Brookhaven she spends her days lying in a bed surrounded with barred metal panels. The bars have been padded with foam rubber. Although most of the time Juli is curled tightly in a fetal position, she sometimes flails around wildly and makes guttural sounds. The padding keeps her from injuring herself.

Juli's body is thin and underdeveloped, with sticklike arms and legs. She is blind and deaf and has no control over her bowels and bladder. She is totally dependent on others to clean her and care for her. She can swallow the food put into her mouth, but she cannot feed herself. She makes no response to the people or events around her.

There is no hope that Juli will walk or talk, laugh or cry, or even show the slightest sign of intelligence or awareness. She is the victim of one of the forms of Schilder's disease. The nerve fibers that make up her central nervous system have mostly degenerated. The cause of the degeneration is not fully known, nor is it known how to halt the process. The condition is irreversible, and Juli will never be better than she is.

At birth Juli seemed perfectly normal and healthy, but at three months she began to lose her sight and hearing. She made the gurgling noises typical of babies less and less frequently. By the end of her first year, she made no sounds at all and was completely blind and deaf. Also, she was losing control of her muscles, and her head lolled on her shoulders, like a doll with a broken neck.

She became highly subject to infections, and more than once she had pneumonia. Once when she was on the critical list, a specialist suggested to her mother that it would be pointless to continue treating her. Even if she recovered from the pneumonia, she would remain hopelessly impaired. Mrs. Meyers angrily rejected the suggestion and insisted that everything possible be done to save Juli's life.

Although not wealthy, the family bore the high cost of hospitalization and treatments. Mrs. Meyers devoted herself almost totally to caring for Juli at home, and the other four children in the family received little of her attention. Eventually, Mrs. Meyers began to suffer from severe depression, and when Juli was eight and a half her parents decided she would have to be placed in an institution. Since then, Juli has changed little. No one expects her to change. Her mother visits her three times a month and brings Juli freshly laundered and ironed clothes.

> *Would Robertson's arguments support Mrs. Meyer's decision not to allow Juli to die? How might a utilitarian criticize the decision?*

> *Would treatment for pneumonia in Juli's case be considered "normal medical measures" on the Roman Catholic view?*

> *Are there any grounds for supposing that Juli is being made to suffer what Engelhardt calls "the injury of continued existence?"*

> *Would your decision have been the same as Mrs. Meyers's?*

> *Is it possible to justify using society's limited medical resources to keep Juli alive?*

> *Evaluate the following argument. Opponents of abortion oppose spending public funds for abortion on the grounds that they (the opponents) are being forced to support murder, which is a serious moral evil. Keeping Juli alive is a serious moral evil. Therefore, no public funds should be used for this purpose.*

Decision Scenario 3 ••

Susan Roth was looking forward to being a mother. She had quit her secretarial job three months before her baby was due so she could spend the time getting everything ready. Her husband David was equally enthusiastic, and they spent many hours happily speculating about the way things would be when their baby came. It was their first child.

"I hope they don't mix her up with some other baby," Mrs. Roth said to her husband after delivery.

She didn't know yet that there was little chance of confusion. The Roth infant was seriously deformed. Her arms and legs had failed to develop, her skull was misshapen, and her face deformed. Her large intestine emptied through her vagina, and she had no muscular control over her bladder.

When she was told, Mrs. Roth said, "We cannot let it live, for her sake and ours." On the day she left the hospital with the child, Mrs. Roth mixed a lethal dose of a tranquilizing drug with the baby's formula and fed it to her. The child died that evening.

Mrs. Roth and her husband were charged

with infanticide. During the court proceedings, Mrs. Roth admitted to the killing but said she was satisfied she had done the right thing. "I know I could not let my baby live like that," she said. "If only she had been mentally abnormal, she would not have known her fate. But she had a normal brain. She would have known. Placing her in an institution might have helped me, but it wouldn't have helped her."

The jury, after deliberating for two hours, found Mrs. Roth and her husband guilty of the charge.

> *Are laws against infanticide unjust?*

> *Does the fact that the intelligence of the child is normal support the mother's claim that killing was justifiable? Might normal intelligence make the "injury of continued existence" even greater than subnormal intelligence?*

> *Why might Robertson consider the mother's action morally wrong?*

> *Would the "best interest" of the infant standard, as presented by Arras, offer any support for the mother's action?*

Decision Scenario 4 ••

I can't believe God has done this to me, Mike Chovo said to himself. Tears came to his eyes and his nose started running.

His wife Carol handed him a tissue from the box by her bed. "It's all right, Mikey," she said. "We'll make it all right."

Mike wiped his eyes and blew his nose. The yellow tissue struck him as being absurdly cheerful. Given the circumstances, it seemed totally out of place in the hospital room.

"I know," he said. "But it's going to be so hard, so very hard. And it's going to be terrible for Chris and Jan."

"They'll adjust," Carol said. "In some ways it will be good for them to have a brother like Terry. They'll learn somebody doesn't have to be perfect for you to love them."

"Oh, Jesus," Mike said. "Maybe we should have told them not to do anything. He's in such bad shape. The doctors told me they're not sure he has enough of a brain even to learn who we are. I mean, it may be like he's unconscious all of his life."

Mike pulled another tissue out of the box and held it over his eyes. He pressed hard with his fingertips. He wanted Terry to die, but he couldn't tell Carol that. He could barely allow himself to think it. He wished he hadn't given permission for the operation to drain the fluid from Terry's head. But he couldn't oppose Carol at a time like this.

"But we'll love him anyway," Carol said. "We'll take care of him until God calls him away."

"I wonder if we're doing him a favor. I wonder if he's really fit for this world."

"We couldn't just stand by and let him die," Carol said.

"No, I guess we couldn't." Mike hesitated, then went on. "You know, this one operation won't be the end of them. Dr. Flanners told me

that it's not unusual to have to operate ten or twelve times in cases like this."

"It's going to be expensive."

"That's right, and I don't know where we're going to get the money."

"We can probably borrow some from my parents. And if we have to, I guess we can get a second mortgage on the house."

"I guess so," Mike admitted.

Carol looked at Mike and smiled at him. After a moment, he smiled back.

Would the line of reasoning taken by Robertson tend to support the decision made by Carol Chovo?

Might the considerations mentioned by Engelhardt be used to argue that it would have been better for the Chovos to allow their son to die?

Does the natural law view require treatment in such a case?

On what grounds might Kantian principles be appealed to in order to justify a decision not to treat Terry Chovo?

In what ways, if any, are such considerations as the financial status of the Chovos and the likely influence on the other two children of having a wholly dependent and impaired brother relevant to the decision that faced the parents?

Would the "best interest" standard discussed by Arras provide grounds for justifying a decision to withhold medical treatment?

Decision Scenario 5 ....

Irene Towers had been a nurse for almost twelve years; for the last three of those years she had worked in the Neonatal Unit of Halifax County Hospital. It was a job she loved. Even when the infants were ill or required special medical or surgical treatment, she found the job of caring for them immensely rewarding. She knew that without her efforts many of the babies would simply die.

Irene Towers was on duty the night that Siamese twins were born to Corrine Couchers and brought at once to the Neonatal Unit. Even Irene, with all her experience, was distressed to see

them. The twin boys were joined at their midsections in a way that made it impossible to separate them surgically. Because of the position of the single liver and the kidneys, not even one twin could be saved at the expense of the life of the other. Moreover, both children were severely deformed, with incompletely developed arms and legs and misshapen heads. As best as the neurologist could determine, both suffered severe brain damage.

The father of the children was Dr. Harold Couchers. Dr. Couchers, a slightly built man in his early thirties, was a specialist in internal medicine with a private practice.

Irene felt sorry for him the night the children were born. When he went into the room with the obstetrician to examine his sons, he had already been told what to expect. He showed no signs of grief as he stood over the slat-sided crib, but the corners of his mouth were drawn tight, and his face was almost unnaturally empty of expression. Most strange for a physician, Irene thought, he merely looked at the children and did not touch them. She was sure that in some obscure way he must be blaming himself for what had happened to them.

Later that evening, Irene saw Dr. Couchers sitting in the small conference room at the end of the hall with Dr. Cara Rosen, Corrine Couchers's obstetrician. They were talking earnestly and quietly when Irene passed the open door. Then while she was looking over the assignment sheet at the nursing station, the two of them walked up. Dr. Rosen took a chart from the rack behind the desk and made a notation. After returning the chart, she shook hands with Dr. Couchers, and he left.

It was not until the end of her shift that Irene read the chart; Dr. Rosen's note said that the twin boys were to be given neither food nor water. At first, Irene couldn't believe the order. But when she asked her supervisor, she was told that the supervisor had telephoned Dr. Rosen and that the obstetrician had confirmed the order.

Irene said nothing to the supervisor or to anyone else, but she made her own decision. She believed it was wrong to let the children die, particularly in such a horrible way. They deserved every chance to fight for their lives, and she was going to help them the way she had helped hundreds of other babies in the unit.

For the next week and a half, Irene saw to it that the children were given water and fed the standard infant formula. She did it all herself, on her own initiative. Although some of the other nurses on the floor saw what she was doing, none of them said anything to her. One even smiled and nodded to her when she saw Irene feeding the children.

Apparently someone else also disapproved of the order to let the twins die. Thirteen days after their birth, an investigator from the state Family Welfare Agency appeared in the neonatal ward. The rumor was that his visit had been prompted by an anonymous telephone call.

Late in the afternoon of the day of that visit, the deformed twins were made temporary wards of the Agency, and the orders on the chart were changed—the twins were now to be given food and water. On the next day, the county prosecutor's office announced publicly that it would conduct an investigation of the situation and decide whether criminal charges should be brought against Dr. Couchers or members of the hospital staff.

Irene was sure that she had done the right thing. Nevertheless, she was glad to be relieved of the responsibility.

> *Might a utilitarian argument be offered in defense of Dr. Couchers's decision to allow the twins to die?*
>
> *What criticism of such an argument might Robertson offer?*
>
> *Is there a morally relevant distinction between not treating (and allowing to die) and not providing such minimal needs as food and water (and allowing to die)?*
>
> *Does Engelhardt's line of reasoning support the action taken by Irene Towers?*
>
> *Did Irene Towers exceed the limits of her responsibility, or did she act in a morally heroic way?*
>
> *Proposed federal regulations require that impaired infants be given food and water, even if medical treatment can justifiably be withheld. Are there any moral grounds for making the distinction between treatment and nutritional support?*

Decision Scenario 6 ....

Dr. Daniel McKay and his wife Carol had only a few moments of joy at the birth of their son. They learned almost immediately that the child was severely impaired. Half an hour later, the infant was dead—Dr. McKay, a veterinarian, had slammed him onto the floor of the delivery room.

Mrs. McKay had had problems during pregnancy. An ultrasound test indicated excessive fluid in the uterus, a sign that something might be wrong. Dr. Joaquin Ramos assured the McKays that everything was all right and that the pregnancy should continue. On June 27, 1983, he ordered Mrs. McKay admitted to the Markham, Illinois, hospital so that labor could be induced.

"Don't do any heroic measures," Dr. McKay told Dr. Ramos when Dr. McKay learned that the infant was impaired. Dr. Ramos explained that that was not his choice, for hospital policy required that everything possible be done for babies, even ones like the McKay baby that might not live more than a few months. The child had webbed fingers, heart and lung malfunctions, and missing testicles. It was suspected that the child also had a genetic disorder that might mean kidney malfunctions, mental retardation, and death within months.

Dr. McKay smashed the infant's head against the floor several times, splattering the wall and floor with brain tissue and blood. "Dan, what have you done?" a nurse shouted. Dr. McKay later said that while holding the child he asked himself, "Can I accept and love this child or would it be better off dead?" He had just talked to his wife. "I said to Dan, 'Is it a boy or a girl?' He said it was a little boy. I said, 'Oh, Dan, we got our boy!' Dan really wasn't saying anything. He had tears in his eyes." She then realized that the baby was not crying and asked her husband to go see what was wrong.

Dr. McKay was charged with murder. Two defense psychiatrists testified that he had been temporarily insane. Two others said that he had succumbed to stress. A prosecution psychiatrist said that he was legally sane but that "he made a decision that he had a moral imperative to do what he did." The jury could not agree whether Dr. McKay was guilty, not guilty, guilty but not mentally ill, or not guilty by reason of insanity. A mistrial was declared, but another trial was scheduled.

How might the hospital policy of "doing everything possible" for all impaired infants be criticized in terms of the two standards presented by Arras?

Would any of the authors here endorse such a policy? If so, on what grounds?

Would Arras's relational potential standard justify withholding medical care from the McKay infant?

Might one argue that Dr. McKay's action was morally right, whether or not it was legally justifiable?

Under what conditions, if any, ought the parents of an impaired infant be allowed to decide how the child is to be treated?

CHAPTER 3

EUTHANASIA

CASE PRESENTATION
Karen Quinlan

At two in the morning on Tuesday, April 14, 1975, Mrs. Julie Quinlan was awakened by a telephone call. When she hung up she was crying. "Karen is very sick," Mrs. Quinlan said to her husband Joseph. "She's unconscious, and we have to go to Newton Hospital right away."

The Quinlans thought that their twenty-one-year-old adopted daughter might have been in an automobile accident. But the doctor in the intensive care unit told them that wasn't so. Karen was in a critical comatose state of unknown cause and was being given oxygen through a mask taped over her nose and mouth. She had been brought to the hospital by two friends who had been with her at a birthday party. After a few drinks, she had started to pass out, and her friends decided she must be drunk and put her to bed. Then a girl checked on her later in the evening and found that Karen wasn't breathing. Her friends gave her mouth-to-mouth resuscitation and took her to the nearest hospital.

Blood and urine tests showed that Karen had not consumed a dangerous amount of alcohol. They also showed the presence of .6 milligram percent of aspirin and the tranquilizer Valium. Two milligrams would have been toxic, and five lethal. Why Karen stopped breathing was mysterious. But it was during that time that part of her brain died from oxygen depletion.

After Karen had been unconscious for about a week, she was moved to St. Clare's Hospital in nearby Denville, where testing and life-support facilities were better. Dr. Robert J. Morse, a neurologist, and Dr. Arshad Javed, a pulmonary internist, became her physicians. Additional tests were made. Extensive brain damage was confirmed, and several possible causes of the coma were ruled out.

During the early days, the Quinlans were hopeful. Karen's eyes opened and closed, and her mother and her nineteen-year-old sister, Mary Ellen, thought that they detected signs that she recognized them. But Karen's condition began to deteriorate. Her weight gradually droppped from one hundred twenty pounds to seventy. Her body began to contract into a rigid fetal position, until her five-foot two-inch frame was bent into a shape hardly longer than three feet. She was now breathing mechanically, by means of an MA-1 respirator that pumped air through a tube in her throat.

By early July, Karen's physicians and her mother, sister, and brother had come to believe it was hopeless to expect her ever to regain consciousness. Only her father continued to believe it might be possible. But when he told Dr. Morse about some encouraging sign he had noticed, Dr. Morse said to him "Even if God did perform a miracle so that Karen would live, her damage is so extensive she would spend the rest of her life in an institution." Mr. Quinlan then realized that Karen would never again be as he remembered her. He now agreed with Karen's sister: "Karen would never want to be kept alive on machines like this. She would hate this."

The Quinlan's parish priest, Father Thomas Trapasso, had also assured them that the moral doctrines of the Roman Catholic Church did not require the continuation of extraordinary measures to support a hopeless life. Before making his decision, Mr. Quinlan asked the priest, "Am I playing God?" Father Thomas said, "God has made the decision that Karen is going to die. You're just agreeing with God's decision, that's all."

On July 31, after Karen had been unconscious

for three and a half months, the Quinlans gave Drs. Morse and Jared their permission to take Karen off the respirator. The Quinlans signed a letter authorizing the discontinuance of extraordinary procedures and absolving the hospital from all legal liability. "I think you have come to the right decision," Dr. Morse said to Mr. Quinlan.

But the next morning Dr. Morse called Mr. Quinlan. "I have a moral problem about what we agreed on last night," he said. "I feel I have to consult somebody else and see how he feels about it." The next day, Dr. Morse called again. "I find I will not do it," he said. "And I've informed the administrator at the hospital that I will not do it."

The Quinlans were upset and bewildered by the change in Dr. Morse. Later, they talked with the hospital attorney and were told by him that because Karen was over twenty-one, they were no longer her legal guardians. The Quinlans would have to go to court and be appointed to guardianship. After that, the hospital might or might not remove Karen from the respirator.

Mr. Quinlan consulted attorney Paul Armstrong. Because Karen was an adult without income, Mr. Quinlan explained, Medicare was paying the four hundred and fifty dollars a day it cost to keep her alive. The Quinlans thus had no financial motive in asking that the respirator be taken away. Mr. Quinlan said that his belief that Karen should be allowed to die rested on his conviction that it was God's will, and it was for this reason that he wanted to be appointed Karen's guardian.

Mr. Armstrong filed a plea with Judge Robert Muir of the New Jersey Superior Court on September 12, 1975. He explicitly requested that Mr. Quinlan be appointed Karen's guardian so that he would have "the express power of authorizing the discontinuance of all extraordinary means of sustaining her life." Later, on October 20, Mr. Armstrong argued the case on three constitutional grounds. First, he claimed that there is an implicit right to privacy guaranteed by the Constitution and that this right permits individuals or others acting for them to terminate the use of extraordinary medical measures, even when death may result. This right holds, Armstrong said, unless there are compelling state interests that set it aside.

Second, Armstrong argued that the First Amendment guarantee of religious freedom ex-

tended to the Quinlan case. If the Court did not allow them to act in accordance with the doctrines of their church, their religious liberty would be infringed. Finally, Armstrong appealed to the "cruel and unusual punishment" clause of the Eighth Amendment. He claimed that "for the state to require that Karen Quinlan be kept alive, against her will and the will of her family, after the dignity, beauty, promise and meaning of earthly life have vanished, is cruel and unusual punishment."

Karen's mother, sister, and a friend testified that Karen had often talked about not wanting to be kept alive by machines. An expert witness, a neurologist, testified that Karen was in a "chronic vegetative state" and that it was unlikely that she would ever regain consciousness. Doctors testifying for St. Clare's hospital and Karen's physicians agreed with this. But, they argued, her brain still showed patterns of electrical activity, and she still had a discernible pulse. Thus, she could not be considered dead by legal or medical criteria.

On November 10, Judge Muir ruled against Joseph Quinlan. He praised Mr. Quinlan's character and concern, but he decided that Mr. Quinlan's anguish over his daughter might cloud his judgment about her welfare so he should not be made her guardian. Furthermore, Judge Muir said, because Karen is still medically and legally alive, "the Court should not authorize termination of the respirator. To do so would be homicide and an act of euthanasia."

Mr. Armstrong appealed the decision to the New Jersey Supreme Court. On January 26, 1976, the Court convened to hear arguments, and Mr. Armstrong argued substantially as before. But this time the Court's ruling was favorable. The Court agreed that Mr. Quinlan could assert a right of privacy on Karen's behalf and that whatever he decided for her should be accepted by society. It also set aside any criminal liability for removing the respirator, claiming that if death resulted it would not be homicide and that, even if it were homicide, it would not be unlawful. Finally, the Court stated that if Karen's physicians believed that she would never emerge from her coma, they should consult an ethics committee to be established by St. Clare's Hospital. If the committee accepted their prognosis, then the respirator could be removed. If Karen's present physicians were then unwilling to take her off the respirator, Mr. Quinlan was free to find a physician who would.

Six weeks after the court decision, the respirator still had not been turned off. In fact, another machine, one for controlling body temperature, had been added. Mr. Quinlan met with Morse and Jared and demanded that they remove the respirator. They agreed to "wean" Karen from the machine, and soon she was breathing without mechanical assistance. Dr. Morse and St. Clare's Hospital were determined that Karen would not die while under their care. Although she was moved to a private room, it was next door to the intensive care unit. They intended to put her back on the respirator at the first sign of breathing difficulty.

Because Karen was still alive, the Quinlans began a long search for a chronic-care hospital. Twenty or more institutions turned them away, and physicians expressed great reluctance to become involved in the case. Finally, Dr. Joseph Fennelly volunteered to treat Karen, and on June 9 she was moved from St. Clare's to the Morris View Nursing Home.

Karen Quinlan continued to breathe. She received high-nutrient feedings and regular doses of antibiotics to ward off infections. During some periods she was more active than at others, making reflexive responses to touch and sound.

On June 11, 1985, at 7:01 in the evening, nine years after she lapsed into a coma, Karen Quinlan finally died. She was thirty-one years old.

CASE PRESENTATION
Elizabeth Bouvia's Demand to Starve

On September 3, 1983, Elizabeth Bouvia was admitted, at her own request, to Riverside General Hospital in Riverside, California. She sought admission on the grounds that she was suicidal. She was twenty-six years old, a victim of cerebral palsy, and almost totally paralyzed. She had the partial use of one arm, could speak, and could chew her food if someone fed it to her. In addition to her paralysis, she suffered almost constant pain from arthritis.

Despite the severity of her handicap, Mrs. Bouvia had earned a degree in social work, been married, and lived independently with the assistance of relatives and others. Then matters became particularly difficult for her. She had not been successful in an attempt to have a child, her husband left her, and she lost the state grant that paid for her special transportation needs.

After her admission, Mrs. Bouvia announced to the hospital staff that she wished to starve herself to death. She asked to be provided with hygienic care and painkilling medicines but no food. She explained that she wanted the hospital to be a place where she would "just be left alone and not bothered by friends or family or anyone else" so that she could "ultimately starve to death" and be free from her "useless body."

Mrs. Bouvia refused to eat the solid food offered to her, and her attending physician declared that, if she did not eat, he would have her declared mentally ill and a danger to herself. She could then be force-fed. She responded by calling local newspapers and asking for legal assistance. The American Civil Liberties Union agreed to provide her an attorney, and Richard Stanley Scott became her legal representative.

Mr. Scott convinced her to allow herself to be fed while he made efforts to secure a court order restraining the hospital from either discharging her or force-feeding her. At the court hearing, Mrs. Bouvia testified as to her reasons for refusing nourishment:

> I hate to have someone care for every personal need . . . it's humiliating. It's disgusting, and I choose to no longer do that, no longer to be dependent on someone to take care of me in that manner . . . I am choosing this course of action due to my physical limitation and disability.

Dr. Donald E. Fisher, head of psychiatry at the hospital, testified that he would force-feed Mrs. Bouvia, even if the court ordered him not to.

On behalf of his client, Mr. Scott argued that her decision to refuse nourishment was "exactly medically and morally analogous to the patient deciding to forego further kidney dialysis," knowingly accepting death as the consequence.

Judge John H. Hews refused to grant the restraining order. He expressed the view that Mrs. Bouvia was a competent, rational, and sincere person whose decision was based on her physical condition and not upon her recent misfortunes. Nevertheless, allowing her to starve herself to death in the hospital would "have a profound effect" on the staff, other patients, and other handicapped people. Mrs. Bouvia, Judge Hews held, was "not terminal" and might expect to live another fifteen to twenty years. Accordingly, he held that "the established ethics of the medical profession clearly outweigh and overcome her own rights of self-determination," and "forced feeding, however invasive, would be administered for the purpose of saving the life of an otherwise nonterminal patient and should be permitted. There is no other reasonable option." In effect, in Judge Hews's view, Mrs. Bouvia had a right to commit suicide, but she did not have the right to have others assist her.

Mrs. Bouvia later refused to eat, and Judge Hews authorized the hospital to feed her against her will. Her attorney argued that this was an unlawful invasion of her privacy and appealed to the California Supreme Court. The Court unanimously refused to grant a hearing on the appeal, thus allowing the lower court ruling to stand.

In February 1986, Mrs. Bouvia was back in court. Through her attorney, she sought an injunction to stop High Desert Hospital of Lancaster, California, where she had become a patient, from using a nasogastric tube to feed her against her wishes. In a public statement, she accounted that she had no intention to attempt to starve herself to death, but wished only to receive a liquid diet. The hospital's physicians and lawyers maintained that a liquid diet would be a form of starvation and that the law precluded them from agreeing to her demand. The eventual court decision was again in favor of Mrs. Bouvia, and in April the feeding tube was removed.

However, the controversy between Mrs. Bouvia and the hospital did not end. Because of her constant pain, Mrs. Bouvia was receiving a steady infusion of morphine by means of an implanted pump. The hospital informed her that, because morphine is "too addictive," she would be withdrawn from the drug, and other non-narcotic drugs prescribed.

Mrs. Bouvia expressed fear and dismay at the prospect. Morphine, she said, was the only drug that had helped ease her pain and keep her comfortable for a long period of time. Also, detoxification would be agonizing. In her view, the hospital intended to withdraw the morphine in order to punish her for her lawsuit.

S. J. Carnevale, the hospital's attorney, denied that this was so. "I know she says this is in retaliation for her lawsuit. But the hospital has been planning this for a while. She was told of the decision a few days before the appeals court ruled." Furthermore, Mr. Carnevale said, "According to the appeals court, Mrs. Bouvia won the right to refuse medical treatment. But I know of no law that says she is entitled to prescribe her own medicine."

The hospital proceeded with its plan, but on April 24, 1986, the California Superior Court ordered the hospital to restore Mrs. Bouvia's dosage of morphine. A hearing on the matter was scheduled.

CASE PRESENTATION
The Death of J. K. Collums

On November 16, 1981, sixty-nine-year-old Woodrow Collums went into the Oak Hills Care Center in the small town of Poteet, Texas, to visit his seventy-two-year-old brother J. K. Collums. J. K. was a victim of Alzheimer's disease, a poorly understood illness in which the brain undergoes progressive degeneration. J. K. had already reached the point of being unable to care for any of his bodily needs, and he could no longer speak or respond to others. A nasogastric tube fed him the nutrients needed to keep him alive.

"I just stood there and looked at him a few minutes," Woody Collums said about his brother. "He was beyond saying anything to me. So I left and went back to the car, thinking I'd just go on and let the Lord take care of it. But I got to the car, and this gun was in the car."

Mr. Collums decided to shoot his brother, and took the gun back into the room. But once there, he changed his mind. "So I started to leave, and I looked back at him, and I just couldn't go off and leave him like that. I turned around and shot him five times, just as fast as I could shoot him. He never moved. He was the most peaceful looking guy you've ever seen."

Mr. Collums then checked his brother's pulse to be sure that he was dead. He put the pistol down on a bedside tray, and waited for someone to call the police. While waiting, he said to a staff member, "I've killed horses, cows, and dogs that were suffering. He's suffered long enough."

Mr. Collums freely admitted shooting his brother, but he refused to acknowledge that he had murdered him. "I feel like he's been dead since he's been in this condition," he said.

A Bexar County, Texas, grand jury indicted Mr. Collums for the shooting of his brother. But even the county prosecutors regarded the action as a clear case of mercy killing. The two brothers had been very close all their lives, and, although J. K. Collums had not signed an actual "living will," which is legal in Texas, he had written a letter to his physician in which he expressed his views about being kept alive by extraordinary means. According to J. K. Collums's wife Helen, he said that "if they couldn't do something to help his brain, to please put him to sleep forever." The letter was written before the disease had progressed to the point that he was no longer able to reason and communicate.

When asked if she blamed her brother-in-law for his actions, Helen Collums said, "Oh, no! God, no, no!" She went on to say, "I thank God Jim's out of his misery. I hate to think it had to be done the way it was done, but I understand it. I couldn't ever have shot him. I could have asked for the life supports to be taken away, because I don't believe

in life supports. I just think it's cruelty for someone who's terminally ill, to stuff a tube down his nose from May to November. That's agony and cruelty. People don't know about these things. I just hope it helps somebody else, so they don't have to go through what he went through."

Helen Collums now believes she should not have allowed the stomach tube to be put into place. But once it had been, other members of the family refused to allow it to be removed. They thought removing it would constitute murder. Besides, it was not clear that the nursing home would agree to its removal. Court decisions allow the removal of support systems that are "extraordinary means" of prolonging life when the patient has "clearly and convincingly" rejected the use of such means beforehand. But is a feeding tube "extraordinary"?

Woodrow Collums received much public sympathy, but not everyone approved of his action. Theresa Brock, the administrator of the Oak Hills Care Center, expressed the opposition view. "None of us knows," she said, "and nobody here can tell you, nobody on this earth can tell you, what Jim was able to feel, or perceive, or think or know, and it's not up to any of us to end somebody's life for them."

Everyone agreed that J. K. Collums could still recognize his wife and could still pucker his lips as if to kiss her. He did just that on the day that he died.

In February of 1982, Woodrow Collums pleaded guilty to a charge of murder. He waived a jury trial, and at a punishment hearing he told Judge Tom Rickhoff about what he had done. Mr. Collums said of his brother, "He looked like he was just begging me to get him out of his misery. I regret having to do what I did, but I don't regret doing it. I felt he would have done it himself if he could have."

Mr. Collums's lawyer, Roy Barrera, expressed the hope that the hearing would help people understand the need for euthanasia. "If we can do mercy killings for animals to relieve pain and suffering," he said, "I just can't see where under the proper conditions a human being would be given any less than what we give animals."

Judge Rickhoff was faced with the decision of whether to send Mr. Collums to jail or to put him on probation. On March 4, Judge Rickhoff ruled that Mr. Collums was to be placed on probation for a period of ten years. During that time, he would be required to spend ten hours each week working at homes for the elderly.

INTRODUCTION

Death comes to us all. We hope that when it comes it will be swift and allow us to depart without prolonged suffering, our dignity intact. We also hope that it will not force burdens on our family and friends, making them pay both financially and emotionally by our lingering and hopeless condition.

Such considerations give euthanasia a strong appeal. Should we not be able to snip the thread of life when the weight of suffering and hopelessness grows too heavy to bear? The answer to this question is not so easy as it may seem, for hidden within it are a number of complicated moral issues.

Just what is euthanasia? The word comes from the Greek for "good death," and in English it has come to have the meaning "easy death." But this does very little to help us understand the concept. For consider this: if we give ourselves an easy death, are we committing suicide? If we assist someone else to an easy death (with or without that person's permission), are we committing murder? Anyone who opposed killing (either of one's self or of others) on moral grounds might also consider it necessary to object to euthanasia.

It may be, however, that the answer to both of these questions is no. But if it is, then it is necessary to specify the conditions that distinguish euthanasia from both suicide and murder. Only then would it be possible to argue, without contradiction, that euthanasia is morally acceptable but the other two forms of killing are not. (Someone believing that suicide is morally legitimate would not object to euthanasia carried out by the person herself, but he would still have to deal with the problem posed by the euthanasia/murder issue.)

ACTIVE AND PASSIVE EUTHANASIA

We have talked of euthanasia as though it involved directly taking the life of a person, either one's own life or the life of another. However, some philosophers distinguish between "active euthanasia" and "passive euthanasia," which in turn rests on a distinction between *killing* and *letting die*. To kill someone (including one's self) is to take a definite action to end his or her life (administering a lethal injection, for example). To allow someone to die, by contrast, is to take no steps to prolong a person's life when those steps seem called for (failing to give an injection of antibiotics, for example). Active euthanasia, then, is direct killing and is an act of commission. Passive euthanasia is an act of omission.

This distinction is used in most contemporary codes of medical ethics (that of the American Medical Association, for example) and is also recognized in the Anglo-American tradition of law. Except in special circumstances, it is illegal to deliberately cause the death of another person. It is not, however, illegal (except in special circumstances) to allow a person to die. Clearly, one might consider active euthanasia morally wrong while recognizing passive euthanasia as morally legitimate.

Some philosophers, however, have argued that the active-passive distinction is morally irrelevant with respect to euthanasia. Both are cases of causing death, and it is the circumstances in which death is caused, not the manner of causing it, that is of moral importance. (This is the claim defended by James Rachels in his essay "Active and Passive Euthanasia," included in this chapter.) Furthermore, the active-passive distinction is not always clear-cut. If a person dies after special life-sustaining equipment has been withdrawn, is this a case of active or passive euthanasia? Or is it a case of euthanasia at all?

VOLUNTARY AND NONVOLUNTARY EUTHANASIA

Philosophers and other writers on euthanasia have often thought it important to distinguish between *voluntary* and *nonvoluntary* euthanasia. Voluntary euthanasia includes cases in which a person takes his or her own life, either directly or by refusing treatment. But it also includes cases in which a person deputizes another to act in accordance with his wishes. Thus, a person might instruct her family not to permit the use of artificial support systems, should she become unconscious, suffer from brain damage, and be unable to speak for herself. Or a person might request that he be given a lethal injection, after suffering third-degree burns over most of his body and being told that he has virtually no hope of recovery. That the individual explicitly consents to death is a necessary feature of voluntary euthanasia.

Nonvoluntary (or involuntary) euthanasia includes those cases in which the decision about death is not made by the person who is to die. Here the person gives no specific consent or instructions, and the decision is made by family, friends, or physician. The distinction between voluntary and nonvoluntary euthanasia is not always a clear one. Physicians sometimes assume that people are "asking" to die, even when no explicit request has been made. Also the wishes and attitudes that people express when they are *not* in extreme life-threatening medical situations may be too vague for us to be certain that they would choose death when they are in such a situation. Is "I never want to be hooked up to one of those machines" an adequate indication that the person who says

this does not want to be put on a respirator should he meet with an accident and fall into a comatose state?

If the distinctions we have made are considered legitimate and relevant, it is clear that there are six cases in which euthanasia becomes a moral decision:

1. Self-administered euthanasia
    a. active
    b. passive

2. Other-administered euthanasia
    a. active and voluntary
    b. active and nonvoluntary
    c. passive and voluntary
    d. passive and nonvoluntary

Even these possibilities do not exhaust the cases that euthanasia presents us with. For example, notice that the voluntary/nonvoluntary distinction does not appear in connection with self-administered euthanasia in our scheme. It might be argued that it should, for a person's decision to end his life (actively or passively) may well not be a wholly voluntary or free decision. People who are severely depressed by their illness and decide to end their lives, for example, might not be thought of as having made a voluntary choice. Hence, one might approve of self-administered voluntary euthanasia, yet think that the nonvoluntary form should not be permitted. It should not be allowed not because it is necessarily morally wrong, but because it would not be a genuine decision by the person. The person might be thought of as suffering from a psychiatric disability.

ETHICAL THEORIES AND EUTHANASIA

Roman Catholicism explicitly rejects all forms of euthanasia as against the natural law duty to preserve life. It considers euthanasia as morally identical with either suicide or murder. This position is not as rigid as it may seem, however. As we have already seen in the introductory chapter and in the last chapter, the principle of double effect makes it morally acceptable to give medication for the relief of pain—even if the indirect result of the medication will be to shorten the life of the recipient. The intended result is not the death of the person but the relief of suffering. The difference in intention is thus considered to be a morally significant one. Those not accepting the principle of double effect would be likely to classify the administration of a substance that would relieve pain but would also cause death as a case of euthanasia.

Furthermore, on the Catholic view there is no moral obligation to continue treatment when a person is medically hopeless. It is legitimate to allow people to die as a result of their illness or injury, even though their lives might be lengthened by the use of extraordinary means. Additionally, we may legitimately make the same decisions about ourselves that we make about others who are in no condition to decide. Thus, without intending to kill ourselves, we may choose measures for the relief of pain that may secondarily hasten our end. Or we may refuse extraordinary treatment and let "nature" take its course, let "God's will" determine the outcome. (See the introductory chapter for a fuller discussion of the Roman Catholic position on euthanasia and extraordinary means of sustaining life.)

At first sight, utilitarianism would seem to endorse euthanasia in all of its forms. Whenever suffering is great and the condition of the person is one without legitimate medical hope, then the principle of utility might be invoked to approve putting the person to death. After all, in such a case we seem to be acting to end suffering and to bring about a state of affairs in which happiness exceeds unhappiness. Thus, whether the person concerned is ourself or another, euthanasia would seem to be a morally right action.

A utilitarian might argue in this way, but this is not the only way in which the principle of utility might be applied. It could be argued, for example, that, since life is a necessary condition for happiness, it is wrong to destroy that condition, because, by doing so, the possibility of all future happiness is lost. Furthermore, a rule utilitarian might well argue that a rule like "The taking of a human life is permissible when suffering is intense and the condition of the person permits no legitimate hope" would be open to abuse. Consequently, in the long run the rule would actually work to increase the amount of unhappiness in the world. Obviously, it is not possible to say there is such a thing as "the utilitarian view of euthanasia. The principle of utility supplies a guide for an answer, but it is not itself an answer.

Euthanasia presents a considerable difficulty for Kant's ethics. For Kant, an autonomous rational being has a duty to preserve his or her life. Thus, one cannot rightly refuse needed medical care or commit suicide. Yet our status as autonomous rational beings also endows us with an inherent dignity. If that status is destroyed or severely compromised, as it is when people become comatose and unknowing because of illness or injury, then it is not certain that we have a duty to maintain our lives under such conditions. It may be more in keeping with our freedom and dignity for us to instruct others either to put us to death or to take no steps to keep us alive should we ever be in such a state. Voluntary euthanasia may be compatible with (if not required by) Kant's ethics.

By a similar line of reasoning, it may be that nonvoluntary euthanasia might be seen as a duty that we have to others. We might argue that by putting to death a comatose and hopeless person we are recognizing the dignity that person possessed in his or her previous state. Also, as we mentioned in the last chapter, it might also be argued that a human being in a vegetative state is not a person in the relevant moral sense. Thus, our ordinary duty to preserve life does not hold.

According to Ross, we have a strong prima facie obligation not to kill a person except in justifiable self-defense—unless we have an even stronger prima facie moral obligation to do something that cannot be done without killing. Since active euthanasia typically requires taking the life of an innocent person, there is a moral presumption against it. However, another of Ross's prima facie obligations is that we keep promises made to others. Accordingly, if someone who is now in an irreversible coma with no hope of recovery has left instructions that in case of such an event's happening she wishes her life to be ended, then we are under a prima facie obligation to follow her instructions. Thus, in such a case, we may be justified in overriding the presumption against taking an innocent life.

What if there are no such instructions? It could be argued that our prima facie obligation of acting beneficently toward others requires us to attempt to determine what someone's wishes would be from what we know about him as a person. We would then treat him the way that we believe that he would want us to. In the absence of any relevant information, we might make the decision on the basis of how a rational person would want to be treated in similar circumstances. Of course, if anyone has left instructions that his life is to be maintained, if possible, under any circumstances, then we have a prima facie obligation to respect this preference also.

THE SELECTIONS

The selections that make up this chapter represent the diversity of issues and responses the problem of euthanasia poses. Peter Singer argues for the moral rightness of voluntary euthanasia, even in those cases in which it is fundamentally the same as assisted suicide. He attempts to show that classical and preference utilitarianism, a theory

of what it is to have a right to life, and a respect for the autonomy of rational agents all count as reasons favoring euthanasia. Technical objections to legalizing even active euthanasia, he believes, can be met by employing particular procedural safeguards.

J. Gay-Williams's "The Wrongfulness of Euthanasia" presents a statement of the conservative view. He defines "euthanasia" as intentionally taking the life of a person who is believed to be suffering from some illness or injury from which recovery cannot reasonably be expected. Gay-Williams rejects passive euthanasia as a *name* for actions that are usually designated by the phrase but seems to approve of the actions themselves. He argues that euthanasia as intentional killing goes against natural law because it violates the natural inclination to preserve life. Furthermore, both self-interest and possible practical consequences of euthanasia provide reasons for rejecting it.

The traditional view that there is an important moral difference between active and passive euthanasia is one accepted by J. Gay-Williams. Active euthanasia involves killing, and passive euthanasia letting die, and this fact has led many physicians and philosophers to reject active euthanasia as morally wrong, even while approving of passive euthanasia. James Rachels's essay challenges both the use and moral significance of the distinction. Since both forms of euthanasia result in the death of a person, Rachels argues that active euthanasia ought to be preferred to passive. It is more humane because it allows suffering to be brought to a speedy end. Furthermore, Rachels claims, the distinction itself can be shown to be morally irrelevant. Is there, he asks, any genuine moral difference between drowning a child and merely watching a child drown and doing nothing to save it?

Finally, Rachels attempts to show that the bare fact that there is a difference between killing and letting die doesn't make active euthanasia wrong. Killing of any kind is right or wrong depending on the intentions and circumstances in which it takes place, and, if the intentions and circumstances are of a certain kind, then active euthanasia can be morally right.

For these reasons, Rachels suggests that the approval given to the active-passive euthanasia distinction in the Code of Ethics of the American Medical Association is unwise. He encourages physicians to rely upon the distinction only to the extent that they are forced to do so by law but not to give it any significant moral weight. In particular, they should not make use of it when writing new policies or guidelines.

Because of Rachels's concern with the active-passive distinction, he focuses most attention on nonvoluntary euthanasia. By contrast, Peter Singer, in the selection presented here, is concerned exclusively with voluntary euthanasia. Nonvoluntary euthanasia, as characterized by Singer, involves the killing of "a merely conscious being," whereas voluntary euthanasia involves "the killing of a person, a rational and self-conscious being." Hence, according to Singer, it is a more serious matter.

The presumption against killing a person is supported by the classical utilitarian claim that to kill someone puts others in fear of their lives and the preference utilitarian claim that the desire of a person to live is a reason not to kill her. Further, the presumption is supported by the notion that having a right to life means being able to desire one's continued existence and by the respect we have for the decisions of autonomous agents to maintain their lives.

Singer argues that these four grounds for holding that it is usually wrong to kill a person do not prohibit killing in cases in which a competent person is suffering from a painful and incurable disease. Indeed, these same considerations show that voluntary euthanasia is fully justified. In Singer's view, the objections to legalizing voluntary active eutha-

nasia are basically technical ones that can be met by employing certain procedural safeguards. Hence, Singer supports the general thesis that active voluntary euthanasia is morally permissible, even in those cases in which it is fundamentally the same as assisted suicide.

The 1976 decision of the New Jersey Supreme Court in the case of Karen Quinlan was significant in establishing that a legally based right of privacy permits a patient to decide to refuse medical treatment. The Court also held that this right can be exercised by a parent or guardian when the patient herself is in no position to do so. Thus, in the opinion of the Court, removal of life-sustaining equipment would not be a case of homicide (or any other kind of wrongful killing), even if the patient should die as a result.

The ruling in the Quinlan case has had an enormous impact on decisions about discontinuing extraordinary medical measures. However, the ruling has been generally construed rather narrowly so as to apply only to mentally incompetent patients who are brain-dead, comatose, or in an irreversible coma.

The 1985 decision of the New Jersey Supreme Court in the Conroy case is regarded by some observers as setting a precedent comparable in significance to that in the Quinlan case. Although, like the Quinlan decision, the ruling is binding only in New Jersey, it too is likely to have an impact on court decisions and medical practices throughout the country.

In particular, the Conroy decision broadens the class of patients from whom it may be legitimate to withdraw or withhold life-sustaining medical care. Patients who are terminally ill and mentally incompetent, although not brain-dead or comatose, may have care discontinued. Further, and of equal significance, the Court rejects the distinction between ordinary and extraordinary measures and so permits artificial feeding to be discontinued. (Thus, the principle of the ruling would have allowed Karen Quinlan's nutritional support to be withdrawn also.) The decision was limited to incompetent, elderly patients in nursing homes, and it is not yet clear how much influence it is likely to have in connection with patients in other circumstances.

Justice Sidney Schreiber, the author of the majority opinion, bases the decision on the common law and constitutional right of a competent individual to accept or reject any medical treatment, even treatment necessary to preserve one's life. In this, he follows the Quinlan decision. The issue for individuals who are no longer mentally competent becomes one of substituted judgment. If their right to self-determination is to be exercised, then someone else must make a decision on their behalf. Justice Schreiber outlines three "tests" that may be employed to determine whether treatment may be withheld or discontinued. All three require considering evidence relevant to determining the patient's past desires and attitudes and present experiences of pain and enjoyment. The Court specifically disapproved of any decision to withdraw treatment based on an assessment of the "personal worth" or "social utility" of a patient's life.

Justice Schreiber also expresses the view that the type of treatment involved in a particular case is irrelevant to the decision. He rejects as "unpersuasive" the distinctions between active and passive actions, withholding and withdrawing treatment, ordinary and extraordinary measures, and artificial feeding and medical treatment.

Like so many issues, euthanasia has traditionally been discussed only in the back rooms of medicine. Often decisions about whether to allow a patient to die are made by physicians acting on their own authority. Such decisions do not represent so much an arrogant claim to godlike wisdom as an acknowledgment of the physician's obligation to do what is best for the patient. Most physicians admit that allowing or helping a patient to die is sometimes the best assistance that can be given. Decisions made in this fashion depend on the beliefs and judgment of particular physicians. Because these may differ from those of the patient concerned, it is quite possible that the physician's decision may differ from the wishes of the patient.

But covert decisions made by a physician acting alone are becoming practices of the past as euthanasia is discussed more widely and openly. Court cases, such as Quinlan and now Conroy, have both widened the scope of legally permissible actions and reinforced the notion that an individual has a right to refuse or discontinue life-sustaining medical treatment. Such cases have also made it clear that there are limits to the benefits that can be derived from medicine, and that under some conditions, individuals may be better off if everything that technologically can be done is not done. Increasingly, people want to be sure that they have some say in what happens to them should they fall victim to hopeless injury or illness.

One indication of this newly developing interest is the California "Natural Death Act," passed by the California legislature on August 30, 1977. The act permits a competent adult to sign a directive that will authorize physicians to withhold or discontinue "mechanical" or "artificial" life-support equipment if the person is judged to be "terminal" and if "death is imminent."

The strength of the bill is that it allows a person to express in an explicit manner how he or she wishes to be treated before treatment is needed. In this way, the autonomy of the individual is recognized. Even though unconscious or comatose, a person can continue to exert control over his or her life. This, in turn, means that physicians need not—and should not—be the decisive voice in deciding upon the continuation or use of special medical equipment.

But some critics of the bill claim that it

does not go far enough in protecting autonomy and making death easier, where this is what is wanted. They point out the directive specified in the bill would have made no difference in the case of Karen Quinlan. She had not been diagnosed as having a "terminal condition" at least two weeks prior to being put on a respirator, yet this is one of the requirements of the act. Consequently, the directive would have been irrelevant to her condition.

Nor, for that matter, would those people be allowed to die who wish to, if their disease or injury does not involve treatment by "artificial" or "mechanical" means. Thus, a person suffering from throat cancer would simply have to bear the pain and wait for a "natural" death. Also, it is not clear that all courts or physicians are likely to follow the lead of Justice Schreiber and consider provision of nutrition a form of artificial treatment.

However, in favor of such directives, it should be said that had J. K. Collums signed the one that is legal in the state of Texas, then he could have avoided being attached to a life-support system.

Whatever may be thought of the merits of the Natural Death Act, that it exists at all is a sure indication that more public attention is being given to euthanasia than ever before.

Although the California bill was the first of its kind, a number of other states have now also adopted "right-to-die" legislation.

Another sign of change is the recent concern with the medical circumstances in which people die. The medical ideal of a "hospital death," one in which the patient's temperature, pulse rate, and respiration are brought within normal limits by medication and machinery, is being severely challenged. This is reflected in the policy adopted in 1986 by the AMA that holds that it may be morally appropriate to withhold "all means of life prolonging medical treatment," including artificial feeding, from patients in irreversible comas.

A new ideal of natural death also seems to be emerging. In this view, the kind of support a dying patient needs is psychological counseling and contact with family and friends, rather than heroic medical efforts. An acceptance of death as a normal end of life and the development of new means of caring for the dying may ease the problem of euthanasia. If those who are hopeless and near death are offered an alternative to either euthanasia or an all-out medical effort to preserve their lives, they may choose that alternative. "Death with dignity" need not always mean choosing a lethal injection.

The Wrongfulness of Euthanasia

J. Gay-Williams

My impression is that euthanasia—the idea, if not the practice—is slowly gaining acceptance within our society. Cynics might attribute this to an increasing tendency to devalue human life, but I do not believe this is the major factor. The acceptance is much more likely to be the result of unthinking sympathy and benevolence. Well-publicized, tragic stories like that of Karen Quinlan

elicit from us deep feelings of compassion. We think to ourselves, "She and her family would be better off if she were dead." It is an easy step from this very human response to the view that if someone (and others) would be better off dead, then it must be all right to kill that person.[1] Although I respect the compassion that leads to this conclusion, I believe the conclusion is wrong. I want to show that euthanasia is wrong. It is inherently wrong, but it is also wrong judged from the standpoints of self-interest and of practical effects.

Before presenting my arguments to support this claim, it would be well to define "euthanasia." An essential aspect of euthanasia is that it involves taking a human life, either one's own or that of another. Also, the person whose life is taken must be someone who is believed to be suffering from some disease or injury from which recovery cannot reasonably be expected. Finally, the action must be deliberate and intentional. Thus, euthanasia is intentionally taking the life of a presumably hopeless person. Whether the life is one's own or that of another, the taking of it is still euthanasia.

It is important to be clear about the deliberate and intentional aspect of the killing. If a hopeless person is given an injection of the wrong drug by mistake and this causes his death, this is wrongful killing but not euthanasia. The killing cannot be the result of accident. Furthermore, if the person is given an injection of a drug that is believed to be necessary to treat his disease or better his condition and the person dies as a result, then this is neither wrongful killing nor euthanasia. The intention was to make the patient well, not kill him. Similarly, when a patient's condition is such that it is not reasonable to hope that any medical procedures or treatments will save his life, a failure to implement the procedures or treatments is not euthanasia. If the person dies, this will be as a result of his injuries or disease and not because of his failure to receive treatment.

The failure to continue treatment after it has been realized that the patient has little chance of benefitting from it has been characterized by some as "passive euthanasia." This phrase is misleading and mistaken.[2] In such cases, the person involved is not killed (the first essential aspect of euthanasia), nor is the death of the person intended by the withholding of additional treatment (the third essential aspect of euthanasia). The aim may be to spare the person additional and unjustifiable pain, to save him from the indignities of hopeless manipulations, and to avoid increasing the financial and emotional burden on his family. When I buy a pencil it is so that I can use it to write, not to contribute to an increase in the gross national product. This may be the unintended consequence of my action, but it is not the aim of my action. So it is with failing to continue the treatment of a dying person. I intend his death no more than I intend to reduce the GNP by not using medical supplies. His is an unintended dying, and so-called "passive euthanasia" is not euthanasia at all.

1. The Argument from Nature

Every human being has a natural inclination to continue living. Our reflexes and responses fit us to fight attackers, flee wild animals, and dodge out of the way of trucks. In our daily lives we exercise the caution and care necessary to protect ourselves. Our bodies are similarly structured for survival right down to the molecular level. When we are cut, our capillaries seal shut, our blood clots, and fibrogen is produced to start the process of healing the wound. When we are invaded by bacteria, antibodies are produced to fight against the alien organisms, and their remains are swept out of the body by special cells designed for clean-up work.

Euthanasia does violence to this natural goal of survival. It is literally acting against nature because all the processes of nature are bent towards the end of bodily survival. Euthanasia defeats these subtle mechanisms in a way that, in a particular case, disease and injury might not.

It is possible, but not necessary, to make an appeal to revealed religion in this connection.[3] Man as trustee of his body acts against God, its rightful possessor, when he takes his own life. He also violates the commandment to hold life sacred and never to take it without just and compelling cause. But since this appeal will persuade only those who are prepared to accept that religion has access to revealed truths, I shall not employ this line of argument.

It is enough, I believe, to recognize that the organization of the human body and our patterns of behavioral responses make the continuation of life a natural goal. By reason alone, then, we can recognize that euthanasia sets us against our own nature.[4] Furthermore, in doing so, euthanasia does violence to our dignity. Our dignity comes from seeking our ends. When one of our goals is survival, and actions are taken that eliminate that goal, then our natural dignity suffers. Unlike animals, we are conscious through reason of our nature and our ends. Euthanasia involves acting as if this dual nature—inclination towards survival and awareness of this as an end—did not exist. Thus, euthanasia denies our basic human character and requires that we regard ourselves or others as something less than fully human.

2. The Argument from Self-Interest

The above arguments are, I believe, sufficient to show that euthanasia is inherently wrong. But there are reasons for considering it wrong when judged by standards other than reason. Because death is final and irreversible, euthanasia contains within it the possibility that we will work against our own interest if we practice it or allow it to be practiced on us.

Contemporary medicine has high standards of excellence and a proven record of accomplishment, but it does not possess perfect and complete knowledge. A mistaken diagnosis is possible, and so is a mistaken prognosis. Consequently, we may believe that we are dying of a disease when, as a matter of fact, we may not be. We may think that we have no hope of recovery when, as a matter of fact, our chances are quite good. In such circumstances, if euthanasia were permitted, we would die needlessly. Death is final and the chance of error too great to approve the practice of euthanasia.

Also, there is always the possibility that an experimental procedure or a hitherto untried technique will pull us through. We should at least keep this option open, but euthanasia closes it off. Furthermore, spontaneous remission does occur in many cases. For no apparent reason, a patient simply recovers when those all around him, including his physicians, expected him to die. Euthanasia would just guarantee their expectations and leave no room for the "miraculous" recoveries that frequently occur.

Finally, knowing that we can take our life at any time (or ask another to take it) might well incline us to give up too easily. The will to live is strong in all of us, but it can be weakened by pain and suffering and feelings of hopelessness. If during a bad time we allow ourselves to be killed, we never have a chance to reconsider. Recovery from a serious illness requires that we fight for it, and anything that weakens our determination by suggesting that there is an easy way out is ultimately against our own interest. Also, we may be inclined towards euthanasia because of our concern for others. If we see our sickness and suffering as an emotional and financial burden on our family, we may feel that to leave our life is to make their lives easier.[5] The very presence of the possibility of euthanasia may keep us from surviving when we might.

3. The Argument from Practical Effects

Doctors and nurses are, for the most part, totally committed to saving lives. A life lost is, for them, almost a personal failure, an insult to their skills and knowledge. Euthanasia as a practice might well alter this. It could have a corrupting influence so that in any case that is severe doctors and nurses might not try hard enough to save the patient. They might decide that the patient would simply be "better off dead" and take the steps necessary to make that come about. This attitude could then carry over to their dealings with patients less seriously ill. The result would be an overall decline in the quality of medical care.

Finally, euthanasia as a policy is a slippery slope. A person apparently hopelessly ill may be allowed to take his own life. Then he may be permitted to deputize others to do it for him should he no longer be able to act. The judgment of others then becomes the ruling factor. Already at this point euthanasia is not personal and voluntary, for others are acting "on behalf of" the patient as they see fit. This may well incline them to act on behalf of other patients who have not authorized them to exercise their judgment. It is only a short step, then, from voluntary euthanasia (self-inflicted or authorized), to directed euthanasia administered to a patient who has given no authorization, to involuntary euthanasia conducted as part of a social policy.[6] Recently many psychiatrists and sociologists have argued that we define as "mental illness" those forms of behavior that we disapprove of.[7] This gives us license then to lock up those who display the behavior. The category of the "hopelessly ill" provides the possibility of even worse abuse. Embedded in a social policy, it would give society or its representatives the authority to eliminate all those who might be considered too ''ill'' to function normally any longer. The dangers of euthanasia are too great to all to run the risk of approving it in any form. The first slippery step may well lead to a serious and harmful fall.

I hope that I have succeeded in showing why the benevolence that inclines us to give approval of euthanasia is misplaced. Euthanasia is inherently wrong because it violates the nature and dignity of human beings. But even those who are not convinced by this must be persuaded that the potential personal and social dangers inherent in euthanasia are sufficient to forbid our approving it either as a personal practice or as a public policy.

Suffering is surely a terrible thing, and we have a clear duty to comfort those in need and to ease their suffering when we can. But suffering is also a natural part of life with values for the individual and for others that we should not overlook. We may legitimately seek for others and for ourselves an easeful death, as Arthur Dyck has pointed out.[8] Euthanasia, however, is not just an easeful death. It is a wrongful death. Euthanasia is not just dying. It is killing.

Notes

1. For a sophisticated defense of this position see Philippa Foot, ''Euthanasia,'' *Philosophy and Public Affairs*, vol. 6 (1977), pp. 85–112. Foot does not endorse the radical conclusion that euthanasia, voluntary and involuntary, is always right.

2. James Rachels rejects the distinction between active and passive euthanasia as morally irrelevant in his ''Active and Passive Euthanasia,'' *New England Journal of Medicine*, vol. 292, pp. 78–80. But see the criticism by Foot, pp. 100–103.

3. For a defense of this view see J. V. Sullivan, ''The Immorality of Euthanasia,'' in *Beneficent Euthanasia*, ed. Marvin Kohl (Buffalo, New York: Prometheus Books, 1975), pp. 34–44.

4. This point is made by Ray V. McIntyre in ''Voluntary Euthanasia: The Ultimate Perversion,'' *Medical Counterpoint*, vol. 2, pp. 26–29.

5. See McIntyre, p. 28.

6. See Sullivan, ''Immorality of Euthanasia,'' pp. 34–44, for a fuller argument in support of this view.

7. See, for example, Thomas S. Szasz, *The Myth of Mental Illness*, rev. ed. (New York: Harper & Row, 1974).

8. Arthur Dyck, ''Beneficent Euthanasia and Benemortasia,'' Kohl, op. cit., pp. 117–129.

Active and Passive Euthanasia

James Rachels

The distinction between active and passive euthanasia is thought to be crucial for medical ethics. The idea is that it is permissible, at least in some cases, to withhold treatment and allow a patient to die, but it is never permissible to take any direct action designed to kill the patient. This doctrine seems to be accepted by most doctors, and it is endorsed in a statement adopted by the House of Delegates of the American Medical Association on December 4, 1973:

> The intentional termination of the life of one human being by another—mercy killing—is contrary to that for which the medical

profession stands and is contrary to the policy of the American Medical Association.

The cessation of the employment of extraordinary means to prolong the life of the body when there is irrefutable evidence that biological death is imminent is the decision of the patient and/or his immediate family. The advice and judgment of the physician should be freely available to the patient and/or his immediate family.

However, a strong case can be made against this doctrine. In what follows I will set out some of the relevant arguments, and urge doctors to reconsider their views on this matter.

Reprinted by permission from the New England Journal of Medicine 292, no. 2 (January 9, 1975): 78–80.

To begin with a familiar type of situation, a patient who is dying of incurable cancer of the throat is in terrible pain, which can no longer be satisfactorily alleviated. He is certain to die within a few days, even if present treatment is continued, but he does not want to go on living for those days since the pain is unbearable. So he asks the doctor for an end to it, and his family joins in the request.

Suppose the doctor agrees to withhold treatment, as the conventional doctrine says he may. The justification for his doing so is that the patient is in terrible agony, and since he is going to die anyway, it would be wrong to prolong his suffering needlessly. But now notice this. If one simply withholds treatment, it may take the patient longer to die, and so he may suffer more than he would if more direct action were taken and a lethal injection given. This fact provides strong reason for thinking that, once the initial decision not to prolong his agony has been made, active euthanasia is actually preferable to passive euthanasia, rather than the reverse. To say otherwise is to endorse the option that leads to more suffering rather than less, and is contrary to the humanitarian impulse that prompts the decision not to prolong his life in the first place.

Part of my point is that the process of being "allowed to die" can be relatively slow and painful, whereas being given a lethal injection is relatively quick and painless. Let me give a different sort of example. In the United States about one in 600 babies is born with Down's syndrome. Most of these babies are otherwise healthy—that is, with only the usual pediatric care, they will proceed to an otherwise normal infancy. Some, however, are born with congenital defects such as intestinal obstructions that require operations if they are to live. Sometimes, the parents and the doctor will decide not to operate, and let the infant die. Anthony Shaw describes what happens then:

> . . . When surgery is denied [the doctor] must try to keep the infant from suffering while natural forces sap the baby's life away. As a surgeon whose natural inclination is to use the scalpel to fight off death, standing by and watching a salvageable baby die is the most emotionally exhausting experience I know. It is easy at a conference, in a theoretical discussion, to decide that such infants should be allowed to die. It is altogether different to

stand by in the nursery and watch as dehydration and infection wither a tiny being over hours and days. This is a terrible ordeal for me and the hospital staff—much more so than for the parents who never set foot in the nursery.[1]

I can understand why some people are opposed to all euthanasia, and insist that such infants must be allowed to live. I think I can also understand why other people favor destroying these babies quickly and painlessly. But why should anyone favor letting "dehydration and infection wither a tiny being over hours and days"? The doctrine that says that a baby may be allowed to dehydrate and wither, but may not be given an injection that would end its life without suffering, seems so patently cruel as to require no further refutation. The strong language is not intended to offend, but only to put the point in the clearest possible way.

My second argument is that the conventional doctrine leads to decisions concerning life and death made on irrelevant grounds.

Consider again the case of the infants with Down's syndrome who need operations for congenital defects unrelated to the syndrome to live. Sometimes, there is no operation, and the baby dies, but when there is no such defect, the baby lives on. Now, an operation such as that to remove an intestinal obstruction is not prohibitively difficult. The reason why such operations are not performed in these cases is, clearly, that the child has Down's syndrome and the parents and doctor judge that because of that fact it is better for the child to die.

But notice that this situation is absurd, no matter what view one takes of the lives and potentials of such babies. If the life of such an infant is worth preserving, what does it matter if it needs a simple operation? Or, if one thinks it better that such a baby should not live on, what difference does it make that it happens to have an unobstructed intestinal tract? In either case, the matter of life and death is being decided on irrelevant grounds. It is the Down's syndrome, and not the intestines, that is the issue. The matter should be decided, if at all, on that basis, and not be allowed to depend on the essentially irrelevant question of whether the intestinal tract is blocked.

What makes this situation possible, of course, is the idea that when there is an intestinal blockage, one can "let the baby die," but when there is no such defect there is nothing that can be done, for one must not "kill" it. The fact that this idea leads to such results as deciding life or death on irrelevant grounds is another good reason why the doctrine should be rejected.

One reason why so many people think that there is an important moral difference between active and passive euthanasia is that they think killing someone is morally worse than letting someone die. But is it? Is killing, in itself, worse than letting die? To investigate this issue, two cases may be considered that are exactly alike except that one involves killing whereas the other involves letting someone die. Then, it can be asked whether this difference makes any difference to the moral assessments. It is important that the cases be exactly alike, except for this one difference, since otherwise one cannot be confident that it is this difference and not some other that accounts for any variation in the assessments of the two cases. So, let us consider this pair of cases:

In the first, Smith stands to gain a large inheritance if anything should happen to his six-year-old cousin. One evening while the child is taking his bath, Smith sneaks into the bathroom and drowns the child, and then arranges things so that it will look like an accident.

In the second, Jones also stands to gain if anything should happen to his six-year-old cousin. Like Smith, Jones sneaks in planning to drown the child in his bath. However, just as he enters the bathroom Jones sees the child slip and hit his head, and fall face down in the water. Jones is delighted; he stands by, ready to push the child's head back under if it is necessary, but it is not necessary. With only a little thrashing about, the child drowns all by himself, "accidentally," as Jones watches and does nothing.

Now Smith killed the child, whereas Jones "merely" let the child die. That is the only difference between them. Did either man behave better, from a moral point of view? If the difference between killing and letting die were in itself a morally important matter, one should say that Jones's behavior was less reprehensible than Smith's. But does one really want to say that? I think not. In the first place, both men acted from the same motive, personal gain, and both had exactly the same end

in view when they acted. It may be inferred from Smith's conduct that he is a bad man, although that judgment may be withdrawn or modified if certain further facts are learned about him—for example, that he is mentally deranged. But would not the very same thing be inferred about Jones from his conduct? And would not the same further considerations also be relevant to any modification of this judgment? Moreover, suppose Jones pleaded, in his own defense, "After all, I didn't do anything except just stand there and watch the child drown. I didn't kill him; I only let him die." Again, if letting die were in itself less bad than killing, this defense should have at least some weight. But it does not. Such a "defense" can only be regarded as a grotesque perversion of moral reasoning. Morally speaking, it is no defense at all.

Now, it may be pointed out, quite properly, that the cases of euthanasia with which doctors are concerned are not like this at all. They do not involve personal gain or the destruction of normal healthy children. Doctors are concerned only with cases in which the patient's life is of no further use to him, or in which the patient's life has become or will soon become a terrible burden. However, the point is the same in these cases: the bare difference between killing and letting die does not, in itself, make a moral difference. If a doctor lets a patient die, for humane reasons, he is in the same moral position as if he had given the patient a lethal injection for humane reasons. If his decision was wrong—if, for example, the patient's illness was in fact curable—the decision would be equally regrettable no matter which method was used to carry it out. And if the doctor's decision was the right one, the method used is not in itself important.

The AMA policy statement isolates the crucial issue very well; the crucial issue is "the intentional termination of the life of one human being by another." But after identifying this issue, and forbidding "mercy killing," the statement goes on to deny that the cessation of treatment is the intentional termination of a life. This is where the mistake comes in, for what is the cessation of treatment, in these circumstances, if it is not "the intentional termination of the life of one human being by another"? Of course it is exactly that, and if it were not, there would be no point to it.

Many people will find this judgment hard to

accept. One reason, I think, is that it is very easy to conflate the question of whether killing is, in itself, worse than letting die, with the very different question of whether most actual cases of killing are more reprehensible than most actual cases of letting die. Most actual cases of killing are clearly terrible (think, for example, of all the murders reported in the newspapers), and one hears of such cases every day. On the other hand, one hardly ever hears of a case of letting die, except for the actions of doctors who are motivated by humanitarian reasons. So one learns to think of killing in a much worse light than of letting die. But this does not mean that there is something about killing that makes it in itself worse than letting die, for it is not the bare difference between killing and letting die that makes the difference in these cases. Rather, the other factors—the murderer's motive of personal gain, for example, contrasted with the doctor's humanitarian motivation—account for different reactions to the different cases.

I have argued that killing is not in itself any worse than letting die; if my contention is right, it follows that active euthanasia is not any worse than passive euthanasia. What arguments can be given on the other side? The most common, I believe, is the following:

"The important difference between active and passive euthanasia is that, in passive euthanasia, the doctor does not do anything to bring about the patient's death. The doctor does nothing, and the patient dies of whatever ills already afflict him. In active euthanasia, however, the doctor does something to bring about the patient's death: he kills him. The doctor who gives the patient with cancer a lethal injection has himself caused his patient's death; whereas if he merely ceases treatment, the cancer is the cause of the death."

A number of points need to be made here. The first is that it is not exactly correct to say that in passive euthanasia the doctor does nothing, for he does do one thing that is very important: he lets the patient die. "Letting someone die" is certainly different, in some respects, from other types of action—mainly in that it is a kind of action that one may perform by way of not performing certain other actions. For example, one may let a patient die by way of not giving medication, just as one may insult someone by way of not shaking his hand. But for any purpose of moral assessment, it is a type of action nonetheless. The decision to let a patient die is subject to moral appraisal in the same way that a decision to kill him would be subject to moral appraisal: it may be assessed as wise or unwise, compassionate or sadistic, right or wrong. If a doctor deliberately let a patient die who was suffering from a routinely curable illness, the doctor would certainly be to blame for what he had done, just as he would be to blame if he had needlessly killed the patient. Charges against him would then be appropriate. If so, it would be no defense at all for him to insist that he didn't "do anything." He would have done something very serious indeed, for he let his patient die.

Fixing the cause of death may be very important from a legal point of view, for it may determine whether criminal charges are brought against the doctor. But I do not think that this notion can be used to show a moral difference between active and passive euthanasia. The reason why it is considered bad to be the cause of someone's death is that death is regarded as a great evil—and so it is. However, if it has been decided that euthanasia—even passive euthanasia—is desirable in a given case, it has also been decided that in this instance death is no greater an evil than the patient's continued existence. And if this is true, the usual reason for not wanting to be the cause of someone's death simply does not apply.

Finally, doctors may think that all of this is only of academic interest—the sort of thing that philosophers may worry about but that has no practical bearing on their own work. After all, doctors must be concerned about the legal consequences of what they do, and active euthanasia is clearly forbidden by the law. But even so, doctors should also be concerned with the fact that the law is forcing upon them a moral doctrine that may well be indefensible, and has a considerable effect on their practices. Of course, most doctors are not now in the position of being coerced in this matter, for they do not regard themselves as merely going along with what the law requires. Rather, in statements such as the AMA policy statement that I have quoted, they are endorsing this doctrine as a central point of medical ethics. In that statement, active euthanasia is condemned not merely as illegal but as "contrary to that for which the medical profession stands," whereas passive euthanasia is approved. However, the preceding considerations suggest that there is really no moral difference between the two, considered in themselves (there may be important moral differences in some cases in their *consequences*, but, as I pointed out, these differences may make active euthanasia, and not passive euthanasia, the morally preferable option). So, whereas doctors may have to discriminate be-

tween active and passive euthanasia to satisfy the law, they should not do any more than that. In particular, they should not give the distinction any added authority and weight by writing it into official statements of medical ethics.

Note

1. A. Shaw, "Doctor, Do We Have a Choice?" *The New York Times Magazine,* January 30, 1972, p. 54.

Justifying Voluntary Euthanasia

Peter Singer

Most of the groups currently campaigning for changes in the law to allow euthanasia are campaigning for voluntary euthanasia—that is, euthanasia carried out at the request of the person killed.

Sometimes voluntary euthanasia is scarcely distinguishable from assisted suicide. In *Jean's Way*, Derek Humphry has told how his wife Jean, when dying of cancer, asked him to provide her with the means to end her life swiftly and without pain. They had seen the situation coming and discussed it beforehand. Derek obtained some tablets and gave them to Jean, who took them and died soon afterwards.

In other cases, people wanting to die may be unable to kill themselves. In 1973 George Zygmaniak was injured in a motorcycle accident near his home in New Jersey. He was taken to hospital, where he was found to be totally paralysed from the neck down. He was also in considerable pain. He told his doctor and his brother, Lester, that he did not want to live in this condition. He begged them both to kill him. Lester questioned the doctor and hospital staff about George's prospects of recovery: he was told that they were nil. He then smuggled a gun into the hospital, and said to his brother: 'I am here to end your pain, George. Is it all right with you?' George, who was now unable to speak because of an operation to assist his breathing, nodded affirmatively. Lester shot him through the temple.

The Zygmaniak case appears to be a clear in-

stance of voluntary euthanasia, although without some of the procedural safeguards that advocates of the legalization of voluntary euthanasia propose. For instance, medical opinions about the patient's prospects of recovery were obtained only in an informal manner. Nor was there a careful attempt to establish, before independent witnesses, that George's desire for death was of a fixed and rational kind, based on the best available information about his situation. The killing was not carried out by a doctor. An injection would have been less distressing to others than shooting. But these choices were not open to Lester Zygmaniak, for the law in New Jersey, as in most other places, regards mercy killing as murder, and if he had made his plans known, he would not have been able to carry them out.

Euthanasia can be voluntary even if a person is not able, as Jean Humphry and George Zygmaniak were able, to indicate the wish to die right up to the moment the tablets are swallowed or the trigger pulled. A person may, while in good health, make a written request for euthanasia if, through accident or illness, she should come to be incapable of making or expressing a decision to die, in pain, or without the use of her mental faculties, and there is no reasonable hope of recovery. In killing a person who has made such a request, has re-affirmed it from time to time, and is now in one of the states described, one could truly claim to be acting with her consent. . . .

. . . Under existing laws people suffering unrelievable pain or distress from an incurable illness who ask their doctors to end their lives are asking their doctors to become murderers. Although juries are extremely reluctant to convict in cases of this kind the law is clear that neither the request, nor the degree of suffering, nor the incurable condition of the person killed, is a defence to a charge of murder. Advocates of voluntary euthanasia propose that this law be changed so that a doctor could legally act on a patient's desire to die without further suffering.

The case for voluntary euthanasia has some common ground with the case for nonvoluntary euthanasia, in that the reason for killing is to end suffering. The two kinds of euthanasia differ, however, in that voluntary euthanasia involves the killing of a person, a rational and self-conscious being and not a merely conscious being. (To be strictly accurate it must be said that this is not always so, because although only rational and self-conscious beings can consent to their own deaths, they may not be rational and self-conscious at the time euthanasia is contemplated—the doctor may, for instance, be acting on a prior written request for euthanasia if, through accident or illness, one's rational faculties should be irretrievably lost. For simplicity we shall, henceforth, disregard this complication.)

We have seen [in an earlier section] that it is possible to justify nonvoluntary euthanasia, when the being killed lacks the capacity to consent. We must now ask in what way the ethical issues are different when the being is capable of consenting, and does in fact consent.

Let us return to the general principles about killing proposed in Chapter 4 [of *Practical Ethics*]. I argued there that the wrongness of killing a conscious being which is not self-conscious, rational or autonomous, depends on utilitarian considerations. It is on this basis that I have defended nonvoluntary euthanasia. On the other hand it is, as we saw, plausible to hold that killing a self-conscious being is a more serious matter than killing a merely conscious being. We found four distinct grounds on which this could be argued:

i. The classical utilitarian claim that since self-conscious beings are capable of fearing their own death, killing them has worse effects on others.

ii. The preference utilitarian calculation which counts the thwarting of the victim's desire to go on living as an important reason against killing.

iii. A theory of rights according to which to have a right one must have the ability to desire that to which one has a right, so that to have a right to life one must be able to desire one's own continued existence.

iv. Respect for the autonomous decisions of rational agents.

Now suppose we have a situation in which a person suffering from a painful and incurable disease wishes to die. If the individual were not a person—not rational or self-conscious—euthanasia would, as I have said, be justifiable. Do any of the four grounds for holding that it is normally worse to kill a person provide reasons against killing when the individual is a person?

The classical utilitarian objection does not apply to killing that takes place only with the genuine consent of the person killed. That people are killed under these conditions would have no tendency to spread fear or insecurity, since we have no cause to be fearful of being killed with our own genuine consent. If we do not wish to be killed, we simply do not consent. In fact, the argument from fear points in favour of voluntary euthanasia, for if voluntary euthanasia is not permitted we may, with good cause, be fearful that our deaths will be unnecessarily drawn-out and distressing.

Preference utilitarianism also points in favour of, not against, voluntary euthanasia. Just as preference utilitarianism must count a desire to go on living as a reason against killing, so it must count a desire to die as a reason for killing.

Next, according to the theory of rights we have considered, it is an essential feature of a right that one can waive one's rights if one so chooses. I may have a right to privacy; but I can, if I wish, film every detail of my daily life and invite the neighbours to my home movies. Neighbours sufficiently intrigued to accept my invitation could do so without violating my right to privacy, since the right has on this occasion been waived. Similarly, to say that I have a right to life is not to say that it would be wrong for my doctor to end my life, if she does so at my request. In making this request I waive my right to life.

Lastly, the principle of respect for autonomy tells us to allow rational agents to live their own lives according to their own autonomous decisions, free from coercion or interference; but if rational agents should autonomously choose to die, then respect for autonomy will lead us to assist them to do as they choose.

So, although there are reasons for thinking that killing a self-conscious being is normally worse than killing any other kind of being, in the special case of voluntary euthanasia most of these reasons count for euthanasia rather than against. Surprising as this result might at first seem, it really does no more than reflect the fact that what is special about self-conscious beings is that they can know that they exist over time and will, unless they die, continue to exist. Normally this continued existence is fervently desired; when the foreseeable continued existence is dreaded rather than desired however, the desire to die may take the place of the normal desire to live, reversing the reasons against killing based on the desire to live. Thus the case for voluntary euthanasia is arguably much stronger than the case for nonvoluntary euthanasia.

Some opponents of the legalization of voluntary euthanasia might concede that all this follows, if we have a genuinely free and rational decision to die: but, they add, we can never be sure that a request to be killed is the result of a free and rational decision. Will not the sick and elderly be pressured by their relatives to end their lives quickly? Will it not be possible to commit outright murder by pretending that a person has requested euthanasia? And even if there is no pressure or falsification, can anyone who is ill, suffering pain, and very probably in a drugged and confused state of mind, make a rational decision about whether to live or die?

These questions raise technical difficulties for the legalization of voluntary euthanasia, rather than objections to the underlying ethical principles; but they are serious difficulties nonetheless. Voluntary euthanasia societies in Britain and elsewhere have sought to meet them by proposing that euthanasia should be legal only for a person who:

i.   is diagnosed by two doctors as suffering from an incurable illness expected to cause severe distress or the loss of rational faculties;

and

ii. has, at least 30 days before the proposed act of euthanasia, and in the presence of two independent witnesses, made a written request for euthanasia in the event of the situation described in (i) occurring.

Only a doctor could administer euthanasia, and if the patient was at the time still capable of consenting, the doctor would have to make sure that the patient still wished the declaration to be acted upon. A declaration could be revoked at any time.

These provisions, though in some respects cumbersome, appear to meet most of the technical objections to legalization. Murder in the guise of euthanasia would be far-fetched. Two independent witnesses to the declaration, the 30 day waiting period, and—in the case of a mentally competent person—the doctor's final investigation of the patient's wishes would together do a great deal to reduce the danger of doctors acting on requests which did not reflect the free and rational decisions of their patients.

It is often said, in debates about euthanasia, that doctors can be mistaken. Certainly some patients diagnosed by competent doctors as suffering from an incurable condition have survived. Possibly the legalization of voluntary euthanasia would, over the years, mean the deaths of one or two people who would otherwise have recovered. This is not, however, the knockdown argument against euthanasia that some imagine it to be. Against a very small number of unnecessary deaths that might occur if euthanasia is legalized we must place the very large amount of pain and distress that will be suffered by patients who really are terminally ill if euthanasia is not legalized. Longer life is not such a supreme good that it outweighs all other considerations. (If it were, there would be many more effective ways of saving life—such as a ban on smoking, or on cars that can drive faster than 10 m.p.h.—than prohibiting voluntary euthanasia.) The possibility that two doctors may make a mistake means that the person who opts for euthanasia is deciding on the balance of probabilities, and giving up a very slight chance of survival in order to avoid suffering that will almost certainly end in death. This may be a perfectly rational choice. Probability is, as Bishop Butler said, the guide of life, and we must follow its guidance right to the end. Against this, some will reply that improved care for the terminally ill has eliminated pain and made voluntary euthanasia unnecessary. Elisabeth Kübler-Ross, whose *On Death and Dying* is perhaps the best-known book on care for the dying, has claimed that none of her patients request euthanasia. Given personal attention and the right medication, she says, people come to accept their deaths and die peacefully without pain.

Kübler-Ross may be right. It may be possible, now, to eliminate pain. It may even be possible to do it in a way which leaves patients in possession of their rational faculties and free from vomiting, nausea, or other distressing side-effects. Unfortunately only a minority of dying patients now receive this kind of care. Nor is physical pain the only problem. There can also be other distressing conditions, like bones so fragile they fracture at sudden movements, slow starvation due to a cancerous growth, inability to control one's bowels or bladder, difficulty in breathing and so on.

Take the case of Jean Humphry, as described in *Jean's Way*. This is not a case from the period before effective painkillers: Jean Humphry died in 1975. Nor is it the case of someone unable to get good medical care: she was treated at an Oxford hospital and if there were anything else that could have been done for her, her husband, a well-connected Fleet Street journalist, would have been better placed than most to obtain it. Yet Derek Humphry writes:

> when the request for help in dying meant relief from relentless suffering and pain and I had seen the extent of this agony, the option simply could not be denied . . . and certainly Jean deserved the dignity of selecting her own ending. She must die soon—as we both now realized—but together we would decide when this would be.

Perhaps one day it will be possible to treat all terminally ill patients in such a way that no one requests euthanasia and the subject becomes a non-issue; but this still distant prospect is no reason to deny euthanasia to those who die in less comfortable conditions. It is, in any case, highly paternalistic to tell dying patients that they are now so well looked after they need not be offered the option of euthanasia. It would be more in keeping with respect for individual freedom and autonomy to legalize euthanasia and let patients decide whether their situation is bearable—let them, as Derek Humphry puts it, have the dignity of selecting their own endings. Better that voluntary euthanasia be an unexercised legal right than a prohibited act which, for all we know, some might desperately desire.

Finally, do these arguments for voluntary euthanasia perhaps give too much weight to individual freedom and autonomy? After all, we do not allow people free choices on matters like, for instance, the taking of heroin. This is a restriction of freedom but, in the view of many, one that can be justified on paternalistic grounds. If preventing people becoming heroin addicts is justifiable paternalism, why isn't preventing people having themselves killed?

The question is a reasonable one, because respect for individual freedom can be carried too far. John Stuart Mill thought that the state should never interfere with the individual except to prevent harm to others. The individual's own good, Mill thought, is not a proper reason for state intervention. But Mill may have had too high an opinion of the rationality of a human being. It may occasionally be right to prevent people making choices which are obviously not rationally based and which we can be sure they will later regret. The prohibition of voluntary euthanasia cannot be justified on paternalistic grounds, however, for voluntary euthanasia is, by definition, an act for which good reasons exist. Voluntary euthanasia occurs only when, to the best of medical knowledge, a person is suffering from an incurable and painful or distressing condition. In these circumstances one cannot say that to choose to die quickly is obviously irrational. The strength of the case for voluntary euthanasia lies in this combination of respect for the preferences, or autonomy, of those who decide for euthanasia; and the clear rational basis of the decision itself.

In the Matter of Karen Quinlan, an Alleged Incompetent

The Supreme Court of New Jersey

Background Note. The decision of the court was issued on March 31, 1976. It was delivered by Chief Justice Hughes. The following abridgement omits references and case citations.

Constitutional and Legal Issues

I. The Free Exercise of Religion

Simply stated, the right to religious beliefs is absolute but conduct in pursuance thereof is not wholly immune from governmental restraint. So it is that, for the sake of life, courts sometimes (but not always) order blood transfusions for Jehovah's Witnesses (whose religious beliefs abhor such procedure), forbid exposure to death from handling virulent snakes or ingesting poison (interfering with deeply held religious sentiments in such regard), and protect the public health as in the case of compulsory vaccination (over the strongest of religious objections). . . . The Public interest is thus considered paramount, without essential dissolution of respect for religious beliefs.

We think, without further examples, that, ranged against the State's interest in the preservation of life, the impingement of religious belief, much less religious "neutrality" as here, does not reflect a constitutional question, in the circumstances at least of the case presently before the Court. Moreover, like the trial court, we do not recognize an independent parental right of religious freedom to support the relief requested.

II. Cruel and Unusual Punishment

Similarly inapplicable to the case before us is the Constitution's Eighth Amendment protection against cruel and unusual punishment which, as held by the trial court, is not relevant to situations other than the imposition of penal sanctions. Historic in nature, it stemmed from punitive excesses in the infliction of criminal penalties. We find no precedent in law which would justify its extension to the correction of social injustice or hardship, such as, for instance, in the case of poverty. The latter often condemns the poor and deprived to horrendous living conditions which could certainly be described in the abstract as "cruel and unusual punishment." Yet the constitutional base of protection from "cruel and unusual punishment" is plainly irrelevant to such societal ills which must be remedied, if at all, under other concepts of constitutional and civil right.

So it is in the case of the unfortunate Karen Quinlan. Neither the State, nor the law, but the accident of fate and nature, has inflicted upon her conditions which though in essence cruel and most unusual, yet do not amount to "punishment" in any constitutional sense.

Neither the judgment of the court below, nor the medical decision which confronted it, nor the law and equity perceptions which impelled its action, nor the whole factual base upon which it was predicated, inflicted "cruel and unusual punishment" in the constitutional sense.

III. The Right of Privacy

It is the issue of the constitutional right of privacy that has given us most concern, in the exceptional circumstances of this case. Here a loving parent, *qua* parent and raising the rights of his incompetent and profoundly damaged daughter, probably irreversibly doomed to no more than a biologically vegetative remnant of life, is before the court. He seeks authorization to abandon specialized technological procedures which can only maintain for a time a body having no potential for resumption or continuance of other than a "vegetative" existence.

We have no doubt, in these unhappy circumstances, that if Karen were herself miraculously lucid for an interval (not altering the existing prognosis of the condition to which she would soon return) and perceptive of her irreversible condition, she could effectively decide

From In the Matter of Karen Quinlan, an Alleged Incompetent. *Supreme Court of New Jersey, 70 N.J. 10, 355 A. 2d 647.*

upon discontinuance of the life-support apparatus, even if it meant the prospect of natural death. To this extent we may distinguish [a case] which concerned a severely injured young woman (Delores Heston), whose life depended on surgery and blood transfusion; and who was in such extreme shock that she was unable to express an informed choice (although the Court apparently considered the case as if the patient's own religious decision to resist transfusion were at stake), but most importantly a patient apparently salvable to long life and vibrant health;—a situation not at all like the present case.

We have no hesitancy in deciding, in the instant diametrically opposite case, that no external compelling interest of the State could compel Karen to endure the unendurable, only to vegetate a few measurable months with no realistic possibility of returning to any semblance of cognitive or sapient life. We perceive no thread of logic distinguishing between such a choice on Karen's part and a similar choice which, under the evidence in this case, could be made by a competent patient terminally ill, riddled by cancer and suffering great pain; such a patient would not be resuscitated or put on a respirator in the example described by Dr. Korein, and *a fortiori* would not be kept *against his will* on a respirator.

Although the Constitution does not explicitly mention a right of privacy, Supreme Court decisions have recognized that a right of personal privacy exists and that certain areas of privacy are guaranteed under the Constitution. The Court has interdicted judicial intrusion into many aspects of personal decision, sometimes basing this restraint upon the conception of a limitation of judicial interest and responsibility, such as with regard to contraception and its relationship to family life and decision.

The Court in *Griswold* found the unwritten constitutional right of privacy to exist in the penumbra of specific guarantees of the Bill of Rights "formed by emanations from those guarantees that help give them life and substance." Presumably this right is broad enough to encompass a patient's decision to decline medical treatment under certain circumstances, in much the same way as it is broad enough to encompass a woman's decision to terminate pregnancy under certain conditions.

The claimed interests of the State in this case

are essentially the preservation and sanctity of human life and defense to the right of the physician to administer medical treatment according to his best judgment. In this case the doctors say that removing Karen from the respirator will conflict with their professional judgment. The plaintiff answers that Karen's present treatment serves only a maintenance function; that the respirator cannot cure or improve her condition but at best can only prolong her inevitable slow deterioration and death; and that the interests of the patient, as seen by her surrogate, the guardian, must be evaluated by the court as predominant, even in the face of an option *contra* by the present attending physicians. Plaintiff's distinction is significant. The nature of Karen's care and the realistic chances of her recovery are quite unlike those of the patients discussed in many of the cases where treatments were ordered. In many of those cases the medical procedure required (usually a transfusion) constituted a minimal bodily invasion and the chances of recovery and return to functioning life were very good. We think that the State's interest *contra* weakens and the individual's right to privacy grows as the degree of bodily invasion increases and the prognosis dims. Ultimately there comes a point at which the individual's rights overcome the State interest. It is for that reason that we believe Karen's choice, if she were competent to make it, would be vindicated by the law. Her prognosis is extremely poor,—she will never resume cognitive life. And the bodily invasion is very great,—she requires 24-hour intensive nursing care, antibiotics, and the assistance of a respirator, a catheter and feeding tube.

Our affirmance of Karen's independent right of choice, however, would ordinarily be based upon her competency to assert it. The sad truth, however, is that she is grossly incompetent and we cannot discern her supposed choice based on the testimony of her previous conversation with friends, where such testimony is without sufficient probative weight. Nevertheless we have concluded that Karen's right of privacy may be asserted on her behalf by her guardian under the peculiar circumstances here present.

If a putative decision by Karen to permit this non-cognitive, vegetative existence to terminate by natural forces is regarded as a valuable incident of her right of privacy, as we believe it to be, then it should not be discarded solely on the basis that her condition prevents her conscious exercise of the choice. The only practical way to prevent destruction of the right is to permit the guardian and family of Karen to render their best judgment, subject to the qualifications hereinafter stated, as to whether she would exercise it in these circumstances. If their conclusion is in the affirmative this decision should be accepted by a society the overwhelming majority of whose members would, we think, in similar circumstances, exercise such a choice in the same way for themselves or for those closest to them. It is for this reason that we determine that Karen's right of privacy may be asserted in her behalf, in this respect, by her guardian and family under the particular circumstances presented by this record. [Sections IV (Medical Factors), V (Alleged Criminal Liability), and VI (Guardianship of the Person) omitted.]

Declaratory Relief

We thus arrive at the formulation of the declaratory relief which we have concluded is appropriate to this case. Some time has passed since Karen's physical and mental condition was described to the Court. At that time her continuing deterioration was plainly projected. Since the record has not been expanded we assume that she is now even more fragile and nearer to death than she was then. Since her present treating physicians may give reconsideration to her present posture in the light of this opinion, and since we are transferring to the plaintiff as guardian the choice of the attending physician and therefore other physicians may be in charge of the case who may take a different view from that of the present attending physicians, we herewith declare the following affirmative relief on behalf of the plaintiff. Upon the concurrence of the guardian and family of Karen, should the responsible attending physicians conclude that there is no reasonable possibility of Karen's ever emerging from her present comatose condition to a cognitive, sapient state and that the life-support apparatus now being administered to Karen should be discontinued, they shall consult with the hospital "Ethics Committee" or like body of the institution in which Karen is then hospitalized. If that consultative body agrees that there is no reasonable possibility of Karen's ever emerging from her present comatose condition to a cognitive, sapient state, the present life-support system may be withdrawn and said action shall be without any civil or criminal liability therefor on the part of any participant, whether guardian, physician, hospital or others. We herewith specifically so hold.

In the Matter of Claire C. Conroy

The Supreme Court of New Jersey

Background Note. In 1979 Claire Conroy, age 80, was admitted to a nursing home. She suffered from an organic brain syndrome, and because of periodic mental confusion, she was declared incompetent, and her nephew was appointed as her guardian. In 1982 during her treatment in a hospital, a nasogastric feeding tube was inserted to improve her nutrition, and when she was returned to the nursing home, the tube was left in place. Although attempts were made to remove it, Ms. Conroy was incapable of swallowing sufficient amounts of food and water to meet her needs. Her guardian asked that the tube be removed. When her physician refused, the guardian petitioned the New Jersey Superior Court to order it done.

By this time, Ms. Conroy was confined to her bed and unable to move from a semifetal position. She suffered arteriosclerotic heart disease, hypertension, and diabetes. Her left leg was gangrenous, she was unable to control her bladder or bowels, and she could not speak. Trial testimony indicated that although she was not brain dead, comatose, or in a chronic vegetative state, she was demented, unable to respond to words, and showed no signs of having any consciousness or higher brain functions. This condition was judged to be permanent. Testimony as to whether she might be in pain was inconclusive.

It also emerged that Ms. Conroy was a Roman Catholic, that she feared and avoided physicians, had never con-

From In the Matter of Claire C. Conroy. *Supreme Court of New Jersey, 98 N.J. 321, 486 A.2d 1209.*

sulted a physician when she was competent, and once when taken to an emergency room in a semiconscious state, she left immediately when she realized where she was. Her guardian testified that he was certain that she would never have consented to the insertion of the feeding tube.

The court granted the request to remove the tube, but the decision was stayed pending appeal. Meanwhile, Ms. Conroy died on February 15, 1983. The Appeals Court reversed the original decision, but the New Jersey Supreme Court agreed to review the case.

The decision of the court was issued on January 17, 1985. The 6–1 majority opinion was written by Associate Justice Sidney M. Schreiber. The following abridgment omits references and case citations. Headings have been added.

Rights of a Competent Patient

The starting point in analyzing whether life-sustaining treatment may be withheld or withdrawn from an incompetent patient is to determine what rights a competent patient has to accept or reject medical care. It is therefore necessary at the outset of this discussion to identify the nature and extent of a patient's rights that are implicated by such decisions.

The right of a person to control his own body is a basic societal concept, long recogized in the common law:

No right is held more sacred, or is more carefully guarded by the common law, than the right of every individual to the possession and control of his own person, free from all restraint or interference of others, unless by clear and unquestionable authority of law. As well said by *Judge* Cooley, "The right to one's person may be said to be a right of complete immunity: to be let alone." Cooley on Torts, 29. . . .

The doctrine of informed consent is a primary means developed in the law to protect this personal interest in the integrity of one's body. "Under this doctrine, no medical procedure may be performed without a patient's consent, obtained after explanation of the nature of the treatment, substantial risks, and alternative therapies." Cantor, "A Patient's Decision to Decline Life-Saving Medical Treatment: Bodily Integrity Versus the Preservation of Life," 26 *Rutgers L.Rev.* 228, 237 (1973). . . .

The patient's ability to control his bodily integrity through informed consent is significant only when one recognizes that this right also encompasses a right to informed refusal. Thus, a competent adult person generally has the right to decline to have any medical treatment initiated or continued. . . .

The right to make certain decisions concerning one's body is also protected by the federal constitutional right of privacy. The Supreme Court first articulated the right of privacy in *Griswold v. Connecticut*, which held that married couples have a constitutional right to use contraceptives. The Court in *Roe v. Wade* further extended its recognition of the privacy right to protect a woman's decision to abort a pregnancy although the woman's right to choose abortion directly conflicted with the state's legitimate and important interest in preserving the potentiality of fetal life. Finally, in *Quinlan*, we indicated that the right of privacy enunciated by the Supreme Court "is broad enough to encompass a patient's decision to decline medical treatment under certain circumstances," even if that decision might lead to the patient's death. While this right of privacy might apply in a case such as this, we need not decide that issue since the right to decline medical treatment is, in any event, embraced within the common-law right to self-determination.

Whether based on common-law doctrines or on constitutional theory, the right to decline life-sustaining medical treatment is not absolute. In some cases, it may yield to countervailing societal interests in sustaining the person's life. Courts and commentators have commonly identified four state interests that may limit a person's right to refuse medical treatment: preserving life, preventing suicide, safeguarding the integrity of the medical profession, and protecting innocent third parties. . . .

On balance, the right to self-determination ordinarily outweighs any countervailing state interests, and competent persons generally are permitted to refuse medical treatment, even at the risk of death. Most of the cases that have held otherwise, unless they involved the interest in protecting innocent third parties, have concerned the patient's competency to make a rational and considered choice of treatment. . . .

In view of the case law, we have no doubt that Ms. Conroy, if competent to make the decision and if resolute in her determination, could have chosen to have her nasogastric tube withdrawn. Her interest in freedom from nonconsensual invasion of her bodily integrity would outweigh any state interest in preserving life or in safeguarding the integrity of the medical profession. In addition, rejecting her artificial means of feeding would not constitute attempted suicide, as the decision would probably be based on a wish to be free of medical intervention rather than a specific intent to die, and her death would result, if at all, from her underlying medical condition, which included her inability to swallow. Finally, removal of her feeding tube would not create a public health or safety hazard, nor would her death leave any minor dependents without care or support. . . .

The Issue with Incompetent Patients

The *Quinlan* decision dealt with a special category of patients: those in a chronic, persistent vegetative or comatose state. In a footnote, the opinion left open the question whether the principles it enunciated might be applicable to incompetent patients in "other types of terminal medical situations * * *, not necessarily involving the hopeless loss of cognitive or sapient life." We now are faced with one such situation: that of elderly, formerly competent nursing-home residents who, unlike Karen Quinlan, are awake and conscious and can interact with their environment to a limited extent, but whose mental and physical functioning is severely and permanently impaired and whose life expectancy, even with the treatment, is relatively short. The capacities of such people, while significantly diminished, are not as limited as those of irreversibly comatose persons, and their deaths, while no longer distant, may not be imminent. Large numbers of aged, chronically ill, institutionalized persons fall within this general category. . . .

Since the condition of an incompetent patient makes it impossible to ascertain definitively his present desires, a third party acting on the patient's behalf often cannot say with confidence that his treatment decision for the patient will further rather than frustrate the patient's right to control his own body. Nevertheless, the goal of decision-making for incompetent patients should be to determine and effectuate, insofar as possible, the decision that the patient would have made if competent. Ideally, both aspects of the patient's right to bodily integrity—the right to consent to medical intervention and the right to refuse it—should be respected.

The Subjective Standard

In light of these rights and concerns, we hold that life-sustaining treatment may be withheld or withdrawn from an incompetent patient when it is clear that the particular patient would have refused the treatment under the circumstances involved. The standard we are enunciating is a subjective one, consistent with the notion that the right that we are seeking to effectuate is a very personal right to control one's own life. The question is not what a reasonable or average person would have chosen to do under the circumstances but what the particular patient would have done if able to choose for himself.

The patient may have expressed, in one or more ways, an intent not to have life-sustaining medical intervention. Such an intent might be embodied in a written document, or "living will," stating the person's desire not to have certain types of life-sustaining treatment administered under certain circumstances. It might also be evidenced in an oral directive that the patient gave to a family member, friend, or health care provider. It might consist of a durable power of attorney or appointment of a proxy authorizing a particular person to make the decisions on the patient's behalf if he is no longer capable of making them for himself. It might take the form of reactions that the patient voiced regarding medical treatment administered to others.

It might also be deduced from a person's religious beliefs and the tenets of that religion, or from the patient's consistent pattern of conduct with respect to prior decisions about his own medical care. Of course, dealing with the matter in advance in some sort of thoughtful and explicit way is best for all concerned.

Any of the above types of evidence, and any other information bearing on the person's intent, may be appropriate aids in determining what course of treatment the patient would have wished to pursue. In this respect, we now believe that we were in error in *Quinlan* to diregard the evidence of statements that Ms. Quinlan made to friends concerning artificial prolongation of the lives of others who were terminally ill. Such evidence is certainly relevant to shed light on whether the patient would have consented to the treatment if competent to make the decision. . . .

Medical evidence bearing on the patient's condition, treatment, and prognosis, like evidence of the patient's wishes, is an essential prerequisite to decision-making under the subjective test. The medical evidence must establish that the patient fits within the Claire Conroy pattern: an elderly, incompetent nursing-home resident with severe and permanent mental and physical impairments and a life expectancy of approximately one year or less. In addition, since the goal is to effectuate the patient's right of informed consent, the surrogate decision-maker must have at least as much medical information upon which to base his decision about what the patient would have chosen as one would expect a competent patient to have before consenting to or rejecting treatment. Such information might include evidence about the patient's present level of physical, sensory, emotional, and cognitive functioning; the degree of physical pain resulting from the medical condition, treatment, and termination of treatment, respectively; the degree of humiliation, dependence, and loss of dignity probably resulting from the condition and treatment; the life expectancy and prognosis for recovery with and without treatment; the various treatment options; and the risks, side effects, and benefits of each of those options. Particular care should be taken not to base a decision on a premature diagnosis or prognosis.

We recognize that for some incompetent patients it might be impossible to be clearly satisfied as to the patient's intent either to accept or reject the life-sustaining treatment. Many people may have spoken of their desires in general or casual terms, or, indeed, never considered or resolved the issue at all. In such cases, a surrogate decision-maker cannot presume that treatment decisions made by a third party on the patient's behalf will further the patient's right to self-determination, since effectuating another person's right to self-determination presupposes that the substitute decision-maker knows what the person would have wanted. Thus, in the absence of adequate proof of the patient's wishes, it is naive to pretend that the

right to self-determination serves as the basis for substituted decision-making.

We hesitate, however, to foreclose the possibility of humane actions, which may involve termination of life-sustaining treatment, for persons who never clearly expressed their desires about life-sustaining treatment but who are now suffering a prolonged and painful death. An incompetent, like a minor child, is a ward of the state, and the state's *parens patriae* power supports the authority of its courts to allow decisions to be made for an incompetent that serve the incompetent's best interests, even if the person's wishes cannot be clearly established. This authority permits the state to authorize guardians to withhold or withdraw life-sustaining treatment from an incompetent patient if it is manifest that such action would further the patient's best interests in a narrow sense of the phrase, even though the subjective test that we articulated above may not be satisfied. We therefore hold that life-sustaining treatment may also be withheld or withdrawn from a patient in Claire Conroy's situation if either of two "best interest" tests—a limited-objective or a pure-objective test—is satisfied.

The Limited-Objective and Pure-Objective Tests

Under the limited-objective test, life-sustaining treatment may be withheld or withdrawn from a patient in Claire Conroy's situation when there is some trustworthy evidence that the patient would have refused the treatment, and the decision-maker is satisfied that it is clear that the burdens of the patient's continued life with the treatment outweigh the benefits of that life for him. By this we mean that the patient is suffering, and will continue to suffer throughout the expected duration of his life, unavoidable pain, and that the net burdens of his prolonged life (the pain and suffering of his life with the treatment less the amount and duration of pain that the patient would likely experience if the treatment were withdrawn) markedly outweigh any physical pleasure, emotional enjoyment, or intellectual satisfaction that the patient may still be able to derive from life. This limited-objective standard permits the termination of treatment for a patient who had not unequivocally expressed his desires before becoming incompetent, when it is clear that the treatment in question would merely prolong the patient's suffering.

Medical evidence will be essential to establish that the burdens of the treatment to the patient in terms of pain and suffering outweigh the benefits that the patient is experiencing. The medical evidence should make it clear that the treatment would merely prolong the patient's suffering and not provide him with any net benefit. Information is particularly important with respect to the degree, expected duration, and constancy of pain with and without treatment, and the possibility that the pain could be reduced by drugs or other means short of terminating the life-sustaining treatment. The same types of medical evidence that are relevant to the subjective analysis, such as the patient's life expectancy, prognosis, level of functioning, degree of humiliation and dependency, and treatment options, should also be considered.

This limited-objective test also requires some trustworthy evidence that the patient would have wanted the treatment terminated. This evidence could take any one or more of the various forms appropriate to prove the patient's intent under the subjective test. Evidence that, taken as a whole, would be too vague, casual, or remote to constitute the clear proof of the patient's subjective intent that is necessary to satisy the subjective test—for example, informally expressed reactions to other people's medical conditions and treatment—might be sufficient to satisfy this prong of the limited-objective test.

In the absence of trustworthy evidence, or indeed any evidence at all, that the patient would have declined the treatment, life-sustaining treatment may still be withheld or withdrawn from a formerly competent person like Claire Conroy if a third, pure-objective test is satisfied. Under that test, as under the limited-objective test, the net burdens of the patient's life with the treatment should clearly and markedly outweigh the benefits that the patient derives from life. Further, the recurring, unavoidable and severe pain of the patient's life with the treatment should be such that the effect of administering life-sustaining treatment would be inhumane. Subjective evidence that the patient would not have wanted the treatment is not necessary under this pure-objective standard. Nevertheless, even in the context of severe pain, life-sustaining treatment should not be withdrawn from an incompetent patient who had previously expressed a wish to be kept alive in spite of any pain that he might experience.

Although we are condoning a restricted evaluation of the nature of a patient's life in terms of pain, suffering, and possible enjoyment under the limited-objective and pure-objective tests, we expressly decline to authorize decision-making based on assessments of the personal worth or social utility of another's life, or the value of that life to others. We do not believe that it would be appropriate for a court to designate a person with the authority to determine that someone else's life is not worth living simply because, to that person, the patient's "quality of life" or value to society seems negligible. The mere fact that a patient's functioning is limited or his prognosis dim does not mean that he is not enjoying what remains of his life or that it is in his best interests to die. More wide-ranging powers to make decisions about other people's lives, in our view, would create an intolerable risk for socially isolated and defenseless people suffering from physical or mental handicaps. . . .

The surrogate decision-maker should exercise extreme caution in determining the patient's intent and in evaluating medical evidence of the patient's pain and possible enjoyment, and should not approve withholding or withdrawing life-sustaining treatment unless he is manifestly satisfied that one of the three tests that we have outlined has been met. When evidence of a person's wishes or physical or mental condition is equivocal, it is best to err, if at all, in favor of preserving life.

Active–Passive and Withholding–Withdrawing

We emphasize that in making decisions whether to administer life-sustaining treatment to patients such as Claire Conroy, the primary focus should be the patient's desires and experience of pain and enjoyment—not the type of treatment involved. Thus, we reject the distinction that some have made between actively hastening death by terminating treatment and passively allowing a person to die of a disease as one of limited use in a legal analysis of such a decision-making situation.

Characterizing conduct as active or passive is often an elusive notion, even outside the context of medical decision-making. . . . The distinction is particularly nebulous, however, in the context of decisions whether to withhold or withdraw life-sustaining treatment. In a case like that of Claire Conroy, for example, would a physician who discontinued nasogastric feeding be actively causing her death by removing her primary source of nutrients; or would he merely be omitting to continue the artificial form of treatment, thus passively allowing her medical condition, which includes her inability to swallow, to take its natural course?

For a similar reason, we also reject any distinction between withholding and withdrawing life-sustaining treatment. . . .

This distinction is more psychologically compelling than logically sound. As mentioned above, the line between active and passive conduct in the context of medical decisions is far too nebulous to constitute a principled basis for decision-making. Whether necessary treatment is withheld at the outset or withdrawn later on, the consequence—the patient's death—is the same. Moreover, from a policy standpoint, it might well be unwise to forbid persons from discontinuing a treatment under circumstances in which the treatment could permissibly be withheld. Such a rule could discourage families and doctors from even attempting certain types of care and could thereby force them into hasty and premature decisions to allow a patient to die.

Ordinary–Extraordinary and Feeding–Treatment

We also find unpersuasive the distinction relied upon by some courts, commentators, and theologians between "ordinary" treatment, which they would always require, and "extraordinary" treatment, which they deem optional. . . .

The distinction between ordinary and extraordinary treatment is frequently phrased as one between common and unusual, or simple and complex, treatment; "extraordinary" treatment also has been equated with elaborate, artificial, heroic,

aggressive, expensive, or highly involved or invasive forms of medical intervention. Depending on the definitions applied, a particular treatment for a given patient may be considered both ordinary and extraordinary. Further, since the common/unusual and simple/complex distinctions among medical treatments "exist on continuums with no precise dividing line," and the continuum is constantly shifting due to progress in medical care, disagreement will often exist about whether a particular treatment is ordinary or extraordinary. In addition, the competent patient generally could refuse even ordinary treatment; therefore, an incompetent patient theoretically should also be able to make such a choice when the surrogate decision-making is effectuating the patient's subjective intent. In such cases, the ordinary/extraordinary distinction is irrelevant except insofar as the particular patient would have made the distinction. . . .

Some commentators have made yet a fourth distinction, between the termination of artificial feedings and the termination of other forms of life-sustaining medical treatment. . . .

Once one enters the realm of complex high-technology medical care, it is hard to shed the "emotional symbolism" of food. However, artificial feedings such as nasogastric tubes, gastrostomies, and intravenous infusions are significantly different from bottle-feeding or spoonfeeding—they are medical procedures with inherent risks and possible side effects, instituted by skilled health-care providers to compensate for impaired physical functioning. Analytically, artificial feeding by means of a nasogastric tube or intravenous infusion can be seen as equivalent to artificial breathing by means of a respirator. Both prolong life through mechanical means when the body is no longer able to perform a vital bodily function on its own.

Furthermore, while nasogastric feeding and other medical procedures to ensure nutrition and hydration are usually well tolerated, they are not free from risks or burdens; they have complications that are sometimes serious and distressing to the patient. Nasogastric tubes may lead to pneumonia, cause irritation and discomfort, and require arm restraints for an incompetent patient. Finally, dehydration may well not be distressing or painful to a dying patient. For patients who are unable to sense hunger and thirst, withholding of feeding devices such as nasogastric tubes may not result in more pain than the termination of any other medical treatment. Indeed, it has been observed that patients near death who are not receiving nourishment may be more comfortable than patients in comparable conditions who are being fed and hydrated artificially. Thus, it cannot be assumed that it will always be beneficial for an incompetent patient to receive artificial feeding or harmful for him not to receive it.

Under the analysis articulated above, withdrawal or withholding of artificial feeding, like any other medical treatment, would be permissible if there is sufficient proof to satisfy the subjective, limited-objective, or pure-objective test. A competent patient has the right to decline any medical treatment, including artificial feeding, and should retain that right when and if he becomes incompetent.

Natural Death Act

The State of California

Legislative Counsel's Digest

AB 3060, Keene. Cessation of medical care for terminal patients.

No existing statute prescribes a procedure whereby a person may provide in advance for the withholding or withdrawal of medical care in the event the person should suffer a terminal illness or mortal injury.

This bill would expressly authorize the withholding or withdrawal of life-sustaining procedures, as defined, from adult patients afflicted with a terminal condition, as defined, where the patient has executed a directive in the form and manner prescribed by the bill. Such a directive would generally be effective for 5 years from the date of execution unless sooner revoked in a specified manner. This bill would relieve physicians, licensed health professionals acting under the direction of a physician, and health facilities from civil liability, and would relieve physicians and licensed health professionals acting under the direction of a physician from criminal prosecution or charges of unprofessional conduct, for withholding or withdrawing life-sustaining procedures in accordance with the provisions of the bill.

The bill would provide that such a withholding or withdrawal of life-sustaining procedures shall not constitute a suicide nor impair or invalidate life insurance, and the bill would specify that the making of such a directive shall not restrict, inhibit, or impair the sale, procurement, or issuance of life insurance or modify existing life insurance. The bill would provide that health insurance carriers, as prescribed, could not require execution of a directive as a condition for being insured for, or receiving, health care services.

The bill would make it a misdemeanor to willfully conceal, cancel, deface, obliterate, or damage the directive of another without the declarant's consent. Any person, not justified or excused by law, who falsifies or forges the directive of another or willfully conceals or withholds personal knowledge of a prescribed revocation with the intent to cause a withholding or withdrawal of life-sustaining procedures contrary to the wishes of the declarant and thereby causes life-sustaining procedures to be withheld or withdrawn, and death to thereby be hastened, would be subject to prosecution for unlawful homicide.

The people of the State of California do enact as follows:

CHAPTER 3.9. NATURAL DEATH ACT

7188. Any adult person may execute a directive directing the withholding or withdrawal of life-sustaining procedures in a terminal condition.

From California Health and Safety Code, Part I, Division 7, Chapter 3.9, Section 7188. Approved by the Governor on the 30th of September, 1976.

The directive shall be signed by the declarant in the presence of two witnesses not related to the declarant by blood or marriage and who would not be entitled to any portion of the estate of the declarant upon his decease under any will of the declarant or codicil thereto then existing or, at the time of the directive, by operation of law then existing. In addition, a witness to a directive shall not be the attending physician, an employee of the attending physician or a health facility in which the declarant is a patient, or any person who has a claim against any portion of the estate of the declarant upon his decease at the time of the execution of the directive. The directive shall be in the following form:

DIRECTIVE TO PHYSICIANS

Directive made this _____ day of _____ _____ (month, year).

I _____ , being of sound mind, willfully, and voluntarily make known my desire that my life shall not be artificially prolonged under the circumstances set forth below, do hereby declare:

1. If at any time I should have an incurable injury, disease, or illness certified to be a terminal condition by two physicians, and where the application of life-sustaining procedures would serve only to artificially prolong the moment of my death and where my physician determines that my death is imminent whether or not life-sustaining procedures are utilized, I direct that such procedures be withheld or withdrawn, and that I be permitted to die naturally.

2. In the absence of my ability to give directions regarding the use of such life-sustaining procedures, it is my intention that this directive shall be honored by my family and physician(s) as the final expression of my legal right to refuse medical or surgical treatment and accept the consequences from such refusal.

3. If I have been diagnosed as pregnant and that diagnosis is known to my physician, this directive shall have no force or effect during the course of my pregnancy.

4. I have been diagnosed and notified at least 14 days ago as having a terminal condition by _____ M.D., whose address is _____ , and whose telephone number is _____ . I understand that if I have not filled in the physician's name and address, it shall be presumed that I did not have a terminal condition when I made out this directive.

5. This directive shall have no force or effect five years from the date filled in above.

6. I understand the full import of this directive and I am emotionally and mentally competent to make this directive.

Signed _____

City, County and State of Residence_____

The declarant has been personally known to me and I believe him or her to be of sound mind.

Witness _____

Witness _____

Decision Scenario 1 ··

"Apparently he was inside the tank with an oxygen hose to provide ventilation," Dr. Mangel said. "There was some oil residue on the walls. When Mr. Golenga struck an arc to weld the seam, there was a flash fire."

Mrs. Golenga gripped the hand of her nineteen-year-old son Cervando. Both had been crying, but now listening was so important that they forced back their tears.

"How badly hurt is he?" Mrs. Golenga asked.

"Very badly," Dr. Mangel said. "Most of his body is covered with severe burns, and his lungs are damaged from breathing in the fire and smoke."

"Will he live?" Cervando asked.

"I have to be honest with you and say that I don't think he will," Dr. Mangel said. "We are giving him plasma and saline solutions to rehydrate him and antibiotics to try to stop infections. But he hasn't got much of a chance."

"The pain, what about the pain?" asked Mrs. Golenga.

"There's only so much we can do."

"There's really no hope?" Cervando asked.

"I wouldn't say that," Dr. Mangel said. "There is always hope. But in this case it is very limited. He might die in a few hours or he might die tomorrow or the next day."

"Please," Mrs. Golenga said. "Can you help him die? I know he doesn't want to suffer if he has no real hope. He told me often, 'If something happens to me, don't let them stick me full of needles and keep me alive. Tell them to put me out of my misery.' Can you do that, Doctor?"

"Are you sure that's what he would want?" Dr. Mangel asked.

"My mother is right," Cervando said. "I've heard my father say that many times. He said he never wanted to just lie around and suffer, being a burden to himself and everyone. We want to do as he wanted us to."

"We could stop treating him," Dr. Mangel said. "Then let nature take its course."

"That sounds terrible," Mrs. Golenga said. "To make a man fight for his life when he has no hope and no help. It is cold and cruel."

"I'm sorry," said Dr. Mangel. "It is all that the law permits me to do."

Would Rachels regard this as the kind of case in which active euthanasia would be more humane than passive?

Using Justice Schreiber's tests, would it be legitimate to withhold additional treatments?

According to the conservative view of Gay-Williams, is there anything that might be done to put an end to Mr. Golenga's life that would also be morally acceptable?

Would the line of reasoning taken by Chief Justice Hughes in the Quinlan case make Mrs. Golenga and Cervando the appropriate people to decide whether Mr. Golenga receives additional treatment, is allowed to die, or is killed?

Decision Scenario 2 ....

Mr. Jeffry Box was eighty-one years old when he was brought to Doctor's Hospital. His right side was paralyzed, he spoke in a garbled way, and he had trouble understanding even the simplest matters. His only known relative was a sister four years younger, and she lived half a continent away. When a hospital social worker called to tell her about her brother's condition, she was quite uninterested. "I haven't seen him in fifteen years," she said. "I thought he might already be dead. Just do whatever you think best for him. I'm too old to worry about him."

Neurological tests and x-ray studies showed Mr. Box was suffering from a brain hemorrhage caused by a ruptured blood vessel.

"Can you fix it?" asked Dr. Hollins. She was the resident responsible for Mr. Box's primary care. The man she addressed was Dr. Carl Oceana, the staff's only neurosurgeon.

"Sure," said Dr. Oceana. "I can repair the vessel and clean out the mess. But it won't do much good, you know."

"You mean he'll still be paralyzed?"

"That's right. And he'll still be mentally incoherent. After the operation he'll have to be put in a nursing home or some other chronic-care place, because he won't be able to see to his own needs."

"And if you don't operate?" Dr. Hollins asked.

Dr. Oceana shrugged. "He'll be dead by tomorrow. Maybe sooner, depending on how long it takes for the pressure in his skull to build up."

"What would you do?"

"I know what I would want done to me if I were the patient," said Dr. Oceana. "I'd want people to keep their knives out of my head and let me die a nice, peaceful death."

"But we don't know what he would want," Dr. Hollins said. "He's never been our patient before, and the social worker hasn't been able to find any friends who might tell us what he'd want done."

"Let's just put ourselves in his place," said Dr. Oceana. "Let's do unto others what we would want done unto us."

"That means letting Mr. Box die."

"Exactly."

Would the pure-objective test in the Conroy decision support the view taken by Dr. Oceana?

On what grounds might Gay-Williams object?

Would Rachels's principles justify active euthanasia?

Would the natural law view make the operation discussed a moral mandate?

Decision Scenario 3 ....

On April 8, 1984, Mr. William Bartling was admitted to the Glendale Adventist Medical Center in Los Angeles. He was seventy years old and suffered from five ordinarily fatal diseases: emphysema, diffuse arteriosclerosis, coronary arteriosclerosis, an abdominal aneurysm, and inoperable lung cancer. During the performance of a biopsy to diagnose the lung cancer, Mr. Bartling's left lung collapsed. He was placed in the ICU, and a chest tube and mechanical respirator were used to assist his breathing.

Mr. Bartling complained about the pain the respirator caused him, and he repeatedly asked to have it removed. When his physician refused, he pulled out the chest tube himself. This happened so often that eventually Mr. Bartling's hands were tied to the bed to keep him from doing it. He had signed a living will in an attempt to avoid just such a situation.

Although after discussions with Richard S. Scott, Mr. Bartling's attorney, Mr. Bartling's physician and the hospital administration agreed to disconnect the respirator, the hospital's attorney refused to permit it. He argued that since Mr. Bartling was not terminally ill, brain dead, nor in a persistent vegetative state, the hospital might be open to legal action.

Mr. Scott took the case to Los Angeles Superior Court. He argued that Mr. Bartling was legally competent to make a decision about his welfare and that, although he did not want to die, he understood that disconnecting the respirator might lead to his death. The hospital's attorney took the position that Mr. Bartling was ambivalent on the question of his death. His statements "I don't want to die" and "I don't want to live on the respirator" were taken as inconsistent and so as evidence of ambivalence. Removing the respirator, the attorney argued, would be tantamount to aiding suicide or even committing homicide.

The court refused either to allow the respirator to be removed or to order that Mr. Bartling's hands be freed. To do so, the court ruled, would be to take a positive step to end treatment, and the only precedents for doing so were in cases in which the patients were comatose, brain dead, or in a chronic vegetative state.

The case was then taken to the California Court of Appeal, which ruled: "If the right of a patient to self-determination as to his own medical treatment is to have any meaning at all, it must be paramount to the interests of the patient's hospitals and doctors. The right of a competent adult patient to refuse medical treatment is a constitutionally guaranteed right which must not be abridged."

The rule came too late for Mr. Bartling. He died twenty-three hours before the court heard his appeal.

Is there any merit to the hospital's position that to remove Mr. Bartling's respirator or to free his hands would be equivalent to assisting suicide? How might Singer's arguments apply to this position?

On the natural law view, would the request to remove the respirator be, in effect, a request for assistance in committing suicide?

How can the reasoning in the Quinlan and Conroy cases be extended to Mr. Bartling's case?

Can the arguments offered by Gay-Williams be used to support the view that it would be morally wrong even to untie Mr. Bartling's hands?

Decision Scenario 4 ....

When two plainclothes detectives arrived at Virginia Crawford's suburban apartment at 6:30 on a Sunday morning to arrest her for murder, she was not terribly surprised to see them.

She cried when they insisted on putting her in handcuffs before transporting her to the jail in the county court building. Yet she had more or less expected to be arrested eventually.

For almost a month, a police investigation had been conducted at Mercy Hospital, where Ms. Crawford worked as a nurse in the intensive care unit. The entire hospital staff knew about the investigation, and Ms. Crawford herself had been questioned on three occasions by officers conducting the inquiry. At the time, her answers had seemed to be satisfactory to the police, and there was no hint that she was under suspicion. Still, she always believed that eventually they would catch up with her.

The investigation centered on the deaths of four elderly patients during the period February 1979 to March 1980. All of the patients were in the intensive care unit at the times of their deaths. Each had been diagnosed as suffering from a terminal illness, and the chart notation on each case indicated that they had all suffered irreversible brain damage and were totally without higher brain functions.

The three women and one man were all unmarried and had no immediate family to take an interest in their welfare. All of them were being kept alive by respirators, and their deaths were caused directly by their respirators being turned off. In each instance of death, Ms. Crawford had been the person in charge of the ICU.

After securing the services of an attorney, Ms. Crawford was released on bail, and a time was set for her appearance in court. Through her attorney, Marvin Washington, she made a statement to the media.

"My client has asked me to announce that she fully and freely admits that she was the one who turned off the respirators of the four patients in question at Mercy Hospital. She acted alone and without the knowledge of any other individual. She is prepared to take full responsibility for her actions."

Mr. Washington went on to say that he would request a jury trial for his client. "I am sure," he said, "that no jury will convict Ms. Crawford of murder merely for turning off the life-support systems of people who were already dead."

When asked what he meant by that, Mr. Washington explained. "These patients were no longer people," he said. "Sometime during the course of the treatment, their brains simply stopped functioning in a way that we associate with human life."

Ms. Crawford was present during the reading of her statement, and after a whispered conversation with her attorney, she spoke once for herself. "I consider what I did an act of compassion and humanity," she said. "I consider it altogether moral, and I feel no guilt about it. I did for four people what they would have wanted done, if they had only been in a condition to know."

Does the natural law view offer grounds for removing life-support systems for people who are beyond a reasonable hope of recovery? If so, what are they?

Why would Gay-Williams's arguments lead us to condemn the actions of Ms. Crawford?

Can Singer's arguments favoring voluntary active euthanasia be extended to justify Ms. Crawford's actions?

Could any of the three "tests" described by Justice Schreiber be appealed to in defending Ms. Crawford?

Decision Scenario 5 ·····················

"I'm ready to die now," Zema Radford said to the physician who stood by her hospital bed.

"I don't think you really mean that," Dr. Carl Tang said. "You're very ill, so you aren't really in a position to make a decision like that."

"My mind is quite clear at the moment. I'll admit it isn't always, but now I know what I want. I want you to take away all these nasty tubes and wires."

"We really can't do that, Mrs. Radford. Without them you would die, and none of us wants to be responsible for your death."

Mrs. Radford was eighty-three years old, and disease had wasted her body. She lay curled on the narrow bed, her frail left arm outside the sheets so the line from the IV bag would not be obstructed. Thin green wires leading to the machine monitoring her heart rate snaked across a corner of the bed.

"Can't a patient refuse treatment?" she asked Dr. Tang.

"Ordinarily, yes. But usually only ambulatory patients do that. And, of course, we have to be sure the patient is mentally competent."

"I'm really too weak to argue," Mrs. Radford said. "If I had any of my family with me, I would ask them to help me die. I don't, so I have to ask you."

"I'll take it up with your other doctors. I can't promise what we'll do, but we'll discuss it."

If Dr. Tang believes that removing the equipment will result in the death of Mrs. Radford, would he be right, according to Gay-Williams, in refusing to remove it?

If Dr. Tang holds such a belief, then according to Rachels, would he be equally justified in killing Mrs. Radford as in removing the equipment?

Would the reasoning in the court decisions in the Quinlan and Conroy cases tend to support Mrs. Radford's request?

Why, according to Singer, would it be wrong for Dr. Tang to deny Mrs. Radford's demand?

Decision Scenario 6 ....

Consider the following four cases.

1. Harvey Shick of Tyler, Texas, on June 1, 1983, shot his wife in the head twice with a .22 caliber pistol. Mrs. Marie Shick had suffered from severe arteriosclerosis since the late 1970s and, according to her physician, suffered extreme pain in her lower legs. The couple had been happily married for forty-five years. Although Mr. Shick was charged with murder, the charges were dismissed by the state district court judge. "I found nothing would be gained in this case by further punishing this man," Judge Donald Carroll said. "This was an act motivated by love," Mr. Shick's attorney said. "He was distressed at the sickness, and additional treatment would have brought only a precarious and burdensome prolonging of life." Mrs. Shick's family supported the action.

2. On September 14, 1984, Mr. Thomas P. Engel, a registered nurse, removed the respirator from Joseph Dohr, a seventy-eight-year-old stroke victim at St. Michael Hospital in Milwaukee. Mr. Engel said that Mr. Dohr's family asked that treatment be stopped. Mr. Dohr's physician said that he had refused the request because he believed that death was imminent.

Mr. Engel described the bedside scene with Mr. Dohr's daughter that had led him to act:

> She was standing there by her father's bed, stroking his arm and cheek and crying and talking to him. He was in a coma, in a steady decline. The only thing keeping him alive was the ventilator breathing for him. "This isn't right," she said. Then she looked across the bed at me, right in my eyes, and she said, "If I could do this thing, I would." Now, what would you do?

Mr. Engel was charged with practicing medicine without a license. He pleaded guilty and received a twenty-month suspended sentence. His nursing license was revoked for one year by the state nursing board.

3. On August 8, 1985, seventy-nine-year-old Abel Montigny walked into the intensive care unit of Worcester Memorial Hospital in Worcester, Massachusetts, and shot his wife in the head. He then shot himself. Both died from the injuries. Mrs. Leona Montigny, seventy-six, had been in the hospital for several months. She suffered from serious stomach and blood disorders and was recovering from surgery. Her illnesses were considered treatable, and she was in no immediate danger of death from them.

4. Roswell Gilbert, a seventy-five-year-old retired engineer, was convicted in Ft. Lauderdale, Florida, on May 9, 1985, for killing his incurably ill seventy-three-year-old wife. The couple had been married fifty-one years. Emily Gilbert had a debilitating bone disease and Alzheimer's disease, and as a consequence, she suffered both severe pain and mental disorientation. According to a witness, on the day of the killing Mrs. Gilbert had said to her husband, "I'm in pain. I want to die." Mr. Gilbert said later, "Who's that somebody but me? I guess I got cold as ice. I took the gun off the shelf, put a bullet in it and shot her. Then I felt her pulse. I thought, 'Oh, my God, I loused it up.' I put in another bullet and shot her again."

Mr. Gilbert was sentenced to twenty-five years in prison with no chance of parole. As he left the courtroom, his daughter cried out, sobbing, "Daddy, Daddy, I don't want to see my daddy in jail—he'll die in jail."

Mr. Gilbert lost a chance for clemency when two of the members of the Florida Cabinet rejected the governor's recommendation that he be freed while the case is appealed. "The law does not give one person the right to kill another because of illness or age," said Gerald Lewis, one of those who voted against clemency.

> Compare the issues that are raised in these four cases. In what ways are the cases the same, in what ways different?

Decision Scenario 7 ....

In 1984 the Netherlands Supreme Court held that an individual who suffers from a permanent mental or physical condition that he or she finds unendurable may request assistance in dying from a physician. The patient's decision to die must be informed and irrevocable, and there must be no other solution acceptable to the patient that would improve the situation.

The decision to help the patient die must involve the physician from whom help is sought and at least one other professional. The court also held that the time and manner of death should not cause avoidable misery to others.

> Can the arguments offered by Singer be used to support a public policy of this kind?

> Are the procedural safeguards adopted in the Netherlands and those advocated by Singer ade-

> In which cases, if any, could the action taken be justified by Singer's arguments in favor of voluntary euthanasia?

> In which cases, if any, could the action be justified by the reasoning in the Conroy case?

> Is it likely that the arguments presented by Rachels could be used to justify any of the actions taken?

> quate to prevent deliberate homicide? Are they adequate to prevent people who are temporarily depressed or irrational from harming themselves?

> What danger does such a policy pose, according to Gay-Williams?

> Does the right of an individual to refuse life-sustaining medical treatment imply that an individual has a right to terminate his life by active means? If so, does this mean that society has a duty to provide assistance?

> On what grounds might Elizabeth Bouvia have been permitted to starve herself to death under medical supervision? On what grounds might her request have been refused?

PART II

RIGHTS

CHAPTER 4

PATERNALISM, TRUTH TELLING, AND CONFIDENTIALITY

SOCIAL CONTEXT: AIDS AND ITS THREATS

In the spring of 1981, the federal Centers for Disease Control began receiving reports from physicians in New York and Los Angeles that they were seeing patients with an unusual form of pneumonia caused by a protozoan, *Pneumocystis carinii*. The patients also showed signs of having damaged immune systems, leaving them prey to so-called opportunistic infections that may include bacterial and viral diseases and rare forms of cancer. In fact, the CDC soon learned that a number of the reported cases of the unusual pneumonia also had developed Kaposi's sarcoma, a rare form of cancer of the skin and internal organs. Until then it had been found almost exclusively in elderly Jewish and Mediterranean males.

The most striking aspect of the cases was that all the patients were homosexual males. When the CDC checked its records for similar cases in the past, it discovered that the first cases were in New York in 1978 and 1979—also gay males. A rapid survey of several major cities led to the discovery of almost 100 cases. The almost exclusive occurrence of the disease—whatever it might be—among gay men led to the question "What characteristic do male homosexuals have that might be responsible for the disease they are getting?"

Out of the identified cases, investigators from the CDC intensively interviewed the thirty people known to be alive.

The interviews produced information that led to the first hypothesis. Amyl and butyl nitrites ("poppers") are stimulants that when inhaled produce a temporary high. They are used almost exclusively by gay men, and more than 90 percent of those interviewed said that they had used them. This suggested that perhaps the nitrites might damage the immune system in some direct or indirect way. Or perhaps some bad batches of poppers had got on the market, and whatever was in them caused damage. The CDC began experiments with mice, collected samples of the various brands of nitrites, and conducted more interviews about their use.

Meanwhile, additional cases were being reported. The class of those affected grew to include intravenous drug users and Haitian immigrants. The fact that Haiti had a reputation for being a vacation spot for gay men suggested that the disease might have spread from there, but not all the Haitians were homosexuals. Some intravenous drug users were homosexuals, but by no means all of them. The facts were not falling into any neat and obvious pattern. The names that had been given to the disease, such as "the gay plague" and "gay-related immunological deficiency" or GRID, seemed somewhat inappropriate.

Another syndrome that seemed connected with the disease was identified. Called lymphadenopathy, it was characterized by fatigue, sudden weight loss, swollen lymph nodes, fever, chills, and night sweats. The diseases that commonly cause such generalized symptoms were all absent. This led physicians and researchers to speculate that the syndrome might be the disease at early stage.

Other hypotheses were proposed. A promising one was the "immune system overload" theory. According to it, the frequency with which gay men engage in sexual activity and the nature of activity expose them to a great variety of foreign substances, and the immune systems of some simply break down from repeated assault. The obvious difficulty with the hypothesis was that such sexual activity had been going on for thousands of years, and there was no particular reason for such immunological assaults suddenly to produce a new disease.

Some researchers favored viewing the disease as an infectious disease caused by a mutated virus or by an existing virus that was gaining wider circulation. The virus, according to the hypothesis, would in some way attack and destroy the immune system and leave its victims open to the opportunistic infections that people with an intact immune system are not prey to.

The hypothesis gained support when two cases of the disease were diagnosed in hemophiliacs. The only way in which they could have been exposed was through the injection of blood factors they required to control their hemophilia. Both had received injections of the blood-clotting protein called factor VIII. It is so chemically unstable that it cannot be subjected to the usual purification

process of pasteurization without being destroyed. That, plus the fact that a single injection may contain the factor from as many as 2,500 people, means that hemophiliacs are exposed to an unusual extent to bloodborne viruses. It began to look more certain that the mysterious disease was caused by an infectious agent, probably a virus.

The disease soon received the more neutral name of Acquired Immune Deficiency Syndrome—AIDS. Laboratory work began to reveal some of the characteristics of AIDS at the biological and molecular level. Although AIDS patients have a normal or elevated level of antibodies in their blood, researchers discovered that the patients lack a normal number of white blood cells known as "helper T-cells" or T-4 lymphocytes that play a crucial role in making antibodies effective. Furthermore, white blood cells known as "suppressor T-cells" or T-8 lymphocytes that inhibit the antibody system are present in increased numbers. The immune system is thus rendered very ineffective. (It is now known that this condition is not specific for AIDS, but it was more evidence that a virus-like organism that attacks the immune system might be responsible for the disease.)

In the spring of 1984, Robert C. Gallo of the National Cancer Institute and Luc Montagnier of the Pasteur Institute in Paris independently reported the identification of a virus that is almost certainly the cause of AIDS. The American name for the virus is HTLV-III (Human T-cell Lymphotropic Virus-III), and the French name is LAV (Lymphadenopathy-Associated Virus).

Additional research has done much to identify the mechanism by which the AIDS virus works. When it is introduced into the body, it enters the T-cell and becomes a part of the DNA in the cell's nucleus. When the T-cell is activated in the presence of an infection, the virus reproduces itself and kills the T-cell, and this releases new virus to infect other T-cells.

Epidemiologists currently believe that the disease originated in Central Africa, most likely in Zaire. It then spread to the Caribbean, was acquired by American homosexuals in Haiti, then began to spread in the United States, probably from New York. Cases in Europe still number in the hundreds, and some cases have been reported in the USSR and the People's Republic of China. Larger numbers of cases have been reported in South America. The spread of the disease is a worldwide phenomenon.

The way in which the virus is transmitted is not well understood. The virus is most concentrated in the blood and semen of those infected, and the introduction of the virus directly into the blood seems the most certain mode of transmission. Thus, drug users who share a syringe with a carrier are at most risk of infection, as are those who receive blood products contaminated with the virus.

The virus seems most often transmitted by sexual relations in which semen comes into contact with mucous membrane. Thus, in the case of male homosexuals, the virus may enter the bloodstream through the lining of the rectum during anal intercourse. In heterosexual intercourse, the vaginal membrane may be the means of entry. Anal sex seems to pose the greatest risk for both men and women, for the rectal membrane is delicate, and small tears may allow entry of the virus. Because of the presence of the virus in semen, transmission seems more likely from male to female than vice versa. Pregnant women who carry the virus may pass it on to the fetus through the maternal–fetal circulatory system.

The virus has been discovered in low concentrations in the saliva and tears of those infected. Kissing in which saliva is exchanged is thought to be a slight risk, but sneezing, coughing, touching, and so on are not considered likely means of transmission. Even food handlers with AIDS are not thought to pose a significant risk to others.

Outside a host, the AIDS virus seems to be quite fragile, and this means it is unlikely anyone could become infected by using dishes, eating utensils, books, toilet seats, or other articles touched by a carrier. In short, there is strong evidence to believe that AIDS is not spread by means of ordinary social contact in the way that, for example, cold viruses are spread.

Since the discovery of the virus, the most important result has been the development of a blood test to determine exposure to the virus. The test works by detecting the presence of antibodies to the virus in a blood sample. Blood collection agencies now routinely screen blood donors. Since there is normally a six-week period between an individual's becoming infected and developing antibodies, the test cannot eliminate all potential donors who might be carriers. However, public health officials claim that the blood supply is safer than it has ever been.

No effective treatment for AIDS has yet been devised. Nor is a vaccine to protect against it available. In the view of some, it may be as long as ten years before a vaccine is developed. Meanwhile, according to most experts, the only practical means to slow the spread of the virus and keep the number of cases from increasing is public education. Thus, people are advised to limit their sexual contacts, avoid anal intercourse, use condoms, avoid using unsterilized syringes, avoid sexual relations with anyone who might have AIDS, and make an effort to determine the sexual history of a potential sex partner.

Although statistics will change as more information about the disease and its spread accumulates, here is what is known and projected for the next five years as of June 1986:

> About 21,500 cases of AIDS have been reported. Some 12,000 people have died from the disease. No one has been known to recover.

It is estimated that 1 to 1.5 million people in the United States have been exposed to the virus and may be assumed to be carriers. That is, they may be able to pass on the virus to others.

The Public Health Service estimates that by 1991 there will be a cumulative total of 270,000 cases and 179,000 deaths.

In 1986, about 9,000 people died of AIDS. The 1991 figure is expected to be 54,000. (For comparison, in 1982 45,800 people died in automobile accidents.)

Fewer than 400 cases of AIDS have been diagnosed in children. The figure is expected to rise to 3,000 by 1991.

It takes an average of four years for an infected person to develop the disease. Many now infected may appear healthy, but 20 to 30 percent will become ill.

Currently 31 percent of AIDS cases are in New York, and 10 percent are in San Francisco. Within five years, the two cities will account for less than 20 percent of the cases.

About 1,400 cases have been diagnosed in women. Nearly half deny being intravenous drug abusers.

Homosexual or bisexual men now account for about 73 percent of AIDS cases. This figure is not expected to change sharply. About 25 percent of new cases is expected to involve intravenous drug use.

In 1986, 1,100 cases involved heterosexual men and women, about 7 percent of the total. By 1991, the figure is projected to rise to 7,000 or 9 percent of the total number.

AIDS and Social Issues

In the view of some observers, AIDS poses a public health threat that is more serious than those of the infamous plagues of the past. In part this is due to the long incubation period of the virus, which may be on the order of two to five years, so those who are infected can infect others without being sick themselves. In the years since the disease was identified, the number of victims has at least doubled every year.

Public concern has increased to match the spread of the disease, and a recent poll indicates that over sixty percent believe that it is likely that AIDS will eventually become an epidemic threatening the public at large.

An issue that has become a matter of controversy in several states is whether children with AIDS should be allowed to attend public school. In Kokomo, Indiana, for example, thirteen-year-old Ryan White, a hemophiliac who acquired the virus from blood transfusion, was allowed to enroll in the seventh grade only after a long court battle. Officials were afraid he would spread the disease to other children.

School officials in New Jersey and New York City have decided that most children with AIDS should be allowed to attend regular classes. In New York, the city has set up a panel to review each child with the disease in a case-by-case fashion. Children with open sores, those who lack control over their bodily functions, or those who show a tendency to bite will be dealt with under special programs and not allowed to enter ordinary classrooms. In proceeding in this fashion, the school officials are following the advice of the CDC, which has recommended that most children with AIDS be allowed in the classroom and that officials do their best to protect the privacy of such pupils.

Some parents of unaffected children see any risk at all as too much, when the disease in question is invariably fatal. In the New York borough of Queens, eleven thousand elementary and junior high school students were kept out of class to protest the admission of AIDS children. "They send children home if they have lice or chicken pox, but they want to let them in if they have AIDS," one of the demonstrating parents said. "Now what kind of reasoning is that?"

Another issue generated by the AIDS epidemic has been raised by the insurance industry. The cost of medical care for each AIDS patient has been estimated to be over $150,000, and insurance companies are considering ways of discovering whether an applicant is likely to get the disease. Some say they may add a blood test to the application procedure, while others say an applicant's medical history is enough to indicate whether he is a higher-than-average risk.

Homosexual rights groups are fearful that the insurers will make use of questions about AIDS to discriminate against male homosexuals in general. Further, there is the possibility that all unmarried males might find it difficult to get insurance. An indication of this is the memo from Lincoln National advising its underwriters to flag applications "if life style, habits or medical history suggests a person is in one of the AIDS risk groups." The memo also suggested using marital status as an indicator of possible homosexuality, particularly those 20 to 49 who live in such cities as New York and Los Angeles.

Critics of plans to screen for AIDS have also pointed out that the antibody test indicates only exposure to the virus, and not everyone who has been exposed gets the disease. The insurance industry contends that the tests are reliable. "If we can't use the test, it will adversely affect our other applicants," an industry spokesman said. California and Wisconsin have forbidden the use of the test to determine insurability, as have state regulatory agencies in New York and Michigan.

A third issue concerns discrimination against AIDS victims. Many have become the lepers of our time. Some have been unable to rent apartments or to renew leases. Others have lost their jobs and been unable to find another. Some have been refused admission to health care facilities. Even undertakers have been unwilling to accept the bodies of AIDS victims or have charged higher prices to bury them. In one case, an entire jury refused to hear a case because the defendant was an AIDS sufferer.

Various municipalities have under consideration ordinances that would require a blood test for applicants for certain jobs, such as schoolteacher and restaurant worker, and would refuse employment to anyone who showed evidence of having been exposed to the AIDS virus. The U.S. armed forces now requires the test for all new recruits and turns down those who test positive. A policy to extend testing to those who are already members has recently been put into effect.

No one doubts the obligation of government, through its laws and agencies, to protect the welfare of citizens. Protection from infectious disease sometimes requires restricting or abridging the rights of those likely to spread the disease. Thus, those with tuberculosis are not allowed to come into contact with schoolchildren or to hold jobs that may permit the bacillus to be passed on to others.

The difficulty with AIDS is that, although it is clearly an infectious disease, it is not a highly infectious disease, and many aspects of its modes of transmission remain obscure. On the basis of what is currently known, a complete quarantine of those who may be carriers of the HTLV-III virus is hardly justifiable. Furthermore, if it is true that as many as 1.5 million people in the United States may be carriers, isolating them from the general population is a practical impossibility.

However, balanced against these obvious considerations is another that is equally obvious—namely, AIDS is a very serious disease, with a mortality rate that seems to be one hundred percent, for which there is no effective treatment. It can be argued that the disease is so serious that extraordinary measures must be taken to prevent its spread.

The practical and moral problem that is most pressing is the discovery of the measures to take that will provide most protection for the public, while avoiding the unnecessary abridgment of the rights of those who either have AIDS or may be carriers of the AIDS virus.

The Continuing Effort

In September of 1986, researchers announced results showing some success in treating AIDS with the drug AZT (azidothymidine). The investigators were also quick to point out that this did not mean that a cure for the disease is now available. At best, AZT appears to halt the reproduction of the virus and prolong the life of AIDS patients. It does not reverse the damage to the immune system caused by the virus, and its long-term effects are still unknown. Still, it is the only therapy known to have any degree of success.

In an initial test in 1985, most of nineteen AIDS patients who received AZT showed improvements in health and no serious toxic side effects. These results encouraged the National Institutes of Health, in cooperation with the Burrough Wellcome Company, manufacturers of the drug, to initiate clinical trials. In April 1986, the first of 280 patients with AIDS or AIDS-related complex were enrolled in trials at twelve research centers. The trials were double-blind, in that neither the patients nor the physicians treating them knew whether the drug administered was AZT or an inactive placebo. An independent panel of anonymous experts was established to assess the data.

From the beginning, there were plans to stop the trials if the data indicated that either the placebo or the AZT group was doing so poorly or so well that it would be morally wrong to continue the experiment. (See Chapter 5 for a discussion of the issues involved in human experimentation.) The initial results of a six-month study showed that AZT was relatively effective in the treatment of AIDS patients with *Pneumocystis carinii* pneumonia and those in an advanced stage of the disease. This outcome was judged to be so significant that the use of placebos in the treatment of the 64 percent of patients who fall into these categories is now considered to be unjustifiable. However, researchers fear that once AZT becomes generally available for prescription, it will be difficult to recruit experimental subjects. AIDS patients may be reluctant to enroll in studies that involve other drugs, even if the patients have a form of the disease that places them in a different category from the one for which AZT was shown to be effective.

Another development holding some promise was the announcement in December 1986 that a vaccine for AIDS was being tested in Zaire by a team headed by Daniel Zagury of the University of Paris. Most American experts had expected that it would be at least a year later before clinical trials with a vaccine could be initiated. When interviewed, Dr. Zagury said that he was "under oath" to the government of Zaire not to disclose anything about the experiment until the results were published. Other scientists suggested that the vaccine would be administered to those who are carriers of the AIDS virus but have not yet developed the disease. The vaccine, which may be made out of fragments of the viral membrane, is supposed to trigger the production of great quantities of "killer lymphocytes" that will eliminate a larger group of variations in the virus than would a specific antibody. That the vaccine itself might produce the disease in those free of symptoms is a genuine danger.

Research into the prevention and treatment of AIDS is proceeding with a speed unprecedented in the history of medicine. Yet to those who are ill with the disease or who know they are carriers of the virus and to their families and friends, the pace of advancement must seem glacially slow.

SOCIAL CONTEXT: UNAPPROVED DRUGS AND PERSONAL FREEDOM

The public first became aware that actor Rock Hudson was an AIDS victim when his press representative announced that he was in Paris to seek treatment for the disease. A drug rumored to have some chance of success against AIDS was not legally available in the United States. After treatment, Hudson returned to his home in California where he died a few weeks later.

Every year hundreds, perhaps even thousands, of Americans travel to foreign countries to seek medical treatments that are not available to them at home. They go to clinics in Mexico, West Germany, Switzerland, Brazil, Greece, the Bahamas, and a number of other places. Mostly they are cancer patients, but more recently they include a growing number of AIDS patients. Most have learned that they can reasonably expect to live only a few more weeks or months. Whatever their disease, they all share a sense of desperation. They are trying to save their lives.

According to the American Cancer Society, some of the clinics are simply outright frauds that are operated by unscrupulous physicians to profit from the desperation of their patients. A week's treatment can sometimes cost as much as ten thousand dollars, although most cost less. Even those clinics that are operated by physicians who are sincere do not provide treatments that are considered effective by the standards of the U.S. Food and Drug Administration.

One such clinic is located in Athens, Greece. The owner, Dr. Heriton Alvizatos, claims to have developed a serum that is sixty percent effective in halting the growth of most types of cancer, except in very advanced cases. In an interview with reporter Robert Lindsey, Dr. Alvizatos said that the serum attacks a substance that surrounds cancer cells and weakens the body's ability to keep the disease from spreading. He regards the content of the serum a "medical secret."

Both Greek and American experts have rejected such claims as ridiculous. The Minister of Social Services called Dr. Alvizatos a "merchant charlatan selling hope." However, Greek courts acquitted him of fraud charges, on the grounds that his patients took the serum willingly and it caused no bad side effects.

The American Cancer Society said in a statement that it has no evidence that the Alvizatos treatment produces any objective benefits. Lacking such evidence, the Society "would strongly urge individuals affected with cancer not to participate in Dr. Alvizatos's treatment."

Despite such warnings, dozens of Americans receive treatment in the clinic each week. In interviews with Robert Lindsey, some of them claimed that their cancer went into remission after Alvizatos treated them. All reported that their American physicians had told them that the treatment had nothing to do with the remission and that they would have recovered anyway.

Why are Americans required to travel to distant countries and spend large amounts of money just to get treatments they want? Why are such treatments not available in their own communities? Why should desperate and dying people be forced to make personal and financial sacrifices to gain access to therapies that they believe might be of benefit to them?

One answer to these questions lies in the responsibilities assigned to the federal Food and Drug Administration. The FDA has the task of approving for use all new drugs and medical devices. Even before a drug is used experimentally in clinical trials, it must have FDA approval for experimental use. Applications for approval must include data about the use of the drug in experimental animals. Only after such approval can clinical studies of the drug be initiated. Randomized clinical trials of the drug in patient populations are conducted, and the significance of the results is established through statistical analysis. In general, an effort is made to design studies that possess the formal features of any good scientific experiment.

Before a drug is approved by the FDA for use in medical therapy, the experimental evidence must show that the drug is safe and effective as a treatment for a particular disease or class of diseases. Once approval is granted, the drug may then be legally prescribed by physicians.

Drugs that have not been granted.FDA approval cannot be legally prescribed. Thus, a drug such as Dr. Alvizatos's serum cannot be legally obtained in the United States and could be approved only if it went through the testing process required by the FDA.

The testing required by the FDA is extensive and ordinarily takes a long time—a period of years is not uncommon. Also, the FDA has historically been reluctant to accept the data produced in foreign studies. Consequently, the agency has often been criticized for slowing down the introduction of effective drugs in this country. Often a drug is available in Europe long before it is available in the United States.

However, the slow and rigorous process required by the FDA also has its advantages. Patients in the United States are provided with a great deal of protection from the harmful effects of new and poorly-tested drugs. Perhaps the most dramatic instance of this is the FDA's refusal to approve the drug thalidomide. Even though it was widely prescribed as a tranquilizer in several European countries and some studies of its safety had been done, its effects when taken by pregnant women had not been studied. The tragic outcome was that the children born to women who had taken the drug were severely malformed, blind or deaf, or had seriously defective internal organs. The United States was saved from having a "thalidomide generation" by FDA requirements.

Certainly no one wishes to run unknown risks from the effects of drugs under ordinary circumstances. However, those who have been told that they have terminal diseases for which approved therapies are of limited effectiveness can hardly be said to be in ordinary circumstances. Should they not be allowed access to whatever drug they might wish to try? Should they not be permitted to experiment on themselves if they choose to do so? Is it not paternalistic to the point of absurdity to attempt to protect people who believe themselves beyond protection and wish only the freedom to attempt to save their lives?

It would certainly be possible to pass laws that would allow anyone diagnosed as having an ordinarily terminal illness to request treatment of any sort. Thus, anyone who wished to use an untested drug merely rumored to be effective would have the freedom to do so.

Although such legislation would promote individual freedom, it would also have some serious negative consequences. Perhaps the most serious result would be that the integrity and effectiveness of the medical care system would be threatened. The system is supported to a considerable extent by current drug regulations, and if any and all drugs were legalized for even restricted therapeutic use, the way would be opened for the development of various forms of quackery. It is easy to imagine that clinics specializing in the treatment of "hopeless" patients would soon spring up.

The existence of such clinics would have the effect of encouraging patients to place their trust in worthless but well-publicized drugs. Patients who might derive benefits from established therapies would be likely to turn away from them in favor of unproved remedies. The very fact of legalization would serve to give an air of legitimacy to virtually any kind of treatment. Those desperately attempting to lengthen their lives might actually shorten them.

It cannot be denied that placing restrictions on the type of therapy an individual is free to choose can be construed as a form of paternalism. We legitimately assume that individuals want to protect themselves from therapies judged by ordinary scientific standards as useless and potentially harmful. Thus we are usually not inclined to regard drug regulations and standards of medical practice as paternalistic. However, from the point of view of someone with a terminal illness who is desperate enough to try any remedy, such restrictions may be viewed as blatantly paternalistic. But can we safely make exceptions for such people without subjecting the rest of the population to unacceptable risks?

CASE PRESENTATION
Juan Gonzalez and the Prediction of Dangerousness

In July of 1986, while the Staten Island ferry was making its run across New York harbor, Juan Gonzalez unsheathed a two-foot souvenir sword and began slashing and stabbing the people around him. Shouting incoherently, Gonzalez continued his attack until Edward del Pino, a retired police officer, fired a shot into the air and ordered Gonzalez to drop to the deck. By that time, two people were dead and nine others were wounded.

"The Father, the Son, and the Holy Spirit made me do it," Mr. Gonzalez told the police as he was charged with murder and assault. He was later taken to a hospital for a psychiatric evaluation. Only a few days before, Gonzalez had undergone another evaluation. Police had taken him into custody after he had been reported wandering the streets and making threats like "I'm going to kill! God told me so." At Presbyterian Hospital, psychiatrists had diagnosed his illness as a psychotic paranoid disorder and released him after two days.

After events aboard the ferry, the question asked by the Mayor, physicians, and ordinary citizens was, Why was such an obviously dangerous person released? A brief investigation showed that Mr. Gonzalez had responded well to treatment, that no hospital space was available, and that he had been given antipsychotic drugs to take. He had also agreed to report as an outpatient, although he never did.

The Gonzalez case raised in combination two issues that have been the subjects of dispute in recent years—the right of the state to restrict the liberties of mentally ill individuals and the ability of psychiatry to predict dangerous behavior.

For almost thirty years, in response to court decisions, states have moved away from forcibly confining the mentally ill. More effective drugs to control psychoses and the movement to protect the civil rights of the mentally ill are two major factors responsible for this change in legal and social policies. In most states, the grounds for involuntary civil commitment and psychiatric treatment require that an individual be shown to be dangerous to himself or to others or to suffer from a condition that renders him mentally disabled. After a period of time, typically amounting to only a few days, a court hearing is then required to determine whether commitment and treatment may legitimately continue.

Some critics are of the opinion that the movement to keep the majority of mentally ill people out of institutions has gone too far. By some estimates, more than thirty percent of the homeless people on the streets of larger cities suffer from some kind of psychiatric illness that would warrant their being confined to an institution. The liberty of these people has been protected only by imposing on them a burden of responsibility they are unable to bear.

Furthermore, critics charge, a new standard of involuntary commitment and treatment is needed to prevent incidents like the one on the Staten Island ferry. Those who are judged to pose a *potential*, as well as an immediate, threat to others should be institutionalized and treated. The safety of the public demands no less.

However, the difficulty with adopting such a standard is that it is not possible to make reliable predictions about the dangerousness of an individual. This is a matter on which psychiatric experts are in general agreement. John Monahan, the author of *Predicting Violent Behavior*, points out that "No psychological test has any proven ability, not even the crudest accuracy, in forecasting violence." Furthermore, there is no apparent connection between a particular psychiatric diagnosis and violent behavior. For example, schizophrenics as a group are no more likely to be violent than are other people. Violence is associated with a wide range of both chronic and acute mental problems.

Whether an individual has been violent in the past is something of an indicator of how he is likely to behave in the future. But unless the individual is able to reveal this information and chooses to do so, it is often not known to the psychiatrist who is called upon to make an evaluation. Also, an individual who has "command hallucinations," voices that command him to act in certain ways, may be presumed to be more inclined to violence than others, if the hallucinations have a violent content. (It was the manifestation of command hallucinations that led Mr. Gonzalez to be taken to Presbyterian Hospital for his first psychiatric evaluation.) However, not all who have such hallucinations will admit to them, and a psychiatrist may have little or no objective reason to believe that such a patient may be dangerous.

The dilemma facing the psychiatrist is neatly summed up by Samuel Perry of the Payne-Whitney Clinic. "The decision to hold someone because he is dangerous is psychiatry's Scylla and Charybdis. On one hand, if you hold a patient against his will and there is no good medical reason, you are violating his civil rights. On the other hand, if you fail to keep someone who is disturbed and dangerous, and he harms someone, the victim can sue you for negligence."

INTRODUCTION

Consider the following cases:

1. A state decides to require that all behavioral therapists (that is, all who make use of psychological conditioning techniques to alter behavior patterns) be either licensed psychologists or psychiatrists.

2. A member of the Plymouth Brethren sect is opposed to the "shedding of blood" and refuses to consent to a needed appendectomy, but when his appendix ruptures and he lapses into unconsciousness, the surgical resident operates and saves his life.

3. A physician decides not to tell the parents of an infant who died shortly after birth that the cause of death was an unpredictable birth defect because he does not wish to influence their desire to have a child.

4. A janitor employed in an elementary school consults a psychiatrist retained by the school board and tells her that he has on two occasions molested young children; the psychiatrist decides that it is her duty to inform the school board.

There is perhaps no single moral issue that is present in all these cases. Rather, there is a complex of related issues. Each case involves acting on the behalf of someone else— the public, a patient, or a special group. And each action comes into conflict with the desires, rights, or expectations of some person or persons. Even though the issues are related, it is most fruitful to discuss them separately.

PATERNALISM

Exactly what paternalism is, is itself a matter of dispute. Roughly speaking, we can say that paternalism consists in acting in a way that is believed to protect or advance the interest of a person although acting in this way goes against the person's own immediate desires or limits the person's freedom of choice. (Oversimplifying, paternalism is the view that "Father knows best.") Thus, the first three cases presented above are instances of paternalistic behavior.

It is useful to distinguish what we can call "state paternalism" from "personal paternalism." State paternalism, as the name suggests, is the control exerted by a legislature, agency, or other governmental body over particular kinds of practices or procedures. Such control is typically exercised through laws, licensing requirements, technical specifications, and operational guidelines and regulations. (The first case above is an example of state paternalism.)

By contrast, personal paternalism consists in an individual's deciding, on the basis of his own principles or values, that he knows what is best for another person. The individual then acts in a way that deprives the other person of genuine and effective choice. (Cases two and three are examples of this.) Paternalism is personal when it is not a matter of public or semipublic policy but is a result of private, moral decision making.

State Paternalism in Medical and Health Care

At first sight, state paternalism seems wholly unobjectionable in the medical context. We are all certain to feel more confident in consulting a physician when we know that she or he has had to meet the standards for education, competence, and character set by a state licensing board and medical society. We feel relatively sure that we aren't putting ourselves in the hands of an incompetent quack.

Indeed, that we can feel such assurance can be regarded as one of the marks of the social advancement of medicine. As late as the early twentieth century in the United States, the standards for physicians were low, and licensing laws were either nonexistent or poorly enforced. It was possible to qualify as a physician with as little as four

months formal schooling and a two-year apprenticeship. Even these requirements were enforced only at prestigious medical schools such as Yale's. Privately owned schools that were run for profit were not overly stringent in their admissions policies or graduation requirements.

In addition, many people practiced a form of medicine not taught in the medical schools. Thompsonists claimed that herbs of the right kind would cure all ailments, and homeopaths believed that minute doses of drugs that would cause disease symptoms in a healthy person would also eliminate those symptoms in a sick person. Hydropaths relied upon externally and internally applied water as a basic treatment modality, and naturopaths emphasized the curative power of proper diet and exercise.

Virtually all of the nonstandard medicine practiced in the nineteenth century we would now regard as quackery. Most of those who practiced it were sincere in their beliefs, but the theories on which their practices were based are ones that we consider to be completely false. Ironically, the irregular practitioners were often more successful than their orthodox counterparts. Whereas standard medicine relied on such "heroic" measures as bleeding and purging, the "quacks" generally stressed minimum intervention and the healing power of nature. Nature quite often turned out to be a better physician than even the best trained physician.

Strict licensing laws and the upgrading of medical schools eventually led to the triumph of a standard medicine based on the theories of the natural sciences. Irregular medicine virtually disappeared from the American scene. Confidence in the scientific basis of medicine was increased with the widespread acceptance of the germ theory of disease, the identification of particular disease-causing bacterial agents, and the development of specific drug therapies that could bring about almost miraculous cures in some diseases. The

Pure Food and Drug Laws reflected this confidence, and their enforcement was used as a weapon to protect consumers from practitioners who used therapies that were unproved scientifically. The laws are still used for this purpose.

There is little doubt that rigorous standards and strictly enforced laws have done much to improve medical care in this country. At the very least, they have made it less dangerous to consult a physician. At the same time, however, they have also placed close restrictions on individual freedom of choice. In the nineteenth century, a person could choose among a variety of medical viewpoints. That is no longer so today.

It is no longer the case because we now recognize that some medical viewpoints are wrong and if implemented, may endanger a patient. At the very least, people treated by those who espouse such views run the risk of not getting the best kind of medical care available. Unlike people in the nineteenth century, we are confident that we know (within limits) what kinds of medical therapies are effective and what kinds are useless or harmful. The scientific character of contemporary medicine gives us this confidence.

Secure in these beliefs, our society generally endorses paternalism by the state in the regulation of medical practice. We believe it is important to protect sick people from quacks and charlatans, from those who raise false hopes and take advantage of human suffering. We generally accept, then, that the range of choice of health therapy ought to be limited to what we consider to be legitimate and scientific.

This point of view is not one that everyone is pleased to endorse. In particular, those seeking treatment for cancer or for AIDS have sometimes wanted to try drugs rumored to be effective but not approved by the Food and Drug Administration. Such drugs cannot be legally prescribed in the United States, and those wishing to gain access to them

must travel to foreign clinics, often at considerable discomfort and expense. (See the Social Context above for additional discussion of the situation.) Some have claimed that FDA regulations make it impossible for them to choose the therapy that they wish and that this is an unwarranted restriction of their rights. It should be enough, they claim, for the government to issue a warning if it thinks one is called for. But after that, people should be free to act as they choose.

The debate about unapproved therapies raises a more general question: To what extent is it legitimate for a government to restrict the actions and choices of its citizens for their own good? It is perhaps not possible to give a wholly satisfactory general answer to this question. No one objects that he is not permitted to drink polluted water from the city water supply or that he is not able to buy candy bars contaminated with insect parts. Yet some do object if they have to drink water that contains fluorides or if they cannot buy candy bars that contain saccharine. But all such limitations result from governmental attempts to protect the health of citizens.

Seeing to the well-being of its citizens certainly has to be recognized as one of the legitimate aims of a government. And such functioning may easily include seeing to their physical health. State paternalism with respect to health seems, in general, to be justifiable. Yet the laws and regulations through which the paternal concern is expressed are certain to come into conflict with the exercise of individual liberties. Perhaps the only way in which conflicts can be resolved is on an issue-by-issue basis. Later, we will discuss some of the limitations that moral theories place on state paternalism.

It is worth noticing that state paternalism in medical and health-care matters may be more pervasive than it seems at first sight. Laws regulating medical practice, the licensing of physicians and medical personnel, regulations governing the licensing and testing of drugs, and guidelines that must be followed in scientific research are some of the more obvious expressions of paternalism. Less obvious is the fact that government research funds can be expended only in prescribed ways and that only certain approved forms of medical care and therapy will be paid for under government-sponsored health programs. For example, it was a political and social triumph for chiropractors and Christian Science Readers when some of their services were included under Medicare coverage. Thus, government money, as well as laws and regulations, can be used in paternalistic ways.

Personal Paternalism in Medical and Health Care

That patients occupy a dependent role with respect to their physicians seems to be true historically, sociologically, and psychologically. The patient is sick, the physician is well. The patient is in need of the knowledge and skills the physician possesses, but the physician does not need those possessed by the patient. The patient seeks out the physician to ask for help, but the physician does not seek out the patient. The patient is a single individual, while the physician represents the institution of medicine with its hospitals, nurses, technicians, consultants, and so on.

In his dependence on the physician, the patient willingly surrenders some of his autonomy. Explicitly or implicitly, he agrees to allow the physician to make certain decisions for him that he would ordinarily make for himself. The physician tells him what to eat and drink and what to avoid, what medicine he should take and when to take it, how much exercise he should get and what kind it should be. The patient consents to run at least part of his life by "doctor's orders" in the hope that he will regain his health or at least improve his condition.

The physician acquires a great amount of power in this relationship. But he also acquires a great responsibility. It has been recognized at least since the time of Hippocrates that the physician has an obligation to act in the best interest of his patient. The patient is willing to transfer part of his autonomy because he is confident that the physician will act in this way.

If this analysis of the present form of the physician-patient relationship is roughly correct, two questions are appropriate.

First, should the relationship be one in which the patient is so dependent on the paternalism of the physician? Perhaps it would be better if patients did not think of themselves as transferring *any* of their autonomy to physicians. Physicians might better be thought of as people offering advice, rather than as ones issuing orders. Thus, patients, free to accept or reject advice, would retain fully their power to govern their own lives. If this is a desirable goal, it is clear that the present nature of the physician-patient relationship needs to be drastically altered.

The problem with this point of view is that the patient is ordinarily not in a position to judge the advice that is offered. The reason for consulting a physician in the first place is to gain the advantage of his knowledge and judgment. Moreover, courses of medical therapy are often complicated ones involving many interdependent steps. A patient could not expect the best treatment if he insisted on accepting some of the steps and rejecting others. As a practical matter, a patient who expects good medical care must pretty much put himself in the hands of his physician.

For this reason, the second question is perhaps based on a more realistic assessment of the nature of medical care: How much autonomy must be given up by the patient? The power of the physician over the patient cannot be absolute. The patient cannot become the slave or creature of the physician—this is not what a patient consents to when he agrees to place himself under the care of a physician. What, then, are the limits of the paternalism that can be legitimately exercised by the physician?

TRUTH TELLING IN MEDICINE

This question arises most forcefully when physicians deceive patients. When, if ever, is it justifiable for a physician to deceive her or his patient?

The paternalistic answer, of course, is that deception by the physician is justified when it is in the best interest of the patient. Suppose, for example, that a transplant surgeon detects signs of tissue rejection in a patient who has just received a donor kidney. The surgeon is virtually certain that within a week the kidney will have to be surgically removed and the patient transferred to dialysis equipment again. Although in no immediate clinical danger, the patient is suffering from postoperative depression. It is altogether possible that if the patient is told at this time that the transplant appears to be a failure, his depression will become more severe. This, in turn, might lead to a worsening of the patient's physical condition, perhaps even to a life-threatening extent.

Eventually the patient will have to be told of the need for another operation. But by the time that need arises, his psychological condition may have improved. Is the surgeon justified in avoiding giving a direct and honest answer to the patient when he asks about his condition? In the surgeon's assessment of the situation, the answer is likely to do the patient harm. His duty as a physician, then, seems to require that he deceive the patient, either by lying to him (an act of commission) or by allowing him to believe (an act of omission) that his condition is satisfactory and the transplant was successful.

Yet doesn't the patient have a right to know the truth from his physician? After all, it is his life that is being threatened. Should he not be told how things stand with him so

that he will be in a position to make decisions that affect his own future? Is the surgeon not exceeding the bounds of the powers granted to him by the patient? The patient surely had no intention of completely turning over his autonomy to the surgeon.

This issue is one of "truth telling." Does the physician always owe it to the patient to tell the truth? Some writers make a distinction between lying to the patient and merely being nonresponsive or evasive. But is this really a morally relevant distinction? In either case, the truth is being kept from the patient. Both are instances of medical paternalism.

The use of placebos (from the Latin *placebo* meaning "I shall please") in medical therapy is another issue that raises questions about the legitimate limits of paternalism in medicine. The "placebo effect" is a well-documented psychological phenomenon: even patients who are seriously ill will sometimes show improvement when they are given *any* kind of medication (a sugar pill, for example) or treatment. This can happen even when the medication or treatment is irrelevant to their condition.

The placebo effect can be exploited by physicians for the (apparent) good of their patients. Many patients cannot accept a physician's well-considered judgments. When they come to a physician with a complaint and are told that there is nothing organically wrong with them, that no treatment or medication is called for, they continue to ail. They may then lose confidence in their physician or their inclination to seek medical advice for more serious complaints.

One way to avoid these consequences is for the physician to prescribe a placebo for the patient. Since the patient (we can assume) suffers from no organic disease condition, he is not in need of any genuine medication. And because of the placebo effect, he may actually find himself relieved of the symptoms that caused him to seek medical help. Moreover, the patient feels satisfied that he has been treated, and his confidence in his physician and in medicine in general remains intact.

Since the placebo effect is not at all likely to be produced if the patient knows he is being given an ineffective medication, the physician cannot be candid about the "treatment" prescribed. She must either be silent, say something indefinite like "I think this might help your condition," or lie. Since the placebo effect is more likely to be achieved if the medication is touted as being amazingly effective against complaints like those of the patient, there is a reason for the physician to lie outright. Because the patient may stand to gain a considerable amount of good from placebo therapy, the physician may think of herself as acting in the best interest of her patient.

Despite its apparent advantages, placebo therapy may be open to two ethical criticisms. First, we can ask whether giving placebos is really in the best interest of a patient. It encourages many patients in their belief that drugs can solve their problems. Patients with vague and general complaints may need some kind of psychological counseling, and giving them placebos merely discourages them from coming to grips with their genuine problems. Also, not all placebos are harmless (see the discussion in the introduction to Chapter 5). Some contain active chemicals that produce side effects (something likely to enhance the placebo effect) so the physician who prescribes placebos may be subjecting her patient to some degree of risk.

Second, by deceiving her patient, the physician is depriving him of the chance to make genuine decisions about his own life. Because the person is not genuinely sick, it does not seem legitimate to regard him as having deputized his physician to act in his behalf or as having transferred any of his power or autonomy to the physician. In Kant's terms, the physician is not acknowledging the patient's status as an autonomous rational agent. She is not according him the dignity that he possesses simply by virtue of being human. (A utilitarian who wished to claim that telling the truth to patients is a policy that will produce the best overall benefits could offer essentially the same criticism.)

Deception is not the only issue raised by the general question of the legitimacy of medical paternalism. Another of some importance is difficult to state precisely, but it has to do with the general attitude of physicians toward their patients. Patients often feel that physicians deal with them in a way that is literally paternalistic—that physicians treat them like children.

The physician, like the magician or shaman, is often seen as a figure of power and mystery, one who controls the forces of nature and, by doing so, relieves suffering and restores health. Some physicians like this role and act in accordance with it. They resent having their authority questioned and fail to treat their patients with dignity and respect.

For example, many physicians call their patients by their first names while expecting patients to refer to them as "Dr. X." In our society, women in particular have been most critical of such condescending attitudes displayed by physicians.

More serious is the fact that many physicians do not make a genuine effort to educate patients about the state of their health, the significance of laboratory findings, or the reasons why medication or other therapy is being prescribed. Patients are not only expected to follow orders, but they are expected to do so blindly.

The issue here is not one of informed consent (which we will discuss in detail in the next chapter). For in informed consent, a patient must give permission for a procedure of a special sort to be performed. Here we are talking only about the ordinary medical situation—someone consults a physician because of a shoulder pain or just to get a yearly checkup.

The amount of time that it takes to help a patient understand his medical condition and the reason for the prescribed therapy is, of course, one reason why physicians do not attempt to provide such information. A busy physician in an office practice might see thirty or forty patients a day, and it is difficult to give each of them the necessary amount of attention. Also, patients without a medical background obviously can find it hard to understand medical explanations—particularly in the ways in which they are often given.

The result, for whatever reasons, is a situation in which physicians make decisions about patients without allowing patients to know the basis for them. Explanations are not given, it is sometimes said, because patients "wouldn't understand" or "might draw the wrong conclusions about their illness" or "might worry needlessly." Patients are thus not only *not* provided information, they are discouraged from asking questions or revealing their doubts.

The moral questions here concern the responsibility of the physician. Is it ultimately useful for patients that physicians should play the role of a distant and mysterious figure of power? If so, then it may be that physicians should cultivate the role. Do patients have a right to ask that physicians treat them with the same dignity as physicians treat one another? Should a physician attempt to educate her or his patients about their illnesses? Or is a physician's only real responsibility to provide patients with needed medical treatment?

Furthermore, is it always obvious that the physician knows what will count as the all-around best treatment for a patient? Patients, being human, have values of their own, and they may well not rank their best chance for effective medical treatment above all else. A woman with breast cancer, for example, may wish to avoid having a breast surgically removed (mastectomy) and so prefer another mode of treatment, even though her physician may consider it less effective. Can her physician legitimately withhold from her knowledge of alternate modes of treatment and so allow her no choice? Can he make the decision about treatment himself on the grounds that it is a purely medical matter, one about which the patient has no expert knowledge?

CONFIDENTIALITY

"Whatever I see or hear, professionally or privately, which ought not be divulged, I will keep secret and tell no one," runs one of the pledges in the Hippocratic Oath.

The tradition of medical practice in the West has taken this injunction very seriously. That it has done so is not entirely due to the high moral character of physicians, for the pledge to secrecy also serves an important practical function. Physicians need to have information of an intimate and highly personal sort in order to make diagnoses and prescribe courses of therapy. If physicians were known to reveal such personal information, then patients would be reluctant to cooperate, and the practice of medicine would be adversely affected. Furthermore, because psychological factors play a role in medical therapy, the chances of success in medical treatment are improved when patients can place trust and confidence in their physicians. This aspect of the physician-patient relationship actually forms a part of medical therapy. Of course this is particularly so of the "talking cures" characteristic of some forms of psychiatry.

A number of states recognize the need for "privileged communication" between physician and patient and have laws to protect physicians from being compelled to testify about their patients in court. Yet physicians are also members of a society, and the society must attempt to protect the general interest. This sometimes places the physician in the middle of a conflict between the interest of the individual and the interest of society.

For example, physicians are often required by law to act in ways that force them to reveal certain information about their patients. The best instance of this is perhaps the legal obligation to report to health departments the names of those patients who are carriers of such communicable diseases as syphilis and tuberculosis. This permits health authorities to warn those with whom the carriers have come into contact and to guard against the spread of the diseases. Thus, the interest of the society is given precedence over physician-patient confidentiality.

Few people would question society's right to demand that physicians violate a patient's confidence when the issue is that of protecting the health of great numbers of people. More open to question are laws that require physicians to report gunshot wounds or other injuries that might be connected with criminal actions. (In some states, before abortion became legal, physicians were required to report cases of attempted abortion.) Furthermore, physicians as citizens have a legal duty to report any information they may have about a crime unless they are protected by a privileged-communication law.

Thus, the physician is placed in a position of conflict. If he acts to protect the patient's confidences, then he runs the risk of acting illegally. If he acts in accordance with the law, then he must violate the confidence of his patients. What needs to be decided from a moral point of view is to what extent the laws that place a physician in such a situation are justified.

The physician who is not in private practice but is employed by a government agency or a business organization also encounters similar conflicts. Her obligations run in two directions: to her patients and to her employer. Should a physician who works for a government agency tell her superiors that an employee has confided in her that he is a drug addict? If she does not, the man may be subject to blackmail or bribery. If she does, then she must violate the patient's confidence. Or what if a psychiatrist retained by a company decides that one of the employees is so psychologically disturbed that she cannot function effectively in her job? Should the psychiatrist inform the employer of this, even it is means going against the wishes of the patient? (Consider also the fourth case cited at the beginning of this chapter.)

Even more serious problems arise in psychiatry. Suppose that a patient expresses to his psychiatrist feelings of great anger against someone and even announces that he intends to go out and kill that person. What should the psychiatrist do? Is it his obligation to warn the person being threatened? Should he report the threat to the police? This is fundamentally the issue that was dealt with by the California Supreme Court in the case of *Tarasoff* v. *Regents of the University of California.* (See the selection in this chapter by William J. Curran for a discussion.)

The basic question about confidentiality concerns the extent to which we are willing to go to protect it. It is doubtful that anyone would want to assert that confidentiality should be absolutely guaranteed. But if not, then under what conditions is it better to violate it than to preserve it?

ETHICAL THEORIES: PATERNALISM, TRUTH TELLING, CONFIDENTIALITY

What we have called state paternalism and personal paternalism are compatible with utilitarian ethical theory. But whether they are justifiable is a matter of controversy. If the principle of utility shows that governmental laws, policies, practices, or regulations increase the general happiness, then they are justified. It can be argued that they are justified even if they restrict the individual's freedom of choice or action because for utilitarianism such freedom has no absolute value. Personal paternalism is justified in a similar way. If a physician believes that she can protect her patient from unnecessary suffering or can relieve his pain by keeping him in ignorance, by lying to him, by giving him placebos or by otherwise deceiving him, then these actions are morally legitimate.

However, John Stuart Mill did not take this view of paternalism. Mill argued that freedom of choice is of such importance that it can be justifiably restricted only when it can be shown that unregulated choice would cause harm to other people. Mill claimed that compelling people to act in certain ways "for their own good" is never legitimate. This position, Mill argued, is one that is justified by the principle of utility. Gerald Dworkin, in the selection included in this chapter, provides an analysis of Mill's position, and there is no need for us to repeat it here. We should note, however, that utilitarianism does not offer a straightforward answer to the question of the legitimacy of paternalism.

What we have said about paternalism also applies more or less to the issue of confidentiality. Generally speaking, if violating confidentiality seems necessary to produce a state of affairs in which happiness is increased, then the violation is justified. This might be the case when, for example, someone's life is in danger or someone is being tried for a serious crime and the testimony of a physician is needed to help establish her innocence. Yet it also might be argued from the point of view of rule utilitarianism that confidentiality is such a basic ingredient in the physician-patient relationship that, in the long run, more good will be produced if confidentiality is never violated.

The Kantian view of paternalism, truth telling, and confidentiality is more clear-cut. Every person is a rational and autonomous agent. As such he or she is entitled to make decisions that affect his or her own life. This means that a person is entitled to receive information relevant to making such decisions and is entitled to the truth, no matter how painful it might be. The use of placebos or any other kind of deception in medicine is morally illegitimate because this would involve denying a person the respect and dignity to which he or she is entitled. The categorical imperative also rules out lying, for the maxim involved in such an action produces a contradiction. (There are special difficulties in applying the categorical imperative that we discussed in the introductory chapter. When these are taken into account, Kant's view is perhaps not quite so straightforward and definite as it first appears.)

It can be argued that Kant's principles also establish that confidentiality should be regarded as absolute. When a person becomes a patient, she does so with the expectation that what she tells her physician will be kept confidential. Thus, in the physician-patient relationship there is an implicit promise. The physician implicitly promises that he will not reveal any information about his patient, either what he has been told or what he has learned for himself. If this analysis is correct, then the physician is under an obligation to preserve confidentiality because keeping promises is an absolute duty. (Here, as in the case of lying, there are difficulties connected with the way in which a maxim is stated. See the introductory chapter for a discussion.)

Ross's principles recognize that everyone has a moral right to be treated as an autonomous agent who is entitled to make decisions affecting his own life. Also, everyone is entitled to know the truth and to be educated in helpful ways. Similarly, if confidentiality is a form of promise keeping, everyone is entitled to expect that it will be kept. Thus, paternalism, lying, and violation of confidence are prima facie morally objectionable. But, of course, it is possible to imagine circumstances in which they would be justified. The right course of action that a physician must follow is one that can be determined only on the basis of the physician's knowledge of the patient, the patient's problem, and the general situation. Thus, Ross's principles rule out paternalism, deception, and violations of confidence as general policies, but they do not make them morally illegitimate in an absolute way.

Rawls's theory of social and political morality is compatible with state paternalism of a restricted kind. No laws, practices, or policies can legitimately violate the rights of individuals. At the same time, however, a society, viewing arrangements from the original position, might decide to institute a set of practices that would promote what they agreed to be their interests. If, for example, health is agreed to be an interest, then they might be willing to grant to the state the power to regulate a large range of matters connected with the promotion of health. Establishing standards for physicians would be an example of such regulation. But they might also go so far as to give the state power to decide (on the advice of experts) what medical treatments are legitimate, what drugs are safe and effective to use, what substances should be controlled or prohibited, and so on. So long as the principles of justice are not violated and so long as the society can be regarded as imposing these regulations on itself for the promotion of its own good, then such paternalistic practices are unobjectionable. With respect to personal paternalism, deception, and confidentiality, Rawls's general theory offers no specific answers. But since Rawls endorses Ross's account of prima facie duties (while rejecting Ross's intuitionism), it seems reasonable to believe that Rawls's view on these matters would be the same as Ross's.

The natural law doctrine of Roman Catholicism suggests that paternalism in both of its forms is legitimate. When the state is organized to bring about such "natural goods" as health, then laws and practices that promote those goods are morally right. Individuals do have a worth in themselves and should be free to direct and organize their own lives. But at the same time, individuals may be ignorant of relevant information, lack the intellectual capacities to determine what is really in their best interest, or be moved by the momentary passions and circumstances. For these reasons, the state may act so that people are protected from their own shortcomings, and yet their genuine desires, their "natural ends," are satisfied.

Thus, natural law doctrine concludes that because each individual has an inherent worth, she is entitled to be told the truth in medical situations (and others) and not deceived. But it reasons too that because a physician has superior knowledge, he may often perceive the interest of the patient better than the patient herself. Accordingly, natural law doctrine indicates that although he should avoid lying, a physician is still under an obligation to act for the best interest of his patient. This may mean allowing the patient to believe something that is not so (as in placebo therapy) or withholding information from the patient. In order for this to be morally legitimate, however, the physician's motive must always be that of advancing the welfare of the patient.

In the matter of confidentiality, the natural law doctrine of Roman Catholicism recognizes that the relationship between physician and patient is one of trust, and a physician has a duty not to betray the confidences of her patients. But the relationship is not sacrosanct and the duty is not absolute. When the physician finds herself in a situation in which a greater wrong will be done if she does not reveal a confidence entrusted to her by a patient, then she has a duty to reveal the confidence. If, for example, the physician possesses knowledge that would save someone from death or unmerited suffering, then it is her duty to make this knowledge available, even if by doing so she violates a patient's trust.

We have been able merely to sketch an outline of possible ways in which our ethical theories might deal with the issues involved in paternalism, truth telling, and confidentiality. Some of the views presented are open to challenge, and none of them has been worked out in a completely useful way. That is one of the tasks that remains to be performed.

THE SELECTIONS

In his essay included in this chapter, Gerald Dworkin attempts to show that even if we place an absolute value on individual choice, then a variety of paternalistic policies can still be justified. In consenting to a system of representative government, we understand that it may act to safeguard our interests in certain ways. But, Dworkin asks, what are the "kinds of conditions which make it plausible to suppose that rational men could reach agreement to limit their liberty even when other men's interests are not affected?"

Dworkin suggests that such conditions are satisfied in cases in which there is a "good" such as health involved—one that everybody needs to pursue other goods. Rational people would agree that attaining such a good should be promoted by the government even when individuals don't recognize it as a good at a particular time. There is a sense, Dworkin argues, in which we are not really imposing such a good on people. What we are really saying is that if everyone knew the facts and assessed them properly, this is what they would choose. Also, we are sometimes influenced by immediate alternatives that look more attractive, or we are careless or depressed and so do not act for what we acknowledge as a good. Thus, we might approve of laws such as ones against cigarette smoking because we know we should not smoke cigarettes.

It is plausible, Dworkin suggests, that rational people would grant to a legislature the right to impose such restrictions on their conduct. But the government has to demonstrate the exact nature of the harmful effects to be avoided. Also, if there is an alternative way of accomplishing the end without restricting liberty, then the society should adopt it.

In "About AIDS" David A. Conway uses the dialogue form to explore the extent to which individual freedom may be restricted in the name of protecting the public from the disease. Is it legitimate to close down gay meeting places? Should children with the disease be kept out of school? Should carriers of the antibody be prohibited from working in restaurants? Most important, should those with AIDS be identified in some public way so that people wishing to avoid contact with them might do so? As one of Conway's speakers makes clear, there is always the danger that restrictions proposed in the name of public health may be no more than an expression of widespread dislike and disapproval of homosexuals. Some proposed policies are not so much paternalistic as covertly prejudicial.

Perhaps the most common form of paternalism in medicine consists in withholding information from patients. Physician Mack Lipkin, in "On Telling Patients the Truth," provides a defense of the practice. It is usually a practical impossibility to tell patients "the whole truth," he claims. Patients usually simply do not possess enough information about how their bodies work to understand the nature of their disease, and their understanding of the terms used by a physician is likely to be quite different from the meaning intended. Besides, some patients do not wish to be told the truth about their illness. Whether it is a matter of telling the truth or of deceiving patients by giving them placebos, the crucial question, according to Lipkin, is "whether the deception was intended to benefit the patient or the doctor."

Sissela Bok, in "Lies to the Sick and Dying," reviews three arguments that physicians frequently use to justify not telling the truth to their parents. All three are arguments appealed to be Lipkin. However, Bok finds each of them faulty and unpersuasive.

Bok points out that the first of the arguments trades on a confusion between telling "the truth" (that is, everything that is true about a situation) and "truthfulness" (being honest). In effect, the argument asserts that since it is impossible to tell "the truth" to people who are not medical experts, then there is no clear distinction between what is true and what is false. Anything medical said to them is, at best, partially true. When this argument is accepted, Bok claims, the way is open for the physician to decide just how much of "the truth" will be revealed to serve the best interest of the patient.

Are physicians correct in claiming that patients don't want to know the truth? This is an issue that is open to empirical tests. Bok cites studies which show that a large majority of people say they want to be told the truth about themselves, even if they should be diagnosed as having a catastrophic illness.

The last argument examined by Bok holds that information given to a patient might damage the patient (or at least not help the patient), thus proper health care demands that information not be supplied. This argument also has an empirical aspect and is open to challenge on factual grounds. As Bok observes, the harm associated with the disclosure of bad news and risks is probably greatly overestimated. What is more, very real benefits (such as increased cooperation) are never mentioned.

Bok is not willing to go so far as to say that lying to a patient is never justified. She is primarily concerned with showing that withholding the truth is a serious matter that requires justification in each case. Like Ross, she sees telling the truth to be a prima facie obligation that can be set aside only for the sake of some more weighty obligation.

In "Confidentiality in Medicine—A Decrepit Concept," Mark Siegler calls attention to the impossibility of preserving the confidentiality traditionally associated with the physician-patient relationship. In the modern hospital, a great many people have legitimate access to a patient's chart and so to all medical, social, and financial information the patient has provided. Yet the loss of confidentiality is a threat to good medical care. Confidentiality protects a patient at a time of vulnerability and promotes the trust that is necessary for effective diagnosis and treatment. Siegler concludes by suggesting some possible solutions for preserving confidentiality, while meeting the needs of others to know certain things about the patient.

William J. Curran, in the last selection, discusses a case decided by the California Supreme Court that has been of particular concern to psychiatrists. The court ruled that therapists at the student health service of the University of California at Berkeley were negligent in their duty to warn a woman named Tarasoff that her life had been threatened by one of their parents. Although the therapists had reported the threat to the police, Ms. Tarasoff was murdered by the patient. The question that Curran addresses is whether or not the therapists had done all they were obligated to do to protect both their patient and the community by reporting the case to the police. But more general issues are also involved here: Does a psychiatrist have a duty to warn at all? Should a patient be told that not everything he tells his psychiatrist will beheld in confidence? Is a psychiatrist obliged to seek a court order committing a patient involuntarily to an institution if the patient utters a threat that the psychiatrist judges to be seriously motivated? (See the Juan Gonzalez Case Presentation for a recent example of these issues.)

Paternalism, truth telling, and confidentiality are bound together in a complicated web of moral issues. We have not identified all of the strands of the web, nor have we traced out their connections with one another. We have, however, mentioned enough difficulties to reveal the seriousness of the issues.

Some of the issues are social ones and require that we decide about the moral legitimacy of certain kinds of laws, practices, and policies. Others are matters of personal morality, ones that concern our obligations to society and to other people. Our ethical theories, we can hope, will provide us with the means of arriving at workable and justifiable resolutions of the issues. But before this point is reached, much intellectual effort and ingenuity will have to be invested.

Paternalism

Gerald Dworkin

Neither one person, nor any number of persons, is warranted in saying to another human creature of ripe years, that he shall not do with his life for his own benefit what he chooses to do with it. *Mill*

I do not want to go along with a volunteer basis. I think a fellow should be compelled to become better and not let him use his discretion whether he wants to get smarter, more healthy or more honest. *General Hershey*

I take as my starting point the "one very simple principle" proclaimed by Mill in *On Liberty* . . . "That principle is, that the sole end for which mankind are warranted, individually or collectively, in interfering with the liberty of action of any of their number, is self-protection. That the only purpose for which power can be rightfully exercised over any member of a civilized community, against his will, is to prevent harm to others. He cannot rightfully be compelled to do or forbear because it will be better for him to do so, because it will make him happier, because, in the opinion of others, to do so would be wise, or even right."[1]

This principle is neither "one" nor "very simple." It is at least two principles; one asserting that self-protection or the prevention of harm to others is sometimes a sufficient warrant and the other claiming that the individual's own good is *never* a sufficient warrant for the exercise of compulsion either by the society as a whole or by its individual members. I assume that no one with the possible exception of extreme pacifists or anarchists questions the correctness of the first half of the principle. This essay is an examination of the negative claim embodied in Mill's principle—the objection to paternalistic interferences with a man's liberty.

I

By paternalism I shall understand roughly the interference with a person's liberty of action justified by reasons referring exclusively to the welfare, good, happiness, needs, interests or values of the person being coerced. One is always well-advised to illustrate one's definitions by examples but it is not easy to find "pure" examples of paternalistic interferences. For almost any piece of legislation is justified by several different kinds of reasons and even if historically a piece of legislation can be shown to have been introduced for purely paternalistic motives, it may be that advocates of the legislation with an anti-paternalistic outlook can find sufficient reasons justifying the legislation without appealing to the reasons which were originally adduced to support it. Thus, for example, it may be that the original legislation requiring motorcyclists to wear safety helmets was introduced for purely paternalistic reasons. But the Rhode Island Supreme Court recently upheld such legislation on the grounds that it was "not persuaded that the legislature is powerless to prohibit individuals from pursuing a course of conduct which could conceivably result in their becoming public charges," thus clearly introducing reasons of a quite different kind. Now I regard this decision as being based on reasoning of a very

Reprinted from The Monist, *LaSalle, IL, Vol. 56, no. 1, with the permission of the author and the publisher.*

dubious nature but it illustrates the kind of problem one has in finding examples. The following is a list of the kinds of interferences I have in mind as being paternalistic.

II

1. Laws requiring motorcyclists to wear safety helmets when operating their machines.

2. Laws forbidding persons from swimming at a public beach when lifeguards are not on duty.

3. Laws making suicide a criminal offense.

4. Laws making it illegal for women and children to work at certain types of jobs.

5. Laws regulating certain kinds of sexual conduct, e.g. homosexuality among consenting adults in private.

6. Laws regulating the use of certain drugs which may have harmful consequences to the user but do not lead to anti-social conduct.

7. Laws requiring a license to engage in certain professions with those not receiving a license subject to fine or jail sentence if they do engage in the practice.

8. Laws compelling people to spend a specified fraction of their income on the purchase of retirement annuities. (Social Security)

9. Laws forbidding various forms of gambling (often justified on the grounds that the poor are more likely to throw away their money on such activities than the rich who can afford to).

10. Laws regulating the maximum rates of interest for loans.

11. Laws against duelling.

In addition to laws which attach criminal or civil penalties to certain kinds of action there are laws, rules, regulations, decrees, which make it either difficult or impossible for people to carry out their plans and which are also justified on paternalistic grounds. Examples of this are:

1. Laws regulating the types of contracts which will be upheld as valid by the courts, e.g. (an example of Mill's to which I shall return) no man may make a valid contract for perpetual involuntary servitude.

2. Not allowing as a defense to a charge of murder or assault the consent of the victim.

3. Requiring members of certain religious sects to have compulsory blood transfusions. This is made possible by not allowing the patient to have recourse to civil suits for assault and battery and by means of injunctions.

4. Civil commitment procedures when these are specifically justified on the basis of preventing the person being committed from harming himself. (The D.C. Hospitalization of the Mentally Ill Act provides for involuntary hospitalization of a person who "is mentally ill, and because of that illness, is likely to injure *himself* or others if allowed to remain at liberty." The term injure in this context applies to unintentional as well as intentional injuries.)

5. Putting fluorides in the community water supply.

All of my examples are of existing restrictions on the liberty of individuals. Obviously one can think of interferences which have not yet been imposed. Thus one might ban the sale of cigarettes, or require that people wear safety-belts in automobiles (as opposed to merely having them installed) enforcing this by not allowing motorists to sue for injuries even when caused by other drivers if the motorist was not wearing a seat-belt at the time of the accident.

I shall not be concerned with activities which though defended on paternalistic grounds are not interferences with the liberty of persons, e.g. the giving of subsidies in kind rather than in cash on the grounds that the recipients would not spend the money on the goods which they really need, or not including a $1000 deductible provision in a basic protection automobile insurance plan on the ground that the people who would elect it could least afford it. Nor shall I be concerned with measures such as "truth-in-advertising" acts and the Pure Food and Drug legislation which are often attacked as paternalistic but which should not be considered so. In these cases all that is provided—it is true by the use of compulsion—is information which it is presumed that rational persons are interested in having in order to make wise decisions. There is no interference with the liberty of the consumer unless one wants to stretch a point beyond good sense and say that his liberty to apply for a loan without knowing the true rate of interest is diminished. It is true that sometimes there is sentiment for going further than providing information, for example when laws against usurious interest are passed preventing those who might wish to contract loans at high rates of interest from doing so, and these measures may correctly be considered paternalistic.

III

Bearing these examples in mind let me return to a characterization of paternalism. I said earlier that I meant by the term, roughly, interference with a person's liberty for his own good. But as some of the examples show the class of persons whose good is involved is not always identical with the class of persons whose freedom is restricted. Thus in the case of professional licensing it is the practitioner who is directly interfered with and it is the would-be patient whose interests are presumably being served. Not allowing the consent of the victim to be a defense to certain types of crime primarily affects the would-be aggressor but it is the interests of the willing victim that we are trying to protect. Sometimes a person may fall into both classes as would be the case if we banned the manufacture and sale of cigarettes and a given manufacturer happened to be a smoker as well.

Thus we may first divide paternalistic interferences into "pure" and "impure" cases. In "pure" paternalism the class of persons whose freedom is restricted is identical with the class of persons whose benefit is intended to be promoted by such restrictions. Examples: the making of suicide a crime, requiring passengers in automobiles to wear seat-belts, requiring a Christian Scientist to receive a blood transfusion. In the case of "impure" paternalism in trying to protect the welfare of a class of persons we find that the only way to do so will involve restricting the freedom of other persons besides those who are benefitted. Now it might be thought that there are no cases of "impure" paternalism since any such case could always be justified on non-paternalistic grounds, i.e. in terms of preventing harms to others. Thus we might ban cigarette manufacturers from continuing to manufacture their product on the

grounds that we are preventing them from causing illness to others in the same way that we prevent other manufacturers from releasing pollutants into the atmosphere, thereby causing danger to the members of the community. The difference is, however, that in the former but not the latter case the harm is of such a nature that it could be avoided by those individuals affected if they so chose. The incurring of the harm requires, so to speak, the active co-operation of the victim. It would be mistaken theoretically and hypocritical in practice to assert that our interference in such cases is just like our interference in standard cases of protecting others from harm. At the very least someone interfered with in this way can reply that no one is complaining about his activities. It may be that impure paternalism requires arguments or reasons of a stronger kind in order to be justified since there are persons who are losing a portion of their liberty and they do not even have the solace of having it be done "in their own interest." Of course in some sense, if paternalistic justifications are ever correct then we are protecting others, we are preventing some from injuring others, but it is important to see the differences between this and the standard case.

Paternalism then will always involve limitations on the liberty of some individuals in their own interest but it may also extend to interferences with the liberty of parties whose interests are not in question.

IV

Finally, by way of some more preliminary analysis, I want to distinguish paternalistic interferences with liberty from a related type with which it is often confused. Consider, for example, legislation which forbids employees to work more than, say, 40 hours per week. It is sometimes argued that such legislation is paternalistic for if employees desired such a restriction on their hours of work they could agree among themselves to impose it voluntarily. But because they do not the society imposes its own conception of their best interests upon them by the use of coercion. Hence this is paternalism.

Now it may be that some legislation of this nature is, in fact, paternalistically motivated. I am not denying that. All I want to point out is that there is another possible way of justifying such measures which is not paternalistic in nature. It is not paternalistic because as Mill puts it in a similar context such measures are "required not to overrule the judgment of individuals respecting their own interest, but to give effect to that judgment: they being unable to give effect to it except by concert, which concert again cannot be effectual unless it receives validity and sanction from the law."[2]

The line of reasoning here is a familiar one first found in Hobbes and developed with great sophistication by contemporary economists in the last decade or so. There are restrictions which are in the interests of a class of persons taken collectively but are such that the immediate interest of each individual is furthered by his violating the rule when others adhere to it. In such cases the individuals involved may need the use of compulsion to give effect to their collective judgment of their own interest by guaranteeing each individual compliance by the others. In these cases compulsion is not used to achieve some benefit which is not recognized to be a benefit by those concerned, but rather because it is the only feasible means of achieving some benefit which *is* recognized as such by all concerned. This way of viewing matters provides us with another characterization of paternalism in general. Paternalism might be thought of as the use of coercion to achieve a good which is not recognized as such by those persons for whom the good is intended. Again while this formulation captures the heart of the matter—it is surely what Mill is objecting to in *On Liberty*—the matter is not always quite like that. For example when we force motorcyclists to wear helmets we are trying to promote a good—the protection of the person from injury—which is surely recognized by most of the individuals concerned. It is not that a cyclist doesn't value his bodily integrity; rather, as a supporter of such legislation would put it, he either places, perhaps irrationally, another value or good (freedom from wearing a helmet) above that of physical well-being or, perhaps, while recognizing the danger in the abstract, he either does not fully appreciate it or he underestimates the likelihood of its occurring. But now we are approaching the question of possible justifications of paternalistic measures and the rest of this essay will be devoted to that question.

V

I shall begin for dialectical purposes by discussing Mill's objections to paternalism and then go on to discuss more positive proposals.

An initial feature that strikes one is the absolute nature of Mill's prohibitions against paternalism. It is so unlike the carefully qualified admonitions of Mill and his fellow Utilitarians on other moral issues. He speaks of self-protection as the *sole* end warranting coercion, of the individual's own goals as *never* being a sufficient warrant. Contrast this with his discussion of the prohibition against lying in *Util[itarianism]*.

> Yet that even this, rule, sacred as it is, admits of possible exception, is acknowledged by all moralists, the chief of which is where the with-holding of some fact . . . would save an individual . . . from great and unmerited evil.[3]

The same tentativeness is present when he deals with justice.

> It is confessedly unjust to break faith with any one: to violate an engagement, either express or implied, or disappoint expectations raised by our own conduct, at least if we have raised these expectations knowingly and voluntarily. Like all the other obligations of justice already spoken of, this one is not regarded as absolute, but as capable of being overruled by a stronger obligation of justice on the other side.[4]

This anomaly calls for some explanation. The structure of Mill's argument is as follows:

1. Since restraint is an evil the burden of proof is on those who propose such restraint.

2. Since the conduct which is being considered is purely self-regarding, the normal appeal to the protection of the interests of others is not available.

3. Therefore we have to consider whether reasons involving reference to the individual's own good, happiness, welfare, or interests are sufficient to overcome the burden of justification.

4. We either cannot advance the interests of the individual by compulsion, or the attempt to do so involves evil which outweighs the good done.

5. Hence the promotion of the individual's own interests does not provide a sufficient warrant for the use of compulsion.

Clearly the operative premise here is 4 and it is bolstered by claims about the status of the individual as judge and appraiser of his welfare, interests, needs, etc.

> With respect to his own feelings and circumstances, the most ordinary man or woman has means of knowledge immeasurably surpassing those that can be possessed by any one else.[5]
>
> He is the man most interested in his own well-being: the interest which any other person, except in cases of strong personal attachment, can have in it, is trifling, compared to that which he himself has.[6]

These claims are used to support the following generalizations concerning the utility of compulsion for paternalistic purposes.

> The interferences of society to overrule his judgment and purposes in what only regards himself must be grounded on general presumptions; which may be altogether wrong, and even if right, are as likely as not to be misapplied to individual cases.[7]
>
> But the strongest of all the arguments against the interference of the public with purely personal conduct is that when it does interfere, the odds are that it interferes wrongly and in the wrong place.[8]
>
> All errors which the individual is likely to commit against advice and warning are far outweighed by the evil of allowing others to constrain him to what they deem his good.[9]

Performing the utilitarian calculation by balancing the advantages and disadvantages we find that:

> Mankind are greater gainers by suffering each other to live as seems good to themselves, than by compelling each other to live as seems good to the rest.[10]

From which follows the operative premise 4.

This classical case of a utilitarian argument with all the premises spelled out is not the only line of reasoning present in Mill's discussion. There are asides, and more than asides, which look quite different and I shall deal with them later. But this is clearly the main channel of Mill's thought and it is one which has been subjected to vigorous attack from the moment it appeared—most often by fellow Utilitarians. The link that they have usually seized on is, as Fitzjames Stephen put it, the absence of proof that the "mass of adults are so well acquainted with their own interests and so much disposed to pursue them that no compulsion or restraint put upon them by any others for the purpose of promoting their interest can really promote them."[11] Even so sympathetic a critic as Hart is forced to the conclusion that:

> In Chapter 5 of his essay Mill carried his protests against paternalism to lengths that may now appear to us as fantastic. . . . No doubt if we no longer sympathise with this criticism this is due, in part, to a general decline in the belief that individuals know their own interest best.[12]
>
> Mill endows the average individual with "too much of the psychology of a middle-aged man whose desires are relatively fixed, not liable to be artificially stimulated by external influences; who knows what he wants and what gives him satisfaction of happiness; and who pursues these things when he can."[13]

Now it is interesting to note that Mill himself was aware of some of the limitations on the doctrine that the individual is the best judge of his own interests. In his discussion of government intervention in general (even where the intervention does not interfere with liberty but provides alternative institutions to those of the market) after making claims which are parallel to those just discussed, e.g.

> People understand their own business and their own interests better, and care for them more, than the government does, or can be expected to do.[14]

He goes on to an intelligent discussion of the "very large and conspicuous exceptions" to the maxim that:

> Most persons take a juster and more intelligent view of their own interest, and of the means of promoting it than can either be prescribed to them by a general enactment of the legislature, or pointed out in the particular case by a public functionary.[15]

Thus there are things

> of which the utility does not consist in ministering to inclinations, nor in serving the

daily uses of life, and the want of which is least felt where the need is greatest. This is peculiarly true of those things which are chiefly useful as tending to raise the character of human beings. The uncultivated cannot be competent judges of cultivation. Those who most need to be made wiser and better, usually desire it least, and, if they desired it, would be incapable of finding the way to it by their own lights.

. . . . A second exception to the doctrine that individuals are the best judges of their own interest, is when an individual attempts to decide irrevocably now what will be best for his interest at some future and distant time. The presumption in favor of individual judgment is only legitimate, where the judgment is grounded on actual, and especially on present, personal experience; not where it is formed antecedently to experience, and not suffered to be reversed even after experience has condemned it.[16]

The upshot of these exceptions is that Mill does not declare that there should never be government interference with the economy but rather that

. . . in every instance, the burden of making out a strong case should be thrown not on those who resist but on those who recommend government interference. Letting alone, in short, should be the general practice: every departure from it, unless required by some great good, is a certain evil.[17]

In short, we get a presumption not an absolute prohibition. The question is why doesn't the argument against paternalism go the same way?

I suggest that the answer lies in seeing that in addition to a purely utilitarian argument Mill uses another as well. As a Utilitarian Mill has to show, in Fitzjames Stephen's words, that:

Self-protection apart, no good object can be attained by any compulsion which is not in itself a greater evil than the absence of the object which the compulsion obtains.[18]

To show this is impossible; one reason being that it isn't true. Preventing a man from selling himself into slavery (a paternalistic measure which Mill himself accepts as legitimate), or from taking heroin, or from driving a car without wearing seatbelts may constitute a lesser evil than allowing him to do any of these things. A consistent Utilitarian can only argue against paternalism on the grounds

that it (as a matter of fact) does not maximize the good. It is always a contingent question that may be refuted by the evidence. But there is also a non-contingent argument which runs through *On Liberty*. When Mill states that "there is a part of the life of every person who has come to years of discretion, within which the individuality of that person ought to reign uncontrolled either by any other person or by the public collectively" he is saying something about what it means to be a person, an autonomous agent. It is because coercing a person for his own good denies this status as an independent entity that Mill objects to it so strongly and in such absolute terms. To be able to choose is a good that is independent of the wisdom of what is chosen. A man's "mode of laying out his existence is the best, not because it is the best in itself, but because it is his own mode."[19]

It is the privilege and proper condition of a human being, arrived at the maturity of his faculties, to use and interpret experience in his own way.[20]

As further evidence of this line of reasoning in Mill consider the one exception to his prohibition against paternalism.

In this and most civilised countries, for example, an engagement by which a person should sell himself, or allow himself to be sold, as a slave, would be null and void; neither enforced by law nor by opinion. The ground for thus limiting his power of voluntarily disposing of his own lot in life, is apparent, and is very clearly seen in this extreme case. The reason for not interfering, unless for the sake of others, with a person's voluntary acts, is consideration for his liberty. His voluntary choice is evidence that what he so chooses is desirable, or at least endurable, to him, and his good is on the whole best provided for by allowing him to take his own means of pursuing it. But by selling himself for a slave, he abdicates his liberty; he foregoes any future use of it beyond that single act.

He therefore defeats, in his own case, the very purpose which is the justification of allowing him to dispose of himself. He is no longer free; but is thenceforth in a position which has no longer the presumption in its favour, that would be afforded by his voluntarily remaining in it. The principle of freedom cannot require that he should be free not to be free. It is not freedom to be allowed to alienate his freedom.[21]

Now leaving aside the fudging on the meaning of freedom in the last line it is clear that part of this argument is incorrect. While it is true that *future* choices of the slave are not reasons for thinking that what he chooses then is desirable for him, what is at issue is limiting his immediate choice; and since this choice is made freely, the individual may be correct in thinking that his interests are best provided for by entering such a contract. But the main consideration for not allowing such a contract is the need to preserve the liberty of the person to make future choices. This gives us a principle—a very narrow one—by which to justify some paternalistic interferences. Paternalism is justified only to preserve a wider range of freedom for the individual in question. How far this principle could be extended, whether it can justify all the cases in which we are inclined upon reflection to think paternalistic measures justified remains to be discussed. What I have tried to show so far is that there are two strains of argument in Mill—one a straight-forward Utilitarian mode of reasoning and one which relies not on the goods which free choice leads to but on the absolute value of the choice itself. The first cannot establish any absolute prohibition but at most a presumption and indeed a fairly weak one given some fairly plausible assumptions about human psychology; the second while a stronger line of argument seems to me to allow on its own grounds a wider range of paternalism than might be suspected. I turn now to a consideration of these matters.

VI

We might begin looking for principles governing the acceptable use of paternalistic power in cases where it is generally agreed that it is legitimate. Even Mill intends his principles to be applicable only to mature individuals, not those in what he calls "non-age." What is it that justifies us in interfering with children? The fact that they lack some of the emotional and cognitive capacities required in order to make fully rational decisions. It is an empirical question to just what extent children have an adequate conception of their own present and future interests but there is not much doubt that there are many deficiencies. For example it is very difficult for a child to defer gratification for any considerable period of time. Given these deficiencies and given the very real and permanent dangers that may befall the child it becomes not only permissible but even a duty of the parent to restrict the child's freedom in various ways. There is however an important moral limitation on the exercise of such parental power which is provided by the notion of the child eventually coming to see the correctness of his parent's interventions. Parental paternalism may be thought of as a wager by the parent on the child's subsequent recognition of the wisdom of the restrictions. There is an emphasis on what could be called future-oriented consent—on what the child will come to welcome, rather than on what he does welcome.

The essence of this idea has been incorporated by idealist philosophers into various types of "real-will" theory as applied to fully adult persons. Extensions of paternalism are argued for by claiming that in various respects, chronologically mature individuals share the same deficiencies in knowledge, capacity to think rationally, and the ability to carry out decisions that children possess. Hence in interfering with such people we are in effect doing what they would do if they were fully rational. Hence we are not really opposing their will, hence we are not really interfering with their freedom. The dangers of this move have been sufficiently exposed by Berlin in his Two Concepts of Liberty. I see no gain in theoretical clarity nor in practical advantage in trying to pass over the real nature of the interferences with liberty that we impose on others. Still the basic notion of consent is important and seems to me the only acceptable way of trying to delimit an area of justified paternalism.

Let me start by considering a case where the consent is not hypothetical in nature. Under certain conditions it is rational for an individual to agree that others should force him to act in ways in which, at the time of action, the individual may not see as desirable. If, for example, a man knows that he is subject to breaking his resolves when temptation is present, he may ask a friend to refuse to entertain his requests at some later stage.

A classical example is given in the Odyssey when Odysseus commands his men to tie him to the mast and refuse all future orders to be set free, because he knows the power of the Sirens to enchant men with their songs. Here we are on relatively sound ground in later refusing Odysseus' request to be set free. He may even claim to have changed his mind but since it is just such changes that he wished to guard against we are entitled to ignore them.

A process analogous to this may take place on a social rather than individual basis. An electorate may mandate its representatives to pass legislation which when it comes time to "pay the price" may be unpalatable. I may believe that a tax increase is necessary to halt inflation though I may resent the lower pay check each month. However in both this case and that of Odysseus the measure to be enforced is specifically requested by the party involved and at some point in time there is genuine consent and agreement on the part of those persons whose liberty is infringed. Such is not the case for the paternalistic measures we have been speaking about. What must be involved here is not consent to specific measures but rather consent to a system of government, run by elected representatives, with an understanding that they may act to safeguard our interests in certain limited ways.

I suggest that since we are all aware of our irrational propensities, deficiencies in cognitive and emotional capacities and avoidable and unavoidable ignorance it is rational and prudent for us to in effect take out "social insurance policies." We may argue for and against proposed paternalistic measures in terms of what fully rational individuals would accept as forms of protection. Now, clearly since the initial agreement is not about specific measures we are dealing with a more-or-less blank check and therefore there have to be carefully defined limits. What I am looking for are certain kinds of conditions which make it plausible to suppose that rational men could reach agreement to limit their liberty even when other men's interests are not affected.

Of course as in any kind of agreement schema there are great difficulties in deciding what rational individuals would or would not accept. Particularly in sensitive areas of personal liberty, there is always a danger of the dispute over agreement and rationality being a disguised version of evaluative and normative disagreement.

Let me suggest types of situations in which it seems plausible to suppose that fully rational individuals would agree to having paternalistic restrictions imposed upon them. It is reasonable to suppose that there are "goods" such as health which any person would want to have in order to pursue his own good—no matter how that good is conceived. This is an argument that is used in connection with compulsory education for children but it seems to me that it can be extended to other goods which have this character. Then one could agree that the attainment of such goods should be promoted even when not recognized to be such, at the moment, by the individuals concerned.

An immediate difficulty that arises stems from the fact that men are always faced with competing goods and that there may be reasons why even a value such as health—or indeed life—may be overridden by competing values. Thus the problem with the Christian Scientist and blood transfusions. It may be more important for him to reject "impure substances" than to go on living. The difficult problem that must be faced is whether one can give sense to the notion of a person irrationally attaching weights to competing values.

Consider a person who knows the statistical data on the probability of being injured when not wearing seat belts in an automobile and knows the types and gravity of the various injuries. He also insists that the inconvenience attached to fastening the belt every time he gets in and out of the car outweighs for him the possible risks to himself. I am inclined in this case to think that such a weighing is irrational. Given his life-plans which we are assuming are those of the average person, his interests and commitments already undertaken, I think it is safe to predict that we can find inconsistencies in his calculations at some point. I am assuming that this is not a man who for some conscious or unconscious reasons is trying to injure himself nor is he a man who just likes to "live dangerously." I am assuming that he is like us in all the relevant respects but just puts an enormously high negative value on inconvenience—one which does not seem comprehensible or reasonable.

It is always possible, of course to assimilate this person to creatures like myself. I, also, neglect to fasten my seat belt and I concede such behavior is not rational but not because I weigh the inconvenience differently from those who fasten the belts. It is just that having made (roughly) the same calculation as everybody else I ignore it in my actions. [Note: a much better case of weakness of the will than those usually given in ethics texts.] A plausible explanation for this deplorable habit is that although I know in some intellectual sense what the probabilities and risks are I do not fully appreciate them in an emotionally genuine manner.

We have two distinct types of situation in which a man acts in a non-rational fashion. In one case he attaches incorrect weights to some of his values; in the other he neglects to act in accordance with his actual preferences and desires. Clearly there is a stronger and more persuasive argument for paternalism in the latter situation. Here we are really not—by assumption—imposing a good on another person. But why may we not extend our interference to what we might call evaluative delusions? After all in the case of cognitive delusions we are prepared, often, to act against the expressed will of the person involved. If a man believes that when he jumps out the window he will float upwards—Robert Nozick's example—would not we detain him, forcibly if necessary? The reply will be that this man doesn't wish to be injured and if we could convince him that he is mistaken as to the consequences of his action he would not wish to perform the action. But part of what is involved in claiming that a man who doesn't fasten his seat-belts is attaching an irrational weight to the inconvenience of fastening them is that if he were to be involved in an accident and severely injured he would look back and admit that the inconvenience wasn't as bad as all that. So there is a sense in which if I could convince him of the consequences of his action he also would not wish to continue his present course of action. Now the notion of consequences being used here is covering a lot of ground. In one case it's being used to indicate what will or can happen as a result of a course of action and in the other it's making a prediction about the future evaluation of the consequences—in the first sense—of a course of action. And whatever the difference between facts and values—whether it be hard and fast or soft and slow—we are genuinely more reluctant to consent to interferences where evaluative differences are the issue. Let me now consider another factor which comes into play in some of these situations which may make an important difference in our willingness to consent to paternalistic restrictions.

Some of the decisions we make are of such a character that they produce changes which are in one or another way irreversible. Situations are created in which it is difficult or impossible to return to anything like the initial stage at which the decision was made. In particular some of these changes will make it impossible to continue to make reasoned choices in the future. I am thinking specifically of decisions which involve taking drugs that are physically or psychologically addictive and those which are destructive of one's mental and physical capacities.

I suggest we think of the imposition of paternalistic interferences in situations of this kind as being a kind of insurance policy which we take out against making decisions which are far-reaching, potentially dangerous and irreversible. Each of these factors is important. Clearly there are many decisions we make that are relatively irreversible. In deciding to learn to play chess I could predict in view of my general interest in games that some portion of my free-time was going to be pre-empted and that it would not be easy to give up the game once I acquired a certain competence. But my whole life-style was not going to be jeopardized in an extreme manner. Further it might be argued that even with addictive drugs such as heroin one's normal life plans would not be seriously interfered with if an inexpensive and adequate supply were readily available. So this type of argument might have a much narrower scope than appears to be the case at first.

A second class of cases concerns decisions which are made under extreme psychological and sociological pressures. I am not thinking here of the making of the decision as being something one is pressured into—e.g. a good reason for making duelling illegal is that unless this is done many people might have to manifest their courage and integrity in ways in which they would rather not do so—but rather of decisions such as that to commit suicide which are usually made at a point where the individual is not thinking clearly and calmly about the nature of his decision. In addition, of course, this comes under the previous heading of all-too-irrevocable decision. Now there are practical steps which a society could take if it wanted to decrease the possibility of suicide—for example not paying social security benefits to the survivors or as religious institutions do, not allowing such persons to be buried with the same status as natural deaths. I think we may count these as interferences with the liberty of persons to attempt suicide and the question is whether they are justifiable.

Using my argument schema the question is whether rational individuals would consent to such limitations. I see no reason for them to consent to an absolute prohibition but I do think it is reasonable for them to agree to some kind of enforced waiting period. Since we are all aware of the possibility of temporary states, such as great fear or depression, that are inimical to the making of well-informed and rational decisions, it would be prudent for all of us if there were some kind of institutional arrangement whereby we were restrained from making a decision which is (all too) irreversible. What this would be like in practice is difficult to envisage and it may be that if no practical arrangements were feasible then we would have to conclude that there should be no restriction at all on this kind of action. But we might have a "cooling off" period, in much the same way that we now require couples who file for divorce to go through a waiting period. Or, more far-fetched, we might imagine a Suicide Board composed of a psychologist and another member picked by the applicant. The Board would be required to meet and talk with the person proposing to take his life, though its approval would not be required.

A third class of decisions—these classes are not supposed to be disjoint—involves dangers which are either not sufficiently understood or appreciated correctly by the persons involved. Let me illustrate, using the example of cigarette smoking, a number of possible cases.

1. A man may not know the facts—e.g. smoking between 1 and 2 packs a day shortens life expectancy 6.2 years, the costs and pain of the illness caused by smoking, etc.

2. A man may know the facts, wish to stop smoking, but not have the requisite will-power.

3. A man may know the facts but not have them play the correct role in his calculation because, say, he discounts the danger psychologically because it is remote in time and/or inflates the attractiveness of other consequences of his decision which he regards as beneficial.

In case 1 what is called for is education, the posting of warnings, etc. In case 2 there is no theoretical problem. We are not imposing a good on someone who rejects it. We are simply using coercion to enable people to carry out their own goals. (Note: There obviously is a difficulty in that only a subclass of the individuals affected wish to be prevented from doing what they are doing.) In case 3 there is a sense in which we are imposing a good on someone since given his current appraisal of the facts he doesn't wish to be restricted. But in another sense we are not imposing a good since what is being claimed—and what must be shown or at least argued for—is that an accurate accounting on his part would lead him to reject his current course of action. Now we all know that such cases exist, that we are prone to disregard dangers that are only possibilities, that immediate pleasures are often magnified and distorted.

If in addition the dangers are severe and far-reaching we could agree to allowing the state a certain degree of power to intervene in such situations. The difficulty is in specifying in advance, even vaguely, the class of cases in which intervention will be legitimate.

A related difficulty is that of drawing a line so that it is not the case that all ultra-hazardous activities are ruled out, e.g. mountain-climbing, bull-fighting, sports-car racing, etc. There are some risks—even very great ones—which a person is entitled to take with his life.

A good deal depends on the nature of the deprivation—e.g. does it prevent the person from engaging in the activity completely or merely limit his participation—and how important to the nature of the activity is the absence of restriction when this is weighed against the role that the activity plays in the life of the person. In the case of automobile seat belts, for example, the restriction is trivial in nature, interferes not at all with the use or enjoyment of the activity, and does, I am assuming, considerably reduce a high risk of serious injury. Whereas, for example, making mountain-climbing illegal prevents completely a person engaging in an activity which may play an important role in his life and his conception of the person he is.

In general the easiest cases to handle are those which can be argued about in the terms which Mill thought to be so important—a concern not just for the happiness or welfare, in some broad sense, of the individual but rather a concern for the autonomy and freedom of the person. I suggest that we would be most likely to consent to paternalism in those instances in which it preserves and enhances for the individual his ability to rationally consider and carry out his own decisions.

I have suggested in this essay a number of types of situations in which it seems plausible that rational men would agree to granting the legislative powers of a society the right to impose restrictions on what Mill calls "self-regarding" conduct. However, rational men knowing something about the resources of ignorance, ill-will and stupidity available to the law-makers of a society—a good case in point is the history of drug legislation in the United States—will be concerned to limit such intervention to a minimum. I suggest in closing two principles designed to achieve this end.

In all cases of paternalistic legislation there must be a heavy and clear burden of proof placed on the authorities to demonstrate the exact nature of the harmful effects (or beneficial consequences) to be avoided (or achieved) and the probability of their occurrence. The burden of proof here is twofold—what lawyers distinguish as the burden of going forward and the burden of persuasion. That the authorities have the burden of going forward means that it is up to them to raise the question and bring forward evidence of the evils to be avoided. Unlike the case of new drugs where the manufacturer must produce some evidence that the drug has been tested and found not harmful, no citizen has to show with respect to self-regarding conduct that it is not harmful or promotes his best interests. In addition the nature and cogency of the evidence for the harmfulness of the course of action must be set at a high level. To paraphrase a formulation of the burden of proof for criminal proceedings—better 10 men ruin

themselves than one man be unjustly deprived of liberty.

Finally I suggest a principle of the least restrictive alternative. If there is an alternative way of accomplishing the desired end without restricting liberty then although it may involve great expense, inconvenience, etc. the society must adopt it.

Notes

1. J. S. Mill, *Utilitarianism* and *On Liberty* (Fontana Library Edition, ed. by Mary Warnock, London, 1962), p. 135. All further quotes from Mill are from this edition unless otherwise noted.

2. J. S. Mill, *Principles of Political Economy* (New York: P. F. Collier and Sons, 1900), p. 442.

3. Mill, *Utilitarianism* and *On Liberty*, p. 174.

4. *Ibid.*, p. 299.

5. *Ibid.*, p. 207.

6. *Ibid.*, p. 206.

7. *Ibid.*, p. 207.

8. *Ibid.*, p. 214.

9. *Ibid.*, p. 207.

10. *Ibid.*, p. 138.

11. J. F. Stephen, *Liberty, Equality, Fraternity* (New York: Henry Holt & Co., n.d.), p. 24.

12. H. L. A. Hart, *Law, Liberty and Morality* (Stanford: Stanford University Press, 1963), p. 32.

13. *Ibid.*, p. 33.

14. Mill, *Principles*, II, 448.

15. *Ibid.*, II, 458.

16. *Ibid.*, II, 459.

17. *Ibid.*, II, 451.

18. Stephen, p. 49.

19. Mill, *Utilitarianism* and *On Liberty*, p. 197.

20. *Ibid.*, p. 186

21. *Ibid.*, pp. 235–236.

About AIDS: A Dialogue

David A. Conway

There can be no question that Acquired Immune Deficiency Syndrome poses crucial scientific problems for the medical community. It is a disease that is lethal and is spreading at a rapid rate. Thus medical problems regarding its prevention and cure are matters of first importance. In addition, AIDS gives rise to numerous non-scientific problems, many of which turn on ethical, social, and political considerations. These problems may well be no less difficult and no less important than the scientific ones. In the dialogue that follows some of these problems are discussed.

I: The Threat to Society—Catastrophe or Overrated?

BASCOMBE: Have you two been paying attention to the AIDS news? It is terrifying. If we don't take more strenuous measures right away, none of us will be safe. AIDS may be the greatest threat to mankind since the bubonic plague.

FITCH: That is utter nonsense. AIDS is hardly the bubonic plague. What it is is the perfect media disease. Sex. Drugs. Death. The glamour of Hollywood stars. What titillation! You can't check out of a supermarket without seeing lurid tabloid headlines about Ms. X holding hands with Mr. Y in movie Z and will she get AIDS? Or about whether a good deep French kiss can spread AIDS. Or about whether a large number of prostitutes are carriers and did they get it from their Johns or from sharing each others' drug needles? If AIDS didn't exist, it would have been invented by the tabloids. It has everything. The people love it.

SHERWOOD: "The people" are terrified of it.

FITCH: Of course they are. They are terrified of it and they love it. There's no incompatibility in that. The weird, the terrifying, the perverted, the bizarre, the deadly. The *fascinating*.

Suppose that some other new disease had been first named about four years ago and six thousand people in the United States had died of it since then. That would be like AIDS. But suppose that this disease were transmitted by breathing viruses in from the air. What do you think would have happened? I can tell you what. It would have been noted in the media every once in a while, but for the most part no one would have paid any attention to it. Here we would have had just another disease to try to get rid of. A celebrity or two might have come on in the cheap television slots at 2:00 A.M. pleading for a few dollars for research, but that's about all that would have happened.

With AIDS what we have is a whole society in

a kind of vulgar awe for fear that its six-year-olds will get a disease that is spread by anal intercourse and druggies sharing hypodermic needles.

BASCOMBE: AIDS is a hideous disease. Your attempt to make light of it is in extremely bad taste, to say the least.

FITCH: I'm not making light of it at all. It is a hideous disease. People who get it suffer and die. But as a killer AIDS is small potatoes compared to cancer, heart disease, diabetes, and a few dozen other causes of death we could name. Do you know that last year 50,000 people died of pneumonia and influenza in the United States? That's something like fifteen times the number of people who died of AIDS.

BASCOMBE: But people who have pneumonia or influenza don't *always* die. They don't even usually die. It is the fact that getting AIDS is a sure death sentence that makes it so much more horrible than pneumonia or flu.

FITCH: You know I don't think that I have ever had a five-minute conversation about AIDS without someone bringing that up. It's true that AIDS is always lethal, and flu, pneumonia, and even cancer are not. But what is this supposed to show?

SHERWOOD: At least it helps to explain why people are so much more frightened of AIDS than they are of other diseases. It's for basically the same reason that a lot of people find flying a lot more frightening than being in a car. If the plane goes down, you are almost certainly dead as a stone. If you are in an auto accident, you will probably walk away with a few bruises at most. It's not hard to understand that this makes flying much more frightening to a lot of people.

FITCH: It makes it understandable that we might think this way, but it is still a mistake. A plane crash is much more likely to be lethal than is an auto accident, but the fact remains that your life is safer getting into an airplane than into your car because there are so many *more* car accidents and *some* of them will be fatal. So if we are going to be afraid of something we ought to be more afraid of riding in an automobile than in an airplane.

In exactly the same way we should be more afraid of a disease that strikes one thousand people and kills twenty of those than of a much more "lethal" disease that strikes only ten people but kills all of them. The bite of the green mamba is a lot more deadly than the sting of a bee. But the average citizen of the U.S. has a lot more reason to fear death from bee stingers than from green mamba fangs.

BASCOMBE: You are really just wrong if you think that there is no good reason to be very much afraid of AIDS. The number of people who have died or who actually have the disease is not nearly so important as the fact that the number of cases has been doubling each year. If that continues all you need is a few punches on a calculator to tell you that within about four years there will be one hundred thousand cases. And if we extrapolate to fifteen years or so everyone in the United States will be dead of it.

FITCH: You don't really believe that is going to happen, do you?

BASCOMBE: It could.

SHERWOOD: It could, but it surely won't. For one thing, there may be medical breakthroughs that will give us means of preventing, controlling, or even curing the disease.

FITCH: And we don't have to depend entirely on medical breakthroughs anyway. Even at the past rate of spread, the projection that everybody would have it in the foreseeable future is just silly. At most we could project that a very large number of people within the highest risk groups would get it. And even that isn't likely to happen. There seem to have been changes in sexual behavior among male homosexuals. In particular, many are having relations with fewer partners. This by itself should slow the spread of the disease considerably.[1]

SHERWOOD: You know, Bascombe, Fitch has really made a pretty good case. AIDS doesn't seem to be much at all like the bubonic plague.

FITCH: It's lethal if you get it, but only a handful of people have gotten it. It's spreading, but there is no good reason to think it will continue to spread in ways that will result in huge numbers of people getting it. Bascombe, you are just another victim of AIDS hysteria.

BASCOMBE: You two are just hiding your heads in the sand. The thing is . . .

II: AIDS, Gays, and God

SHERWOOD: Let me interrupt you, Bascombe. I want to go back a bit. Fitch, you explicitly mentioned male homosexuals a minute ago, and before that you said something about "the highest risk groups," referring again, I take it, to gay males.

FITCH: To gay males and intravenous drug users. These are the people we are essentially concerned with here. Facts are facts, and it does no good politely to pretend they are not.

SHERWOOD: But you have to be careful here, Fitch. It almost sounds as if you mean that since AIDS is largely confined to these groups, society need not be concerned about it.

FITCH: Did I say anything like that? What I meant was only that projections about cases doubling every year are more frightening than realistic.

SHERWOOD: Still there are dangers in emphasizing that most AIDS victims have been male homosexuals. It encourages seeing AIDS as "the gay plague." One result of this is that the intolerant right, posing as the voice of morality, tells us we should see it as God's retribution for "unnatural acts." That's what Jerry Falwell said it was.[2] Patrick Buchanan, a man who is now director of communications at the White House, wrote that homosexuals "have declared war upon nature, and now nature is exacting an awful retribution." This is a dangerous view, because if AIDS is really God's retribution justly meted out to those who are deserving, then why should we try to put a stop to it? That would be interfering with God's justice.

FITCH: The view is not just dangerous. It's also clearly false. That is, it is false that only "sinful" gays and drug users can get it or have gotten it. Is "nature exacting [its] awful retribution" on the thirteen-year-old hemophiliac who has AIDS and is not allowed to go to school? Or on the baby born with AIDS whose life will be only torment?

SHERWOOD: Actually there is a kind of elementary school theology involved in what Falwell and Buchanan say. Who, since Job's friends anyway, has been willing to claim that it is the wicked who do the suffering in this world?

FITCH: Maybe Falwell and Buchanan think God put AIDS here to punish sinners and it just happened to spill over on some innocents.

SHERWOOD: If so, that's a pretty incompetent God they have there.

FITCH: Even a moderately knowing one should have recognized that a disease caused by a virus would not be so well-behaved as to always stay within some prescribed boundaries. Using drugs and indulging in anal intercourse don't *cause* AIDS. A virus causes it. A clever God surely would have fixed it so the "nasty practices" themselves cause it. *Then* it would just hit those who deserve it, according to these moralizers' version of who deserves what. But it doesn't work this way, so either we are dealing with an incredibly deficient God or the whole notion of AIDS as punishment is just nonsense. Let the Falwells and the Buchanans decide which of these they want to embrace.

SHERWOOD: Okay, so clearly the notion of AIDS as punishment does not really make any sense. And most people probably don't really think it does. Or at least they don't quite consciously think of AIDS as a punishment for sinners. Still, insofar as there is a close connection in the public mind between AIDS and homosexuality, those who have AIDS are not thought of as victims in the way those who have other terrible diseases are. There are too many horror stories about the way AIDS victims are treated, ways in which people with cancer or heart disease are never treated.

BASCOMBE: That is just fear of contagion. When hospitalized victims are left unwashed, lying in their own excrement,[3] it is horrible but understandable.

SHERWOOD: That may be understandable. But it isn't the sort of thing I had in mind. I was thinking more of the kind of incident reported in *Newsweek*.[4] "After he made television appearances to explain that AIDS patients should not be pariahs, Baltimore activist Don Miller, a victim of the disease, was taunted by neighborhood children with cries of 'You're going to die!'" On the same

date *Time* had a similar horror story: "Just over a week ago, a carload of people threw a vial of acid at a woman employee [of the Edmund D. Edelman Health Center of the Gay and Lesbian Community Services Center in Los Angeles], burning her face, shoulder, and arm. The victim said one of the attackers screamed, 'Die, you AIDS faggots!'"[5] Here it isn't even an AIDS sufferer who is a victim of such horrible actions. So homophobia contributes to the misery of those with AIDS and even attaches to those who attempt to help them. And AIDS in turn increases the level of homophobia as gays are perceived not only as perverts but as sort of modern-day lepers.

FITCH: You accused me of taking a position that would encourage such homophobia when I was emphasizing the degree to which AIDS has been a disease of gays and intravenous drug users. But to put it bluntly, and I suppose rather obnoxiously, it *is* a druggies' disease and a "gay plague." It actually appears to be hard to transmit, and now that blood for transfusion is being tested for it, those outside these groups seem to be at very small risk. So I ask you, what will do more to encourage homophobia? Making clear, as I do, that the risk for most people is small or carrying on about how it was initially a disease that was spread by homosexuals but now is about to get us all? It is the latter that makes homosexuality responsible for the imminent destruction of all mankind. Spreading that message is hardly going to discourage homophobia.[6] Who do you think is likely to be more homophobic? People who know that they are not at risk of getting the disease from the gays who have it or people like the clown who was out spraying insecticide in his backyard because his gay neighbor had a barbecue and he wanted to kill any mosquitoes that might have bitten one of the guests?[7] What we really need is a lot less of the sort of hype that has led to inordinant fear of sexual activity of any sort and that threatens to give us a society of paranoid mosquito sprayers.

III: AIDS and the Classroom— The Nature of the Risks

BASCOMBE: Sherwood, if you had children, would you let them go to school with a child that has AIDS?

SHERWOOD: It would be a hard decision. I think I would but I would probably feel uneasy about it.

FITCH: Why would you even feel uneasy? You know perfectly well that there are no known cases of AIDS being spread by casual contact, by the sort of contact that school children have with each other. Even siblings who live together in the same house with all the normal sibling contacts have never contracted AIDS from one another. This evidence is absolutely clear. On the other side all we have are empty "maybe's." *Maybe* AIDS can be spread by just touching another person and *maybe* you can get it by sharing a drinking glass or eating at the same table or just breathing the same air as someone who has it. That's a pretty easy game to play. *Maybe* Howard Hughes was really an alien from another planet, and *maybe* the world will end next Thursday. Maybe . . . but there is no reason to think so, and you know what we think of people who take such possibilities seriously.

BASCOMBE: Come now, Fitch. You know it isn't that simple. Even if there are not any cases in which it is *known* to have been spread by casual contact, this disease is not noncommunicable in the way that, say, multiple sclerosis is. We don't know all that much about it, but we do know that it is caused by a virus. We also know that viruses can be spread from one person to another and that some of them are spread by casual contact. Add to this that the AIDS virus has been found not just in semen but in blood, mucus, and even tears. With all that in mind are you really going to tell me that we can discount the possibility that one child can get AIDS from another in a classroom setting? It's hardly rare to see blood, mucus, or tears when children are together. It is much more than a mere abstract possibility that AIDS can be communicated to well children by the sorts of contacts that children have in schools.

FITCH: The fact remains that there are no known cases of it being communicated by those sorts of contacts. And that is the very best evidence that it cannot be communicated in those ways.

BASCOMBE: You sound awfully certain about this. Statements from the scientific community about AIDS are hardly ever so unqualified. Scientists tell us things like—"there is *little risk* of contracting AIDS through kissing" and "it is *very unlikely* that one would get AIDS from a toilet seat" and "it is *improbable* that one would get AIDS from contact with a victim's tears." These aren't good enough. You don't fool around with "probably" and "little risks" when your children are concerned.

Anyway, why should I place such faith in the scientists' evaluations of what the risks are? They could just be wrong, and it would not be the first time. It is foolish to believe in the infallibility of science. Those who do so have fallen prey to a modern superstition.

FITCH: Of course science can be wrong. But that doesn't mean that we should ignore the evidence. And the evidence is that it cannot be spread by casual contact. In fact it very clearly looks as if it can only be caught if the virus is directly introduced into the blood.[8]

BASCOMBE: I am *not* ignoring the evidence. I am saying that the evidence leaves room for a risk that I am not willing to take. You know that there are school board members in various places around the country who do not want AIDS children in the public schools. They too are often accused of simply being ignorant of the evidence about how AIDS is spread or of ignoring the evidence. Maybe some of them are guilty of these things. But if you listen you will hear many of them saying what I am saying. It is their responsibility to look out for the welfare of the greatest number of children under their jurisdictions, and they do not think it is justifiable to subject the great majority to even a small risk of AIDS for the benefit of the unfortunate few who suffer from the disease.

FITCH: I'm not sure you aren't giving most of the school board people too much credit for clear thinking. Anyway, that approach is much too conservative. It basically amounts to a policy of *take no risks*. And that is a policy that nobody should follow, that nobody does follow, that nobody *can* follow. In some sense or the other everything we do in this world involves risk. You could choke while brushing your teeth or drown while taking a bath. And if you send your children to school any number of bad things could happen to them. They could be poisoned in the cafeteria or break their necks on the playground. Some of these risks are not farfetched. The school could burn with children trapped inside; the school bus could plunge into a ravine. Why should you be willing to send your children to school and accept these risks but not be willing to accept the alleged risk of allowing AIDS children to attend the school?

BASCOMBE: You have a flair for overgeneralizing. First you wrongly accuse me of being committed to a policy of taking *no* risks. Then you leap from the near truism that we have to take many risks in this life to the conclusion that I ought to be willing to take *just any* risk. The fact is that it makes perfectly good sense for me to be willing to take the risk of putting my child on the school bus every day and yet not be willing to put her into a school with AIDS victims. Some risks are worth taking and others aren't. I put my child on the bus every day because the good of her being in school outweighs the rather small risk that the bus will crack up. The risk is one that is worth taking. But allowing the AIDS child to be in school is just not a great enough good to make it worth the risk that my child *and many other children* will contract that hideous affliction. That risk isn't worth it.

FITCH: If you are that sure it isn't worth it you must be thinking of the AIDS child's being allowed to live as normal a life as possible as not being of much value. The really important thing, though, is that no matter what you say about other viruses being communicable from drinking cups or from touching of hands, the AIDS virus is not some other virus. There is no good reason to think that this particular virus can be passed on by casual contact. The risk of doing so really should be considered to be zero. There is just no risk worth taking into consideration. Let the child into the school and don't worry about it. If you are inclined to worry, just chalk it up to AIDS hysteria.

BASCOMBE: I'm not convinced. There is enough uncertainty to make it a risk.

FITCH: I keep telling you: your supposed risks are entirely too abstract. They are based on nothing but the sheerest "maybe's." There is nothing here that would count as any genuine "risk." Let the children all go to school without further ado.

BASCOMBE: And I am telling you that you cannot take chances with children.

IV. Bathhouses, AIDS, and Legal Paternalism

FITCH: I keep hearing about calls to close down the so-called gay bathhouses. I suppose you're in favor of that, Bascombe.

BASCOMBE: It's a damned good idea. Those places are regular AIDS virus breeding farms.

FITCH: People who want to close the bathhouses are intrusive busybodies. I am tired of government trying to protect individuals from themselves. If I want to read dirty books or commit suicide or ride a motorcycle without wearing a helmet, it's my own business. I don't want the government or anybody else telling me I cannot do these things because they are immoral or because they will harm me.

SHERWOOD: You are against paternalism.

FITCH: Exactly. And closing down the bathhouses is a clear case of paternalism.[9]

BASCOMBE: No it isn't. Paternalism is abridging a person's own liberty to keep him from being immoral or from harming *himself*. Closing down the baths is abridging the bath owners' liberty to keep someone *else* from the harm of contracting AIDS. So that isn't paternalism.

FITCH: Don't be silly. You would close the baths so that a person cannot go to one if he chooses, and you would do this to protect that person from himself, from his own choices. The fact that you protect him from his own choices by closing the bath rather than by locking *him* up so that he cannot go to an open one is irrelevant. That is just a different means of protecting him from himself, and so its aim is clearly paternalistic.[10]

SHERWOOD: You know, Fitch, it's really not entirely obvious that paternalism is always such a bad thing. But let's suppose it is for now. What would that come to? It would mean that any regulation of the individual that can be justified *only* on paternalistic grounds would be wrong. If some other justification of a regulation can be given, the fact that it also protects an individual from himself doesn't matter one way or another.

Now, suppose that the only justification for closing the bathhouses went this way: If they are left open more men will patronize them, even though they know the risk of doing so. Some of these men will contract AIDS and will suffer and die. Therefore, to protect them from this horrible fate we should close the baths. This reasoning is as clearly paternalistic as anything can be. Close the baths to protect these people from themselves—if this were the only justification that could be given for closing the baths, then anyone opposed to paternalism would have to oppose closing them.

FITCH: I bet I know where you are going with this. You are going to say that a lot of the bath patrons who get AIDS will not be rich and it will fall to society to take care of them. And when this is included, the rationale for closing the baths isn't entirely paternalistic. The point of closing them is not just to protect the patrons from becoming sick; it is also to protect society from the burden of caring for them when they do become sick.

SHERWOOD: I wasn't going to say that at all. That sort of reasoning bothers me. If we are going to have a policy of "we won't interfere with your choices for the sake of protecting you from yourself," then it seems we should also have the policy that "we won't save you from the consequences of your stupid choices."

BASCOMBE: But does anybody stick to that resolve? We see the sick and the old people who chose not to make provision for themselves, and we adopt the burden of care anyway.

FITCH: Not often enough or well enough.

SHERWOOD: The thing is that we can avoid these hard issues entirely. We get into them only if we take it that the reason for closing the bathhouses has to do primarily with the welfare of those who would choose to frequent them and knowingly take the risk of contracting AIDS.

We avoid these issues when we realize that there is a legitimate rationale for closing the baths that does not center around the welfare of those who choose to use them. Suppose that we were talking about the common cold. I tell you that you can't kiss your boyfriend who has a cold because you might catch it. My concern here could be for your welfare—in which case you can accuse me of paternalism—but it need not be. If you catch the cold you are likely to sneeze in public or otherwise spread it to others who certainly don't want it.

This rationale for preventing you from kissing your friend is not at all paternalistic. It is a straightforward matter of protecting others in the society from a minor but annoying harm that you may inflict on them very much against their will.

In a similar way the rationale for closing the baths need not be the protection of those who deliberately choose to frequent them and to take the risk of contracting AIDS. It is for the protection of society from the general spread of the AIDS virus. It's like the case of the common cold, in that respect.

FITCH: Hold on there, Sherwood. It is like the case of the common cold *if* you assume that AIDS can be spread by sneezing or by other casual and inadvertent contact the way the cold can be. Then the rationale for closing the baths is that people in society at large are protected from having the AIDS virus inflicted on them through no choices of their own. And I certainly agree that that is clearly not a paternalistic rationale.

But the problem here is that you and I both know perfectly well that AIDS is not spread in such ways. Since it is entirely, or nearly entirely, spread by sharing drug needles and by sexual activity, then those who are at significant risk are those who choose to act in certain ways. It doesn't matter whether we consider the people who frequent the baths or those who might get AIDS directly or indirectly from the ones who do—in either case we are dealing with people who *choose* to do the things that may result in the harm to themselves. So closing the baths would still only protect from risk those who would choose to take the risk. And that is paternalism.

SHERWOOD: If the only harm in question here were actually getting AIDS then that would be right. One can indeed choose whether to take the risk of suffering this harm. But as the virus spreads, as more and more people actually have the disease and more and more others become carriers, the more it will become a universal choice between celibacy and risking AIDS. Any of us can choose whether to risk the harm of getting AIDS or be celibate, but none of us will have the choice of whether to be faced with only these miserable alternatives. And being faced with them is itself a very real harm. The existence of gay baths may well contribute significantly to this harm.

FITCH: So we close the baths so that people will not be forced to face the choice of being celibate or risk contracting AIDS. And since being faced with that choice is itself a harm, closing the baths is justified on the ground that it prevents bringing harm to others. And that is a nonpaternalistic justification for closing them.

SHERWOOD: Exactly. And this isn't some trumped-up nonpaternalistic rationale for doing what we really want to do on paternalistic grounds. The genuine threat here is that we would have to refrain from sex or risk getting AIDS. Living in a society in which those are the alternatives would be an extremely frightening harm for any of us to face.

BASCOMBE: I am with you completely. Close the baths. I have to admit, though, Sherwood, I didn't expect you to be on my side in this.

SHERWOOD: I didn't say I was on your side. I really do not have any convictions about whether or not it is a good idea to close the baths. My claim is just that leaving the baths open may well bring harm to people who do not choose to take the risk of that harm. To that extent there is some nonpaternalistic ground for closing the baths, but there still may not be a *good overall case* for closing them. It would not be hard to come up with some nonpaternalistic grounds for prohibiting chewing tobacco in public, lying about having had a vasectomy, or having an annual income of over one hundred thousand dollars. But so far at least we haven't thought there to be a sufficient overall case for prohibiting any of these things. Maybe laws against baths or bath-like gay meeting places would be unenforceable or could be enforced only by quadrupling the number of police, which we don't have the dollars to do; maybe the kind of investigative powers we would have to grant would be too much of a threat to everyone's civil liberties; maybe it just wouldn't do much good since it might have only a minuscule effect on the spread of AIDS.

So even for a devout antipaternalistic, it is not illegitimate to consider closing the baths. Whether it is a good idea overall is something else. And we are not going to answer that question by debating about paternalism. Really, Fitch, I think talk about paternalism is pretty much of a red herring here.

V: Quarantines, Tattoos, and Other Practical Solutions

FITCH: I would like to know what else you have in mind, Bascombe. You want to keep children with AIDS out of school and close the baths, but I'm sure you wouldn't stop there. What do we do next?

BASCOMBE: We do whatever is necessary to prevent the further spread of the disease. First, there are other simple practical measures we can take. For instance, we can see to it that people with AIDS are not allowed to work in restaurants or as hairdressers, manicurists, or masseurs. Dentists and doctors who have the disease will not be allowed to practice. All medical practitioners and anyone else who may come into close physical contact with other people should wear masks and gloves. These and a lot of other common sense precautions could be implemented right away.

SHERWOOD: I suppose they could be, but none of them would be likely to make any difference. Even you have already admitted that there is no positive reason to think that AIDS can be transmitted in ways that would make any of these people a threat to spread the disease.

FITCH: The only result of your ideas so far is that some people will lose their livelihoods.

BASCOMBE: I haven't really gotten to the heart of my proposal yet.

FITCH: Don't tell us. We take all likely carriers of the disease out in the woods and shoot them. Then we dig a great big hole . . .

SHERWOOD: Let Bascombe go on. I am just afraid that it will be impossible to parody what he actually has in mind.

BASCOMBE: What I have in mind is not at all unreasonable. We close down all places that contribute significantly to behavior that results in the spread of AIDS. That would most obviously be the gay baths. But we also get rid of gay bars and other places such as sections of public parks that serve as liaison spots. Finally and far and away most important we just make it illegal for anyone with AIDS to engage in sexual relations with anyone who does not already have AIDS. And severe penalties are to be attached to breaking this law.

FITCH: I'm agog.

SHERWOOD: How, Bascombe, do you propose to enforce your prohibition on sexual activity by AIDS carriers?

FITCH: Sherwood, have you gone utterly mad? You sound as if you are taking him seriously. The very idea of a law forbidding significant numbers of people from having sex at all except with others who are disease carriers is morally repugnant. It is an infringement on one's right to privacy, to freedom of association, to . . .

BASCOMBE: Very noble, Fitch. But let me read you something.

> There is a homosexual man in Alameda County, Calif., who came down with [AIDS a while back], and since then has been treated several times at the county public-health clinic for gonorrhea. He has sexual relations with three to five different men each week, without telling them of his condition. . . . [H]e apparently is breaking no laws.[11]

He *should* be breaking some laws. I am unimpressed with his right to privacy or anything else in the face of his hideous behavior.

SHERWOOD: I want to go back to my question for Bascombe. How would you enforce a prohibition on AIDS carriers' sexual activity?

BASCOMBE: You think I am going to recommend a quarantine and then you will claim that that is unworkable and I will look like a fool.

FITCH: The thought entered our minds.

BASCOMBE: Let me assure you that I know perfectly well that any restrictions must be imposed on carriers and that not only those who have the disease can be carriers. I also know that there are about 7000 known sufferers from the disease alive in the U.S. now, but maybe a million or even two million carriers of the HTLV-III virus. Does that make a quarantine out of consideration? It isn't as if the million or two cannot be identified. The blood test for the presence of antibodies to the HTLV-III virus tells us who the carriers are. And how you quarantine even two million people is just a logistical problem.

FITCH: If we can put one man on the moon we can put two million on an island.

BASCOMBE: You laugh. But that's right. It could be done. Maybe not literally put them on an island but in some relatively isolated region in the West or some such place.

FITCH: That really is laughable. When you and others like you start talking about islands or places in the West you make it sound as if the problems are just those of transportation and of getting a big enough chunk of land. You can't just dump one or two million people somewhere and say "Here's where you will live now." What do they do for food, clothing, stores, hospitals, roads, fuel, and everything else we have in this society? And what about those whose friends, lovers, husbands, wives, children, parents, and breadwinners are whisked away to your island? Overall the upheaval would be so great that society as we know it would be destroyed. My suggestion would be better: take them out and shoot them.

BASCOMBE: Quarantining all carriers would be extremely difficult. It would not be impossible.

FITCH: Neither would shooting them. Although I grant it would be a little messy.

BASCOMBE: Actually I was not going to suggest a quarantine at all. I don't think such an extreme measure is necessary. My plan is much simpler and would work just as well.

First we identify all carriers by means of the blood test. Then we put some identifying mark on each one. Any sort of indelible mark would do. This would not be in a place where it would be casually seen, but it would be visible if someone were looking for it. It would then be illegal for anyone with the mark to have sexual relations with anyone who does not have the mark. Anyone with the mark who does so would be subject to imprisonment, with other carriers, of course. But probably almost no one would have to be imprisoned, because those without the mark would not choose to have sex with anyone who had it. Under these conditions the disease will not spread, work can proceed on finding a cure, and when it is successful these restrictions would be gradually phased out.

SHERWOOD: You don't find anything unsavory about that scheme?

FITCH: Notice how he very carefully talked about an "indelible mark." What he means is that carriers should be tattooed. Just like in Hitler's Germany.

BASCOMBE: That association is ridiculous. Tattooing for the purpose of identification is completely legitimate in some cases. It has been suggested that children be tattooed as a means of identification and protection against kidnappers. Anyway the German case is entirely different. There it was an ethnic group that was singled out. The issue was racism. Here we are identifying individuals each of whom is in fact a danger. There is no comparison at all.[12]

SHERWOOD: Let's see. What other problems might there be with your scheme? For one thing, the HTLV-III test does apparently show false positives on occasion.

BASCOMBE: That's a shame. But it's one of those unfortunate things we will just have to live with.

SHERWOOD: What about the problems of getting everybody tested? How does one arrange that? Lining up 225 million people, taking their blood, running the tests, getting the positives back to be "marked," being sure that very few people have been missed altogether—the logistical problems are hardly less than in sending carriers off to an island. And what if somebody doesn't have a mark? How does another person know if he was tested negative or was never tested at all?

BASCOMBE: Everybody would get certificates when they are tested. Or there could be two marks, one positive, one negative. Then there would be no doubt. As to the logistical problems, they could be overcome. This society managed to get pretty much everybody vaccinated against smallpox. And, by the way, that leaves a mark.

FITCH: Sherwood, let me ask you again. Why are you listening to this? I see images of storm troopers coming in the night and carrying people off for blood tests so they can be branded and then shunned by former friends and strangers alike. Even if we ended up with a society in which people didn't die of AIDS, we would not have ended up with a society worth living in.

SHERWOOD: I'm listening because AIDS is a serious problem. You are surely right in thinking that there is an intolerable degree of hysteria, paranoia, and sensationalism surrounding it. But it is still something well worth worrying about and doing something about, if we can think of anything sensible to do. Bascombe has a suggestion, and so I listened to it.

FITCH: But the minute he started talking about testing everybody and tattooing people it was obvious that he wasn't worth listening to.

SHERWOOD: I am not exactly crazy about those ideas myself, but they seem a bit better than the suggested alternatives, shipping carriers off to islands or just shooting them.

FITCH: Shooting them was an attempt to parody, but you are right that it is hard to parody some of the things Bascombe says.

SHERWOOD: But why is the shooting suggestion just parody anyway? It *would be* a real solution to the problem of AIDS. I think it would anyway. Of course we would have to not let anyone else into the country for a few years so that the virus wasn't brought in again. But problems like that could be taken care of if we are willing to shoot the carriers as a first step.

BASCOMBE: What are you getting at there, Sherwood? You're not going to endorse the shooting solution. I know that.

SHERWOOD: What I want to get at is that it would be a solution to the problems that AIDS poses, but it isn't something any of us will endorse. That indicates that we are not after whatever would be the most swift and certain means of getting rid of AIDS. So what are we after? What are the criteria for being a good plan?

FITCH: Uh-oh. I think we are about to see the professor come out in Sherwood.

SHERWOOD: I will try to control my pedantic tendencies. I don't really think there is anything to say that isn't pretty obvious. We know what the best thing to do would be—find a cure today. The problem with that is that we can't do it. The first thing required of any plan is that it be possible to carry it out.

The second requirement is that the plan would work if it were carried out. Those who say we should quarantine people who have the full-blown AIDS disease have a plan that fails this simple test, since it just ignores the million or two other carriers.

Beyond this, what we have to consider is whether the good achieved—in this case getting rid of the threat of AIDS—is sufficient to outweigh the costs of the way in which the good is achieved. Would it be *worth it* to get rid of AIDS if the cost was that we had a real police state in which nearly every aspect of one's personal life were subject to state scrutiny?

Finally there is at least one other sort of thing to consider. There may be something we could do, and the good of doing it would outweigh its costs. But this still would not be the way to proceed if there were some other way of getting the same good at smaller cost. Suppose Bascombe's tattoo plan would work and would be worth it; that is, the good achieved would outweigh the costs in civil liberties. It still would not be justified to put his plan into effect if the same good or one near to it could be brought about at less cost, for instance by persuading people to alter their social habits.

BASCOMBE: My plan meets all the criteria. It passes with flying colors.

SHERWOOD: Fitch said your plan fails the test of being "worth it." The cure is worse than the disease. Surely most people will agree with that.

BASCOMBE: My plan is the best plan anyone has come up with that has real promise of stamping out AIDS. It is a lot better than the quarantine plan.

SHERWOOD: But it still isn't worth it. While getting rid of AIDS is something we all want very much, that doesn't mean that we should do just anything that might accomplish this. The price we would have to pay could well be just too high.

BASCOMBE: That all sounds very reasonable in the abstract. But AIDS is a very practical problem. And as far as I can tell you don't want to really do anything that would really protect us from it.

SHERWOOD: Of course I want to do something. But probably it's nothing dramatic enough to satisfy you. Obviously we should support medical research insofar as it is at all likely to produce a cure for AIDS or at least to produce something that would retard its development or spread. In the short run, though, maybe the most important thing we can do is attempt to inhibit the spread of the disease by more intense "safe sex" and "don't share hypodermic needles" educational campaigns.

BASCOMBE: That won't get rid of AIDS.

SHERWOOD: No, but it won't give us a police state, either.

FITCH: There is one other thing we can do. We can wish that the supermarket tabloids, in fact, all the media, would just shut up about AIDS except when there is really something to say.

SHERWOOD: I doubt that there is much hope of that happening.

FITCH: There is one way it could happen. Do you remember what was on the front page of every tabloid before they discovered AIDS?

BASCOMBE: No . . . oh yes I do. It was herpes.

FITCH: You hardly ever hear a mention of herpes since AIDS came along. Now you want to get the morbid and sensationalized news about AIDS off the front pages? Well how about if there were a new and worse . . .

SHERWOOD: Don't even think about it.

BASCOMBE: I know I won't.

FITCH: Good night.

Notes

1. There is some evidence that recent changes in sexual behavior have in fact slowed the spread of AIDS. See Jonathan Lieberson, "The Reality of AIDS," *The New York Review*, January 16, 1986, p. 46.

2. Falwell's and Buchanan's views are frequently cited. Both are mentioned, for instance, in a *Newsweek* cover story of September 23, 1985, pp. 22 and 25.

3. *Newsweek*, September 23, 1985, p. 24; *Time*, September 23, 1985, p. 26.

4. *Newsweek*, September 23, 1985, p. 24.

5. *Time*, September 23, 1985, p. 26.

6. Cf. Lieberson, op. cit.: "Eager to stimulate concern about the disease, [many homosexuals] sought to make people aware that it need not affect only homosexuals. At the same time, when some press reports announced that no one was safe from AIDS, the same homosexuals feared that too much publicity of this kind might lead to

discrimination against them as the 'creators' of the epidemic."

7. *Newsweek*, September 23, 1985, p. 18.

8. "It appears that, in order to infect, [the AIDS] virus must be virtually injected into the blood stream and then encounter cells in which it can multiply." (Mathilde Krim, "AIDS: The Challenge to Science and Medicine," *Hastings Center Report*, Vol. 15, No. 4, August 1985, *Special Supplement*, p. 4. This is quoted by Lieberson, op. cit.)

9. Lieberson is among those who have suggested that to close the baths would be to act paternalistically. (*Op. cit.*, p. 48.)

10. In Gerald Dworkin's terms, closing the baths to protect those who would choose to take the risk of visiting them would be a case of "impure paternalism." ("Paternalism," section III; in this

volume, p. 218.) Cf. John Stuart Mill's classic *On Liberty*: "There is no room for [even considering a prohibition] when a person's conduct affects the interest of no persons besides himself, *or needs not affect them unless they like* . . ." (Indianapolis: Hackett, 1978, pp. 73–74, italics added.)

11. *Newsweek*, September 23, 1985, p. 18.

12. Bascombe's "indelible mark" scheme was written in January 1986. Some time later this fictional proposal became a real one when William F. Buckley, Jr., publicly proposed a nearly identical tattooing scheme. (*New York Times* op. ed., March 18, 1986.) Predictably enough, Buckley's proposal gave rise to sharp reactions, and the association between tattooing and Nazi practice did not go unnoticed.

On Telling Patients the Truth

Mack Lipkin

Should a doctor always tell his patients the truth? In recent years there has been an extraordinary increase in public discussion of the ethical problems involved in this question. But little has been heard from physicians themselves. I believe that gaps in understanding the complex interactions between doctors and patients have led many laymen astray in this debate.

It is easy to make an attractive case for always telling patients the truth. But as L. J. Henderson, the great Harvard physiologist-philosopher of decades ago, commented:

> To speak of telling the truth, the whole truth and nothing but the truth to a patient is absurd. Like absurdity in mathematics, it is absurd simply because it is impossible. . . . The notion that the truth, the whole truth, and nothing but the truth can be conveyed to the patient is a good specimen of that class of fallacies called by Whitehead "the fallacy of misplaced concreteness." It results from neglecting factors that cannot be excluded from the concrete situation and that are of an order of magnitude and relevancy that make it imperative to consider them. Of course, another fallacy is also often involved, the

belief that diagnosis and prognosis are more certain than they are. But that is another question.

Words, especially medical terms, inevitably carry different implications for different people. When these words are said in the presence of anxiety-laden illness, there is a strong tendency to hear selectively and with emphases not intended by the doctor. Thus, what the doctor means to convey is obscured.

Indeed, thoughtful physicians know that transmittal of accurate information to patients is often impossible. Patients rarely know how the body functions in health and disease, but instead have inaccurate ideas of what is going on; this hampers the attempts to "tell the truth."

Take cancer, for example. Patients seldom know that while some cancers are rapidly fatal, others never amount to much; some have a cure rate of 99 percent, others less than 1 percent; a cancer may grow rapidly for months and then stop growing for years; may remain localized for years or spread all over the body almost from the beginning; some can be arrested for long periods of time, others not. Thus, one patient thinks of cancer as curable, the next thinks it means certain death.

How many patients understand that "heart trouble" may refer to literally hundreds of different abnormalities ranging in severity from the trivial to the instantly fatal? How many know that the term "arthritis" may refer to dozens of different types of joint involvement? "Arthritis" may raise a vision of the appalling disease that made Aunt Eulalee a helpless invalid until her death years later; the next patient remembers Grandpa grumbling about the damned arthritis as he got up from his chair. Unfortunately but understandably, most people's ideas about the implications of medical terms are based on what they have heard about a few cases.

The news of serious illness drives some patients to irrational and destructive behavior; others handle it sensibly. A distinguished philosopher forestalled my telling him about his cancer by saying, "I want to know the truth. The only thing I couldn't take and wouldn't want to know about is cancer." For two years he had watched his mother die slowly of a painful form of cancer. Several of my physician patients have indicated they would not want to know if they had a fatal illness.

Most patients should be told "the truth" to the extent that they can comprehend it. Indeed, most doctors, like most other people, are uncomfortable with lies. Good physicians, aware that some may be badly damaged by being told more than they want or need to know, can usually ascertain the patient's preferences and needs.

Discussions about lying often center about the use of placebos. In medical usage, a "placebo" is a treatment that has no specific physical or chemical action on the condition being treated, but is given to affect symptoms by a psychologic mechanism, rather than a purely physical one. Ethicists believe that placebos necessarily involve a partial or complete deception by the doctor, since the patient is allowed to believe that the treatment has a specific effect. They seem unaware that placebos, far from being inert (except in the rigid pharmacological sense), are among the most powerful agents known to medicine.

Placebos are a form of suggestion, which is a direct or indirect presentation of an idea, followed by an uncritical, i.e., not thought-out, acceptance. Those who have studied suggestion or looked at medical history know its almost unbelievable potency; it is involved to a greater or lesser extent in the treatment of every conscious patient. It can induce or remove almost any kind of feeling or thought. It can strengthen the weak or paralyze the strong; transform sleeping, feeding, or sexual patterns; remove or induce a vast array of symptoms; mimic or abolish the effect of very powerful drugs. It can alter the function of most organs. It can cause illness or a great sense of well-being. It can kill. In fact, doctors often add a measure of suggestion when they prescribe even potent medications for those who also need psychologic support. Like all potent agents, its proper use requires judgment based on experience and skill.

Communication between physician and the apprehensive and often confused patient is delicate and uncertain. Honesty should be evaluated not only in terms of a slavish devotion to language often misinterpreted by the patient, but also in terms of intent. *The crucial question is whether the deception was intended to benefit the patient or the doctor.*

Physicians, like most people, hope to see good results and are disappointed when patients do poorly. Their reputations and their livelihood depend on doing effective work; purely selfish reasons would dictate they do their best for their patients. Most important, all good physicians have a deep sense of responsibility toward those who have entrusted their welfare to them.

As I have explained, it is usually a practical impossibility to tell patients "the whole truth." Moreover, often enough, the ethics of the situation, the true moral responsibility, may demand that the naked facts not be revealed. The now popular complaint that doctors are too authoritarian is misguided more often than not. Some patients who insist on exercising their right to know may be doing themselves a disservice.

Judgment is often difficult and uncertain. Simplistic assertions about telling the truth may not be helpful to patients or physicians in times of trouble.

Lies to the Sick and Dying

Sissela Bok

Deception as Therapy

A forty-six-year-old man, coming to a clinic for a routine physical checkup needed for insurance purposes, is diagnosed as having a form of cancer likely to cause him to die within six months. No known cure exists for it. Chemotherapy may prolong life by a few extra months, but will have side effects the physician does not think warranted in this case. In addition, he believes that such therapy should be reserved for patients with a chance for recovery or remission. The patient has no symptoms giving him any reason to believe that he is not perfectly healthy. He expects to take a short vacation in a week.

For the physician, there are now several choices involving truthfulness. Ought he to tell the patient what he has learned, or conceal it? If asked, should he deny it? If he decides to reveal the diagnosis, should he delay doing so until after the patient returns from his vacation? Finally, even if he does reveal the serious nature of the diagnosis, should he mention the possibility of chemotherapy and his reasons for not recommending it in this case? Or should he encourage every last effort to postpone death?

In this particular case, the physician chose to inform the patient of his diagnosis right away. He did not, however, mention the possibility of chemotherapy. A medical student working under him disagreed; several nurses also thought that the patient should have been informed of this possibility. They tried, unsuccessfully, to persuade the physician that this was the patient's right. When persuasion had failed, the student elected to disobey the doctor by informing the patient of the alternative of chemotherapy. After consultation with family members, the patient chose to ask for the treatment.

Doctors confront such choices often and urgently. What they reveal, hold back, or distort will matter profoundly to their patients. Doctors stress with corresponding vehemence their reasons for the distortion or concealment: not to confuse a sick person needlessly, or cause what may well be unnecessary pain or discomfort, as in the case of the cancer patient; not to leave a patient without hope, as in those many cases where the dying are not told the truth about their condition; or to improve the chances of cure, as where unwarranted optimism is expressed about some form of therapy. Doctors use information as part of the therapeutic regimen; it is given out in amounts, in admixtures, and according to timing believed best for patients. Accuracy, by comparison, matters far less.

Lying to patients has, therefore, seemed an especially excusable act. Some would argue that doctors, and *only* doctors, should be granted the right to manipulate the truth in ways so undesirable for politicians, lawyers, and others.[1] Doctors are trained to help patients; their relationship to patients carries special obligations, and they know much more than laymen about what helps and hinders recovery and survival.

Even the most conscientious doctors, then, who hold themselves at a distance from the quacks and the purveyors of false remedies, hesitate to forswear all lying. Lying is usually wrong, they argue, but less so than allowing the truth to harm patients. B. C. Meyer echoes this very common view:

> [O]urs is a profession which traditionally has been guided by a precept that transcends the virtue of uttering truth for truth's sake, and that is, "so far as possible, do no harm."[2]

Truth, for Meyer, may be important, but not when it endangers the health and well-being of patients. This has seemed self-evident to many physicians in the past—so much so that we find very few mentions of veracity in the codes and oaths and writings by physicians through the centuries. This absence is all the more striking as other principles of ethics have been consistently and movingly expressed in the same documents.

The two fundamental principles of doing good and not doing harm—of beneficence and nonmaleficence—are the most immediately relevant to medical practitioners, and the most frequently stressed. To preserve life and good health, to ward off illness, pain, and death—these are the perennial tasks of medicine and nursing. These principles have found powerful expression at all times in the history of medicine. In the Hippocratic Oath physicians promise to:

use treatment to help the sick . . . but never with a view to injury and wrong-doing.[3]

And a Hindu oath of initiation says:

Day and night, however thou mayest be engaged, thou shalt endeavor for the relief of patients with all thy heart and soul. Thou shalt not desert or injure the patient even for the sake of thy living.[4]

But there is no similar stress on veracity. It is absent from virtually all oaths, codes, and prayers. The Hippocratic Oath makes no mention of truthfulness to patients about their condition, prognosis, or treatment. Other early codes and prayers are equally silent on the subject. To be sure, they often refer to the confidentiality with which doctors should treat all that patients tell them; but there is no corresponding reference to honesty toward the patient. One of the few who appealed to such a principle was Amatus Lusitanus, a Jewish physician widely known for his skill, who, persecuted, died of the plague in 1568. He published an oath which reads in part:

If I lie, may I incur the eternal wrath of God and of His angel Raphael, and may nothing in the medical art succeed for me according to my desires.[5]

Later codes continue to avoid the subject. Not even the Declaration of Geneva, adopted in 1948 by the World Medical Association, makes any reference to it. And the Principles of Medical Ethics of the American Medical Association[6] still leave the matter of informing patients up to the physician.

Given such freedom, a physician can decide to tell as much or as little as he wants the patient to know, so long as he breaks no law. In the case of the man mentioned at the beginning of this chapter, some physicians might feel justified in lying for the good of the patient; others might be truthful. Some may conceal alternatives to the treatment they recommend; others not. In each case, they could appeal to the AMA Principles of Ethics. A great many would choose to be able to lie. They would claim that not only can a lie avoid harm for the patient, but that it is also hard to know whether they have been right in the first place in making their pessimistic diagnosis; a "truthful" statement could therefore turn out to hurt patients unnecessarily. The concern for curing and for supporting those who cannot be cured then runs counter to the desire to be completely open. This concern is especially strong where the prognosis is bleak; even more so when patients are so affected by their illness or their medication that they are more dependent than usual, perhaps more easily depressed or irrational.

Physicians know only too well how uncertain a diagnosis or prognosis can be. They know how hard it is to give meaningful and correct answers regarding health and illness. They also know that disclosing their own uncertainty or fears can reduce those benefits that depend upon faith in recovery. They fear, too, that revealing grave risks, no matter how unlikely it is that these will come about, may exercise the pull of the "self-fulfilling prophecy." They dislike being the bearers of uncertain or bad news as much as anyone else. And last, but not least, sitting down to discuss an illness truthfully and sensitively may take much-needed time away from other patients.

These reasons help explain why nurses and physicians and relatives of the sick and dying prefer not to be bound by rules that might limit their ability to suppress, delay, or distort information. This is not to say that they necessarily plan to lie much of the time. They merely want to have the freedom to do so when they believe it wise. And the reluctance to see lying prohibited explains, in turn, the failure of the codes and oaths to come to grips with the problems of truth-telling and lying.

But sharp conflicts are now arising. Doctors no longer work alone with patients. They have to consult with others much more than before; if they choose to lie, the choice may not be met with approval by all who take part in the care of the patient. A nurse expresses the difficulty which results as follows:

From personal experience I would say that the patients who aren't told about their terminal illness have so many verbal and mental questions unanswered that many will begin to realize that their illness is more serious than they're being told. . . .

Nurses care for these patients twenty-four hours a day compared to a doctor's daily brief visit, and it is the nurse many times that the patient will relate to, once his underlying fears become overwhelming. . . . This is difficult for us nurses because being in constant contact with patients we can see the events leading up to this. The patient continually asks you, "Why isn't my pain decreasing?" or "Why isn't the radiation treatment easing the pain?" . . . We cannot legally give these patients an honest answer as a nurse (and I'm sure I wouldn't want to) yet the problem is still not resolved and the circle grows larger and larger with the patient alone in the middle.[7]

The doctor's choice to lie increasingly involves co-workers in acting a part they find neither humane nor wise. The fact that these problems have not been carefully thought through within the medical profession, nor seriously addressed in medical education, merely serves to intensify the conflicts.[8] Different doctors then respond very differently to patients in exactly similar predicaments. The friction is increased by the fact that relatives often disagree even where those giving medical care to a patient are in accord on how to approach the patient. Here again, because physicians have not worked out to common satisfaction the question of whether relatives have the right to make such requests, the problems are allowed to be haphazardly resolved by each physician as he sees fit.

The Patient's Perspective

The turmoil in the medical profession regarding truth-telling is further augmented by the pressures that patients themselves now bring to bear and by empirical data coming to light. Challenges are growing to the three major arguments for lying to patients: that truthfulness is impossible; that patients do not want bad news; and that truthful information harms them.

The first of these arguments . . . confuses "truth" and "truthfulness" so as to clear the way for occasional lying on grounds supported by the second and third arguments. At this point, we can see more clearly that it is a strategic move intended to discourage the question of truthfulness from carrying much weight in the first place, and thus to leave the choice of what to say and how to say it up to the physician. To claim that "since telling the truth is impossible, there can be no sharp distinction between what is true and what is false"[9] is to try to defeat objections to lying before even discussing them. One need only imagine how such an argument would be received, were it made by a car salesman or a real estate dealer, to see how fallacious it is.

In medicine, however, the argument is supported by a subsidiary point: even if people might ordinarily understand what is spoken to them, patients are often not in a position to do so. This is where paternalism enters in. When we buy cars or houses, the paternalist will argue, we need to have all our wits about us; but when we are ill, we cannot always do so. We need help in making choices, even if help can be given only by keeping us in the dark. And the physician is trained and willing to provide such help.

It is certainly true that some patients cannot make the best choices for themselves when weakened by illness or drugs. But most still can. And even those who are incompetent have a right to have someone—their guardian or spouse perhaps—receive the correct information.

The paternalistic assumption of superiority to patients also carries great dangers for physicians themselves—it risks turning to contempt. The following view was recently expressed in a letter to a medical journal:

> As a radiologist who has been sued, I have reflected earnestly on advice to obtain Informed Consent but have decided to "take the risks without informing the patient" and trust to "God, judge, and jury" rather than evade responsibility through a legal gimmick. . . .
>
> [I]n a general radiologic practice many of our patients are uninformable and we would never get through the day if we had to obtain their consent to every potentially harmful study.
>
> . . . We still have patients with language problems, the uneducated and the

unintelligent, the stolid and the stunned who cannot form an Informed Opinion to give an Informed Consent; we have the belligerent and the panicky who do not listen or comprehend. And then there are the Medicare patients who comprise 35 percent of general hospital admissions. The bright ones wearily plead to be left alone. . . . As for the apathetic rest, many of them were kindly described by Richard Bright as not being able to comprehend because "their brains are so poorly oxygenated."[10]

The argument which rejects informing patients because adequate truthful information is impossible in itself or because patients are lacking in understanding must itself be rejected when looked at from the point of view of patients. They know that liberties granted to the most conscientious and altruistic doctors will be exercised also in the "Medicaid Mills"; that the choices thus kept from patients will be exercised by not only competent but incompetent physicians; and that even the best doctors can make choices patients would want to make differently for themselves.

The second argument for deceiving patients refers specifically to giving them news of a frightening or depressing kind. It holds that patients do not, in fact, generally want such information. That they prefer not to have to face up to serious illness and death. On the basis of such a belief, most doctors in a number of surveys stated that they do not, as a rule, inform patients that they have an illness such as cancer.

When studies are made of what patients desire to know, on the other hand, a large majority say that they *would* like to be told of such a diagnosis.[11] All these studies need updating and should be done with larger numbers of patients and nonpatients. But they do show that there is generally a dramatic divergence between physicians and patients on the factual question of whether patients want to know what ails them in cases of serious illness such as cancer. In most of the studies, over 80 percent of the persons asked indicated that they would want to be told.

Sometimes this discrepancy is set aside by doctors who want to retain the view that patients do not want unhappy news. In reality, they claim, the fact that patients say they want it has to be discounted. The more someone asks to know, the more he suffers from fear which will lead to the denial of the information even if it is given. Informing patients is, therefore, useless; they resist and deny having been told what they cannot assimilate. According to this view, empirical studies of what patients say they want are worthless since they do not probe deeply enough to uncover this universal resistance to the contemplation of one's own death.

This view is only partially correct. For some patients, denial is indeed well established in medical experience. A number of patients (estimated at between 15 percent and 25 percent) will give evidence of denial of having been told about their illness, even when they repeatedly ask and are repeatedly informed. And nearly everyone experiences a period of denial at some point in the course of approaching death.[12] Elisabeth Kübler-Ross sees denial as resulting often from premature and abrupt information by a stranger who goes through the process quickly to "get it over with." She holds that denial functions as a buffer after unexpected shocking news, permitting individuals to collect themselves and to mobilize other defenses. She describes prolonged denial in one patient as follows:

> She was convinced that the x-rays were "mixed up"; she asked for reassurance that her pathology report could not possibly be back so soon and that another patient's report must have been marked with her name. When none of this could be confirmed, she quickly asked to leave the hospital, looking for another physician in the vain hope "to get a better explanation for my troubles." This patient went "shopping around" for many doctors, some of whom gave her reassuring answers, others of whom confirmed the previous suspicion. Whether confirmed or not, she reacted in the same manner, she asked for examination and reexamination. . . .[13]

But to say the denial is universal flies in the face of all evidence. And to take any claim to the contrary as "symptomatic" of deeper denial leaves no room for reasoned discourse. There is no way that such universal denial can be proved true or false. To believe in it is a metaphysical belief about man's condition, not a statement about what patients do and do not want. It is true that we can never completely understand the possibility of our own death, any more than being alive in the first place. But people certainly differ in the degree to which they can approach such knowledge, take it into account in their plans, and make their peace with it.

Montaigne claimed that in order to learn both to live and to die, men have to think about death and be prepared to accept it.[14] To stick one's head in the sand, or to be prevented by lies from trying to discern what is to come, hampers freedom— freedom to consider one's life as a whole, with a beginning, a duration, an end. Some may request to be deceived rather than to see their lives as thus finite; others reject the information which would require them to do so; but most say that they want to know. Their concern for knowing about their condition goes far beyond mere curiosity or the wish to make isolated personal choices in the short time left to them; their stance toward the entire life they have lived, and their ability to give it meaning and completion, are at stake.[15] In lying or withholding the facts which permit such discernment, doctors may reflect their own fears (which, according to one study,[16] are much stronger than those of laymen) of facing questions about the meaning of one's life and the inevitability of death.

Beyond the fundamental deprivation that can result from deception, we are also becoming increasingly aware of all that can befall patients in the course of their illness when information is denied or distorted. Lies place them in a position where they no longer participate in choices concerning their own health, including the choice of whether to be a "patient" in the first place. A terminally ill person who is not informed that his illness is incurable and that he is near death cannot make decisions about the end of his life; about whether or not to enter a hospital, or to have surgery; where and with whom to spend his last days; how to put his affairs in order—these most personal choices cannot be made if he is kept in the dark, or given contradictory hints and clues. . . .

The reason why even doctors who recognize a patient's right to have information might still not provide it brings us to the third argument against telling all patients the truth. It holds that the information given might hurt the patient and the concern for the right to such information is therefore a threat to proper health care. A patient, these doctors argue, may wish to commit suicide after being given discouraging news, or suffer a cardiac arrest, or simply cease to struggle, and thus not grasp the small remaining chance for recovery. And even where the outlook for a patient is very good, the disclosure of a minute risk can shock some patients or cause them to reject needed protection such as a vaccination or antibiotics.

The factual basis for this argument has been challenged from two points of view. The damages associated with the disclosure of sad news or risks are rarer than physicians believe; and the *benefits* which result from being informed are more substantial, even measurably so. Pain is tolerated more easily, recovery from surgery is quicker, and cooperation with therapy is greatly improved. The attitude that "what you don't know won't hurt you" is proving unrealistic; it is what patients do not know but vaguely suspect that causes them corrosive worry.

It is certain that no answers to this question of harm from information are the same for all patients. If we look, first, at the fear expressed by physicians that informing patients of even remote or unlikely risks conected with a drug prescription or operation might shock some and make others refuse the treatment that would have been best for them, it appears to be unfounded for the great majority of patients. Studies show that very few patients respond to being told of such risks by withdrawing their consent to the procedure and that those who do withdraw are the very ones who might well have been upset enough to sue the physician had they not been asked to consent beforehand.[17] It is possible that on even rarer occasions especially susceptible persons might manifest physical deterioration from shock; some physicians have even asked whether patients who die after giving informed consent to an operation, but before it actually takes place, somehow expire because of the information given to them.[18] While such questions are unanswerable in any one case, they certainly argue in favor of caution, a real concern for the person to whom one is recounting the risks he or she will face, and sensitivity to all signs of distress.

The situation is quite different when persons who are already ill, perhaps already quite weak and discouraged, are told of a very serious prognosis. Physicians fear that such knowledge may cause the patients to commit suicide, or to be frightened or depressed to the point that their illness takes a downward turn. The fear that great numbers of patients will commit suicide appears to be unfounded.[19] And if some do, is that a response so unreasonable, so much against the patient's best interest that physicians ought to make it a reason for concealment or lies? Many societies have allowed suicide in the past; our own has decriminalized it; and some are coming to make distinctions among the many suicides which ought to be prevented if at all possible, and those which ought to be respected.[20]

Another possible response to very bleak news is the triggering of physiological mechanisms which allow death to come more quickly—a form of giving up or of preparing for the inevitable, depending on one's outlook. Lewis Thomas, studying responses in humans and animals, holds it not unlikely that:

> . . . there is a pivotal movement at some stage in the body's reaction to injury or disease, maybe in aging as well, when the organism concedes that it is finished and the time for dying is at hand, and at this moment the events that lead to death are launched, as a coordinated mechanism. Functions are then shut off, in sequence, irreversibly, and, while this is going on, a neural mechanism, held ready for this occasion, is switched on. . . .[21]

Such a response may be appropriate, in which case it makes the moments of dying as peaceful as those who have died and been resuscitated so often testify. But it may also be brought on inappropriately, when the organism could have lived on, perhaps even induced malevolently, by external acts intended to kill. Thomas speculates that some of the deaths resulting from "hexing" are due to such responses. Levi-Strauss describes deaths from exorcism and the casting of spells in ways which suggest that the same process may then be brought on by the community.[22]

It is not inconceivable that unhappy news abruptly conveyed, or a great shock given to someone unable to tolerate it, could also bring on such a "dying response," quite unintended by the speaker. There is every reason to be cautious and to try to know ahead of time how susceptible a patient might be to the accidental triggering—however rare—of such a response. One has to assume, however, that most of those who have survived long enough to be in a situation where their informed consent is asked have a very robust resistance to such accidental triggering of processes leading to death. . . .

Apart from the possible harm from information, we are coming to learn much more about the benefits it can bring patients. People follow instructions more carefully if they know what their disease is and why they are asked to take medications; any benefits from those procedures are therefore much more likely to come about. Similarly, people recover faster from surgery and tolerate pain with less medication if they understand what ails them and what can be done for them.

Respect and Truthfulness

Taken all together, the three arguments defending lies to patients stand on much shakier ground as a counterweight to the right to be informed than is often thought. The common view that many patients cannot understand, do not want, and may be harmed by, knowledge of their condition, and that lying to them is either morally neutral or even to be recommended, must be set aside. Instead, we have to make a more complex comparison. Over against the right of patients to knowledge concerning themselves, the medical and psychological benefits to them from this knowledge, the unnecessary and sometimes harmful treatment to which they can be subjected if ignorant, and the harm to physicians, their profession, and other patients from deceptive practices, we have to set a severely restricted and narrowed paternalistic view—that *some* patients cannot understand, *some* do not want, and *some* may be harmed by, knowledge of their condition, and that they ought not to have to be treated like everyone else if this is not in their best interest.

Such a view is persuasive. A few patients openly request not to be given bad news. Others give clear signals to that effect, or are demonstrably vulnerable to the shock or anguish such news might call forth. Can one not in such cases infer implied consent to being deceived?

Concealment, evasion, withholding of information may at times be necessary. But if someone contemplates lying to a patient or concealing the truth, the burden of proof must shift. It must rest, here, as with all deception, on those who advocate it in any one instance. They must show why they fear a patient may be harmed or how they know that another cannot cope with the truthful knowledge. A decision to deceive must be seen as a very unusual step, to be talked over with colleagues and others who participate in the care of the patient. Reasons must be set forth and debated, alternatives weighed carefully. At all times, the correct information must go to *someone* closely related to the patient.

The law already permits doctors to withhold information from patients where it would clearly hurt their health. But this privilege has been sharply limited by the courts. Certainly it cannot be interpreted so broadly as to permit a general practice of deceiving patients ''for their own good.'' Nor can it be made to include cases where patients might calmly decide, upon hearing their diagnosis, not to go ahead with the therapy their doctor recommends.[23] Least of all can it justify silence or lies to large numbers of patients merely on grounds that it is not always easy to tell what a patient wants.

For the great majority of patients, on the contrary, the goal must be disclosure, and the atmosphere one of openness. But it would be wrong to assume that patients can therefore be told abruptly about a serious diagnosis—that, so long as openness exists, there are no further requirements of humane concern in such communication. Dr. Cicely Saunders, who runs the well-known St. Christopher's Hospice in England, describes the sensitivity and understanding which are needed:

> Every patient needs an explanation of his illness that will be understandable and convincing to him if he is to cooperate in his treatment or be relieved of the burden of unknown fears. This is true whether it is a question of giving a diagnosis in a hopeful situation or of confirming a poor prognosis.
>
> The fact that a patient does not ask does not mean that he has no questions. One visit or talk is rarely enough. It is only by waiting and listening that we can gain an idea of what we should be saying. Silences and gaps are often more revealing than words as we try to learn what a patient is facing as he

travels along the constantly changing journey of his illness and his thoughts about it.

> . . . So much of the communication will be without words or given indirectly. This is true of all real meeting with people but especially true with those who are facing, knowingly or not, difficult or threatening situations. It is also particularly true of the very ill.
>
> The main argument against a policy of deliberate, invariable denial of unpleasant facts is that it makes such communication extremely difficult, if not impossible. Once the possibility of talking frankly with a patient has been admitted, it does not mean that this will always take place, but the whole atmosphere is changed. We are then free to wait quietly for clues from each patient, seeing them as individuals from whom we can expect intelligence, courage, and individual decisions. They will feel secure enough to give us these clues when they wish.[24]

Above all, truthfulness with those who are suffering does not mean that they should be deprived of all hope: hope that there is a chance of recovery, however small; nor of reassurance that they will not be abandoned when they most need help.

Much needs to be done, however, if the deceptive practices are to be eliminated, and if concealment is to be restricted to the few patients who ask for it or those who can be shown to be harmed by openness. The medical profession has to address this problem.

Notes

1. Plato, *The Republic*, 389 b.
2. B. C. Meyer, ''Truth and the Physician,'' *Bulletin of the New York Academy of Medicine* 45 (1969): 59–71.
3. W. H. S. Jones, trans., *Hippocrates*, Loeb Classical Library (Cambridge, Mass.: Harvard University Press, 1923), p. 164.
4. Reprinted in M. B. Etziony. *The Physician's Creed: An Anthology of Medical Prayers. Oaths and Codes of Ethics* (Springfield, Ill.: Charles C. Thomas, 1973), pp. 15–18.
5. See Harry Friedenwald, ''The Ethics of the Practice of Medicine from the Jewish Point of View,'' *Johns Hopkins Hospital Bulletin*, no. 318 (August 1917), pp. 256–61.

6. "Ten Principles of Medical Ethics," *Journal of the American Medical Association* 164 (1957): 1119–20.

7. Mary Barrett, letter, *Boston Globe*, 16 November 1976, p. 1.

8. Though a minority of physicians have struggled to bring them to our attention. See Thomas Percival, *Medical Ethics*, 3d ed. (Oxford: John Henry Parker, 1849), pp. 132–41; Worthington Hooker, *Physician and Patient* (New York: Baker and Scribner, 1849), pp. 357–82; Richard C. Cabot, "Teamwork of Doctor and Patient Through the Annihilation of Lying." in *Social Service and the Art of Healing* (New York: Moffat, Yard & Co., 1909), pp. 116–70; Charles C. Lund, "The Doctor, the Patient, and the Truth," *Annals of Internal Medicine* 24 (1946): 955; Edmund Davies, "The Patient's Right to Know the Truth," *Proceedings of the Royal Society of Medicine* 66 (1973): 533–36.

9. Lawrence Henderson, "Physician and Patient as a Social System," *New England Journal of Medicine* 212 (1955).

10. Nicholas Demy, Letter to the Editor, *Journal of the American Medical Association* 217 (1971): 696–97.

11. For the views of physicians, see Donald Oken, "What to Tell Cancer Patients," *Journal of the American Medical Association* 175 (1961): 1120–28; and tabulations in Robert Veatch, *Death, Dying, and the Biological Revolution* (New Haven and London: Yale University Press, 1976), pp. 229–38. For the view of patients, see Veatch, ibid; Jean Aitken-Swan and E. C. Easson, "Reactions of Cancer Patients on Being Told Their Diagnosis," *British Medical Journal*, 1959, pp. 779–83; Jim McIntosh, "Patients' Awareness and Desire for Information About Diagnosed but Undisclosed Malignant Disease," *The Lancet* 7 (1976): 300–303; William D. Kelly and Stanley R. Friesen, "Do Cancer Patients Want to Be Told?," *Surgery* 27 (1950): 822–26.

12. See Avery Weisman, *On Dying and Denying* (New York: Behavioral Publications, 1972) Elisabeth Kübler-Ross, *On Death and Dying* (New York: The Macmillan Co., 1969); Ernest Becker, *The Denial of Death* (New York: Free Press, 1973); Philippe Ariès, *Western Attitudes Toward Death*, trans. Patricia M. Ranum (Baltimore and London: Johns Hopkins University Press, 1974); and Sigmund Freud, "Negation," *Collected Papers*, ed. James Strachey (London: Hogarth Press, 1950), 5: 181–85.

13. Kübler-Ross, *On Death and Dying*, p. 34.

14. Michel de Montaigne, *Essays*, bk. I, chap. 20.

15. It is in literature that these questions are most directly raised. Two recent works where they are taken up with striking beauty and simplicity are May Sarton, *As We Are Now* (New York: W. W. Norton & Co., 1973); and Freya Stark, *A Peak in Darien* (London: John Murray, 1976).

16. Herman Feifel et al., "Physicians Consider Death," *Proceedings of the American Psychoanalytical Association*, 1967, pp. 201–2.

17. See Ralph Alfidi, "Informed Consent: A Study of Patient Reaction," *Journal of the American Medical Association* 216 (1971): 1325–29.

18. See Steven R. Kaplan, Richard A. Greenwald, and Arvey I. Rogers, Letter to the Editor, *New England Journal of Medicine* 296 (1977): 1127.

19. Oken, "What to Tell Cancer Patients"; Veatch, *Death, Dying, and the Biological Revolution*; Weisman, *On Dying and Denying*.

20. Norman L. Cantor, "A Patient's Decision to Decline Life-Saving Treatment: Bodily Integrity Versus the Preservation of Life," *Rutgers Law Review* 26: 228–64; Danielle Gourevitch, "Suicide Among the Sick in Classical Antiquity," *Bulletin of the History of Medicine* 18 (1969): 501–18; for bibliography, see Bok, "Voluntary Euthanasia."

21. Lewis Thomas, "A Meliorist View of Disease and Dying," *The Journal of Medicine and Philosophy* 1 (1976): 212–21.

22. Claude Lévi-Strauss, *Structural Anthropology* (New York: Basic Books, 1963), p. 167; See also Eric Cassell, "Permission to Die," in John Behnke and Sissela Bok, eds., *The Dilemmas of Euthanasia* (New York: Doubleday, Anchor Press, 1975), pp. 121–31.

23. See Charles Fried, *Medical Experimentation: Personal Integrity and Social Policy* (Amsterdam and Oxford: North Holland Publishing Co., 1974), pp. 20–24.

24. Cicely M. S. Saunders, "Telling Patients," in S. J. Reiser, W. J. Dyck, A. J. Curran, *Ethics in Medicine* (Cambridge, Massachusetts: M.I.T. Press, 1977), pp. 238–40.

Confidentiality in Medicine—A Decrepit Concept

Mark Siegler

Medical confidentiality, as it has traditionally been understood by patients and doctors, no longer exists. This ancient medical principle, which has been included in every physician's oath and code of ethics since Hippocratic times, has become old, worn-out, and useless; it is a decrepit concept. Efforts to preserve it appear doomed to failure and often give rise to more problems than solutions. Psychiatrists have tacitly acknowledged the impossibility of ensuring the confidentiality of medical records by choosing to establish a separate, more secret record. The following case illustrates how the confidentiality principle is compromised systematically in the course of routine medical care.

A patient of mine with mild chronic obstructive pulmonary disease was transferred from the surgical intensive-care unit to a surgical nursing floor two days after an elective cholecystectomy. On the day of transfer, the patient saw a respiratory therapist writing in his medical chart (the therapist was recording the results of an arterial blood gas analysis) and became concerned about the confidentiality of his hospital records. The patient threatened to leave the hospital prematurely unless I could guarantee that the confidentiality of his hospital record would be respected.

This patient's complaint prompted me to enumerate the number of persons who had both access to his hospital record and a reason to examine it. I was amazed to learn that at least 25 and possibly as many as 100 health professionals and administrative personnel at our university hospital had access to the patient's record and that all of them had a legitimate need, indeed a professional responsibility, to open and use that chart. These persons included 6 attending physicians (the primary physician, the surgeon, the pulmonary consultant, and others); 12 house officers (medical, surgical, intensive-care unit, and "covering"

house staff); 20 nursing personnel (on three shifts); 6 respiratory therapists; 3 nutritionists; 2 clinical pharmacists; 15 students (from medicine, nursing, respiratory therapy, and clinical pharmacy); 4 unit secretaries; 4 hospital financial officers; and 4 chart reviewers (utilization review, quality assurance review, tissue review, and insurance auditor). It is of interest that this patient's problem was straightforward, and he therefore did not require many other technical and support services that the modern hospital provides. For example, he did not need multiple consultants and fellows, such specialized procedures as dialysis, or social workers, chaplains, physical therapists, occupational therapists, and the like.

Upon completing my survey I reported to the patient that I estimated that at least 75 health professionals and hospital personnel had access to his medical record. I suggested to the patient that these people were all involved in providing or supporting his health-care services. They were, I assured him, working for him. Despite my reassurances the patient was obviously distressed and retorted, "I always believed that medical confidentiality was part of a doctor's code of ethics. Perhaps you should tell me just what you people mean by 'confidentiality'!"

Two Aspects of Medical Confidentiality

Confidentiality and Third-Party Interests

Previous discussions of medical confidentiality usually have focused on the tension between a physician's responsibility to keep information divulged by patients secret and a physician's legal and moral duty, on occasion, to reveal such confidences to third parties, such as families, employ-

Supported by a grant (OSS-8018097) from the National Science Foundation and by the National Endowment for the Humanities. The views expressed are those of the author and do not necessarily reflect those of the National Science Foundation or the National Endowment for the Humanities.

ers, public-health authorities, or police authorities. In all these instances, the central question relates to the stringency of the physician's obligation to maintain patient confidentiality when the health, well-being, and safety of identifiable others or of society in general would be threatened by a failure to reveal information about the patient. The tension in such cases is between the good of the patient and the good of others.

Confidentiality and the Patient's Interest

As the example above illustrates, further challenges to confidentiality arise because the patient's personal interest in maintaining confidentiality comes into conflict with his personal interest in receiving the best possible health care. Modern high-technology health care is available principally in hospitals (often, teaching hospitals), requires many trained and specialized workers (a "health-care team"), and is very costly. The existence of such teams means that information that previously had been held in confidence by an individual physician will now necessarily be disseminated to many members of the team. Furthermore, since health-care teams are expensive and few patients can afford to pay such costs directly, it becomes essential to grant access to the patient's medical record to persons who are responsible for obtaining third-party payment. These persons include chart reviewers, financial officers, insurance auditors, and quality-of-care assessors. Finally, as medicine expands from a narrow, disease-based model to a model that encompasses psychological, social, and economic problems, not only will the size of the health-care team and medical costs increase, but more sensitive information (such as one's personal habits and financial condition) will now be included in the medical record and will no longer be confidential.

The point I wish to establish is that hospital medicine, the rise of health-care teams, the existence of third-party insurance programs, and the expanding limits of medicine all appear to be responses to the wishes of people for better and more comprehensive medical care. But each of these developments necessarily modifies our traditional understanding of medical confidentiality.

The Role of Confidentiality in Medicine

Confidentiality serves a dual purpose in medicine. In the first place, it acknowledges respect for the patient's sense of individuality and privacy. The patient's most personal physical and psychological secrets are kept confidential in order to decrease a sense of shame and vulnerability. Secondly, confidentiality is important in improving the patient's health care—a basic goal of medicine. The promise of confidentiality permits people to trust (i.e., have confidence) that information revealed to a physician in the course of a medical encounter will not be disseminated further. In this way patients are encouraged to communicate honestly and forthrightly with their doctors. This bond of trust between patient and doctor is vitally important both in the diagnostic process (which relies on an accurate history) and subsequently in the treatment phase, which often depends as much on the patient's trust in the physician as it does on medications and surgery. These two important functions of confidentiality are as important now as they were in the past. They will not be supplanted entirely either by improvements in medical technology or by recent changes in relations between some patients and doctors toward a rights-based, consumerist model.

Possible Solutions to the Confidentiality Problem

First of all, in all nonbureaucratic, noninstitutional medical encounters—that is, in the millions of doctor-patient encounters that take place in physicians' offices, where more privacy can be preserved—meticulous care should be taken to guarantee that patients' medical and personal information will be kept confidential.

Secondly, in such settings as hospitals or large-scale group practices, where many persons have opportunities to examine the medical record, we should aim to provide access only to those who have "a need to know." This could be accomplished through such administrative changes as dividing the entire record into several sections–for example, a medical and financial section—and permitting only health professionals access to the medical information.

The approach favored by many psychiatrists—that of keeping a psychiatric record separate from the general medical record—is an understandable strategy but one that is not entirely satisfactory and that should not be generalized. The keeping of separate psychiatric records implies that psychiatry and medicine are different undertakings and thus drives deeper the wedge between them and between physical and psychological illness. Furthermore, it is often vitally important for internists or surgeons to know that a patient is being seen by a psychiatrist or is taking a particular medication. When separate records are kept, this information may not be available. Finally, if generalized, the practice of keeping a separate psychiatric record could lead to the unacceptable consequence of having a separate record for each type of medical problem.

Patients should be informed about what is meant by "medical confidentiality." We should establish the distinction between information about the patient that generally will be kept confidential regardless of the interest of third parties and information that will be exchanged among members of the health-care team in order to provide care for the patient. Patients should be made aware of the large number of persons in the modern hospital who require access to the medical record in order to serve the patient's medical and financial interests.

Finally, at some point most patients should have an opportunity to review their medical record and to make informed choices about whether their entire record is to be available to everyone or whether certain portions of the record are privileged and should be accessible only to their principal physician or to others designated explicitly by the patient. This approach would rely on traditional informed-consent procedural standards and might permit the patient to balance the personal value of medical confidentiality against the personal value of high-technology, team health care. There is no reason that the same procedure should not be used with psychiatric records instead of the arbitrary system now employed, in which everything related to psychiatry is kept secret.

Afterthought: Confidentiality and Indiscretion

There is one additional aspect of confidentiality that is rarely included in discussions of the subject. I am referring here to the wanton, often inadvertent, but avoidable exchanges of confidential information that occur frequently in hospital rooms, elevators, cafeterias, doctors' offices, and at cocktail parties. Of course, as more people have access to medical information about the patient the potential for this irresponsible abuse of confidentiality increases geometrically.

Such mundane breaches of confidentiality are probably of greater concern to most patients than the broader issue of whether their medical records may be entered into a computerized data bank or whether a respiratory therapist is reviewing the results of an arterial blood gas determination. Somehow, privacy is violated and a sense of shame is heightened when intimate secrets are revealed to people one knows or is close to—friends, neighbors, acquaintances, or hospital roommates—rather than when they are disclosed to an anonymous bureaucrat sitting at a computer terminal in a distant city or to a health professional who is acting in an official capacity.

I suspect that the principles of medical confidentiality, particularly those reflected in most medical codes of ethics, were designed principally to prevent just this sort of embarrassing personal indiscretion rather than to maintain (for social, political, or economic reasons) the absolute secrecy of doctor-patient communications. In this regard, it is worth noting that Percival's Code of Medical Ethics (1803) includes the following admonition: "Patients should be interrogated concerning their complaint in a tone of voice which cannot be overheard" [Leake, C.D., ed. *Percival's Medical Ethics.* Baltimore: Williams and Wilkins, 1927]. We in the medical profession frequently neglect these simple courtesies.

Conclusion

The principle of medical confidentiality described in medical codes of ethics and still believed in by patients no longer exists. In this respect, it is a decrepit concept. Rather than perpetuate the myth of confidentiality and invest energy vainly to preserve it, the public and the profession would be better served if they devoted their attention to determining which aspects of the original principle of confidentiality are worth retaining. Efforts could then be directed to salvaging those.

Confidentiality and the Prediction of Dangerousness in Psychiatry: The Tarasoff Case

William J. Curran

The California Supreme Court continues to make financial awards to patients in suits against physicians with seemingly little regard for the effect of these awards and decisions upon the practice of medicine and the availability of insurance to cover this largesse of the judiciary, and without regard for the social consequences of this "money-for-everything" attitude.

The particular case, *Tarasoff vs. Regents of the University of California,*[1] has already become infamous among mental-health programs in California and among college and university student medical programs all over the country as it has taken its course through the various levels of trial and appeals courts in the Golden State.

The facts of the situation are undisputed. A student at the University of California's Berkeley campus was in psychotherapy with the student health service on an outpatient basis. He told his therapist, a psychologist, that he wanted to kill an unmarried girl who lived in Berkeley but who was then on a summer trip to Brazil. The psychologist, with the concurrence of another therapist and the assistant director of the Department of Psychiatry, reported the matter orally to the campus police and on their suggestion sent them a letter requesting detention of the student and his commitment for observation to a mental hospital. The campus police picked up the student for questioning but "satisfied" that he was "rational," released him on his "promise to stay away" from Miss Tarasoff. The police reported back to the director of psychiatry, Dr. Powelson. Dr. Powelson asked for the return of the psychologist's letter to the police and directed that all copies of the letter be destroyed. Nothing more was done at the health service about the matter. Two months later, shortly after Miss Tarasoff's return, the student went to her home and killed her.

The parents of Miss Tarasoff brought suit for damages against the University and against the therapists and the campus police, as employees of the University and individually. In suing Dr. Powelson, the plaintiffs sought not only general money damages for negligence in failure to warn the girl and her parents and to confine the student, but exemplary or punitive damages (which could be assessed in huge amounts as multiples of the general damages or in any amount at the determination of the jury) for malicious and oppressive abandonment of a dangerous patient.

The Superior Court dismissed all these grounds for legal action against the defendants. The Supreme Court, in a four-to-two decision, reversed the decision and found that on these facts a cause of action was stated for general damages against all the therapists involved in the case and the assistant director and the director of psychiatry and against the University as their employer for breach of the duty to warn Miss Tarasoff. The Court dismissed the claim for exemplary damages against the therapists. It also dismissed the action against the police as protected from a suit by a statutory immunity, as well as the suit against the therapists for failure to confine the student under a commitment order, again because of a statutory immunity. The Court implied that without the immunity, both these actions might have been meritorious.

It seems to me most physicians would throw up their hands in dismay over this result and the massive contradictions in the assessment of who was and who was not legally responsible for this death. If I were to describe in detail the reasoning

Reprinted by permission from the New England Journal of Medicine 293 *(August 7, 1975): 285–286.*

of the court, the confusion of the medical mind would be compounded a thousand times.

The Court asserted that the *Principles of Medical Ethics of the American Medical Association,* Section 9, did not bar breaching the confidentiality of this patient "in order to protect the welfare of this individual [the patient] or the community." From this premise the Court jumped wholeheartedly to a positive duty to warn Miss Tarasoff. This is not what the *Principles* said. The traditional code of medical ethics allows a physician in his sound discretion to breach the confidentiality, but does not require it. It is almost impossible to draft an ethical principle to force a duty on physicians to breach confidences. Must they always warn of death threats, but have discretion on less dangerous threats? Must they warn if the patient is psychotic, but not if he is less disturbed? Does this case mean that every time a patient makes a threat against an unnamed person, the therapist must take steps to find out who it is and warn him (of anything at all, from vague threats to murder) or suffer money damages in the thousands or tens of thousands if the threat, or an aspect of the threat, is carried out?

This case was greatly confused by the array of immunities from suits created under California law. It can be strongly argued that the thrust of these immunity statutes regarding the duty to warn should also have been applied to the therapists, since the statutes were intended to encourage police and mental-health personnel to release patients and not confine them on the basis of unreliable diagnoses of dangerousness. In the past it was thought that too many mental patients were confined for years and years because of their threats to other people, rarely carried out, and because of the conservatism of mental-health personnel in exercising any doubt about dangerousness in favor of confinement as the safest way to prevent harm to third parties.

It seems clear that the therapists here thought that they had done all they could to protect their patient and the community by reporting the case to the police. They had exercised their discretion to warn the community and to breach the confidence of the patient, for his own sake, and that of the

unknown girl. They could hardly warn her, since she was not even in the country at the time. Also, the threat to Miss Tarasoff might actually have been vaguely directed. The student could well have turned his anger and violence toward another person or toward himself. The only basic recourse was to recommend temporary observational commitment. The practice was to make this to the campus police. It was the police who acted, and they decided to release the student with a warning and a promise to stay away from the girl. How many thousands of such warnings—and releases—do police departments make every year? How many people then proceed to kill? The immunity statute was established to encourage release in these circumstances. But the statutory armor had a hole in it. The director of psychiatry was found by the Court to have a "duty" to warn the girl, irrespective of the police action. The Court utilized some precedents, none clearly applicable to this case, to justify its decision. It seems, however, that the real rationale was the aggravated nature of the case—a killing—in which the family was left without someone else to sue. The therapists, particularly Dr. Powelson, could have warned the girl if they had wanted to go against the police action and if they had thought the specific threat to Miss Tarasoff so serious as to warrant that action. The Court did not apply any test to ascertain the custom of psychiatrists and mental-health programs actually in such situations. The Court declared the duty as a matter of law, regardless of the accepted practices of the profession. As in the *Helling* decision[2] discussed in an earlier column,[3] the Court made the physician a guarantor against harm to this party, here not even a patient, on the basis of its own concept of monetary justice.

Notes

1. 529 P. 2d 553
2. *Helling vs. Carey and Laughlin,* 519 P. 2d 981.
3. Curran W. J. Glaucoma and streptococcal. pharyngitis: diagnostic practices and malpractice liability. N Engl J Med 291:508–509, 1974.

Decision Scenario 1 ....

"I find it incredible that you plan on allowing yourself to be treated by a chiropractor," Martha Redpath said.

"What's the matter with going to a chiropractor?" Roger Smith asked. "I went to an M.D. and that didn't do any good. I haven't felt really good in years, but he told me there wasn't anything wrong with me."

"Chiropractors are frauds," Martha said. "They work on the basis of a false theory because they claim that all illnesses are caused either directly or indirectly by misalignments of the vertebrae. That is just sheer nonsense."

"Maybe so," said Roger. "But why shouldn't I go if it makes me feel better? I think they help a lot of people."

"Maybe they won't do you any harm. But in general they're dangerous. They keep a lot of people from getting competent medical treatment, because the people go see a chiropractor instead of a physician. Also, chiropractors often give a lot of x-rays, even though most of them aren't trained to do that, and that means that a great number of people receive massive doses of harmful radiation."

Ralph shook his head. "I don't say that you're wrong. But it seems to me that everybody ought to be free to choose the kind of treatment that he wants to get. If he thinks a chiropractor can do him some good, then he ought to be able to consult one."

"Look," Martha said, "I'm as much in favor of individual freedom as you are. But a lot of people just aren't well-enough informed to make good choices about their own medical care. I think that we should have laws that make chiropractic 'medicine' illegal. We need to protect people from their own ignorance and from those who take advantage of it."

Using the principles argued for by Dworkin, construct an argument in support of Martha's position.

Is regulation of the sort advocated by Martha compatible with Rawls's theory?

Do such regulations or laws violate the notion of the individual as an autonomous rational agent?

Decision Scenario 2 ....

"I really don't understand you," Dr. Lowell said. "You definitely have cancer of the bladder. We may be able to remove it all surgically, but even if we can't, chemotherapy or radiation treatments have a good chance of success."

"I want none of those," Patricia Jenkins said. "I believe that a high-fiber diet and pure, filtered water are more likely to help me. I don't want to be cut or poisoned or burned."

"You're crazy," Dr. Lowell said. "That won't do anything."

"I intend to try it. Even if I'm wrong, it's my life."

"I won't let you," said Dr. Lowell. "Anybody who thinks the way you do about cancer is out of touch with reality. That's one of the marks of mental illness. And I intend to have you declared mentally incompetent to make decisions about your own welfare. I shall speak to the psychiatrists on our staff and ask the hospital lawyer to arrange for a sanity hearing."

"That's fascism!"

"Call it anything you like. But my duty as a physician is to give you the best medical care possible. If that means having you declared mentally incompetent, then so be it."

Dr. Lowell picked up the telephone.

State and evaluate the argument Dr. Lowell offers to justify her intended course of action.

Dr. Lowell claims that it is her duty as a physician to provide Ms. Jenkins with the best medical care possible. If this is so, is it her only duty as a physician? Is there some other duty that conflicts with this one?

On what grounds might Dr. Lowell be accused of paternalism?

Suppose that Dr. Lowell is successful in her aims and that Ms. Jenkins has surgery and makes a good recovery. Would such an outcome justify her actions? If not, why not?

Decision Scenario 3 ....

In 1986 the Texas Department of Public Health supported legislation that would empower the department to quarantine individuals with AIDS whom it considered to be a threat to the health of the public. Those speaking in favor of such legislation pointed to the case of a Houston man with AIDS who continued to work as a prostitute after the disease was diagnosed and after he had been informed that he could infect others by sexual contact. Public health officials were powerless to take any steps against him.

Critics of the legislation saw it as a potential threat to the civil liberties of homosexuals. They pointed out that it would be possible for the health department to deprive an AIDS victim of his freedom of movement and action, even though he had committed no crime and never been tried for one. The rare case of someone with AIDS acting irresponsibly is not adequate to justify handing over such power to a health department.

After hearings, the Department of Public Health announced that it was no longer pressing for passage of the legislation and asked that it be withdrawn. At the request of its legislative supporters, the bill was dropped.

To what extent does the proposal of such legislation appear to be a reflection of what Conway calls "homophobia" and to what extent does it appear to represent a legitimate response to a genuine problem?

Should those diagnosed as having AIDS be forbidden by law from holding jobs that put them in close contact with people or with food? For example, should it be illegal for them to be school teachers or waiters? Should those who are known to carry the AIDS antibody be treated similarly?

If quarantine controls can be justified in the case of other infectious diseases, why should AIDS be viewed any differently?

Shouldn't someone like the male prostitute described above be made guilty of some crime or other? Shouldn't there be some way to protect unsuspecting sex partners from such a person? Shouldn't there be some social sanction (a law, for example) against someone with AIDS who fails to protect others from the disease or who wantonly disregards the safety of others?

Decision Scenario 4 ....

"You realize that I talked to him for only fifteen or twenty minutes," said Dr. Susan Beck.

"Yeah, but you psychiatrists are supposed to be able to size up a guy just by listening to how he says hello," Dr. Mark Brunetti said.

"Now that I've talked to him, tell me more about him," Beck said.

"I presume you learned his name is T. D. Chang?"

"That was written down for me."

"Fine," said Brunetti. "He's fifty-two years old, a Professor of Asian History at Southwestern University. He's married, has two children in college, and has a solid scholarly reputation."

"What was his complaint?" asked Beck.

"About a month ago he began to experience difficult and painful urination. His attending examined him, found that he had an enlarged prostate, and treated with sulfa. No joy. So the attend-

ing sent him here. We're doing an x-ray scan and a punch biopsy in the morning."

"And you want me to tell you how I think he'll take it if you tell him you suspect cancer?"

"Right," said Brunetti. "I don't like to scare people unless I have to. My inclination here is just to keep quiet until we know for sure."

"I think he would take it all right. He shows no tendency towards hysteria, and his background reveals him to be a person who functions well under normal conditions of stress."

"Good, then if I have to tell him, I won't worry about it."

"Mark, do you mean you're *not* going to tell him?"

"That's right. Not until I know for sure. It's a kindness to him. What he doesn't know won't hurt him, and there's no reason to cause him unnecessary anxiety."

"I don't think I agree with that decision," Beck said. "I think a man like Mr. Chang has a right to know as much about his condition as you do."

"That's silly," Brunetti said. "He can't possibly know as much as I do, and he wouldn't know what to make of the information even if I gave it to him. He would probably figure he's going to die in the next hour."

"So you aren't going to tell him what you suspect or why you're doing the biopsy?"

"I'm not that cruel, even if I am a surgeon."

Do the arguments presented by Lipkin support Brunetti's views? State the arguments explicitly and, if possible, relate them to this example.

Using Bok's line of reasoning, what criticisms might be made of the position taken by Brunetti?

Is it reasonable to believe that Mr. Chang might be able to understand and assess the significance of the medical information relevant to the procedures planned?

What might an act or rule utilitarian say about this situation?

Decision Scenario 5 ....

Multiple sclerosis is a chronic, progressive, neurological disease with symptoms that include loss of coordination, blurred vision, speech difficulties, and severe fatigue. It is most frequent among young adults. A study at Albert Einstein Medical College revealed that MS patients typically had a very hard time getting an explicit diagnosis and explanation from their physicians. Yet the physicians surveyed reported overwhelmingly that they always or usually tell patients the diagnosis.

The researchers learned that a variety of factors account for this discrepancy. Physicians find many reasons for delay—the patient may be under twenty, emotionally unstable, or apparently incapable of understanding the diagnosis. Also, the patient may not ask specifically, a relative may ask that the patient not be told, the patient may be medically unsophisticated or in the midst of an emotional crisis. Most important, there is no cure or wholly effective therapy for MS, and emotional stress seems to aggravate its symptoms. Telling a patient that she or he has a progressive, incurable disease may do no good and may do harm.

Patients are frequently told that they have "a chronic virus infection," "neuritis," and "inflammation of the nervous system," instead of being told they have MS. This sometimes leads patients to consult several physicians in the attempt to get a diagnosis and to undergo expensive and unnecessary diagnostic tests.

Are the physicians who claim they believe in telling MS patients the diagnosis and then not doing so necessarily being hypocritical?

What sort of arguments or considerations might Lipkin offer in their defense?

In what sort of cases, according to Bok's arguments, would it be justifiable to withhold a diagnosis from a patient?

If there is a chance that knowing the diagnosis will make the symptoms of an MS patient worse and if there is no wholly effective therapy for MS, why is it not the duty of a physician to withhold the diagnosis? After all, "Do no harm" is perhaps the most important of the Hippocratic maxims.

Decision Scenario 6 ....

Charles Lofton was a thirty-four-year-old systems analyst who was admitted to Towson Memorial Hospital with a diagnosis of testicular cancer. An intensely private man, Lofton seemed to be as embarrassed by his disease as he was frightened by the impending surgery.

"I want you to guarantee me that an absolute minimum number of people will be told what's wrong with me," he said to Dr. Samuel Shem. "I know the surgeon and the surgical team have to find out, obviously, and maybe three or four nurses, but I would like for that to be all.

I don't want people on the staff talking about me."

"I understand how you must feel," Dr. Shem said. "But I have to be honest with you and tell you that a fairly large number of people will have to know about the disease and the surgery."

"How many are you talking about?"

"I don't know for sure. But there are three nursing shifts with eight nurses on each shift. I can't be here all the time so we're talking about the house staff, and that's another two or three people. Then there are some committee reviews involving several people.

"You must be talking about fifty people," Lofton said.

"I wouldn't be surprised."

"Isn't there anything that can be done to protect my privacy?" Lofton asked.

Why is confidentiality important to good medical practice?

What are some of the more serious threats posed to confidentiality in contemporary medicine?

Does confidentiality have a different meaning in the current medical setting? That is, does it have to be understood as involving something other than a personal and private relationship with a physician?

What proposals does Siegler make in order to resolve some of the problems of maintaining a patient's confidentiality?

If Siegler's proposals were adopted, would confidentiality of the traditional sort be preserved?

Decision Scenario 7 ••

Jane Montrose told herself that it was just one of the things you had to do if you wanted to get promoted. Talking to eleven department heads might be a bore, but so far they had all been quite nice. And it wasn't even a bad idea. If she were going to be working as an Assistant Vice-President, she would have to deal with all of these people frequently. It made sense for them to have an opportunity to say whether they would feel comfortable working with her.

"How did you learn so much about computers?" Art Davis asked her.

It was a question people always asked. For some reason, they invariably seemed surprised to learn that a woman was comfortable dealing with the mysteries of data processing.

"I have a degree in computer science," she said. "Besides, I've been working with computers for about eight years now. You get to know their ways."

David nodded and smiled at her. She was somewhat surprised that he would ask such a naive question. As head of personnel, he more than anyone knew about her educational background and her work history. She wondered if he wasn't just stalling, making polite conversation until he could ask what really interested him.

"How are you doing with your psychiatrist?" Davis asked.

Jane was totally surprised by the question. She had assumed that only her closest friends knew she had been going to a psychiatrist.

"Fine," she said. "I mean, I've been able to work through a lot of problems that were bothering me."

She didn't really want to talk to Davis about her feelings of depression and lack of self-worth that had been troubling her for the last few years. None of it was any of his business.

"Do you think you'll be able to handle new responsibilities? This is a pretty important job you're being considered for, you know."

"I can handle them. I've always done very well at whatever job I've worked at."

"I know you have," Davis said. "But when we see that an employee has been going to a psychiatrist . . . well, that makes us wonder if that person is really to be trusted with a lot of responsibility. I'm sure you understand."

"I don't really. I don't see what my personal problems have to do with my work, assuming they don't get in the way of my doing it. And they never have."

Davis smiled at her in a way that made her

very angry. It was the kind of tolerant but superior smile adults usually reserve for children who are talking about things they don't understand.

"What I want to know," Jane said, "is how you knew about my seeing a psychiatrist. I thought my medical records were all confidential."

"They are, so far as I know. But you did put in an insurance claim for payment, and I have to sign off on all the claims. When I did that, I saw you were getting psychiatric help."

"Are you going to make that public?"

"Not public," Davis said. "But I do feel obliged to mention it to the Executive Planning Group. If they're thinking about promoting you, then that's something they ought to know. I'm surprised you didn't volunteer the information yourself."

"I didn't think it was relevant," Jane said. "I didn't tell them I also suffer from hemorrhoids."

"Well, we'll let them judge whether it's relevant."

Does Davis have an obligation to inform the Executive Planning Group that Jane Montrose is receiving psychiatric treatment?

In New York, employees of the state government have the right to send medical claims for psychiatric or psychological services directly to the insurance company. Should this be made a legal right for all employees in all states?

The so-called Privacy Protection Act of 1980 permits federal law-enforcement agencies to secure search warrants and gain access to all private records, except those of the media. Should the Act be restricted to exclude medical and mental-health records?

Decision Scenario 8 ....

In 1985 investigators from the Massachusetts Attorney General's office secured permission from the state courts to examine the notes taken during patient sessions by psychiatrist Kennard C. Kobrin of Fall River, Massachusetts. Dr. Kobrin was suspected of Medicaid fraud, and the state's Assistant Attorney General Michelle Kacynski argued before the Supreme Judicial Court that the patient's rights to privacy must be set aside in favor of the public's need to know. "We believe that the state should have access to records which may or may not verify that Dr. Kobrin has provided certain services to certain patients on certain dates," she said.

Dr. Kobrin's patients openly protested the violation of their privacy and the fact that some of their records are now in open court files. "I feel kind of humiliated and upset," one of them said. "If you go to see a doctor, and it's supposed to be confidential, that's why you go. If it wasn't, you could tell a friend, and they could blab it all over

the city." Although last names have been deleted from the public records, Fall River is a city of only 92,500, and some of the information in the records would make it possible to identify the patients by name.

Massachusetts state laws protect private conversations between patients and therapists, but the laws regulating Medicaid are federal laws. There are no federal laws protecting a confidential privilege for patient communication.

Is there a solution to the problem posed by Ms. Kacynski? If the public's interest is to be protected, isn't it necessary to set aside the individual's right to privacy?

If it is possible that a therapist's notes might be made part of a public record, what effect is this likely to have on therapy?

Should there be a federal law guaranteeing confidentiality for patient communication?

Decision Scenario 9 ....

"Sometimes I think that what I really want to do is to kill people and drink their blood."

Dr. Allen Wolfe looked at the young man in the chair across from him. The face was round and soft and innocent looking, like that of a large baby. But the body had the powerful shoulders of a college wrestler. There was no doubt that Hal Crane had the strength to carry out his fantasies.

"Any people in particular?" Dr. Wolfe asked.

"Women. Girls about my age. Maybe their early twenties."

"But no one you're personally acquainted with."

"That's right. Just girls I see walking down the street or getting off a bus. I have a tremendous urge to stick a knife into their stomachs and feel the blood come out on my hands."

"But you've never done anything like that?"

Crane shook his head. "No, but I'm afraid I might."

Dr. Wolfe considered Crane a paranoid schizophrenic with compulsive tendencies, someone who might possibly act out his fantasies. He was a potentially dangerous person.

"Would you be willing to take my advice and put yourself in a hospital under my care for a while?"

"I don't want to do that," Crane said. "I don't want to be locked up like an animal."

"But you don't really want to hurt other people, do you?"

"I guess not," Crane said. "But I haven't done anything yet."

"But you might," Dr. Wolfe said. "I'm afraid you might let yourself go and kill someone."

Crane smiled. "That's just the chance the world will have to take, isn't it? I told you I'm not going to let myself be locked up."

Suppose that you are Dr. Wolfe. To take the legal steps necessary to have Mr. Crane committed against his will requires that you violate confidentiality. What justification might a utilitarian offer for doing this?

Might a Kantian oppose commitment on the grounds that it would violate Crane's dignity as a person?

As a physician, how would you justify acting to protect others while going against the wishes of your patient?

Should a physician be required by law to act to protect the welfare of others?

How does this case compare with the Tarasoff case discussed by Curran? What actions, on Curran's view, should be taken by Dr. Wolfe?

CHAPTER 5

MEDICAL EXPERIMENTATION AND [   ]
INFORMED CONSENT

SOCIAL CONTEXT:
THE ARTIFICIAL HEART

On April 4, 1969, Haskell Karp, a forty-seven-year-old printing estimator from Illinois, became the first patient in history to receive an artificial heart. For sixty-three hours the device maintained Karp's blood pressure and circulation; then a transplanted heart was put in its place. Karp died some twenty hours after receiving the transplant.

The surgery was performed at St. Luke's Hospital in Houston by Denton Cooley. Cooley claimed in television interviews after the surgery that he had implanted the artificial device as a desperate measure, because Mr. Karp was dying on the operating table and a donor heart was not available. During the interviews, Cooley made a plea for the donation of a heart to transplant into Mr. Karp.

Almost immediately Cooley's actions became the center of a storm of controversy. In deciding to use the artificial heart, Cooley had consulted no one but his patient. Although a member of the faculty of Baylor University, Cooley had not sought permission from Michael DeBakey, the head of the artificial heart program, nor had he brought the issue before the university's human subjects committee.

In hearings held before various committees charged with investigating the matter, other charges and criticisms emerged. Most seriously, Cooley was said to have acted unethically by implanting "an unproved device . . . into a human being for primary experimentation before its safety and effectiveness"

had been "proved scientifically in animal experiments." Cooley replied that the device had been tested in seven calves, and although all had died, one had lived for forty-four hours. That, Cooley claimed, was enough to justify going forward with using the device in humans. Besides, he said, the device was used because his patient was dying and no other option was available. The artificial heart was there and ready to use. "Everything came together at once," Cooley said.

Cooley insisted that his experience in heart surgery was the only real grounds for his decision: "Based on this experience, I believe I am qualified to judge what is right and proper for my patients. The permission I receive to do what I do, I receive from my patients. It is not received from a government agency or from one of my seniors."

Critics charged that Cooley had actually engineered the whole episode to seek publicity for himself. DeBakey claimed that Cooley had not made an appeal for a donor heart until after he had performed the operation and gone on television. Furthermore, the situation was not the life-or-death one that Cooley claimed. One surgeon said that Cooley had asked him to participate in the surgery days before it took place. Also, Cooley had planned enough in advance to have the console power source for the heart available and to have movie cameras in place to make a complete record of the operation.

At the end of the inquiry, Cooley was

found guilty on eight counts of seeking publicity by the local medical society, but no other disciplinary actions were taken against him. He resigned from Baylor because of his unwillingness to sign National Institutes of Health guidelines on experimental human surgery. He explained that if he did so he would feel that he was giving in to DeBakey, his major critic.

Cooley continued to practice surgery at his Texas Heart Institute, and at medical meetings he was in much demand as a speaker on the Karp operation. Although Karp's widow sued Cooley on the grounds that he had failed to secure a proper consent form for the unprecedented procedure, the courts held that the procedure was primarily therapeutic and not experimental.

The artificial heart program at Baylor was part of a research effort initiated in 1964 by the National Heart, Lung, and Blood Institute of NIH. The initial aim of the federal program was to develop a completely implantable artificial heart by 1970, but this goal turned out to be unrealistic. Research then focused on the development of a reliable, externally powered device as a necessary first step.

The controversy around the Cooley affair had subsided before the next major event occurred. In 1982 Barney Clark, a retired dentist, became the first person to receive an implanted artificial heart intended to be permanent. The surgery was performed with federal Food and Drug Administration approval and only after extensive animal testing had taken place. William C. DeVries of the University of Utah Medical Center was the head of the surgical team. Clark received the Jarvick-7 heart, and despite numerous complications, he lived for 112 days.

Since Barney Clark, DeVries has performed three more permanent implants. An additional implant was made in Sweden so that a total of five have been done at this time. No one given a permanent implant is still alive. The major problem appears to be

that small blood clots form on the surface or valves of the artificial heart, and when these clots break off, they block blood flow to the brain and cause disabling strokes.

William J. Schroeder lived longer than anyone else with an artificial heart—620 days. However, he suffered from three strokes, was often in a coma-like state, and when aroused, was able to say only a few words. Other medical problems, such as recurrent infections due to the suppression of the immune system, internal bleeding, and respiratory difficulties, affected Mr. Schroeder and all other implant recipients.

The very poor quality of life that the artificial heart has provided to patients does not make it a realistic alternative to heart transplants. As DeVries himself, a strong advocate of the artificial heart, remarks, "There is no question that if you have a choice, you have a transplant. Transplants are therapeutic reality and they are good, whereas the artificial heart is still a very highly experimental thing."

DeVries also points out that for patients who are not eligible for transplants because of their age or because of such diseases as pulmonary hypertension, the artificial heart offers the only therapy possible. He mentions William Schroeder as an example of someone who had a poor quality of life but was at least alive and capable of having experiences that otherwise he would have missed. He was able to enjoy the birth of his grandson, celebrate birthdays, and be present at family gatherings. "We lose track of the fact that he would have been dead" without the artificial heart, DeVries reminds us.

Some critics of the artificial heart program are of the opinion that the device should not be used as a permanent implant. In their view, even when the surgery is successful and the device functions properly, the quality of life that it provides for the recipients is so poor that there can be no justification for keeping people alive by such means.

The device should be used only as a temporary measure to keep patients alive until a donor heart for transplant can be secured.

Other critics are even more severe in their strictures and argue for a moratorium on the use of the artificial heart. They point out that even when the device has been used as a temporary bridge to a transplant, results have been mixed. In the past year two of the four patients who have received temporary transplants have died. In part this may be due to the fact that those who receive implants and then transplants must undergo the trauma and risk of major surgery twice. There is also strong evidence that the longer a patient has an implant, the worse his physical condition becomes.

Furthermore, the costs of using the artificial heart are staggeringly high. Even when the device is used as a temporary bridge, treatment costs tens of thousands of dollars per patient. If complications develop or if the patient must remain on the device for an extended period of time, the costs can mount to hundreds of thousands of dollars. Far more lives could be saved by using these resources to prevent heart disease by funding programs aimed at improving diet or eliminating smoking.

Also, critics charge, using the device to keep people alive until transplants can be found is unfair to others who are waiting for transplants. Since those who are implanted with the artificial heart are given priority in receiving donor hearts, others who may actually be better transplant candidates may die as a result.

DeVries, who has now moved to Humana Hospital in Louisville, Kentucky, is the only surgeon currently authorized by the FDA to perform permanent artificial heart implants. (Others have been given permission to implant devices for temporary use.) DeVries has approval to perform three more implants under the current program, and he has announced that he will proceed to do so

as soon as suitable candidates become available.

Ultimately, it will be up to the FDA to decide whether the artificial heart program should be continued and, if so, what direction it should take. The hope of developing a fully implantable, permanent device is still the goal of researchers, and new designs for artificial hearts are being worked on at a number of institutions. For the last twenty-five years, over eleven million dollars a year have been spent on the artificial heart. Whether additional money should be spent in this way or whether it should be turned to other purposes is an issue that must be resolved either by debate or default in the coming years.

Whether public funds should be spent on continuing the artificial heart program is a serious social issue. However, there are also a number of more specific moral issues connected with the use of the device. It is an experimental therapy, and as such it raises questions about consent, participation, and termination.

Since the artificial heart is a therapy that involves so many risks and uncertainties, it is one that is made available only to those who are not likely to benefit from established therapies. It is, indeed, a therapy of last resort. This alone means that candidates who have nominated themselves to be recipients are likely to agree to accept any risks that are spelled out for them. Dr. DeVries reports that all four of his implant patients "told me in their own way that they didn't care" whether they read the consent form or not. "They were not really interested in listening to the long list of horrors that could happen to them," according to Dr. DeVries. "They didn't want to hear that they may have a stroke and be unable to use all mental capabilities. Those are issues that they would rather be left unsaid."

In a sense, such people can be regarded as coerced by their own diseases and their own desperation. In such a circumstance, the very notion of informed consent seems to lose the significance that is ordinarily attached to it. Given that this is so and given the dismal record of outcomes from permanent implant surgery, should we as a society even allow people to agree to become subjects in this experimental therapy? A case can be made for saying that the benefits that can reasonably be expected from an artificial heart implant are so meager that individuals ought not be allowed to consent to it. Of course, this would be equivalent to declaring a moratorium on such surgery.

When should the experimental therapy be ended? That is, when should the power supply to the artificial heart be turned off and the patient allowed to die? Barney Clark was given a key to turn off his power source, and in principle, he would have been able to terminate the experiment at any time of his choosing. However, because of stroke and his deteriorated physical condition, very

soon after the implant he was not considered to be mentally competent to make decisions about his own treatment. Decisions involving consent were made on his behalf by his wife. In practice, his case and others suggest that once a person has agreed to a permanent implant, he is likely to be incapable of exercising any control over the future course of his life.

If this is so, then who should decide when the experiment is to be stopped? Should the patient be allowed to stipulate before the surgery under what conditions he would want the experiment discontinued? Should the physician be allowed to continue the experiment against the wishes of a family member? Furthermore, is turning off an artificial heart no different from turning off a respirator? Or does the certainty of death in the case of the heart make action different in a morally relevant way? These and others like them are basic questions that have apparently not been resolved by those involved in the artificial heart program.

CASE PRESENTATION
Baby Fae

On October 14, 1984, a baby was born in a community hospital in southern California with a malformation known as hypoplastic left-heart syndrome. In such a condition, the mitral valve or aorta on the left side of the heart is underdeveloped, and essentially only the right side of the heart functions properly. Some three hundred to two thousand infants a year are born with this defect, and most die from it within a few weeks.

The infant, who became known to the public as Baby Fae, was taken to the Loma Linda University Hospital Center. There, on October 26, a surgical team headed by Dr. Leonard Bailey performed a heart transplant; and Baby Fae became the first human infant to receive a baboon heart. She died twenty days later.

Baby Fae was not the first human to receive a so-called xenograft or cross-species transplant. In

early 1964, a sixty-eight-year-old man was transplanted with a chimpanzee heart at the University of Mississippi Medical Center. The heart failed after only an hour, and the patient died. Before Baby Fae, three other cross-species transplants had also ended in a quick death.

In the case of Baby Fae, questions about the moral correctness and scientific legitimacy of the transplant were raised immediately. Hospital officials revealed that no effort had been made to find a human donor before implanting the baboon heart, and this led some critics to wonder if research interests were not being given priority over the welfare of the patient. Others questioned whether the parents were adequately informed about alternative corrective surgery, the Norwood procedure, available in Boston and Philadelphia.

Other observers wondered whether the nature of the surgery and its limited value had been properly explained to the parents. Also, some critics raised objections to sacrificing a healthy young animal as part of an experiment no likely to bring any lasting benefit to Baby Fae.

Scientific critics charged that not enough is known about crossing the species barrier to warrant the use of transplant organs at this time. The previous record of failures, with no major advances in understanding, did not make the prospect of another such transplant reasonable. Furthermore, critics said, chimpanzees and gorillas are genetically more similar to humans than baboons, so the choice of a baboon heart was not a wise one. The only advantage of baboons is that they are easier to breed in captivity. Also, one critic suggested that Dr. Bailey was merely engaged in "wishful thinking" in believing that Baby Fae's immune system would not produce a severe rejection response because of its immaturity.

An autopsy on Baby Fae showed that her death was caused by the incompatibility of her blood with that of the baboon heart. Baby Fae's blood was type O, the baboon's type AB. This resulted in the formation of blood clots and the destruction of kidney function. The heart showed mild signs of rejection.

In an address before a medical conference after Baby Fae's death, Dr. Bailey commented on some of the criticisms. He is reported to have said that it was "an oversight on our part not to search for a human donor from the start." Dr. Bailey also told the conference that he and his team believed that the difference in blood types between Baby Fae and the baboon would be less important than other factors and that the immunosuppressive drugs used to prevent rejection would also solve the problem of blood incompatibility. "We came to regret those assumptions," Dr. Bailey said. The failure to match blood types was "a tactical error that came back to haunt us."

On other occasions Dr. Bailey reiterated his view that, because infant donors are extremely scarce, animal-to-human transplants offer a realistic hope for the future. Before the Baby Fae operation, Dr. Bailey had transplanted organs in more than 150 animals. He indicated that he would use the information obtained from Baby Fae to conduct additional animal experiments before attempting another such transplant.

In March of 1985 the National Institutes of Health released a report of a committee that made a site visit to Loma Linda to review the Baby Fae matter. The committee found that the informed consent process was generally satisfactory, in that "the parents were given an appropriate and thorough explanation of the alternatives available, the risks and benefits of the procedure and the experimental nature of the transplant." Moreover, consent was obtained in an "atmosphere which allowed the parents an opportunity to carefully consider, without coercion or undue influence, whether to give permission for the transplant."

The committee also pointed out certain flaws in the consent document. First, it "did not include the possibility of searching for a human heart or performing a human heart transplant." Second, the expected benefits of the procedure "appeared to be overstated," because the consent document "stated that 'long-term survival' is an expected possibility with no further explanation." Finally, the document did not explain "whether compensation and medical treatment was available if injury occurred."

The committee did not question the legitimacy of the cross-species transplant. Moreover, it made no mention of the Norwood procedure, except to say that it had been explained to the mother at the community hospital at the birth of the infant. (The consent document described the procedure as a generally unsuccessful "temporizing operation.")

Although the committee was generally critical of the university's Institutional Review Board in "evaluating the entire informed consent process," it reached the conclusion that "the parents of Baby Fae understood the alternative available as well as the risks and reasonably expected benefits of the transplant."

Officials at Loma Linda University Medical Center promised that before performing another such transplant they would first seek a human infant heart donor.

CASE PRESENTATION
The Willowbrook Hepatitis Experiments

The Willowbrook State School in Staten Island, New York, is an institution devoted to housing and caring for mentally retarded children. In 1956 a research group led by Saul Krugman and Joan P. Giles of the New York University School of Medicine initiated a long-range study of viral hepatitis at Willowbrook. The children confined there were made experimental subjects of the study.

Hepatitis is a disease affecting the liver that is now known to be caused by one of two (possibly more) viruses. Although the viruses are distinct, the results they produce are the same. The liver becomes inflamed and increases in size as the invading viruses replicate themselves. Also, part of the tissue of the liver may be destroyed and the liver's normal functions impaired. Often the flow of bile through the ducts is blocked, and bilirubin (the major pigment in bile) is forced into the blood and urine. This produces the symptom of yellowish or jaundiced skin.

The disease is generally relatively mild, although permanent liver damage can be produced by it. The symptoms are ordinarily flulike—mild fever, tiredness, inability to keep food down. The viruses causing the disease are transmitted orally through contact with the feces and bodily secretions of infected people.

Krugman and Giles were interested in determining the natural history of viral hepatitis—the mode of infection and the course of the disease over time. They also wanted to test the effectiveness of gamma globulin as an agent for inoculating against hepatitis. (Gamma globulin is a protein complex extracted from the blood serum that contains antigens, substances that trigger the production of specific antibodies to counter infectious agents.)

Krugman and Giles considered Willowbrook to be a good choice for investigation because viral hepatitis occurred more or less constantly in the institution. In the jargon of medicine, the disease was endemic. That this was so was recognized in 1949, and it continued to be so as the number of children in the school increased to over five thousand in 1960. Krugman and Giles claimed that "under the chronic circumstances of multiple and repeated exposure . . . most newly admitted children became infected within the first six to twelve months of residence in the institution."

Over a fourteen-year period, Krugman and Giles collected over twenty-five thousand serum specimens from more than seven hundred patients. Samples were taken before exposure, during the incubation period of the virus, and for periods after the infection. In an effort to get the kind of precise data they considered most useful, Krugman and Giles decided to deliberately infect some of the incoming children with the strain of the hepatitis virus prevalent at Willowbrook.

They justified their decision in the following way:

> It was inevitable that susceptible children would become infected in the institution. Hepatitis was especially mild in the 3- to 10-year age group at Willowbrook. These studies would be carried out in a special unit with optimum isolation facilities to protect the children from other infectious diseases such as shigellosis [dysentary caused by a bacillus], and parasitic and respiratory infections which are prevalent in the institution.

Most important, Krugman and Giles claimed to see being an experimental subject as in the best medical interest of the child, for not only would the child receive special care, but infection with the milder form of hepatitis would provide protection against the more virulent and damaging forms. As they say: "It should be emphasized that the artificial induction of hepatitis implies a 'therapeutic' effect because of the immunity which is conferred."

Krugman and Giles obtained what they considered to be adequate consent from the parents of the children used as subjects. Where they were unable to obtain consent, they did not include the child in the experiment. In the earlier phases of the study, parents were provided with relevant information either by letter or orally, and written consent was secured from them. In the later phases, a group procedure was used:

> First, a psychiatric social worker discusses the project with the parents during a preliminary interview. Those who are interested are invited to attend a group session at the institution to discuss the project in greater detail. These sessions are conducted by the staff responsible for the program, including the physician, supervising nurses, staff attendants, and psychiatric social workers. . . . Parents in groups of six to eight are given a tour of the facilities. The purposes, potential benefits, and potential hazards of the program are discussed with them, and they are encouraged to ask questions. Thus, all parents can hear the response to questions posed by the more articulate members of the group. After leaving this briefing session parents have an opportunity to talk with their private physicians who may call the unit for more information. Approximately two weeks after each visit, the psychiatric social worker contacts the parents for their decision. If the decision is in the affirmative, the consent is signed but parents are informed that signed consent may be withdrawn any time before the beginning of the program. It has been clear that the group method has

enabled us to obtain more thorough informed consent. Children who are wards of the state or children without parents have never been included in our studies.

Krugman and Giles point out that their studies have been reviewed and approved by the New York State Department of Mental Hygiene, the New York State Department of Mental Health, the Armed Forces Epidemological Board, and the human experimentation committees of the New York University School of Medicine and the Willowbrook School. They also stress that, although they were under no obligation to do so, they chose to meet the World Medical Association's Draft Code on Human Experimentation.

The value of the research conducted by Krugman and Giles has been recognized as significant in furthering a scientific understanding of viral hepatitis and methods for treating it. Yet serious moral doubts have been raised about the nature and conduct of the experiments. In particular, many have questioned the use of retarded children as experimental subjects, some claiming that children should never be experimental subjects in investigations that are not directly therapeutic. Others have raised questions about the ways in which consent was obtained from the parents of the children, suggesting that parents were implicitly blackmailed into giving their consent. The letters to the British medical journal *Lancet* and the selection from Paul Ramsey's *The Patient as Person* presented in this chapter discuss these issues.

CASE PRESENTATION
The Detroit Psychosurgery Case

Lafayette Clinic is a research facility in Detroit that is part of the Michigan Department of Mental Health. In 1972, the director of the clinic was Dr. J. S. Gottlieb, a psychiatrist, and its chief of neurology was Dr. Ernst Rodin. Both Rodin and Gottlieb had read the book *Violence and the Brain*, by V. H. Mark and F. R. Ervin, shortly after its publication in 1970. They discussed the work and agreed that some of the techniques it described

might be useful in treating patients suffering from uncontrollable sexual and aggressive impulses.

Rodin wrote a description of a research project they might conduct: "Proposal for the Study of the Treatment of Uncontrollable Aggression at Lafayette Clinic." The research was to involve a comparative study of the value of surgical versus drug treatment of aggressive patients. The surgical part of the project proposed implanting depth-electrodes in the brains of twelve subjects to study their brain activity and to attempt to locate areas of electrical abnormality. If such an area was found and if, by brain stimulation, it could be linked to aggressive behavior, then stereotactic surgery would be performed. (Stereotactic surgery involves locating relatively precise areas by using careful measurements.) The target areas would then be either resectioned (cut out) or destroyed by electrocoagulation. The ultimate aim of the project was said to be to restore patients to a "useful life" in the community.

The proposal, which requested $164,000, was submitted to the State Department of Mental Health. It was approved and included in the Department's legislative budget request. Although the state legislature held two hearings, no questions were raised about the Rodin proposal. The money was made available in July 1972.

Even before the allocation of funds, a search was being conducted for suitable subjects. The candidates were those confined in state institutions under the Michigan "Criminal Sexual Psychopath" law. These were people charged with serious sex crimes who were not prosecuted but confined involuntarily for an indeterminate period of time until considered sufficiently "cured" for release.

One such person, identified for the record only as John Doe, was approached by Dr. E. G. Yudashkin, the director of Ionia State Hospital where Doe was confined. Yudashkin described the project to Doe and told him he would probably be released within six months or a year whether or not he participated. But he also pointed out that successful treatment in the research project would lead to an even speedier release.

Doe was not interested in the drug part of the research program but thought he might volunteer for the surgical part. Yudashkin and two staff physicians explained to him on three occasions what this might involve. But the knowledge of the physicians on this topic was not extensive, and Doe later testified that they gave him a misleadingly simple account. But at the time, Doe decided to consent to becoming a subject, and Rodin was informed of this.

Rodin had decided that it was necessary to broaden the population of candidates from which subjects were to be selected. He had gone to Bos-

ton and talked with Vernon Mark about the project, and Mark had been critical of the ethical aspects. Rodin wrote in a memo to Gottlieb:

> When I informed Dr. Mark of our project, namely doing amygdalotomies on patients who do not have epilepsy, he became extremely concerned and stated we had no ethical right in so doing. . . . I then retorted that he was misleading us with his previously cited book and he had no right at all from a scientific point of view to state that in the human, aggression is accompanied by seizure discharges in the amygdala, because he is dealing only with patients who have susceptible brains, namely, temporal lobe epilepsy. . . .
>
> He stated categorically that as far as present evidence is concerned, one has no right to make lesions in a "healthy brain" when the individual suffers from rage attacks only.

Rodin discussed this matter with colleagues, and they decided not to do surgery on patients without verifiable organic brain dysfunctions. They expanded the population to be considered to include retarded, epileptic, and self-mutilating patients.

Lafayette Clinic's Human and Animal Experimentation Committee reviewed the project description and procedures and a draft of the informed-consent form. The committee, charged with protecting the rights and welfare of experimental subjects, raised no questions about the moral issues in the project. They approved it in October of 1972.

The project, as approved, required establishing two review committees to supervise patient selection and to protect patients from unethical practices. The three-member Medical Review Committee was to consider the medical condition and history of potential subjects recommended by Rodin. They were to eliminate patients unsuitable from a medical standpoint. After screening, a three-member Human Rights Review Committee was to determine for each patient whether informed consent was adequate and whether any rights were being infringed. After approval by both committees, a patient would then be given a consent form and a detailed explanation of the procedure to be performed on him. Then he and his family would have a week to consider whether they wished to sign the consent form.

None of this procedure was followed in the case of John Doe. Rodin met with John Doe on October 27. They discussed Doe's medical history for an hour, and at the end Doe indicated that he still wanted to participate in the project as a subject. Rodin read him the consent form, which read in part:

> Since conventional treatment efforts over a period of several years have not enabled me to control my outbursts of rage and anti-social behavior, I submit an application to be a subject in a research project which may offer me a form of effective therapy. This therapy is based upon the idea that episodes of anti-social rage and sexuality might be triggered by a disturbance in certain portions of my brain. I understand that in order to be certain that a significant brain disturbance exists, which might relate to my anti-social behavior, an initial operation will have to be performed. This procedure consists of placing fine wires into my brain, which will record the electrical activity from those structures which play a part in anger and sexuality. These electrical waves can then be studied to determine the presence of an abnormality.
>
> In addition electrical stimulation with weak currents passed through these wires will be done in order to find out if one or several points in the brain can trigger my episodes of violence or unlawful sexuality. In other words this stimulation may cause me to want to commit an aggressive or sexual act, but every effort will be made to have a sufficient number of people present to control me. If the brain disturbance is limited to a small area, I understand that the investigators will destroy this part of my brain with an electrical current. If the abnormality comes from a larger part of my brain, I agree that it

> should be surgically removed, if the doctors determine that it can be done so, without risk of side effects. Should the electrical activity from the parts of my brain into which the wires have been placed reveal that there is no significant abnormality, the wires will simply be withdrawn.

Rodin talked about the meanings of the terms in the form and explained the risks of the surgical procedures.

Later, John Doe was allowed to call his parents. The only explanation they received before signing the consent form was from him. Doe believed that he was agreeing only to implanting depth-electrodes and not to stereotactic surgery. He thought that additional consent would be required for surgery. He and his parents signed the form.

Eventually, after the signing, both committees were given materials relating to John Doe. The members of the committees were all picked by Rodin. The medical committee never met, but each member considered the materials submitted to them by Rodin. The Human Rights Committee also examined the materials individually. Thus, neither committee ever met to discuss Doe's case, nor did any member of either committee talk with Doe.

John Doe was the only patient located to participate in the entire research program. Yet by the end of December, all the committee reviews were completed, and plans were made to implant the electrodes in John Doe's brain in early January.

Before this could happen, the process was brought to a halt. A psychiatric resident at Lafayette Clinic was bothered by the secret way in which the project was being run. He expressed these concerns to Gabe Kaimowitz, an attorney for the Michigan Medical Committee for Human Rights. In early January, Kaimowitz filed a petition and complaint with the Wayne County Circuit Court that asked that the state Department of Mental Health be required to "show cause . . . why they should not be enjoined from performing psychosurgery or using chemotherapy on persons involuntarily confined in the state hospital system in order to study 'uncontrollable aggression' or for any other similar purpose." Kaimowitz also asked that a writ of habeas corpus be issued to release John Doe and others from state hospitals because they were not receiving treatment.

Soon afterwards, the Department of Mental Health decided to cancel funding for the Rodin project. But the court decided that the legal issues were not moot and that the case should be heard. On March 23, the court also decided that the Criminal Sexual Psychopath law, under which John Doe had been committed, was unconstitutional. The court ordered him released, and John Doe was freed from Ionia State Hospital after eighteen years of confinement.

The court then heard arguments on the major legal and moral issues of the complaint. For the first time, a court was being asked to give an opinion on the legitimacy of psychosurgery and other experimental treatment methods involving people involuntarily confined to institutions.

On July 10, 1973, the court ruled that an involuntarily detained adult in a facility of the State Department of Mental Health cannot give legally adequate consent to "an innovative or experimental surgical procedure on the brain." The court was careful to point out that its ruling was based upon the state of knowledge about psychosurgery at the time of the decision. Furthermore, the court emphasized that an involuntary mental patient can give adequate consent to accepted neurological procedures. In the court's view, then, the type of neurosurgery proposed for Doe was not of the character to which he could give proper consent.

INTRODUCTION

In 1947, an international tribunal meeting in Nuremberg convicted fifteen German physicians of "war crimes and crimes against humanity." The physicians were charged with taking part in "medical experiments without the subjects' consent." But the language of the charge fails to indicate the cruel and barbaric nature of the experiments. Here are just some of them:

At the Ravensbrueck concentration camp, experiments were conducted to test the effectiveness of the drug sulfanilamide. Cuts were deliberately made on the bodies of people, then the wounds were infected with bacteria. The infection was worsened by forcing wood shavings and ground glass into the cuts. Then sulfanilamide and other drugs were tested for their effectiveness in combatting the infection.

At the Dachau concentration camp, healthy inmates were injected with extracts from the mucous glands of mosquitos to produce malaria. Various drugs were then used to determine their relative effectiveness.

At Buchenwald, numerous healthy people were deliberately infected with the spotted-fever virus merely for the purpose of keeping the virus alive. Over 90 percent of those infected died as a result.

Also at Buchenwald, various kinds of poisons were secretly administered to a number of inmates to test their efficacy. Either the inmates died or they were killed at once so that autopsies could be performed. Some experimental subjects were shot with poisoned bullets.

At Dachau, to help the German Air Force, investigations were made into the limits of human endurance and existence at very high altitudes. People were placed in sealed chambers then subjected to very high and very low atmospheric pressures. As the indictment puts it, "Many victims died as a result of these experiments and others suffered grave injury, torture, and ill-treatment."

Seven of the physicians convicted were hanged, and the other eight received long prison terms. From the trial there emerged the Nuremberg Code, a statement of the principles that should be followed in conducting medical research with human subjects. (The principles of the code appear as a selection in this chapter.)

Despite the moral horrors that were revealed at Nuremberg, few people doubt the need for medical experimentation involving human subjects. The extent to which contemporary medicine has become effective in the treatment of disease and illness is due almost entirely to the fact that it has become *scientific* medicine. This means that contemporary medicine must conduct inquiries in which data are gathered to test hypotheses and general theories related to disease processes and their treatment. Investigations involving nonhuman organisms are essential, but ultimate tests of the correctness and effectiveness of medical treatments must involve human beings as research subjects. Human physiology and psychology are sufficiently different to make animal studies alone inadequate.

The German physicians tried at Nuremberg were charged with conducting experiments without the consent of their subjects. The notion that consent must be given before a person becomes an experimental subject is still considered to be the basic requirement that must be met for an experiment to be morally legitimate. Ordinarily, it is not merely consent—saying yes—but *informed consent* that is demanded. The basic idea is simply that a person decides to participate in research after he or she has been provided with background information relevant to making the decision.

This same notion of informed consent is also considered a requirement that has to be satisfied before a person can legitimately be subjected to medical treatment. Thus, people are asked to agree to submit themselves to such ordinary medical procedures as blood transfusion or to other procedures such as surgical operations or radiation therapy.

The underlying idea of informed consent in both research and treatment is that people have a right to control what is done to their bodies. The notion of informed consent is thus a recognition of an individual's autonomy—of the right to make decisions governing one's own life. This right is recognized both in practice and in the laws of our society. (Quite often, malpractice suits turn on the issue of whether a patient's informed consent was valid.)

In the abstract, informed consent seems a clear and straightforward notion. After all, we all have an intuitive grasp of what it is to make a decision after we have been supplied with information. Yet in practice informed consent has proved to be a slippery and troublesome concept. In this introduction, we will attempt to identify some of the moral and practical difficulties that make the concept controversial and hard to apply. Our focus will be on informed consent in the context of human experimentation. But most of the issues that arise here also arise in connection with giving and securing informed consent for the application of medical therapies. (They also arise in special forms in abortion and euthanasia.) In effect, then, we will be considering the entire topic.

Before starting our discussion of informed consent, it will be useful to have some idea of what takes place in a typical medical experiment. Perhaps the most common type of research involves the testing of new drugs. Let us consider, then, a sketch of what is involved in such testing.

DRUG TESTING

Traditions of medical research and regulations of the United States Food and Drug Administration more or less guarantee that the development of new drugs follows a set procedure. The procedure consists of two major parts: preclinical and clinical testing.

When it is thought likely that a chemical substance might be useful, animal experiments are conducted to determine how toxic it is. These tests are also used to estimate the drug's therapeutic index (the ratio of a dose producing toxic effects to a dose producing desired effects). The effects of the substance on particular organs and tissues, as well as on the whole animal, are studied. Efforts are made to determine the drug's potential side effects and hazards (whether, for example, it is carcinogenic).

Clinical testing of the substance occurs in three phases. In phase one, normal human volunteers are used to determine whether the drug produces any toxic effects. If these results are acceptable, then in phase two the drug is administered to a limited number of patients who might be expected to benefit from it. If the drug produces desirable results and has no serious side effects, then phase three studies are initiated. The drug is administered to a larger number of patients by a larger number of clinical investigators. Such trials usually take place at teaching hospitals or in large public institutions. Successful results achieved in this phase ordinarily lead to the licensing of the drug for general use.

In the clinical part of testing, careful procedures are followed to attempt to exclude bias in the results. Investigators want their tests to be successful and patients want to get well, and either or both of these factors may influence test results. Investigators may perceive a patient as "improved" just because they want or expect him to be. What is more, all medications produce a "placebo effect." That is, when patients are given inactive substances (placebos), they nevertheless often show improvement.

To rule out these kinds of influences, a common procedure followed in drug testing is the "double-blind" test design. In this design, a certain number of patients are given the drug being tested, and the remainder of the test group are given placebos. (In some cases, an established drug may be used instead of or in addition to placebos.) Neither the investigators nor the patients are allowed to know who is receiving the drug and who is not—both are kept "blind." Sometimes a test group is divided so that part receives placebos all of the time, part only some of the time, and part receives genuine medication all of the time.

Often placebos are no more than just sugar pills. Yet, frequently, substances are prepared to produce side effects like those of the drug being tested. If, for example, the drug causes drowsiness, a placebo will be used that produces drowsiness. In this way, investigators will not be able to learn which patients are being given placebos on the basis of irrelevant observations.

The double-blind test design is employed in many kinds of clinical investigation, not just in drug testing. Thus, the testing of new vaccines and therapies often follows the same form. A major variation is the "single-blind" design, in which those who must evaluate the results of some treatment are kept in ignorance of which patients have received it.

THE "INFORMED" PART OF INFORMED CONSENT

At first sight, consent is no more than agreement. A person consents when he or she says "yes" when asked to be a research subject. But legitimate or valid consent cannot be merely saying yes. If people are to be treated as autonomous agents, they must have the opportunity to *decide* whether they wish to become participants in research. Deciding, whatever else it may be, is a process in which we reason about an issue at hand. We consider such matters as the risks to our participation, its possible advantages to ourselves and others, the risks and advantages of other alternatives that are offered to us, and our own values. In short, valid consent requires that we deliberate before we decide.

But genuine deliberation requires both information and understanding. These two requirements are the source of difficulties and controversies. After all, medical research and treatment are highly technical enterprises. They are based on complicated scientific theories that are expressed in a special vocabulary and involve unfamiliar concepts.

For this reason, some physicians and investigators have argued that it is virtually useless to provide patients with relevant scientific information about research and treatment. Patients without the proper scientific background, they argue, simply don't know what to make of the information. Not only do patients find it puzzling, they find it frightening. Thus, some have suggested, informed consent is at worst a pointless charade and at best a polite fiction. The patient's interest is best served by allowing a physician to make the decision.

This obviously paternalistic point of view (see Chapter 4) implies, in effect, that all patients are incompetent to decide their best interest and that physicians must assume the responsibility of acting for them. An obvious objection to this view is that it assumes that because patients lack a medical background, they cannot be given information in a form they can understand that is at least adequate to allow them to decide how they are to be treated. Thus, it can be argued, proponents of this view confuse the difficulty of communication with the impossibility of communication. It is true that it is often hard to explain technical medical matters to a layperson, but this hardly makes it legitimate to conclude that people should turn over their right to determine what is done to them to physicians. Rather, it imposes on physicians and researchers the obligation to find a way to explain medical matters to their patients.

The information provided to patients must be usable. That is, they must understand enough about the proposed research and treatment in order to deliberate and reach a decision. From the standpoint of the researcher, the problem here is to determine when the patient has an adequate understanding to make informed consent valid. Patients, being people, do not like to appear stupid and say they do not understand an explanation. Also, they may believe they understand an explanation when, as a matter of fact, they do not.

At present, there seems to be no generally accepted solution to the problem of determining when a patient understands the information provided to him or her. It seems reasonable to think that some kind of behavioral criteria—such as answering questions about the research project—would be best. But this is an area that requires empirical investigation.

THE "CONSENT" PART OF INFORMED CONSENT

We have talked so far as though the issue of gaining the legitimate agreement of someone to be a research subject involved only providing information to an ordinary person in ordinary circumstances and then allowing the person to decide. But the matter is more complicated than this because often either the person or the circumstances possess special features. These features can call into question the very possibility of valid consent.

It is generally agreed that in order to be valid, consent must be voluntary. The person must of his or her "own free will" agree to become a research subject. This means that the person must be capable of acting voluntarily. That is, the person must be *competent*.

This is an obvious and sensible requirement that is accepted by virtually everyone. But the difficulty lies in specifying just what it means to be competent. One answer is that a person is competent if he or she is capable of acting rationally. Since we have some idea of what it is to act rationally, this is a movement in the direction of an answer. The problem with it, however, is that people sometimes decide to act for the sake of moral (or religious) principles in ways that may not seem reasonable. For example, someone may volunteer to be a subject in a potentially hazardous experiment because she believes the experiment holds out the promise of helping countless others. In terms of self-interest alone, such an action would not be reasonable.

At present we do not have adequate criteria that can specify who is competent and who is not. Quite apart from this general theoretical problem is the issue of how children, the mentally retarded, and those suffering from psychiatric illnesses are to be considered with respect to consent. Should no person in any of these groups be considered capable of giving consent? If so, then is it ever legitimate to secure the consent from some third party, from a parent or guardian? One possibility is simply to rule out all research that involves such people as subjects. But this has the undesirable consequence of severely hampering efforts to gain the knowledge that might be of use either to the people themselves or to others with similar medical problems.

The questions we have raised here are still matters very much under dispute. Later we will consider some of the special problems that arise with children and other special groups as research subjects.

The circumstances in which research is done can also call into question the voluntariness of consent. This is particularly so with prisons, nursing homes, and mental hospitals. These are all what the sociologist Erving Goffman calls "total institutions," for within them all aspects of a person's life are connected with the social structure. People have a definite place in the structure and particular social roles. Moreover, there are social forces at work that both pressure and encourage an inmate to do what is expected of him.

We will discuss below some of the special problems that arise in research with prisoners. Here we need only to point out that the matter of gaining voluntary consent from inmates in institutions may not be possible at all. If it is possible, then it is necessary to specify the kinds of safeguards that need to be followed in order to free them from the pressures that result from the very fact that they are inmates. Those who suffer from psychiatric illnesses may be considered just as capable intellectually of giving consent, but here too safeguards to protect them from the pressures of the institution need to be specified.

To avoid a misimpression, it is also worth pointing out that ordinary patients in hospitals may also be subject to pressures that call into question the voluntariness of the consent that they give. Patients are psychologically predisposed to act in ways that please physicians. Not only do physicians possess a social role that makes them figures of authority, but an ill person feels very dependent on those who may possess the power to make him well. Thus, he will be inclined to go along with any suggestion or recommendation made by a physician. The ordinary patient, like the inmate in an institution, needs protection from the social and psychological pressures that are exerted by circumstances. Otherwise, the voluntariness of consent will be compromised, and the patient cannot act as a free and autonomous agent.

MEDICAL RESEARCH AND MEDICAL THERAPY

Medical therapy aims at relieving the suffering of people and restoring them to health. It attempts to cure diseases, correct disorders, and bring about normal bodily functioning. Its focus is on the individual patient, and his or her welfare is its primary concern.

Medical research, by contrast, is a scientific enterprise. Its aim is to acquire a better understanding of the chemical and physiological processes that are involved in human functioning. It is concerned with the effectiveness of therapies in ending disease processes and restoring functioning. But this concern is not for the patient as an individual. Rather, it is directed toward establishing theories. The hope, of course, is that this theoretical understanding can be used as a basis for treating individuals. But helping a particular patient get well is not a goal of medical research.

The related but distinct aims of medical research and medical therapy are a source of conflict in human experimentation. It is not unusual for a physician to be acting both as a researcher and as a therapist. This means that although she must be concerned with the welfare of her patient, her aims must also include acquiring data that are important to her research project. It is possible then that she may quite unconsciously encourage her patients to volunteer to be research subjects, provide them with inadequate information on which to base their decisions, or minimize the risks they are likely to be subject to.

The patient, for his part, may be reluctant to question his physician to acquire more information or to help him understand his role and risks in research. Also, as mentioned above, the patient may feel pressured into volunteering for research, just because he wants to do what his physician expects of him.

Medical research is a large-scale operation in this country and affects a great many people. It has been estimated that from four to eight hundred thousand people a year are patients in research programs investigating the effectiveness of drugs and other therapies. Since 1980, the number of clinical studies has increased about 30 percent, from about 3,400 to 4,400. Informed consent is more than an abstract moral issue.

The aims of therapy and the aims of research may also cause moral difficulties for the physician that go beyond the question of consent. This is particularly so in certain kinds of research. Let's look at some of the ethical issues more specifically.

Placebos and Research

As we saw earlier in the description of a typical drug experiment, placebos are considered to be essential in order to determine the true effectiveness of the drug being tested. In practice, this means that during all or some of the time they are being "treated," patients who are also subjects in a research program will not be receiving genuine medication. They are not, then, receiving the best available treatment for their specific condition.

This is one of the risks that a patient needs to know about before consenting to become a research subject. After all, most people become patients in order to be cured, if possible, of their ailments, not to further science or anything of the kind.

The physician-as-therapist will continue to provide medical care to a patient, for under double-blind conditions the physician does not know who is being given placebos and who is not. But the physician-as-researcher will know that a certain number of people will be receiving medication that cannot be expected to help their condition. Thus, the aims of the physician who is also a researcher come into conflict.

This conflict is particularly severe in cases in which it is reasonable to believe (on the basis of animal experimentation, tissue research, and so on) that an effective disease preventative exists, yet to satisfy scientific rigor, tests of its effectiveness involve the giving of placebos. This was the case with the development of a polio vaccine by Thomas Weller, John F. Enders, and Frederick C. Robbins in 1960. The initial phase of the clinical testing involved injecting thirty thousand children with a substance known to be useless in the prevention of polio—a placebo injection. It was realized, statistically, that some of those children would get the disease and die from it.

Since Weller, Enders, and Robbins believed that they had an effective vaccine, they can hardly be regarded as acting in the best interest of these children. As physicians they were not acting to protect the interest and well-being of the children. They did, of course, succeed in proving the safety and effectiveness of the polio vaccine. The moral question is whether they were justified in failing to provide thirty thousand children with a vaccine they believed to be effective, even though it had not been tested on a wide scale with humans. That is, did they correctly resolve the conflict between their role as researchers and their role as physicians?

Placebos also present physician-researchers with another conflict. As we noticed in the earlier discussion, placebos are not always just "sugar pills." They often contain active ingredients that produce in patients effects that resemble those caused by the medication being tested—nervousness, vomiting, loss of appetite, and so on. This means that a patient receiving a placebo is sometimes not only failing to receive any medication for his illness, but also receiving a medication that may do him some harm. Thus, the physician committed to care for the patient and to relieve his suffering is at odds with the researcher who may be harming the patient. Do the aims of scientific research and its potential benefits to others justify treating patients in this fashion? Here is another moral question that the physician must face in particular and we must face in general.

We should not leave the topic of the use of placebos without mentioning that it is possible to make use of an experimental design in research that does not require giving placebos to a control group. An investigator can compare the results of two treatment forms: a standard treatment whose effectiveness is known and a new treatment with a possible but not proven effectiveness. This is not as satisfactory scientifically as the other approach because the researcher must do without a control group that has received no genuine treatment. But it does provide a way out

of the dilemma of both providing medical care and conducting research.

Therapeutic and Nontherapeutic Research

We have mentioned the conflict that faces the physician who is also an investigator. But the patient who has to decide whether or not to consent to become a research subject is faced with a similar conflict.

Some research holds out the possibility of a direct and immediate advantage to those patients who agree to become subjects. For example, a new drug may, on the basis of limited trials, promise to be more effective in treating an illness than those drugs in standard use. Or a new surgical procedure may turn out to give better results than one that would ordinarily be used. By agreeing to participate in research involving such a drug or procedure, a patient may then have a chance of gaining something more beneficial than he or she would gain otherwise.

Yet the majority of medical research projects do not offer any direct therapeutic advantages to patients who consent to be subjects. The research may eventually benefit many patients, but seldom does it bring direct therapeutic benefits to research participants. Ordinarily, the most that participants can expect to gain is advantages such as having the attention of physicians who are more familiar with their illness than most physicians and receiving close observation and supervision in a research ward.

These are matters that ought to be presented to the patient as information relevant to the decision the patient must make. The patient must then decide whether he or she is willing to become a subject even if there are no special therapeutic advantages to be gained. It is in making this decision that one's moral beliefs can play a role. Some people volunteer to become research subjects without hope of reward because they believe that their action may eventually be of help to others.

Let us now turn to examining some of the problems posed by medical research in dealing with special groups. We will also consider some of the related issues that are involved in fetal research.

Research Involving Children

One of the most controversial areas of all medical experimentation has been that involving children as research subjects. The Willowbrook project discussed in the Case Presentation of this chapter is just one among many investigations that have drawn severe criticism and, quite often, court action.

The obvious question is: Why should children ever be made research subjects? Children clearly lack the physical, psychological, and intellectual maturity of adults. It does not seem that they are as capable as adults of giving informed consent because they can hardly be expected to grasp the nature of research and the possible risks to themselves. Furthermore, because they have not yet developed their capacities, it seems wrong to subject children to risks that might alter, for the worse, the course of their lives. They are in a position of relative dependency, relying upon adults to provide the conditions for their existence and development. It seems almost a betrayal of trust to allow children to be subjected to treatment that is of potential harm to them.

Such considerations help explain why we generally regard research involving children with deep suspicion. It is easy to imagine children being exploited and their lives heedlessly blighted by callous researchers. Some writers have been sufficiently concerned by the possibility of dangers and abuses that they have advocated an end to all research with children as subjects.

But there is another side to the coin. Biologically, children are not just small adults.

Their bodies are developing, growing systems. Not only are there anatomical differences; there are also differences in metabolism and biochemistry. For example, some drugs are absorbed and metabolized more quickly in children than in adults, whereas other drugs continue to be active for a longer time. Often some drugs produce different effects when administered to children. Furthermore, just because the bodies of children are still developing, their nutritional needs are different. Findings based on adult subjects cannot simply be extrapolated to children, any more than results based on animal studies can be extrapolated to human beings.

Also, children are prone to certain kinds of diseases (measles, for example) that are either less common in adults or occur in different forms. It is important to know the kinds of therapies that are most successful in the treatment of children afflicted with them. Finally, even familiar surgical procedures cannot be employed in a straightforward way with children. Their developing organ systems are sufficiently different that special pediatric techniques must often be devised.

For many medical purposes, children must be thought of almost as if they were wholly different organisms. Their special biological features set them apart and mark them as subjects requiring special study. To gain the kind of knowledge and understanding required for effective medical treatment of children, it is often impossible to limit research solely to adults.

Failing to conduct research on children raises its own set of ethical issues. It seems likely that if children are excluded from investigations, then the development of pediatric medicine will be severely hindered. In general, this would mean that children would receive medical therapies that are less effective than might be possible. Also, since it is known that children differ significantly from adults in drug reactions, it seems wrong to subject children to the risks of drugs and drug dosages that have been tested only on adults.

Research involving children also seems necessary to avoid causing long-term harm to numerous people. The use of pure oxygen in the environments of prematurely born babies in the early 1940s resulted in blindness and impaired vision in a great number of cases. It was not until a controlled study was done that such damage was traced to the effects of the oxygen. Had the research not been allowed, the chances are very good that the practice would have continued and thousands more infants would have been blinded.

Yet even if we agree that not all research involving children should be forbidden, we still have to face up to the issues that such research generates. Without attempting to be complete, we can mention the following three issues as among the more prominent.

First, who is to be considered a child? For infants and children in elementary school, this question is not a difficult one. But what about people in their teens? Then the line becomes hard to draw. Indeed, perhaps it is not possible to draw a line at all without being arbitrary. The concern behind the question is with the acquisition of autonomy, of self-direction and responsibility. It is obvious on the basis of ordinary experience that people develop at different rates, and some people at sixteen are more capable of taking charge of their own lives than others are at twenty. Some teenagers are more capable of understanding the nature and hazards of a research project than are many people who are much older.

This suggests that many people who are legally children may be quite capable of giving their informed consent. Of course many others probably are not, so that decisions about capability would have to rest on an assessment of the individual. Where medical procedures that have a purely therapeutic aim are concerned, an individual who is capable of deciding whether it is in his or her best interest should probably be the one to decide. The issue may be somewhat different when the aim is not therapy. In such cases, a better policy might be to set a lower limit on the age at which consent can be given, and those below that limit should not be permitted to consent to participate in research. The problem is, of course, what should that limit be?

Second, can anyone else consent on behalf of a child? Parents or guardians have a duty to act for the sake of the welfare of a child under their care. In effect, they have a duty to substitute their judgment for that of the child. We generally agree to this because most often we consider the judgment of an adult more mature and informed than a child's. And because the responsibility for care rests with the adult, we customarily recognize that the adult has a right to decide. It is almost as though the adult's autonomy is being shared with the child—almost as though the child were an extension of the adult.

Society and its courts have recognized limits on the power of adults to decide for children. When it seems that the adult is acting in an irresponsible or unreasonable manner, then society steps in to act as a protector of the child's right to be cared for. Thus, courts have ordered that life-saving procedures or blood transfusions be performed on children even when their parents or guardians have decided against it.

What sort of limits should govern a parent's or guardian's decision to allow a child to become a research subject? Can one person really give informed consent for another? Is it reasonable to believe that if a parent would allow herself to be the subject of an experiment, then it is also right for her to consent to her child's becoming a subject? Or should something more be required before consent for a child's participation can be considered legitimate?

Third, should children be allowed to be

subjects of research that does not offer them a chance of direct therapeutic benefits? Perhaps the "something more" that parents or guardians ought to require before consenting on behalf of a child is the genuine possibility that the research will bring the child direct benefits. This would be in accordance with a parent's duty to seek the welfare of the child. It is also a way of recognizing that the parent's autonomy is not identical with that of the child: one may have the right to take a risk one's self without having the right to impose the risk on someone else.

This seems like a reasonable limitation, and it has been advocated by some writers. (See the Freedman selection in this chapter, for example.) Yet there are difficulties with the position. Some research virtually free from risk (coordination tests, for example) might be stopped because of its lack of a "direct therapeutic value." More important, however, much research promising immense long-term benefits would have to be halted. Research frequently involves the withholding of accepted therapies without any guarantee that what is used in their place will be as effective. Sometimes the withholding of accepted treatment is beneficial. Thus, as it turned out, in the research on the incidence of blindness in premature infants in the 1940s, premature infants who were not kept in a pure oxygen environment were better off than those that received ordinary treatment. But no one could know this in advance, and such research as this is, at best, ambiguous as to the promise of direct therapy. Sheer ignorance imposes restrictions. Yet if the experiment had not been done, the standard treatment would have continued with its ordinary course of (statistically) disastrous results.

Here, at least, there was the possibility of better results from the experimental treatment. But in research that involves the substitution of placebos for medications or vaccines known to be effective, it is known in advance that some children will not receive

medical care considered to be the best. A child who is a subject in such research is then put in a situation in which he or she is subjected to a definite hazard. The limitation on consent that we are considering would rule out such research. But the consequence of doing this would be to restrict the development of new and potentially more effective medications and treatment techniques. That is, future generations of children would be deprived of at least some possible medical advances.

These, then, are some of the issues that we have to face in arriving at a view of the role of children in research. Perhaps the greatest threat to children, however, has to do with social organization. Children, like prisoners, are often grouped together in institutions (schools, orphanages, detention centers, and so on) and are attractive targets for clinical investigators because they inhabit a limited and relatively controlled environment, can be made to follow orders, and do not ask too many questions that have to be answered. It is a misimpression to see researchers in such situations as "victimizing" children, but at the same time, it is clear that careful controls are needed to see that research involving children is legitimate and carried out in a morally satisfactory way.

In response to some of these difficulties, in 1983 the Department of Health and Human Services issued guidelines specifically designed to protect children as research subjects. For children to become subjects, permission must be obtained from parents or guardians, and children must give their "assent." An Institutional Review Board is assigned the responsibility of considering the "ages, maturity, and psychological states" of the children and determining whether they are capable of assenting. (A failure to object cannot be construed as assent.) Children who are wards of the state or of an institution can become subjects only if the research relates to their status as wards or takes place in circumstances in which the majority of subjects are not wards. Each child must also be supplied with an "advocate" to represent her or his interest.

Research Involving Prisoners

Prisoners are in some respects social outcasts. They have been found guilty of breaking the laws of society and, as a consequence, are removed from it. Stigmatized and isolated, prisoners in the relatively recent past were sometimes thought of as less than human. It seemed only reasonable that such depraved and corrupt creatures should be used as the subjects of experiments that might bring benefits to the members of the society that they wronged. It seemed not only reasonable but fitting.

Accordingly, in the early part of this century, tropical medicine expert Richard P. Strong obtained permission from the Governor of the Philippines to inoculate a number of condemned criminals with plague bacillus. The prisoners were not asked for their consent, but they were rewarded by being provided with cigarettes and cigars.

Episodes of this sort were relatively common during the late nineteenth and early twentieth centuries. But as theories about the nature of crime and criminals changed, it became standard practice to use only volunteers and to secure the consent of the prisoners themselves. In the 1940s, for example, the University of Chicago infected over four hundred prisoners with malaria in an attempt to discover new drugs to treat and prevent the disease. A committee set up by the Governor of Illinois recommended that potential volunteers be informed of the risks, be permitted to refuse without fear of such reprisals as withdrawing privileges, and be protected from unnecessary suffering. The committee suggested also that volunteering to be a subject in a medical experiment is a form of good conduct that should be taken into account in deciding whether a prisoner should be paroled or have his sentence reduced.

But the committee also called attention to a problem of great moral significance. They pointed out that if a prisoner's motive for volunteering is the wish to contribute to human welfare, then a reduction in his sentence would be a reward. But if his motive is to obtain a reduction in sentence, then the possibility of obtaining one is really a form of duress. In this case, the prisoner cannot be regarded as making a free decision.

The issue of duress or "undue influence" as it is called in law is central to the question of deciding whether, and under what conditions, valid informed consent can be obtained for research involving prisoners. To avoid undue influence, some ethicists have argued that prisoners should never be promised any substantial advantages for volunteering to be research subjects. If they volunteer, they should do so for primarily moral or humane reasons.

Others have claimed that becoming research subjects offers prisoners personal advantages that they should not be denied. For example, participation in a research project frees them from the boredom of prison life, gives them an opportunity to increase their feelings of self-worth, and allows them to exercise their autonomy as moral agents. It has been argued, in fact, that prisoners have a *right* to participate in research if the opportunity is offered to them and they wish to do so. To forbid the use of prisoners as research subjects is thus to deny to them, without adequate grounds, a right that all human beings possess. As a denial of their basic autonomy, of their right to take risks and control their own bodies, *not* allowing them to be subjects might constitute a form of cruel and unusual punishment.

By contrast, it can also be argued that prisoners do not deserve to be allowed to exercise such autonomy. It is reasoned that because they have been sentenced for crimes, they should be deprived of the right to volunteer to be research subjects: that right belongs to free citizens. Being deprived of the right to act autonomously is part of their punishment. This is basically the position taken in 1952 by the House of Delegates of the American Medical Association. The Delegates passed a resolution expressing disapproval of the use as research subjects of people convicted of "murder, rape, arson, kidnapping, treason, and other heinous crimes."

A more worrying consideration is the question of whether prisoners can be sufficiently free of undue influence or duress to make their consent legitimate. As we mentioned earlier, prisons are total institutions, and the very institutional framework puts pressures on people to do what is desired or expected of them. There need not be, then, promises of rewards (such as reduced sentences) or overt threats (such as withdrawing of ordinary privileges) for coercion to be present. That people may volunteer to relieve boredom is itself an indication that they may be acting under duress. That "good conduct" is a factor in deciding whether to grant parole may function as another source of pressure.

The problem presented by prisoners is fundamentally the same as that presented by inmates in other institutions, such as nursing homes and mental hospitals. In these cases, once it has been determined that potential subjects are mentally competent to give consent, then it must also be decided whether the institutional arrangements allow the consent to be "free and voluntary."

Research Involving the Poor

In the eighteenth century, Princess Caroline of England requested the use of six "charity children" as subjects in the smallpox vaccination experiments she was directing. Then, and until quite recently, charity cases, like prisoners, were regarded by some medical researchers as prime research subjects.

A recent and horrible example of medical research involving the poor is the Tuskegee Syphilis Study that was conducted under the auspices of the U.S. Department of Public Health. From 1932 to 1970, a large but undetermined number of black males suffering from the later stages of syphilis were examined at regular intervals to determine the course their disease was taking. The men in the study were poor and uneducated and believed that they were receiving proper medical care from the state and local public health clinics. As a matter of fact, they were given either no treatment or inadequate treatment, and at least forty of them died as a result of factors connected with their disease. Their consent was never obtained, and the nature of the study, its risks, and the alternatives open to them were never explained. It was known when the study began that those with untreated syphilis have a higher death rate than those whose condition is treated, and although the study was started before the advent of penicillin (which is highly effective against syphilis), other drugs were available but were not used in ways to produce the best results. When penicillin became generally available, it still was not used.

The Tuskegee Study clearly violated the Nuremberg Code, but it was not stopped even after the War Crimes trials. It was reviewed in 1969 by a USPH ad hoc committee and it was decided that the study should be phased out in 1970. The reasons for ending the study were not moral ones. It was simply believed that there was nothing of much scientific value to be gained by continuing the work. In 1973, a USPH Ad Hoc Advisory Panel, which had been established as a result of public and congressional pressure to review the Tuskegee Study, presented its final report. It condemned the study both on moral grounds and because of its lack of worth and rigor.

No one today argues seriously that disadvantaged people ought to be made subjects of research simply as a result of their social or economic status. The "back wards" in hospitals whose poor patients once served as a source of research subjects have mostly disappeared as a result of such programs as Medicare and Medicaid. Each person is now entitled to his or her own physician and is not merely under the care of the state or of a private charity.

Yet many research projects continue to be based in large public or municipal hospitals. And such hospitals have a higher percentage of disadvantaged people as patients than do private institutions. For this reason, such people are still more likely to become research subjects than the educated and wealthy. If society continues to accept this state of affairs, special precautions must be taken to see to it that those who volunteer to become research subjects are genuinely informed and free in their decisions.

Research Involving Fetuses

In 1975 legal charges were brought against several physicians in Boston. They had injected antibiotics into living fetuses that were scheduled to be aborted. The aim of the research was to determine by autopsy, after the death of the fetuses, how much of the drug got into the fetal tissues.

Such information is considered to be of prime importance because it increases our knowledge of how to provide medical treatment for a fetus still developing in its mother's womb. It also helps to determine ways in which drugs taken by a pregnant woman may affect a fetus and so points the way towards improved prenatal care.

Other kinds of research involving the fetus also promise to provide important knowledge. Effective vaccines for preventing viral diseases, techniques for treating children with defective immune-system reactions, and hormonal measurements that indicate the status of the developing fetus are just some of

the potential advances that are partially dependent on fetal research.

But a number of moral questions arise in connection with such research. Even assuming that a pregnant woman consents to allow the fetus she is carrying to be injected with drugs prior to abortion, is such research ethical? Does the fact that the fetus is going to be aborted alter in any way the moral situation? For example, prior to abortion should the fetus be treated with the same respect and concern for its well-being as a fetus which is not scheduled for abortion?

After the fetus is aborted, if it is viable— if it can live separated from the mother—then we seem to be under an obligation to protect its life. But what if a prenatal experiment threatens its viability? The expectation in abortion is that the fetus will not be viable, but this is not in fact always the case. Does this mean that it is wrong to do anything before abortion to threaten the life of the fetus or reduce its chance for life, even though we do not expect it to live?

These are very difficult questions to answer without first settling the question of whether the fetus is to be considered a person. (See the discussion of this issue in the introduction and selections in Chapter 1.) If the fetus is a person, then it is entitled to the same moral considerations that we extend to other persons. If we decide to take its life, if abortion is considered to be at least sometimes legitimate, then we must be prepared to offer justification. Similarly, if we are to perform experiments on a fetus, even one expected to die, then we must also be prepared to offer justification. Whether the importance of the research is adequate justification is a matter that currently remains to be settled.

If the fetus is not a person, then the question of fetal experimentation becomes less important morally. Since, however, the fetus may be regarded as a potential person, we may still believe it is necessary to treat it with consideration and respect. The burden of justification may be somewhat less weighty, but it may still be there.

Let us assume that the fetus is aborted and is apparently not viable. Typically, before such a fetus dies, its heart beats and its lungs function. Is it morally permissible to conduct research on the fetus before its death? The knowledge that can be gained, particularly of lung functions, can be used to help save the lives of premature infants, and the fetus is virtually certain of dying, whether or not it is made a subject of research.

After the death of a fetus that is either deliberately or spontaneously aborted, are there any moral restraints on what is done with the remains? It is possible to culture fetal tissues and use them for research purposes. These tissues might, in fact, be commercially grown and distributed by biological supply companies in the way that a variety of animal tissues are now dealt with. Exactly when a fetus can be considered to be dead so that its tissues and organs are available for experimentation, even assuming that one approves of their use in this manner, is itself an unanswered question.

Scientists have been concerned about proposed federal guidelines and state laws regulating fetal research. Most investigators fear that they will be forced to operate under such rigid restrictions that research will be slowed or even prohibited. Nearly everyone agrees, however, that some important moral and social decisions must be made about fetal research.

Fetal research has to be considered a part of human experimentation. Not only are many fetuses born alive even when deliberately aborted, but they all possess certain human characteristics and potentialities. But who shall give approval to what is done with the fetus? Who is responsible for consent?

It seems peculiar to say that a woman who has decided to have an abortion is also the one who should consent to research involving the aborted fetus. It can be argued that in deciding to have an abortion she has renounced all interest and responsibility with respect to the fetus. Yet if the fetus does live, we would consider her, at least in part, legally and morally responsible for seeing to its continued well-being.

But if the woman (or the parents) is the one who must give consent for fetal experimentation, are there limits to what she can consent to on behalf of the fetus? With this question we are back where we began. It is obvious that fetal research raises both moral and social issues. We need to decide, then, what is right as a matter of personal conduct and what is right as a matter of social policy. At the moment, issues in each of these areas remain unsettled.

Summary

There are other areas of human experimentation that present special forms of moral problems. We have not discussed, for example, research involving military personnel, college and university students, or dying patients. Moreover, we mentioned only a few of the special difficulties presented by the mentally retarded, psychiatric patients, and old people confined to institutions.

We have, however, raised such a multiplicity of questions about consent and human experimentation that it is perhaps worthwhile to attempt to restate some of the basic issues in a general form. Three issues are particularly noteworthy:

1. Who is competent to consent? (Are children? Are mental patients? If a person is not competent, who—if anyone—should have the power to consent for him or her?)

2. When is consent voluntary? (Is any institutionalized person in a position to offer free consent? How can even hospitalized patients be made free of pressures to consent?)

3. When is information and understanding adequate for genuine decision mak-

ing? (Can complicated medical information ever be adequately explained to laypeople? Should we attempt to devise tests for understanding?)

Although we have concentrated on the matter of consent in research, there are other morally relevant matters connected with the character of research that we have not discussed. These often relate to research standards. Among them are the following:

1. Is the research of sufficient scientific and medical worth to justify the human risk involved? Research that involves trivial aims or that is unnecessary (when, for example, it merely serves to confirm what is already well established) cannot be used to justify causing any threat to human well-being.

2. Can the knowledge sought be obtained without human experimentation?

3. Have animal (and other) studies been done to minimize so far as is possible the risk to human subjects? A great deal can be learned about the effects of drugs, for example, by using "animal models," and the knowledge gained can be used to minimize the hazards in human trials. (Ethical issues involving animals in research also call into question some past practices. These issues must also be addressed.)

4. Does the design of the research meet accepted scientific standards? Sloppy research that is scientifically worthless means that people have been subjected to risks for no legitimate purpose.

5. Do the investigators have the proper medical or scientific background to conduct the research effectively?

6. Is the research designed to minimize the risks and suffering of the participants? As we noted earlier, it is sometimes possible to test new drugs without using placebos. Thus, people in need of medi-

cation are not forced to be without treatment for their condition.

7. Have the aims and the design of the research and the qualifications of the investigators been reviewed by a group or committee competent to judge them? Such "peer review" is intended to assure that only research that is worthwhile and that meets accepted scientific standards is conducted. And although such review groups can fail to do their job properly, as they apparently did in the Tuskegee Syphilis Study, they are still necessary instruments of control.

Most writers on experimentation would agree that these are among the questions that must be answered satisfactorily before research involving human subjects is morally acceptable. Obviously, however, a patient who is asked to give his or her consent is in no position to judge whether the research project meets the standards implied by these questions. For this reason, it is important that there be social policies and practices governing research. Everyone should be confident that a research project is, in general, a legitimate one before having to decide whether to volunteer to become a participant.

Special problems are involved in seeing to it that these questions are properly answered. It is enough for our purposes, however, merely to notice that the character of the research and the manner in which it is to be performed are factors that are relevant to determining the moral legitimacy of experimentation involving human subjects.

ETHICAL THEORIES: MEDICAL RESEARCH AND INFORMED CONSENT

We have clearly raised too many issues in too many areas of experimentation to discuss how each of several ethical theories might apply to them all. We must limit ourselves to considering a few suggestions about the general issues of human experimentation and informed consent.

Utilitarianism's principle of utility tells us, in effect, to choose those actions that will produce the greatest amount of benefit. Utilitarianism must approve human experimentation in general since there are cases in which the sacrifices of a few bring great benefits to many. We might, for example, design our social policies to make it worthwhile for people to volunteer for experiments with the view that if people are paid to take risks and are compensated for their suffering or for any damage done to them during the course of a research project, then the society as a whole might benefit.

The principle of utility also tells us to design experiments to minimize suffering and the chance of harm. Also, it forbids us to do research of an unnecessary or trivial kind—research that is not worth its cost in either human or economic resources.

So far as informed consent is concerned, utilitarianism does not seem to require it. If more social good is to be gained by making people research subjects without securing their agreement, then this is morally legitimate. (It is not, of course, necessarily the best procedure to follow. A system of rewards to induce volunteers might be more likely to lead to an increase in general happiness.) Furthermore, the principle of utility suggests that the best research subjects would be "less valuable" members of the society, such as the mentally retarded, the habitual criminal, or the dying. This, again, is not a necessary consequence of utilitarianism, although it is a possible one. If the recognition of rights and dignity would produce a better society in general, then a utilitarian would also say that they must be taken into account in experimentation with human beings.

For utilitarianism, that individual is competent to give consent who is able to balance benefits and risks and then decide what course of action is best for him or her. Thus, if informed consent is taken to be a requirement supported by the principle of utility, those who are mentally ill or retarded or senile have to be excluded from the class of potential experimental subjects. Furthermore, investigators must provide enough relevant information to allow competent people to make a meaningful decision about what is likely to serve their own interests the most.

For Kant, an individual capable of giving consent is one who is rational and autonomous. Kant's principles would thus also rule out as experimental subjects people who are not able to understand experimental procedures, aims, risks, and benefits. People may volunteer for experiments if they expect them to be of therapeutic benefit to themselves, or they may act out of duty and volunteer, thus discharging their imperfect obligation to advance knowledge or to improve human life.

Yet, for Kant, there are limits to the risks that one should take. We have a duty to preserve our lives, so no one should agree to become a subject in an experiment in which the likelihood of death is great. Additionally, no one should subject himself to research in which there is considerable risk that his capacity for rational thought and autonomy will be destroyed. Indeed, Kant's principles appear to require us to regard as morally illegitimate those experiments that seriously threaten the lives or rationality of their subjects. Not only should we not subject ourselves to them, but we should not subject others to them.

Kant's principles also rule out as potential experimental subjects those who are not in a position to act voluntarily, those who cannot exercise their autonomy. This makes it important to determine, from a Kantian point of view, whether children and institutionalized people (including prisoners) can be regarded as free agents capable of moral choice. Also, as in the case of abortion, the status of the fetus must be determined. If the fetus is not a person, then fetal experimentation presents no particular moral problems. But if the fetus is a person, then we must accord it a moral status and act for its sake and not for the sake of knowledge or for others.

Kant's view of people as autonomous rational beings requires that informed consent be obtained for both medical treatment and research. We cannot be forced to accept treatment for "our own good," nor can we be turned into experimental subjects for "the good of others." We must always be treated as ends and never as means only. To be treated in this way requires that others never deliberately deceive us, no matter how good their intentions. In short, we have a right to be told what we are getting into so that we can decide whether we want to go through with it or not.

Ross's theory imposes on researchers prima facie duties to patients that are similar to Kant's requirements. The nature of people as autonomous moral agents requires that their informed consent be obtained. Researchers ought not deceive their subjects, and experiments should be designed in ways in which suffering and the risk of injury or death are minimized.

These are all prima facie duties, of course, and it is possible to imagine situations in which other duties might take precedence over them. In general, however, Ross, like Kant, tells us that human research cannot be based on what is useful, but it must be based on what is right. Ross's principles, like Kant's, do not tell us, however, how we are to deal with such special problems as research involving children or prisoners.

As we saw in the introductory chapter, the principle of double effect and the principle of totality, which are based on the natural law theory of morality, have specific applications to experimentation. Because we hold our bodies in trust, we are responsible for assessing the degree of risk to which we might be put if we agree to become research subjects. Thus, others have an obligation to supply us with the information that we need in order to make our decision. If we decide to give our consent, it must be given freely and not be the consequence of deception or coercion.

If available evidence shows that a sick person may gain benefits from participating in an experiment, then the experiment is justified. But if the evidence shows that the benefits may be slight or if the chance of serious injury or death is relatively great, then the experiment is not justified. In general, the likelihood of a person's benefitting from an experiment must exceed the danger of the person's suffering greater losses. The four requirements that govern the application of the principle of double effect determine what is and what is not an allowable experiment. (See the introductory chapter for a discussion of these.)

People can volunteer for experiments from which they expect no direct benefits. The good they seek in doing so is not their own good but the good of others. But there are limits to what they can subject themselves to. A dying patient, for example, cannot be made the subject of a useless or trivial experiment. The probable value of the knowledge to be gained must balance the risk and suffering the patient is subjected to, and there must be no likelihood that the experiment will seriously injure or kill the patient.

These same restrictions also apply to experiments involving healthy people. The principle of totality forbids a healthy person to submit to an experiment that involves the probability of serious injury, impaired health, mutilation, or death.

The status of the fetus is clear on the Roman Catholic version of the natural law theory: the fetus is a person. As such, the fetus is entitled to the same dignity and respect we accord to other persons. Experiments that involve doing it injury or lessening its chances of life are morally prohibited. But not all fetal research is ruled out. That which may be of therapeutic benefit or which does not directly threaten the fetus's well-being is allowable. Furthermore, research involving fetal tissue or remains is permissible, if it is done for a serious and valuable purpose.

From Rawls's point of view, the difficulty with utilitarianism with respect to human experimentation is that the principle of utility would permit the exploitation of some groups (the dying, prisoners, the retarded) for the sake of others. By contrast, Rawls's principles of justice would forbid all experiments that involve violating a liberty to which a person is entitled by virtue of being a member of society. As a result, all experiments that make use of coercion or deception are ruled out. And since a person has a right to decide what risks she is willing to subject herself to, voluntary informed consent is required of all subjects. Society might, as in utilitarianism, decide to reward those who volunteer to become research subjects. So long as this is a possibility open to all, it is not objectionable.

It would never be right, according to Rawls, to take advantage of those in the society who are least well off to benefit those who are better off. In general, inequalities must be arranged so that they bring benefits (ideally) to everyone or at least to those who are most disadvantaged. Research involving direct therapeutic benefits is clearly acceptable (assuming that there is informed consent), but research that takes advantage of the sick, the poor, the retarded, or the institutionalized and does not benefit them is clearly unacceptable. The status of the fetus—whether or not it is a person in the moral sense—is an issue that has to be resolved before we know how to apply Rawls's principles to fetal research.

We have been able to provide only the briefest sketch here of some of the ways in which our moral theories might apply to the issues in human experimentation. The re-marks are not meant to be anything more than suggestive. Clearly, a satisfactory moral theory of human experimentation requires working out the application of principles to problems in detail, as well as resolving such issues as the status of children and fetuses and whether institutionalized people are capable of acting freely.

THE SELECTIONS

Louis Lasagna in "Some Ethical Problems in Clinical Investigation" discusses some of the issues that face the physician who is in the role of both therapist and researcher. But perhaps the most important aspect of his article is the review of the arguments against informed consent. Lasagna points out that sometimes researchers themselves do not know the risks that may be involved in research, that there are experiments in which information provided to potential subjects can alter the outcome, and that often patients themselves do not wish to be put into a position in which they must make a decision on the basis of information that they are not really competent to evaluate. Taking a basically utilitarian stance, Lasagna suggests that the "greater interest" of society must sometimes be given precedence over the rights of individuals.

This position is in marked contrast to that taken by Hans Jonas in his essay. Jonas argues that if we justify experiments by considering them a right of society, then we are exposing individuals to dangers for the general good. This, for Jonas, is inherently wrong, and no individual should be forced to surrender himself to a social goal.

Any risk that is taken must be voluntary, but obtaining informed consent, Jonas claims, is not sufficient to justify the experimental use of human beings. Two other conditions must be met: subjects must be recruited from those who are most knowledgeable about the circumstances of research and who are intellectually most capable of grasping its purposes and procedures; furthermore, the experiment must be undertaken for an adequate cause. Jonas cautions us that the progress that may come from research is not necessarily worth our efforts or approval, and he reminds us that there are moral values that we ought not to lose in the pursuit of science.

F. J. Ingelfinger claims in "Informed (But Uneducated) Consent" that efforts to secure informed consent from potential patients or subjects are mostly doomed to failure. "The chances are remote," Ingelfinger says, "that the subject really understands what he has consented to—in the sense that the responsible medical investigator understands the goals, nature, and hazards of his study." Nor can the subject be given information that is in any genuine sense complete. In fact, it might even be unethical to present a person with all the contingencies that may be involved in an experiment.

The current procedure, Ingelfinger asserts, is better than ones followed in the past, for then people were not even told that they were going to be research subjects. But beyond this, the process of obtaining informed consent "is no more than an elaborate ritual that, when the patient is uneducated and uncomprehending, confers no more than the semblance of propriety on human experimentation." The subject's only real protection depends on the person directing the research.

Benjamin Freedman claims that an account of what it is to be "free," "informed," and "competent" will allow us to decide when a person is mature enough to give consent and when prisoners are free to consent to participating in experiments. According to Freedman, there is a "right to consent" that arises from our status as persons. To deny someone a right to consent is to deprive him of personhood and autonomy. Also it is often to deprive him of such advantages as direct

therapeutic benefits. For these reasons, we should recognize the possibility that prisoners can give valid consent.

Those who claim that full information can never be given to patients or subjects miss the point, Freedman says. The amount and kind of information are relative to the purpose at hand—namely, to permit the patient to make a meaningful decision. Informed consent, then, is possible. Consent must also be responsible, but the only way to decide this is by considering the character of the patient, Finally, Freedman says, consent must be voluntary, and this condition is met when the "reward" for participating does something more than merely raise a person to the ordinary level of rights and freedoms.

In discussing consent and the incompetent, Freedman rejects as invalid proxy consent for research on children. Children, in his view, have a right to "custody, not liberty." They have a right to be cared for, so consent in adults and proxy consent for children are very different.

"The Willowbrook Letters" by Stephen Goldby, Saul Krugman, M. H. Pappworth, and Geoffrey Edsall concern the moral legitimacy of the study of viral hepatitis that was conducted at the Willowbrook School by Krugman and his associates. (See the Case Presentation for more detail.) Goldby charges that the study was "quite unjustifiable" because it was morally wrong to infect children when no benefit to them could result. Krugman defends himself by claiming that his results demonstrated a "therapeutic effect" for the children involved, as well as for others. He presents four reasons for holding that the infecting of the children was justified.

Pappworth claims that Krugman's defense is presented only after the fact, whereas an experiment is ethical or not in its inception. Moreover, he asserts, consent was obtained through the use of coercion. Parents who wished to put their children in the institution were told there was room only in the "hepatitis unit."

In the final letter, Edsall defends the Krugman study. The experiments, he asserts, involved no greater risk to the children involved than they would have run in any case. What is more, the results obtained were of general benefit.

Paul Ramsey, in the selection included here, reviews the justifications offered for the Willowbrook experiments presented by Krugman. Ramsey observes that there is nothing about hepatitis that requires that research be conducted on children, that no justification except the needs of the experiment is given for withholding gamma globulin from the subjects, that nothing is said about attempting to control the low-grade epidemic by other means. Furthermore, Ramsey questions the morality of consent secured from the parents of the children. His basic recommendation is that the use of captive populations of children ought to be made legally impossible.

The last two articles raise issues more general than consent alone. Thomas Preston

suggests that money currently spent on experimentation with the artificial heart might be better spent on such efforts as reducing infant mortality, for more lives would be saved by doing so. Also, in Preston's view, the therapeutic claims for the artificial heart are unwarranted, and continued promotion of its use may establish a costly public demand. Preston concludes that "What is happening now is not good medicine, is not good science, and is not in the public interest." (See the Case Presentation for details about the artificial heart. Also see the Social Context section of Chapter 9 on health-care costs.)

Alexander Capron raises the question of whether Baby Fae was "hero, victim, or patient." (See the Baby Fae Case Presentation for additional information.) In his view, when a child is a patient and research is involved, then physicians have an obligation never to advance their research "at the expense of the child by foregoing an alternative treatment that offers a better chance." It is possible, Capron suggests, that Baby Fae was indeed "a victim of well-meaning science."

Some Ethical Problems in Clinical Investigation

Louis Lasagna

One potentially important source of tension in clinical investigation is the fundamental discrepancy in outlook between the clinical investigator and the physician. The two positions are rarely identical. One reads that medical experimentation takes place continually in every doctor's office and that the therapy of disease is an experimental aspect of medicine, but in point of fact, the practice of medicine and the pursuit of a scientific problem are not equivalent.

The physician is primarily concerned with the patient *qua* patient, with getting him well as

quickly as possible and with a minimum of discomfort, inconvenience, risk, and cost to the patient. In the practice of his art the doctor has to use any and every measure he considers justified, and he is concerned with what measure (if any) works, not with what contribution (if any) he makes to the body of scientific data.

For the investigator, the primary emphasis is on the research question. This does not mean that he need be callous or lacking in caution; indeed, patients who are in an experiment are likely to be more carefully observed and cared for than if they

Reprinted by permission of the publishers from Human Aspects of Biomedical Innovation, by Everett Mendelsohn, Judith P. Swazey, and Irene Taviss, eds., Cambridge, Mass.: Harvard University Press, Copyright © 1971 by the President and Fellows of Harvard College.

were not research subjects. (In fact, carefully designed experiments result more often in improved patient care than in exciting new scientific information.) There are good reasons for the preferred status of patients in an experiment. Physicians in a research ward or research institution have usually had the advantage of intensive training, experience, and the intellectual discipline of an academic atmosphere. Further, the patient is, paradoxically, often better served by the restraint observed in the therapeutic approach of the critical experimentalist. The uncritical use of many therapeutic measures can be less desirable than the wise use of a few well-chosen ones; in medicine two and two sometimes add up to minus four, as the patient finds his medications working at cross purposes and yielding iatrogenic illness to boot. Often in controlled trials, for example, the placebo-treated patients turn out to be the lucky ones, as the new "remedy" proves to be toxic or therapeutically ineffective.

Notwithstanding the admirable qualities of many research-oriented physicians, however, there still remain important differences in orientation between the physician and the investigator which may affect the individual patient to a significant degree and which deserve discussion. Take, for example, the patient with metastatic cancer. Here is a serious disease for which we lack good treatment. There would seem to be no ethical problem in giving a desperately ill patient a new compound which may do some good. Yet the situation is only superficially simple.

The first cancer patients to receive an investigational drug often fail to obtain significant therapeutic benefit, and the dose exploration and tolerability studies involved in such early pharmacologic trials are likely to entail a certain amount of serious risk because of the powerful drugs generally required to treat malignant disease. In such a situation, therefore, the physician might well say "No" to the earliest trial of a new drug in cases where the investigator might say "Yes." If one then moves to a problem such as the treatment of pain or of insomnia, where we have remedies which, while not perfect, are for most purposes excellent and reasonably safe, what is the physician to say? Statistically, there is no doubt that the patient has a better chance of adequate relief if given a standard and accepted

drug rather than an untried one, no matter how impressive a case for research can be made from the standpoint of society's long-term needs.

Another difficulty stems from the use of both patients and volunteer subjects in medical research. This practice tends to blur the fundamental distinction between these two kinds of subjects. The volunteer (or the patient who is being studied in a way unrelated to his disease) is truly an experimental subject and usually stands to gain little or nothing medically—at least in the near future—from the experience of being exposed to an investigational compound. He may run considerable risk. It seems to me that such a volunteer must be handled quite differently from the patient who is also contributing to research goals but who may derive considerable benefit in the immediate future. To the degree that this distinction is blurred, ethical difficulties will be compounded.

It may be useful to consider the currently controversial issue of obtaining "informed consent" from subjects participating in drug investigation. The new Food and Drug Administration (FDA) regulations governing experimentation on human subjects make it clear that except in rare instances informed written consent must be obtained from anyone who is being given an investigational drug.[1] The FDA has spelled out in great detail the kinds of information that must be supplied to subjects of such experiments. It is interesting to contrast this approach with the usual practice of medicine, in which drug administration also plays an important role, and where patients almost certainly suffer more harm (some avoidable, much of it not) from the use of old drugs than experimental subjects suffer from the prescribing of new drugs by experienced investigators. In ordinary practice, consent is usually not informed, and it is almost never written, except for surgical procedures.

In favor of obtaining informed consent in clinical investigation is the reasonable (and generally held) belief that a person should know what is being done to him and what the risks of participation in an experiment may be. Of course, there are also important legal implications in procedures which—in the absence of consent—may be construed as civil or criminal assault on a person's body. There is a strong common law tradition in this regard which goes back at least as far as Justice Cardozo. In addition, unless a physician or committee other than the investigator is making the final decisions, the patient's informed consent represents a check on the motives of the investigator, motives which may be generally admirable but specifically undesirable, or at least questionable, for the individual patient.

What are the arguments *against* informed consent? To begin with, there are instances in which it would seem clearly not in the patient's best interest to discuss matters with full candor. A person dying of terminal cancer who has been given the few weakly effective available drugs, and whose condition is deteriorating, may gain little from an excessively detailed and frank discussion of the situation when a new drug is available which might possibly provide some benefit. Investigational drug use in psychiatric patients poses similar psychic hazards, including the special risk, if the use of drugs is made to look too much like an experiment, of permanently damaging or destroying the patient-doctor relationship.

One may also argue that obtaining informed consent involves the assumption that the investigator knows the risks of giving the drug, of withholding it, and the alternative risks from the use of other, older agents that might be used instead. The language of the FDA regulations does, it seems to me, imply all this. In fact, this information is available only in small measure.[2] One also assumes that the investigator is capable of the exposition required to present this information to the patient and that the patient is capable of grasping the information. One would also like to think that the patient is capable of making a decision in keeping with his own best interests after hearing the information, although a competent adult should, I suppose, have the freedom to make the wrong decision in the hospital or doctor's office no less than in the voting booth. All of these considerations are not, to be sure, so much arguments against informed consent as examples of the difference between the wish and the achievement.

Some important arguments against consent revolve around the possibility of impeding scientific progress if such consent is routinely obtained. (One could, for "scientific progress," substitute "providing benefit to others, including future generations.") There are some trials that will be impossible if a truly candid explanation has to be provided. One prominent investigator has evinced

his skepticism about convincing people to participate in a trial that will last for years and in which some individuals are given drugs to lower their blood pressure and others receive placebos. Since it is not clear that all patients with hypertension should receive drugs, it would seem unethical *not* to perform the trial, but there is disagreement as to whether it is ethical to inform the patients of the nature of the trial while they are participating in it. With postpartum patients, we found in one experiment that if women were approached while they are actually having pain and asked to sign a consent form to participate in an experiment in which they might also receive inert preparations, some 80 to 85 percent refused to participate. (In work conducted on patients of this sort without written consent over a decade or so, we have never seen any evidence of serious harm or discontent; indeed, it is reasonably certain that these patients have received closer attention and better medical care than they would otherwise have received.) This would result in such an idiosyncratic selection of the population that we refused to conduct the trial, not only because of the time that would be required to complete it but because of the very real possibility that the results in such a minority of the population might not provide legitimate basis for predicting effects in the majority.

There is also the chance—even if patients consent to participate—that one may destroy the validity of a trial by inducing introspection of various kinds, producing a sort of Heisenberg effect. Some patients, when they know they are in a trial, will try to outwit the investigator by guessing which medications they are receiving. Other patients will be troubled by the nontherapeutic aspects of the experience, so that one may have difficulty in relating the responses to the usual clinical situation. Although investigators quite rightly tend to emphasize the difference between clinical practice and rigorous clinical investigation, it is nevertheless true that those studying new drugs experimentally wish very much to collect data applicable to the use of the drugs in patients treated by "ordinary" doctors in "routine" medical practice.

Finally, there are some experiments which lose their entire point if all the cards are laid on the table. Take, for example, the investigation of the impact of a placebo. Although some patients report benefits from placebos even when they are told they are receiving "sugar pills," the full power of suggestibility and the patient-doctor relationship would almost certainly be affected by a discussion of the experiment with the subjects. This would be the medical equivalent of "bugging" a jury room to study the jurors' deliberations and then showing the jury the hidden microphones.[3]

Are there alternatives to "double-blind" placebo trials? (It is assumed that the obtaining of consent will be more feasible if patients do not have to agree to receive placebos.) One possibility, in drug investigation, is to demonstrate differences between a new drug and a standard drug. If the new one is significantly better, there is no problem. But what if it is significantly worse? This could mean that the drug is ineffective or merely that it is a *less* effective one—an important distinction. Another possibility is the use of dose-response relationships. If such relationships can be shown for new and old drugs in the same experiment, potency estimates can be made which are in no way dependent on the use of placebos. This is quite possible in a situation such as alleviation of postoperative pain, where the challenge is severe, the response to powerful analgesics is reasonably predictable, and placebos are thus rarely needed or used. In postpartum pain, however, dose-response relationships are rather difficult to elaborate, and the same may be true in studies of hypnotic drugs. This phenomenon has important implications for the admission of new drugs to the marketplace. If placebo studies are abandoned, will the FDA accept clinical comparisons where no dose-response relationships are evident? Not to do so may keep an effective drug off the market, but accepting at face value experiments where no difference is demonstrated between doses or drugs will surely result in the occasional admission of ineffective agents to the market.

Is some less formidable and stylized consent approach acceptable? It is apparently not, in regard to investigational drugs, unless one is willing to flaunt the FDA regulations. On the other hand, it may be possible to modify these regulations so as to make the consent provisions more flexible. If one eliminates the *written* aspects of the present informed consent regulations and substitutes verbal discussion (perhaps even placed on tape for

the record) it may be possible to avoid some of the threats to experimentation discussed above while at the same time insuring that a certain amount of discussion with the patient has occurred.[4] I believe that the degree of candor utilized in obtaining consent should be related not only to the specific psychological and clinical problems but also to the expected risks of the experiment.

There is also the possibility of monitoring experimentation by use of peer committees or lay-scientific review boards which go over protocols, checking them carefully for flaws of various kinds, including ethical ones. No investigator should be engaged in research that he would be ashamed to have judged by his scientific colleagues or by a responsible group of laymen and scientists. There is at least theoretical advantage to sharing problems of conscience and morality with individuals not directly involved in the research, and of course ample precedent exists in society for delegation of important decision-making powers to others, although I doubt the legal acceptability of such review as an *alternative* to informed patient consent. It should be remembered, however, that a peer review mechanism may safeguard a subject more efficiently than informed consent; some people will agree to undergo risks that an expert committee would veto on their behalf.

It has been suggested that one way of discouraging unethical research is for editors to prevent the publication of data obtained in unsavory experiments by refusing to accept such manuscripts. Although this is an attractive notion at first glance, one wonders whether in fact important data unethically obtained could or should really be buried in this way. If an unscrupulous investigator were to discover a cure for cancer, would it be ethical to keep this knowledge from being used by others for the benefit of cancer patients, in compulsive adherence to "principle"? Although it is often affirmed that the ends do not justify the means, our society often functions as if they do.

One way of improving the present situation would be to acquaint the public, the regulatory agencies, the governmental granting agencies, and hospital committees with the needs and problems of experimentation. The present FDA regulations on informed consent, for example, quite clearly are the result of a particular climate of opinion. The law is susceptible to change. I heard one distinguished Baltimore judge say recently that the purpose of the law is to harmonize progress with stability. Years ago a property owner possessed the land underneath his feet as far as it went and all of the air directly above his property. With the coming of the airplane, this concept has changed. Similarly, educational facilities once considered "separate but equal" are no longer considered "equal." The law reflects the needs and desires of society as society sees these needs and desires, and it is entirely consistent with history to expect an appropriate legal response from society if it becomes educated to the needs of science and the social benefits of research.[5]

One wonders how many of medicine's greatest advances might have been delayed or prevented by the rigid application of some currently proposed principles to research at large. Even physicians were in a sense intellectually and emotionally unprepared for the earliest triumphs of cardiac surgery. What, then, would have been the layman's reaction to a full exposition of the problems involved in the original Blalock-Taussig shunts? And what of cardiac catheterization? The benefits of this technique have, quite appropriately, won Nobel Prizes for three of the physicians who pioneered in its use, but is it difficult to imagine lay journalists dubbing the early experimentation of these men barbaric and Nazi-like? ("and then, dear readers, these monsters have the temerity to thrust a tube down the length of one's arm into the very chambers of the human heart! The mind of anyone not completely brutalized by prolonged immersion in the bloody charnel houses of Science boggles at the thought.") I doubt, on the other hand, that the public would back—provided they had the facts—legislation like that originally proposed by Senator Thaler in New York State, which would have prohibited pediatric research *of all kinds* in the absence of court orders. Others have already pointed out that such legislation would have rendered impossible the development of the poliomyelitis and other vaccines.

If society is to be educated, there are many items that might be put on the agenda for discussion. The desire to involve the patient in the decision-making process in regard to details of medical care implies that there should be fuller and franker discussion about the use of everything from drugs to surgical techniques. Whether the public wants this is a matter for debate; I personally doubt it. In my own experience as a physician and investigator, not only are patients usually incapable of making the decisions in question (which is not surprising) but they are usually not desirous of making such decisions. In considerable anxiety a lay friend once called me to say that his physician had disclosed to him the controversy over the long-term use of anticoagulants in the management of patients who had recovered from a cardiac infarct. My friend protested that he was in no position to judge whether his wife should receive anticoagulants and that he really would have preferred his physician to make this judgment. In many complex decision-making situations in medicine, the patient is really more in the position of being on an airplane that has defective landing gear, is running out of gas, and whose pilot has to make some sort of landing in one of several alternate places than in the position of a passenger who is asked whether he wishes to board a plane whose pilot indicates that he is about to fly for the first time with his eyes closed and "no hands."

How much should be told to a patient by a surgeon who is requesting permission to perform an established operation, but one he personally is attempting for the first time? How much should be told to a patient about the hazards of a debilitating series of diagnostic abdominal X-rays, which may subject him to days of restricted food and fluid intake, as well as repeated cathartics? How much should be told to individuals exposed to radiation of any kind, for diagnosis or therapy, in view of the evidence in both insects and mammals that *no* amount of radiation is innocent in regard to genetic damage?

There are many other points that require consideration. What special safeguards are required for the study of prisoners? Of children? Of the psychiatrically ill? Of the mentally retarded? Of the dying patient? If an experimental live virus vaccine is to be given to subjects, should consent also be obtained from neighbors or schoolmates who may pick up the virus from the volunteers and come down with the disease? Should the patients in the adjoining beds be asked for permission when a new antibiotic is given to a patient, in view of the ability of antibiotics to disturb the ecology of the normal bacteria resident in the body and cause the development of resistant strains which can then spread to these patients?

Should individuals be recompensed for damage suffered in the course of research, without any attempt to establish blame? The patient or volunteer who is injured by an experimental drug and loses his earning power thereby is entitled to compensation. The children of a patient who dies as the result of unanticipated mischief from a new diagnostic technique under investigation perhaps ought to expect financial remuneration. This implies not that the investigator must shoulder this burden alone but that the burden must be borne somehow. Who, then, shall pay the bill? In seeking an answer to this question, we should perhaps ask, "Who reaps the benefits of research?" While it is true that the investigator will gain when research is successful, and that with new drugs the pharmaceutical industry will profit, in the final analysis the beneficiary is really society as a whole. It would therefore seem incumbent on society to seek means of walking safely the narrow ledge between the twin abysses of hampered research and uncompensated patient injury. Scientists must not be reckless in their research; neither can they operate in an atmosphere of perpetual fear of disabling economic loss (or destroyed reputations) if unavoidable harm is the result of a well-planned experiment. Patients must not seek court settlements capriciously; neither must they silently suffer pain, injury, or death in the course of research. The problem is both subtle and complex and deserves an honest and equitable solution.

What should be society's attitude toward harm to the individual in return for benefits to the population as a whole? Mass chest X-ray surveys to detect treatable tuberculosis or other pulmonary diseases may cause leukemia in a few. Is the benefit worth the risk? Who shall decide? What means should be taken to safeguard the rights and health of individuals approached to participate in such a survey? Should a simple majority decide whether an entire community's water supply should be fluoridated? We have become reconciled to the ability of a governmental agency to expropriate our land or homes in order to build a new school or a new bridge, but it is not traditional to force anyone to participate in research. Yet society frequently tramples on the rights of individuals in the "greater interest." One can object, but can we deny the existence of the phenomenon? Should we have different guidelines for individual sacrifice when health or life is at stake, rather than property?

Finally, a word about the effective implantation of an ethical conscience in the minds of physicians and clinical investigators. The doctor becomes increasingly accustomed to a life which does not allow for leisurely contemplation. He is by trade a nonagnostic. Even when he makes a decision not to treat, for example, he is not suspending judgment but expressing the belief that "no treatment" is better than treatment. He must continually choose between remedies even when he has poor basis for making a choice. The doctor is likely to be propelled increasingly in the direction of quick decisions which at times resemble reflex responses. In this pragmatic, frenetic existence he may quickly absorb the moral atmosphere around him without questioning it. It is my conviction, therefore, that ethical problems must be integrated into the doctor's life at the earliest possible moment. I do not believe that it will be effective to bring up such matters relatively late in the medical career, although the doctor will certainly require constant reinforcement throughout his professional life. The medical student must be made, from the beginning, to consider the ethical aspects of medicine, in regard to *both* practice and research. Many a liver biopsy or laboratory test is now performed in the name of science, with little benefit to the patient. A medical student made emotionally immune to the casual performance of risky procedures by the tacit acceptance of such procedures by his mentors is unlikely to be excessively concerned as a physician or investigator with the subtleties of ethical and moral issues. Some way must be found to incorporate these matters so firmly into his moral fabric that he cannot avoid the ethical implications of his acts. I submit that the successful development of such an ethical conscience, combined with professional skill, will protect the patient or experimental subject much more effectively than any laws or regulations.

I have previously said that for the ethical, experienced investigator no laws are needed and for the unscrupulous incompetent no laws will help, except to allow the injured subjects to obtain compensation or to punish the offending scientists.

Between these extremes there still remain many investigators who will unquestionably be constrained in some way by legislation. But it is unlikely that subjects will be *optimally* protected from harm without additional safeguards imposed by the scientific community itself. These safeguards will range all the way from exercise of wisdom and judgment to the invoking of statistical monitoring techniques to halt experiments that were ethical at the outset but cannot ethically be continued.

Some are fond of quoting Claude Bernard when he said, in *An Introduction to the Study of Experimental Medicine*, "The principle of medical and surgical morality, therefore, consists in never performing on man an experiment which might be harmful to him in any extent, even though the result might be highly advantageous to science, i.e., to the health of others."[6] This statement is irrelevant to much of clinical investigation, where patients usually are involved in procedures that may be of considerable benefit to them, although they necessarily involve some risk (like almost everything else in the world). One might point out that Claude Bernard also said, "So, among the experiments that may be tried on man, those that can only harm are forbidden, those that are innocent are permissible, and those that may do good are obligatory."[7] The investigator is responsible not only to the patients currently under his care but also to the many that will never be seen by him. Is this responsibility to mankind less noble than that of the physician concerned with the care of the individual patient?

Bernard's statement is—like my own remarks—full of ambivalence. As J. Bronowski has put it, one of society's major tasks is to reconcile the welfare of man with the welfare of men.[8] In clinical investigation, as in other societal activities, the good of the individual and the good of society are often not identical and sometimes mutually exclusive. I believe it is inevitable that the many will continue to benefit on occasion from the contributions—sometimes involuntary—of the few. The problem is to know when to say "Halt!" There are some societal "gains" that may only be available at an excessively high price. We cannot afford to have the cancer of moral decay that comes from frequent and flagrant disregard of human rights gnawing away at the body of science. We should, therefore, in a very real sense welcome the present and continuing debate on

ethics in clinical investigation. That harm has come from exaggerated stories is unquestioned, as is the possibility that additional harm to patients may occur, but I believe that in the long run both the public and science will benefit from a searching analysis of the roots of our ethical conduct.

Notes

1. While the FDA rules apply only to investigational drugs, the issue of consent is relevant to all clinical investigation because of both legal implications and current National Institutes of Health policies on human experimentation which affect the conduct of grantees.

2. It is surrealistic to read, in an editorial in a leading American medical journal, the statement: "How much more important it is to have informed consent, when the potential risk is unknown!"

3. Dinnerstein et al., in an interesting paper, have reviewed some of the literature on the differential effects of drugs in different experimental settings. Their desire to study the effects of drugs "in a completely concealed form, with the subject not even knowing when he has been drugged" and under situations with different "cover stories" would be out of the question if rigid application of this principle of "total disclosure" were made. Albert J. Dinnerstein, Milton Lowenthal, and Bernard Blitz, "The Interaction of Drugs with Placebos in the Control of Pain and Anxiety," *Perspectives in Biology and Medicine*, 10 (1966), 103–117.

4. It is important to remember that there is no *necessary* relation between a consent procedure that satisfies the law and one that safeguards the patient.

5. John Dewey once warned that part of the public protest against experimentation is related to old misunderstandings and dreads about science. He was talking about animal experimentation, but it may be useful to remember his warning to be "on the alert against every revival of the spirit of animosity to discovery and to the application of the fruits of discovery." One does not need to accuse everyone who is concerned about the ethics of clinical investigation of being antiscientific to believe that at least some of the hue and cry can be traced to antiscientism.

6. Claude Bernard, *An Introduction to the Study of Experimental Medicine* (New York: Dover Publications, 1957), p. 101.

7. Ibid., p. 102.

8. J. Bronowski, *Science and Human Values* (London: Hutchinson & Co., 1961), p. 78.

Philosophical Reflections on Experimenting with Human Subjects

Hans Jonas

Experimenting with human subjects is going on in many fields of scientific and technological progress. It is designed to replace the overall instruction by natural, occasional experience with the selective information from artificial, systematic experiment which physical science has found so effective in dealing with inanimate nature. Of the new experimentation with man, medical is surely the most legitimate; psychological, the most dubious; biological (still to come), the most dangerous. I have chosen here to deal with the first only, where the case *for* it is strongest and the task of adjudicating conflicting claims hardest. . . .

The Peculiarity of Human Experimentation

Experimentation was originally sanctioned by natural science. There it is performed on inanimate objects, and this raises no moral problems. But as soon as animate, feeling beings become the subjects of experiment, as they do in the life sciences and especially in medical research, this innocence of the search for knowledge is lost and questions of conscience arise. The depth to which moral and religious sensibilities can become aroused over these questions is shown by the vivisection issue. Human experimentation must sharpen the issue as it involves ultimate questions of personal dignity and sacrosanctity. One profound difference between the human experiment and the physical (besides that between animate and inanimate, feeling and unfeeling nature) is this: The physical experiment employs small-scale, artificially devised substitutes for that about which knowledge is to be obtained, and the experimenter extrapolates from these models and simulated conditions to nature at large. Something deputizes for the "real thing"—balls rolling down an inclined plane for sun and planets, electric discharges from a condenser for real lightning, and so on. For the most part, no such substitution is possible in the biological sphere. We must operate on the original itself, the real thing in the fullest sense, and perhaps affect it irreversibly. No simulacrum can take its place. Especially in the human sphere, experimentation loses entirely the advantage of the clear division between vicarious model and true object. Up to a point, animals may fulfill the proxy role of the classical physical experiment. But in the end man himself must furnish knowledge about himself, and the comfortable separation of noncommital experiment and definitive action vanishes. An experiment in education affects the lives of its subjects, perhaps a whole generation of schoolchildren. Human experimentation for whatever purpose is always *also* a responsible, nonexperimental, definitive dealing with the subject himself. And not even the noblest purpose abrogates the obligations this involves.

This is the root of the problem with which we are faced: Can both that purpose and this obligation be satisfied? If not, what would be a just compromise? Which side should give way to the other? The question is inherently philosophical as it concerns not merely pragmatic difficulties and their arbitration, but a genuine conflict of values involving principles of a high order. May I put conflict in these terms. On principle, it is felt, human beings *ought* not to be dealt with in that way (the "guinea pig" protest); on the other hand, such dealings are increasingly urged on us by considerations, in turn appealing to principle, that claim to override those objections. Such a claim must be carefully assessed, especially when it is swept along by a mighty tide. Putting the matter thus, we have already made one important assumption rooted in our "Western" cultural tradition: The prohibitive rule is, to that way of thinking, the primary and axiomatic one; the permissive counter-rule, as qualifying the first, is secondary and stands in need of justification. We must justify the infringement of a primary inviolability, which needs no justification itself; and the

Reprinted by permission of Daedalus, *Journal of the American Academy of Arts and Sciences, Spring 1969, Boston, Mass. This essay is included, on pp. 105–131, in a 1980 reedition of Jonas's* Philosophical Essays: From Current Creed to Technological Man, *published by the University of Chicago Press.*

justification of its infringement must be by values and needs of a dignity commensurate with those to be sacrificed.

Health as a Public Good

The cause invoked [for medical experimentation] is health and, in its more critical aspect, life itself—clearly superlative goods that the physician serves directly by curing and the researcher indirectly by the knowledge gained through his experiments. There is no question about the good served or about the evil fought—disease and premature death. But a good to whom and an evil to whom? Here the issue tends to become somewhat clouded. In the attempt to give experimentation the proper dignity (on the problematic view that a value becomes greater by being "social" instead of merely individual), the health in question or the disease in question is somehow predicated on the social whole, as if it were society that, in the persons of its members enjoyed the one and suffered the other. For the purposes of our problem, public interest can then be pitted against private interest, the common good against the individual good. Indeed, I have found health called a national resource, which of course it is, but surely not in the first place.

In trying to resolve some of the complexities and ambiguities lurking in these conceptualizations, I have pondered a particular statement, made in the form of a question, which I found in the *Proceedings* of the earlier *Daedalus* conference: "Can society afford to discard the tissues and organs of the hopelessly unconscious patient when they could be used to restore the otherwise hopelessly ill, but still salvageable individual?" And somewhat later: "A strong case can be made that society can ill afford to discard the tissues and organs of the hopelessly unconscious patient; they are greatly needed for study and experimental trial to help those who can be salvaged."[1] I hasten to add that any suspicion of callousness that the "commodity" language of these statements may suggest is immediately dispelled by the name of the speaker, Dr. Henry K. Beecher, for whose humanity and moral sensibility there can be nothing but admiration. But the use, in all innocence, of this language gives food for thought. Let me,

for a moment, take the question literally. "Discarding" implies proprietary rights—nobody can discard what does not belong to him in the first place. Does society then own my body? "Salvaging" implies the same and, moreover, a use-value to the owner. Is the life-extension of certain individuals then a public interest? "Affording" implies a critically vital level of such an interest—that is, of the loss or gain involved. And "society" itself—what is it? When does a need, an aim, an obligation become social? Let us reflect on some of these terms.

What Society Can Afford

"Can Society afford . . .?" Afford what? To let people die intact, thereby withholding something from other people who desperately need it, who in consequence will have to die too? These other, unfortunate people indeed cannot afford not to have a kidney, heart, or other organ of the dying patient, on which they depend for an extension of their lease on life; but does that give them a right to it? And does it oblige society to procure it for them? What is it that *society* can or cannot afford—leaving aside for the moment the question of what it has a *right* to? It surely can afford to lose members through death; more than that, it is built on the balance of death and birth decreed by the order of life. This is too general, of course, for our question, but perhaps it is well to remember. The specific question seems to be whether society can afford to let some people die whose death might be deferred by particular means if these were authorized by society. Again, if it is merely a question of what society can or cannot afford, rather than of what it ought or ought not to do, the answer must be: Of course, it can. If cancer, heart disease, and other organic, noncontagious ills, especially those tending to strike the old more than the young, continue to exact their toll at the normal rate of incidence (including the toll of private anguish and misery), society can go on flourishing in every way.

Here, by contrast, are some examples of what, in sober truth, society cannot afford. It cannot afford to let an epidemic rage unchecked; a persistent excess of deaths over births, but neither—we must add—too great an excess of births over deaths; too low an average life expectancy even if demographically balanced by fertility, but neither too great a longevity with the necessitated correlative dearth of youth in the social body; a debilitating state of general heath; and things of this kind. These are plain cases where the whole condition of society is critically affected, and the public interest can make its imperative claims. The Black Death of the Middle Ages was a *public* calamity of the acute kind; the life-sapping ravages of endemic malaria or sleeping sickness in certain areas are a public calamity of the chronic kind. Such situations a society as a whole can truly not "afford," and they may call for extraordinary remedies, including, perhaps, the invasion of private sacrosanctities.

This is not entirely a matter of numbers and numerical ratios. Society, in a subtler sense, cannot "afford" a single miscarriage of justice, a single inequity in the dispensation of its laws, the violation of the rights of even the tiniest minority, because these undermine the moral basis on which society's existence rests. Nor can it, for a similar reason, afford the absence or atrophy in its midst of compassion and of the effort to alleviate suffering—be it widespread or rare—one form of which is the effort to conquer disease of any kind, whether "socially" significant (by reasons of number) or not. And in short, society cannot afford the absence among its members of *virtue*, with its readiness for sacrifice beyond defined duty. Since its presence—that is to say, that of personal idealism—is a matter of grace and not of decree, we have the paradox that society depends for its existence on intangibles of nothing less than a religious order, for which it can hope, but which it cannot enforce. All the more must it protect this most precious capital from abuse.

For what objectives connected with the medico-biological sphere should this reserve be drawn upon—for example, in the form of accepting, soliciting, perhaps even imposing the submission of human subjects to experimentation? We postulate that this must be not just a worthy cause, as any promotion of the health of anybody doubtlessly is, but a cause qualifying for transcendent social sanction. Here one thinks first of those cases critically affecting the whole condition, present and future, of the community we have illustrated. Something equivalent to what in the political sphere is called

"clear and present danger" may be invoked and a state of emergency proclaimed, thereby suspending certain otherwise inviolable prohibitions and taboos. We may observe that averting a disaster always carries greater weight than promoting a good. Extraordinary danger excuses extraordinary means. This covers human experimentation, which we would like to count, as far as possible, among the extraordinary rather than the ordinary means of serving the common good under public auspices. Naturally, since foresight and responsibility for the future are of the essence of institutional society, averting disaster extends into long-term prevention, although the lesser urgency will warrant less sweeping licenses.

Society and the Cause of Progress

Much weaker is the case where it is a matter not of saving but of improving society. Much of medical research falls into this category. As stated before, a permanent death rate from heart failure or cancer does not threaten society. So long as certain statistical ratios are maintained, the incidence of disease and of disease-induced mortality is not (in the strict sense) a "social" misfortune. I hasten to add that it is not therefore less of a human misfortune, and the call for relief issuing with silent eloquence from each victim and all potential victims is of no lesser dignity. But it is misleading to equate the fundamentally human response to it with what is owed to society: it is owed by man to man—and it is thereby owed by society to the individuals as soon as the adequate ministering to these concerns outgrows (as it progressively does) the scope of private spontaneity and is made a public mandate. It is thus that society assumes responsibility for medical care, research, old age, and innumerable other things not originally of the public realm (in the original "social contract"), and they become duties toward "society" (rather than directly toward one's fellow man) by the fact that they are socially operated.

Indeed, we expect from organized society no longer mere protection against harm and the securing of the conditions of our preservation, but active and constant improvement in all the domains of life: the waging of the battle against nature, the enhancement of the human estate—in short, the promotion of progress. This is an expansive goal, one far surpassing the disaster norm of our previous reflections. It lacks the urgency of the latter, but has the nobility of the free, forward thrust. It surely is worth sacrifices. It is not at all a question of what society can afford, but of what it is committed to, beyond all necessity, by our mandate. Its trusteeship has become an established, ongoing, institutionalized business of the body politic. As eager beneficiaries of its gains, we now owe to "society," as its chief agent, our individual contributions toward its *continued pursuit*. I emphasize "continued pursuit." Maintaining the existing level requires no more than the orthodox means of taxation and enforcement of professional standards that raise no problems. The more optional goal of pushing forward is also more exacting. We have this syndrome: Progress is by our choosing an acknowledged interest of society, in which we have a stake in various degrees; science is a necessary instrument of progress; research is a necessary instrument of science; and in medical science experimentation on human subjects is a necessary instrument of research. Therefore, human experimentation has come to be a societal interest.

The destination of research is essentially melioristic. It does not serve the preservation of the existing good from which I profit myself and to which I am obligated. Unless the present state is intolerable, the melioristic goal is in a sense gratuitous, and this not only from the vantage point of the present. Our descendants have a right to be left an unplundered planet; they do not have a right to new miracle cures. We have sinned against them, if by our doing we have destroyed their inheritance—which we are doing at full blast; we have not sinned against them if by the time they come around arthritis has not yet been conquered (unless by sheer neglect). And generally, in the matter of progress, as humanity had no claim on a Newton, a Michelangelo, or a St. Francis to appear, and no right to the blessings of their unscheduled deeds, so progress, with all our methodical labor for it, cannot be budgeted in advance and its fruits received as a due. Its coming-about at all and its turning out for good (of which we can never be sure) must rather be regarded as something akin to grace.

The Melioristic Goal, Medical Research, and Individual Duty

Nowhere is the melioristic goal more inherent than in medicine. To the physician, it is not gratuitous. He is committed to curing and thus to improving the power to cure. Gratuitous we called it (outside disaster conditions) as a *social* goal, but noble at the same time. Both the nobility and the gratuitousness must influence the manner in which self-sacrifice for it is elicited, and even its free offer accepted. Freedom is certainly the first condition to be observed here. The surrender of one's body to medical experimentation is entirely outside the enforceable "social contract."

Or can it be construed to fall within its terms—namely, as repayment for benefits from past experimentation that I have enjoyed myself? But I am indebted for these benefits not to society, but to the past "martyrs," to whom society is indebted itself, and society has no right to call in my personal debt by way of adding new to its own. Moreover, gratitude is not an enforceable social obligation; it anyway does not mean that I must emulate the deed. Most of all, if it was wrong to exact such sacrifice in the first place, it does not become right to exact it again with the plea of the profit it has brought me. If, however, it was not exacted, but entirely free, as it ought to have been, then it should remain so, and its precedence must not be used as a social pressure on others for doing the same under the sign of duty.

• • •

The "Conscription" of Consent

The mere issuing of the appeal, the calling for volunteers, with the moral and social pressures it inevitably generates, amounts even under the most meticulous rules of consent to a sort of *conscripting*. And some soliciting is necessarily involved. . . . And this is why "consent," surely a nonnegotiable minimum requirement, is not the full answer to the problem. Granting then that soliciting and therefore some degree of conscripting are part of the situation, who may conscript and who may be conscripted? Or less harshly expressed: Who should issue appeals and to whom?

The naturally qualified issuer of the appeal is the research scientist himself, collectively the main carrier of the impulse and the only one with the technical competence to judge. But his being very much an interested party (with vested interests, indeed, not purely in the public good, but in the scientific enterprise as such, in "his" project, and even in his career) makes him also suspect. The ineradicable dialectic of this situation—a delicate incompatibility problem—calls for particular controls by the research community and by public authority that we need not discuss. They can mitigate, but not eliminate the problem. We have to live with the ambiguity, the treacherous impurity of everything human.

Self-Recruitment of the Community

To whom should the appeal be addressed? The natural issuer of the call is also the first natural addressee: the physician-researcher himself and the scientific confraternity at large. With such a coincidence—indeed, the noble tradition with which the whole business of human experimentation started—almost all of the associated legal, ethical, and metaphysical problems vanish. If it is full, autonomous identification of the subject with the purpose that is required for the dignifying of his serving as a subject—here it is; if strongest motivation—here it is; if fullest understanding— here it is; if freest decision—here it is; if greatest integration with the person's total, chosen pursuit—here it is. With the fact of self-solicitation the issue of consent in all its insoluble equivocality is bypassed per se. Not even the condition that the particular purpose be truly important and the project reasonably promising, which must hold in any solicitation of others, need be satisfied here. By himself, the scientist is free to obey his obsession, to play his hunch, to wager on chance, to follow the lure of ambition. It is all part of the "divine madness" that somehow animates the ceaseless pressing against frontiers. For the rest of society, which has a deep-seated disposition to look with reverence and awe upon the guardians of the mysteries of life, the profession assumes with this proof of its devotion the role of a self-chosen, consecrated fraternity, not unlike the monastic orders of the past, and this would come nearest to the actual, religious origins of the art of healing.

• • •

"Identification" as the Principle of Recruitment in General

If the properties we adduced as the particular qualifications of the members of the scientific fraternity itself are taken as general criteria of selection, then one should look for additional subjects where a maximum of identification, understanding, and spontaneity can be expected—that is, among the most highly motivated, the most highly educated, and the least "captive" members of the community. From this naturally scarce resource, a descending order of permissibility leads to greater abundance and ease of supply, whose use should become proportionately more hesitant as the exculpating criteria are relaxed. An inversion of normal "market" behavior is demanded here —namely, to accept the lowest quotation last (and excused only by the greatest pressure of need); to pay the highest price first.

The ruling principle in our considerations is that the "wrong" of reification can only be made "right" by such authentic identification with the cause that it is the subject's as well as the researcher's cause—whereby his role in its service is not just permitted by him, but *willed*. That sovereign will of his which embraces the end as his own restores his personhood to the otherwise depersonalizing context. To be valid it must be autonomous and informed. The latter condition can, outside the research community, only be fulfilled by degrees; but the higher the degree of understanding regarding the purpose and the technique, the more valid becomes the endorsement of the will. A margin of mere trust inevitably remains. Ultimately, the appeal for volunteers should seek this free and generous endorsement, the appropriation of the research purpose into the person's own scheme of ends. Thus, the appeal is in truth addressed to the one, mysterious, and sacred source of any such generosity of the will— "devotion," whose forms and objects of commitment are various and may invest different motivations in different individuals. The following, for instance, may be responsive to the "call" we are discussing: compassion with human suffering, zeal for humanity, reverence for the Golden Rule, enthusiasm for progress, homage to the cause of knowledge, even longing for sacrificial justification (do not call that "masochism," please). On all these, I say, it is defensible and right to draw when the research objective is worthy enough; and it is a prime duty of the research community (especially in view of what we called the "margin of trust") to see that this sacred source is never abused for frivolous ends. For a less than adequate cause, not even the freest, unsolicited offer should be accepted.

The Rule of the "Descending Order" and its Counterutility Sense

We have laid down what must seem to be a forbidding rule to the number-hungry research industry. Having faith in the transcendent potential of man, I do not fear that the "source" will ever fail a society that does not destroy it—and only such a one is worthy of the blessings of progress. But "elitistic" the rule is (as is the enterprise of progress itself), and elites are by nature small. The combined attribute of motivation and information, plus the absence of external pressures, tends to be socially so circumscribed that strict adherence to the rule might numerically starve the research process. This is why I spoke of a descending order of permissibility, which is itself permissive, but where the realization that it is a *descending* order is not without pragmatic import. Departing from the august norm, the appeal must needs shift from idealism to docility, from high-mindedness to compliance, from judgment to trust. Consent spreads over the whole spectrum. I will not go into the casuistics of this penumbral area. I merely indicate the principle of the order of preference: The poorer in knowledge, motivation, and freedom of decision (and that, alas, means the more readily available in terms of numbers and possible manipulation), the more sparingly and indeed reluctantly should the reservoir be used, and the more compelling must therefore become the countervailing justification.

Let us note that this is the opposite of a social utility standard, the reverse of the order by "availability and expendability": The most valuable and scarcest, the least expendable elements of the social organism, are to be the first candidates for risk and sacrifice. It is the standard of *noblesse oblige;* and with all its counterutility and seeming "wastefulness," we feel a rightness about it and

perhaps even a higher "utility," for the soul of the community lives by this spirit.[2] It is also the opposite of what the day-to-day interests of research clamor for, and for the scientific community to honor it will mean that it will have to fight a strong temptation to go by routine to the readiest sources of supply—the suggestible, the ignorant, the dependent, the "captive" in various senses.[3] I do not believe that heightened resistance here must cripple research, which cannot be permitted; but it may indeed slow it down by the smaller numbers fed into experimentation in consequence. This price—a possibly slower rate of progress—may have to be paid for the preservation of the most precious capital of higher communal life.

Experimentation on Patients

So far we have been speaking on the tacit assumption that the subjects of experimentation are recruited from among the healthy. To the question "Who is conscriptable?" the spontaneous answer is: Least and last of all the sick—the most available of all as they are under treatment and observation anyway. That the afflicted should not be called upon to bear additional burden and risk, that they are society's special trust and the physician's trust in particular—these are elementary responses of our moral sense. Yet the very destination of medical research, the conquest of disease, requires at the crucial stage trial and verification on precisely the sufferers from the disease, and their total exemption would defeat the purpose itself. In acknowledging this inescapable necessity, we enter the most sensitive area of the whole complex, the one most keenly felt and most searchingly discussed by the practitioners themselves. No wonder, it touches the heart of the doctor-patient relation, putting its most solemn obligations to the test. There is nothing new in what I have to say about the ethics of the doctor-patient relation, but for the purpose of confronting it with the issue of experimentation some of the oldest verities must be recalled.

The Fundamental Privilege of the Sick

In the course of treatment, the physician is obligated to the patient and to no one else. He is not the agent of society, nor of the interests of medical science, nor of the patient's family, nor of his cosufferers, nor of future sufferers from the same disease. The patient alone counts when he is under the physician's care. By the simple law of bilateral contract (analogous, for example, to the relation of lawyer to client and its "conflict of interest" rule), the physician is bound not to let any other interest interfere with that of the patient in being cured. But manifestly more sublime norms than contractual ones are involved. We may speak of a sacred trust; strictly by its terms, the doctor is, as it were, alone with his patient and God.

There is one normal exception to this—that is, to the doctor's not being the agent of society vis-à-vis the patient, but the trustee of his interests alone: the quarantining of the contagious sick. This is plainly not for the patient's interest, but for that of others threatened by him. (In vaccination, we have a combination of both: protection of the individual and others.) But preventing the patient from causing harm to others is not the same as exploiting him for the advantage of others. And there is, of course, the abnormal exception of collective catastrophe, the analogue to a state of war. The physician who desperately battles a raging epidemic is under a unique dispensation that suspends in a nonspecifiable way some of the structures of normal practice, including possibly those against experimental liberties with his patients. No rules can be devised for the waiving of rules in extremities. And as with the famous shipwreck examples of ethical theory, the less said about it the better. But what is allowable there and may later be passed over in forgiving silence cannot serve as a precedent. We are concerned with non-extreme, non-emergency conditions where the voice of principle can be heard and claims can be adjudicated free from duress. We have conceded that there are such claims, and that if there is to be medical advance at all, not even the superlative privilege of the suffering and the sick can be kept wholly intact from the intrusion of its needs. About this least palatable, most disquieting part of our subject, I have to offer only groping, inconclusive remarks.

The Principle of "Identification" Applied to Patients

On the whole, the same principles would seem to hold here as are found to hold with "normal subjects": motivation, identification, understanding on the part of the subject. But it is clear that these conditions are peculiarly difficult to satisfy with regard to a patient. His physical state, psychic preoccupation, dependent relation to the doctor, the submissive attitude induced by treatment—everything connected with his condition and situation makes the sick person inherently less of a sovereign person than the healthy one. Spontaneity of self-offering was almost to be ruled out; consent is marred by lower resistance or captive circumstance, and so on. In fact, all the factors that make the patient, as a category, particularly accessible and welcome for experimentation at the same time compromise the quality of the responding affirmation that must morally redeem the making use of them. This, in addition to the primacy of the physician's duty, puts a heightened onus on the physician-researcher to limit his undue power to the most important and defensible research objectives and, of course, to keep persuasion at a minimum.

Still, with all the disabilities noted, there is scope among patients for observing the rule of the "descending order of permissibility" that we have laid down for normal subjects, in vexing inversion of the utility order of quantitative abundance and qualitative "expendability." By the principle of this order, those patients who most identify with and are cognizant of the cause of research—members of the medical profession (who after all are sometimes patients themselves)—come first; the highly motivated and educated, also least dependent, among the lay patients come next; and so on down the line. An added consideration here is seriousness of condition, which again operates in inverse proportion. Here the profession must fight the tempting sophistry that the hopeless case is expendable (because in prospect already expended) and therefore especially usable; and generally the attitude that the poorer the chances of the patient, the more justifiable his recruitment for experimentation (other than for his own benefit). The opposite is true.

Nondisclosure as a Borderline Case

Then there is the case where ignorance of the subject, sometimes even of the experimenter, is of the essence of the experiment (the "double blind"-control group-placebo syndrome). It is said to be a necessary element of the scientific process. Whatever may be said about its ethics in regard to normal subjects, especially volunteers, it is an outright betrayal of trust in regard to the patient who believes that he is receiving treatment. Only supreme importance of the objective can exonerate it, without making it less of a transgression. The patient is definitely wronged even when not harmed. And ethics apart, the practice of such deception holds the danger of undermining the faith in the *bona fides* of treatment, the beneficial intent of the physician—the very basis of the doctor-patient relationship. In every respect it follows that concealed experiment on patients—that is, experiment under the guise of treatment—should be the rarest exception, at best, if it cannot be wholly avoided.

This has still the merit of a borderline problem. The same is not true of the other case of necessary ignorance of the subject—that of the unconscious patient. Drafting him for nontherapeutic experiments is simply and unqualifiedly impermissible; progress or not, he must never be used, on the inflexible principle that utter helplessness demands utter protection.

When preparing this paper, I filled pages with a casuistics of this harrowing field, but then scrapped most of it, realizing my dilettant status. The shadings are endless, and only the physician-researcher can discern them properly as the cases arise. Into his lap the decision is thrown. The philosophical rule, once it has admitted into itself the idea of a sliding scale, cannot really specify its own application. It can only impress on the practitioner a general maxim or attitude for the exercise of his judgment and conscience in the concrete occasions of his work. In our case, I am afraid, it means making life more difficult for him.

It will also be noted that, somewhat at variance with the emphasis in the literature, I have not dwelt on the element of "risk" and very little on that of "consent." Discussion of the first is beyond the layman's competence; the emphasis on the second has been lessened because of its equivocal character. It is a truism to say that one should strive to minimize the risk and to maximize the consent. The more demanding concept of "identification," which I have used, includes "consent" in its maximal or authentic form, and the assumption of risk is its privilege.

No Experiments on Patients Unrelated to Their Own Disease

Although my ponderings have, on the whole, yielded points of view rather than definite prescriptions, premises rather than conclusions, they have led me to a few unequivocal yeses and nos. The first is the emphatic rule that patients should be experimented upon, if at all, *only* with reference to *their disease*. Never should there be added to the gratuitousness of the experiment as such the gratuitousness of service to an unrelated cause. This follows simply from what we have found to be the *only* excuse for infracting the special exemption of the sick at all—namely, that the scientific war on disease cannot accomplish its goal without drawing the sufferers from disease into the investigative process. If under this excuse they become subjects of experiment, they do so *because*, and only because, of *their* disease.

This is the fundamental and self-sufficient consideration. That the patient cannot possibly benefit from the unrelated experiment therapeutically, while he might from experiment related to his condition, is also true, but lies beyond the problem area of pure experiment. I am in any case discussing nontherapeutic experimentation only, where *ex hypothesi* the patient does not benefit. Experiment as part of therapy—that is, directed toward helping the subject himself—is a different matter altogether and raises its own problems but hardly philosophical ones. As long as a doctor can say, even if only in his own thought: "There is no known cure for your condition (or: You have responded to none); but there is promise in a new treatment still under investigation, not quite tested yet as to effectiveness and safety; you will be taking a chance, but all things considered, I judge it in your best interest to let me try it on you"—as long as he can speak thus, he speaks as the patient's physician and may err, but does not transform the patient into a subject of experimentation. Introduction of an untried therapy into the treatment where the tried ones have failed is not "experimentation on the patient."

Generally, and almost needless to say, with all the rules of the book, there is something "experimental" (because tentative) about every individual treatment, beginning with the diagnosis itself; and he would be a poor doctor who would not learn from every case for the benefit of future cases, and a poor member of the profession who would not make any new insights gained from his treatments available to the profession at large. Thus, knowledge may be advanced in the treatment of any patient, and the interest of the medical art and all sufferers from the same affliction as well as the patient himself may be served if something happens to be learned from his case. But his gain to knowledge and future therapy is incidental to the *bona fide* service to the present patient. He has the right to expect that the doctor does nothing to him just in order to learn.

In that case, the doctor's imaginary speech would run, for instance, like this: "There is nothing more I can do for you. But you can do something for me. Speaking no longer as your physician but on behalf of medical science, we could learn a great deal about future cases of this kind if you would permit me to perform certain experiments on you. It is understood that you yourself would not benefit from any knowledge we might gain; but future patients would." This statement would express the purely experimental situation, assumedly here with the subject's concurrence and with all cards on the table. In Alexander Bickel's words: "It is a different situation when the doctor is no longer trying to make [the patient] well, but is trying to find out how to make others well in the future."[4]

But even in the second case, that of the nontherapeutic experiment where the patient does not benefit, at least the patient's own disease is enlisted in the cause of fighting that disease, even if only in others. It is yet another thing to say or think: "Since you are here—in the hospital with its facilities—anyway, under our care and observation anyway, away from your job (or, perhaps, doomed) anyway, we wish to profit from your being available for some other research of great interest we are presently engaged in." From the standpoint of merely medical ethics, which has only to consider risk, consent, and the worth of the objective, there may be no cardinal difference between this case and the last one. I hope that the medical reader will not think I am making too fine a point when I say that from the standpoint of the subject and his dignity there is a cardinal difference that crosses the line between the permissible and the impermissible, and this by the same principle of "Identification" I have been invoking all along. Whatever the rights and wrongs of any experimentation on any patient—in the one case, at least that residue of identification is left him that it is his own affliction by which he can contribute to the conquest of that affliction, his own kind of suffering which he helps to alleviate in others; and so in a sense it is his own cause. It is totally indefensible to rob the unfortunate of this intimacy with the purpose and make his misfortune a convenience for the furtherance of alien concerns.

Conclusion

. . . I wish only to say in conclusion that if some of the practical implications of my reasonings are felt to work out toward a slower rate of progress, this should not cause too great dismay. Let us not forget that progress is an optional goal, not an unconditional commitment, and that its tempo in particular, compulsive as it may become, has nothing sacred about it. Let us also remember that a slower progress in the conquest of disease would not threaten society, grievous as it is to those who have to deplore that their particular disease be not yet conquered, but that society would indeed be threatened by the erosion of those moral values whose loss, possibly caused by too ruthless a pursuit of scientific progress, would make its most dazzling triumphs not worth having. Let us finally remember that it cannot be the aim of progress to abolish the lot of mortality. Of some ill or other, each of us will die. Our mortal condition is upon us with its harshness but also its wisdom—because without it there would not be the eternally renewed promise of the freshness, immediacy, and eagerness of youth; nor would there be for any of us the incentive to number our days and make them count. With all our striving to wrest from our mortality what we can, we should bear its burden with patience and dignity.

Notes

1. *Proceedings of the Conference on the Ethical Aspects of Experimentation on Human Subjects,* November 3–4, 1967 (Boston, Massachusetts; hereafter called *Proceedings*), pp. 50–51.

2. Socially, everyone is expendable relatively—that is, in different degrees; religiously, no one is expendable absolutely: The "image of God" is in

all. If it can be enhanced, then it is not by anyone being expended, but by someone expending himself.

3.   This refers to captives of circumstance, not of justice. Prison inmates are, with respect to our problem, in a special class. If we hold to some idea of guilt, and to the supposition that our judicial system is not entirely at fault, they may be held to stand in a special debt to society, and their offer to serve—from whatever motive—may be accepted with a minimum of qualms as a means of reparation.

4.   *Proceedings,* p. 33.

Informed (But Uneducated) Consent

F. J. Ingelfinger

The trouble with informed consent is that it is not educated consent. Let us assume that the experimental subject, whether a patient, a volunteer, or otherwise enlisted, is exposed to a completely honest array of factual detail. He is told of the medical uncertainty that exists and that must be resolved by research endeavors, of the time and discomfort involved, and of the tiny percentage risk of some serious consequences of the test procedure. He is also reassured of his rights and given a formal, quasi-legal statement to read. No exculpatory language is used. With his written signature, the subject then caps the transaction, and whether he sees himself as a heroic martyr for the sake of mankind, or as a reluctant guinea pig dragooned for the benefit of science, or whether, perhaps, he is merely bewildered, he obviously has given his "informed consent." Because established routines have been scrupulously observed, the doctor, the lawyer, and the ethicist are content.

But the chances are remote that the subject really understands what he has consented to—in the sense that the responsible medical investigator understands the goals, nature, and hazards of his study. How can the layman comprehend the importance of his perhaps not receiving, as determined by luck of the draw, the highly touted new treatment that his roommate will get? How can he appreciate the sensation of living for days with a multi-lumen intestinal tube passing through his mouth and pharynx? How can he interpret the information that an intravascular catheter and radiopaque dye injection have an 0.01 per cent probability of leading to a dangerous thrombosis or cardiac arrhythmia? It is moreover quite unlikely that any patient-subject can see himself accurately within the broad context of the situation, to weigh the inconveniences and hazards that he will have to undergo against the improvements that the research project may bring to the management of his disease in general and to his own case in particular. The difficulty that the public has in understanding information that is both medical and stressful is exemplified by [a report that] only half the families given genetic counseling grasped its impact.[1]

Nor can the information given to the experimental subject be in any sense totally complete. It would be impractical and probably unethical for the investigator to present the nearly endless list of all possible contingencies; in fact, he may not himself be aware of every untoward thing that might happen. Extensive detail, moreover, usually enhances the subject's confusion. Epstein and Lasagna showed that comprehension of medical information given to untutored subjects is inversely correlated with the elaborateness of the material presented.[2] The inconsiderate investigator, indeed, conceivably could exploit his authority and knowledge and extract "informed consent" by overwhelming the candidate-subject with information.

Ideally, the subject should give his consent freely, under no duress whatsoever. The facts are that some element of coercion is instrumental in any investigator-subject transaction. Volunteers for experiments will usually be influenced by

Reprinted by permission from the New England Journal of Medicine *287, 9 (August 31, 1972): 465–466.*
Editor's Note: The notes in this essay have been renumbered.

hopes of obtaining better grades, earlier parole, more substantial egos, or just mundane cash. These pressures, however, are but fractional shadows of those enclosing the patient-subject. Incapacitated and hospitalized because of illness, frightened by strange and impersonal routines, and fearful for his health and perhaps life, he is far from exercising a free power of choice when the person to whom he anchors all his hopes asks, "Say, you wouldn't mind, would you, if you joined some of the other patients on this floor and helped us to carry out some very important research we are doing?" When "informed consent" is obtained, it is not the student, the destitute bum, or the prisoner to whom, by virtue of his condition, the thumb screws of coercion are most relentlessly applied; it is the most used and useful of all experimental subjects, the patient with disease.

When a man or woman agrees to act as an experimental subject, therefore, his or her consent is marked by neither adequate understanding nor total freedom of choice. The conditions of the agreement are a far cry from those visualized as ideal. Jonas would have the subject identify with the investigative endeavor so that he and the researcher would be seeking a common cause: "Ultimately, the appeal for volunteers should seek . . . free and generous endorsement, the appropriation of the research purpose into the person's [i.e., the subject's] own scheme of ends."[3] For Ramsey, "informed consent" should represent a "covenantal bond between consenting man and consenting man [that] makes them . . . joint adventurers in medical care and progress."[4] Clearly, to achieve motivations and attitudes of this lofty type, an educated and understanding, rather than merely informed, consent is necessary.

Although it is unlikely that the goals of Jonas and of Ramsey will ever be achieved, and that human research subjects will spontaneously volunteer rather than be "conscripted,"[3] efforts to promote educated consent are in order. In view of the current emphasis on involving "the community" in such activities as regional planning, operation of clinics, and assignment of priorities, the general public and its political leaders are showing an increased awareness and understanding of medical affairs. But the orientation of this public interest in medicine is chiefly socioeconomic. Little has been done to give the public a basic understanding of medical research and its requirements not only for the people's money but also for their participation. The public, to be sure, is being subjected to a bombardment of sensation-mongering news stories and books that feature "breakthroughs," or that reveal real or alleged exploitations—horror stories of Nazi-type experimentation on abused human minds and bodies. Muckraking is essential to expose malpractices, but unless accompanied by efforts to promote a broader appreciation of medical research and its methods, it merely compounds the difficulties for both the investigator and the subject when "informed consent" is solicited.

The procedure currently approved in the United States for enlisting human experimental subjects has one great virtue: patient-subjects are put on notice that their management is in part at least an experiment. The deceptions of the past are no longer tolerated. Beyond this accomplishment, however, the process of obtaining "informed consent," with all its regulations and conditions, is no more than an elaborate ritual, a device that, when the subject is uneducated and uncomprehending, confers no more than the semblance of propriety on human experimentation. The subject's only real protection, the public as well as the medical profession must recognize, depends on the conscience and compassion of the investigator and his peers.

Notes

1. [Leonard, Claire O., et al. Genetic counseling: a consumer's view. N Engl J Med 287:433–449, 1972.]

2. Epstein, L. C., Lasagna, L. Obtaining informed consent: form or substance. Arch Intern Med 123:682–688, 1969.

3. Jonas, H. Philosophical reflections on experimenting with human subjects. Daedalus 98:219–247, Spring, 1969.

4. Ramsey, P. The ethics of a cottage industry in an age of community and research medicine. N Engl J Med 284:700–706, 1971.

A Moral Theory of Consent

Benjamin Freedman

Most medical codes of ethics, and most physicians, agree that the physician ought to obtain the "free and informed consent" of his subject or patient before attempting any serious medical procedures, experimental or therapeutic in nature. They agree, moreover, that a proxy consent ought to be obtained on behalf of the incompetent subject. And informed consent is seen as not merely a legal requirement, and not merely a formality: it is a substantial requirement of morality.

Acceptance of this doctrine, however, requires the solution of a number of problems. How much information need be imparted? At what age is a person mature enough to consent on his own behalf? Can prisoners give a "free and informed consent" to be experimented upon? Lurking behind these and similar questions there are more fundamental difficulties. What are the functions of consent for the competent and the incompetent? What is the sense in which the patient/subject must be "free," "informed," and "competent?" It is by way of an approach to these latter questions that I shall attempt to respond to the more specific questions.[1]

I. Consent and the Competent

The negative aspects of the doctrine of informed consent have ordinarily been the focus of attention; difficulties in obtaining the informed consent of the subject/patient render the ethics of experimentation and therapeutic measures questionable. Our common view of informed consent is that, when at all relevant, it represents a minimum condition which ethics imposes upon the physician. It is seen as a necessary condition for medical manipulation, but hardly as a sufficient condition.

The reasons why this is so—why it is not sufficient that an experimenter, for instance, have received informed consent from his subject before proceeding—are quite obvious. The scarcity of medical resources (which includes a scarcity of qualified physician-investigators) forbids us from wasting time upon poorly-designed experiments, or upon experiments which merely replicate well-established conclusions. There seems to be, as well, a limit to the dangers which we (ordinarily) allow subjects to face. We do not, as a matter of policy, think it wise to allow would-be suicides to accomplish their end with the aid of a scientific investigator. Many other reasons could be given for the proposition that a person does not have a right to be experimented upon, even when he has given valid consent to the procedure.

The Right to Consent

But there does seem to exist a positive right of informed consent, which exists in both therapeutic and experimental settings. A person who has the capacity to give valid consent, and who has in fact consented to the procedure in question, has a right to have that fact recognized by us. We all have a duty to recognize a valid consent when confronted with it.

From whence derives this right? It arises from the right which each of us possesses to be treated as a person, and in the duty which all of us have, to have respect for persons, to treat a person as such, and not as an object. For this entails that our capacities for personhood ought to be recognized by all—these capacities including the capacity for rational decision, and for action consequent upon rational decision. Perhaps the worst which we may do to a man is to deny him his humanity, for example, by classifying him as mentally incompetent when he is, in fact, sane. It is a terrible thing to be hated or persecuted; it is far worse to be ignored, to be notified that you "don't count."

If an individual is capable of and has given valid consent, I would argue that he has a right, as against the world but more particularly as against his physician, to have it recognized that valid consent has been given. (The same applies, of course, with still greater force, with regard to *refusals* to consent to medical procedures.) The limited force of this claim must be emphasized: it does not entail

Reprinted by permission of the author and publisher from the Hastings Center Report, 5 (August 1975).
©*Institute of Society, Ethics and Life Sciences, 360 Broadway, Hastings-on-Hudson, New York.*

a right to be treated, or to be experimented upon. It is a most innocuous right, one which most of us would have little hesitation about granting.

It is, therefore, curious that the literature on informed consent has failed to recognize this right—has, in fact, tacitly denied this right, at least as regards experimentation. In writings on informed consent it seems to have been assumed that if, under certain conditions, it is *doubtful* that valid consent to an experiment has been granted, it is best to "play it safe" ethically. In cases of doubt, we prefer not to take chances: in this case, we will not take a chance upon violating the canons of ethics by experimenting without being certain that the subject has validly consented to the experiment. Since we do not at present know whether a prisoner can give a valid consent, let us not take chances: we call for a moratorium on prison experimentation. Since we do not know at what age a person has the capacity to give a valid consent, we avoid the problem by setting the age of majority at a point where it is beyond doubt that maturity has been attained. If we must err, we shall ensure that we err in being overly ethical.

The establishment of the innocuous right to have valid consent recognized as such eliminates this expedient. Other writers have conceptualized the conflict as one between a right and, at best, a mere liberty. From the patient's point of view, he has a right to have his health protected by the physician, and a mere liberty to be experimented upon. From the physician-investigator's point of view, he has a duty to protect the subject's health, and a mere liberty to experiment upon the subject (contingent, of course, upon obtaining the subject's consent). A recognition of the claims of personhood and autonomy, however, reveals this to be a conflict between rights and duties. The physician-investigator has a duty to recognize consent when validly offered. When the consent is of doubtful validity, therefore, the physician experiences a conflict between two duties. He will not be ethically well-protected by choosing not to experiment, for there exists the possibility—which, as cases are multiplied, becomes a probability—that he is violating a duty in so choosing. Problems in informed consent present us with a dilemma. It is no longer the case that the burden of proof devolves upon the would-be experimenter. The would-be abstainer-from-experiments may have to prove his case as well.

These considerations give us a new point of departure in investigating problems of informed consent. They show us that there is no "fail-safe" procedure which we can fall back upon in cases of doubt. Rather, what is required is an exhaustive examination of each case and issue, to see whether or not a valid consent has in fact been obtained.

When we fail to recognize a valid consent, of course, more is involved than a denial of personhood. Other benefits may be denied as well. Dr. Vernon Mark, for example, maintains that psychosurgery should not be done on prisoners with epilepsy because of the problem in obtaining a voluntary consent from prisoners.[2] But a resolution of this problem has not been shown to be impossible. Surely, the proper thing to do here would be to see whether prisoners can or cannot give valid consent to such a procedure. To remain satisfied with doubts, to fail to investigate this question, complex though it be, results in a denial of medical treatment for the prisoner, as well as representing a negation of the prisoner's human capacities. In depriving prisoners of the opportunity to serve as subjects in medical experiments, there are losses other than those of human respect.[3] Not the least of these is the loss of an opportunity to be of altruistic service to mankind.[4] Even a child feels at times a need to be useful; in promoting a moratorium on prison experimentation we deny prisoners the satisfaction of this psychic need. We should not need a reminder from John Stuart Mill that there are "higher" as well as "lower" pleasures and needs.

The right to have valid consent recognized as such does not indicate that we must experiment on prisoners. What it does indicate is that we have a moral responsibility to investigate in detail the question of whether prisoners can, under certain conditions, validly consent to experimentation. It also requires that we not prevent a researcher from experimenting on the basis of over-scrupulousness. If prisoners *can* give valid consent, we wrong not only the researcher but the prisoner as well by forbidding prison experimentation.

The Requirement of Information

The most common locution for the requirement which I am discussing is "informed consent"—we require "informed consent" to protect a doctor from legal liability resultant from his therapeutic endeavors, or to ensure the "ethicacy" of an experiment. But I believe "informed consent" to be a serious misnomer for what we do, in fact, want medical practice to conform to.

No lengthy rehearsal of the absurdities consequent upon taking the term "informed consent" at face value is necessary. The claim has been made, and repeated with approval, that "fully informed consent" is a goal which we can never achieve, but toward which we must strive. In order to ensure that fully informed consent has been given, it has seriously been suggested that only medical students or graduate students in the life sciences ought to be accepted as subjects for experimentation. *Reductio ad absurdum* examples of "fully informed consent" have been elaborated, in forms which list all the minutiae of the proposed medical procedure, together with all of its conceivable sequelae. With such a view of "informed consent" and its requirements, it is not surprising to find doctors who claim that since they cannot fully inform patients, they will tell them nothing, but instead will personally assume the responsibility for assuring the subject's safety.

In truth, a *reductio ad absurdum* of this view of "informed consent" need not be constructed; it serves as its own *reductio ad absurdum*. For there is no end to "fully informing" patients. When the doctor wishes to insert a catheter, must he commend to the subject's attention a textbook of anatomy? Although this, of course, would not suffice: he must ensure that the patient understand the text as well. Must he tell the patient the story of Dr. X, that bogey of first-year medical students, who, in a state of inebriation, inserted ("by mistake") his pen-refill instead of the catheter? With, of course, the assurance that *this* physician never gets drunk ("Well, rarely, anyway"). Must the patient be informed of the chemical formula of the catheter? Its melting point?

The basic mistake which is committed by those who harp upon the difficulties in obtaining informed consent (and by critics of the doctrine) is in believing that we can talk about information in the abstract, without reference to any human purpose. It is very likely impossible to talk about "information" in this way; but impossible or not, when we do in fact talk about, or request, information, we do not mean "information in the abstract." If I ask someone to "tell me about those clouds" he will, ordinarily, know what I mean; and he will answer me, in the spirit in which he

was asked, by virtue of his professional expertise as an artist, meteorologist, astronomer, soothsayer, or what-have-you. The meteorologist will not object that he cannot tell you the optical refraction index of the clouds, and therefore that he cannot "fully answer" your question. He knows that you are asking him with a given end in mind, and that much information about the cloud is irrelevant *relative to that purpose*.

That this "abstract information" requirement is not in question in obtaining valid consent is hardly an original point, but it is worth repeating. One of the leading court opinions on human experimentation puts it like this: ". . . the patient's interest in information does not extend to a lengthy polysyllabic discourse on all possible complications. A mini-course in medical science is not required. . . ."[5]

The proper question to ask, then, is not "What information must be given?" That would be premature: we must first know for what purpose information is needed. *Why* must the patient be informed? Put that way, the answer is immediately forthcoming. The patient must be informed so that he will know what he is getting into, what he may expect from the procedure, what his likely alternatives are—in short, what the procedure (and forbearance from it) will mean, so that a responsible decision on the matter may be made. This is the legal stance, as well as, I think, a "common sensical" stance; as Alexander Capron writes, the information component in valid consent derives in law from the recognition that information is "necessary to make meaningful the power to decide."[6] The proper test of whether a given piece of information needs to be given is, then, whether the physician, knowing what he does about the patient/subject, feels that that patient/subject would want to know this before making up his mind. Outré, improbable consequences would not ordinarily, therefore, be relevant information. Exceptionally, they will be: for example, when there is a small risk of impotence consequent upon the procedure which the physician proposes to perform upon a man with a great stake in his sexual prowess. This is only sensible.

Our main conclusion, then, is that valid consent entails only the imparting of that information which the patient/subject requires in order to make a responsible decision. This entails, I think, the possibility of a valid yet ignorant consent.

Consider, first, the therapeutic context. It is, I believe, not unusual for a patient to give his doctor *carte blanche* to perform any medical procedure which the physician deems proper in order to effect a cure. He is telling the doctor to act as his agent in choosing which procedure to follow. This decision is neither unwise nor (in any serious sense) an abdication of responsibility and an unwarranted burden upon the physician. We each of us choose to delegate our power of choice in this way in dealing with our auto mechanic or stockbroker.

It may be harder to accept an ignorant consent as valid in the purely experimental context. I think, however, that much of this difficulty is due to our paucity of imagination, our failure to imagine circumstances in which a person might choose to proceed in this way. We might approach such a case, for example, by imagining a Quaker who chooses to serve society by acting as a research subject, but who has a morbid fear of knives and pointed instruments. The Quaker might say to the physician-investigator that he wants to serve science but is afraid that his phobia would overcome his better judgment. He might consequently request that any experiment which would involve use of scalpels, hypodermic needles, and such, be performed without informing him: while, say, he is asleep or unconscious. He might further ask the doctor not to proceed should the experiment involve considerable risk. In such a case, or one similar, we would find an instance of a valid yet ignorant consent to experimentation.

The ostensible differences between the therapeutic and experimental contexts may be resolved into two components: in the therapeutic context it is supposed that the physician knows what the sequelae to treatment will be, which information, by definition, is not available in the experimental situation; and in the therapeutic context the doctor may be said to be seeking his patient's good, in contrast to the experimental context where some other good is being sought. On the basis of these differences it may be claimed that a valid yet ignorant consent is enough permission for therapy, but not for experimentation.

Closer examination, however, reveals that these differences do not necessarily obtain. First, because I believe it would be granted that a valid yet ignorant consent can be given in the "therapeutic-experimental" situation, where a new drug or procedure is being attempted to aid the patient (in the absence of any traditional available therapy). In the therapeutic-experimental situation, as in the purely experimental situation, the sequelae are not known (although of course in both cases some definite result is expected or anticipated). If a valid yet ignorant consent is acceptable in the one, therefore, it must be acceptable in the other.

Secondly, because it is patently not the case that we can expect there to be no good accruing to the subject of an experiment by reason of his participation. There are, commonly, financial and other "tangible" benefits forthcoming (laboratory training, and so on). And it must once again be said that the pleasures of altruism are not negligible. The proposed differences between experimentation and therapy do not stand up, and so we must say that if a valid yet ignorant consent is acceptable in the one it must be acceptable in the other. It must be remembered that this statement only concerns itself with one part of the consent doctrine, which is, itself, only one of the requirements which the ethical experiment must satisfy.

To mention—without claiming totally to resolve—two problems which may be raised at this point: First, it is said that a doctor often does not know what will happen as a consequence of a recommended procedure, and so cannot tell the patient what the patient wants to know. The obvious response to this seems to be right: the physician should, in that case, tell the patient/subject that he does not know what will happen (which does not exclude an explanation of what the doctor expects to happen, and on what he bases this expectation).

Second, it will be objected that the adoption of a requirement such as I propose would forbid the use of placebos and blind experiments. I am not sure that this is so; sometimes it must be the case that the subjects in an experiment may be asked (without introducing artifacts into the results) to consent to an experiment knowing that some will, and some will not, be receiving placebos. Another alternative would be to inform the subjects that the experiment may or may not involve some subjects receiving placebos.[7] I am aware, however, that these remarks are less than adequate responses to these problems.

Our conclusion, then, is that the informing of the patient/subject is not a fundamental requirement of valid consent. It is, rather, derivative from the requirement that the consent be the expression of a responsible choice. The two requirements which I do see as fundamental in this doctrine are that the choice be responsible and that it be voluntary.

The Requirement of Responsibility

What is meant by saying that the choice must be "responsible"? Does this entail that the physician may at any time override a patient's judgment on the basis that, in the physician's view, the patient has not chosen responsibly? Surely not; to adopt such a criterion would defeat the purpose embodied in the doctrine of consent. It would mean that a person's exercise of autonomy is always subject to review.

Still, some such requirement would appear to be necessary. A small child can certainly make choices.[8] Small children can also be intelligent enough to understand the necessary information. Yet surely we would not want to say that a small child can give valid consent to a serious medical procedure.[9] The reason for this is that the child cannot choose *responsibly*.

We are faced with a dilemma. On the one hand, it appears that we must require that the choice be responsible. To require only that the choice be free would yield counter-intuitive results. On the other hand, if we do require that the choice made be a responsible one, we seem to presuppose some body which shall judge the reasonableness of choices; this represents a paternalism which is antithetical to the doctrine of consent. An elderly patient chooses to forgo further life-saving measures. How are we to judge whether or not this choice is a responsible one?

The path between the horns of this dilemma involves saying that the "responsibility" which we require is to be predicated not on the nature of the particular choice, but on the nature of the patient/subject. What we need to know is whether *he* is a responsible man ("in general," so to speak), not whether the choice which has been made is responsible. In this way, we avoid the danger of upholding as "responsible" only those choices which we ourselves feel are good choices. We can and do admit into the community of responsible persons individuals who make choices with which we do not agree.

In this sense, responsibility is a dispositional characteristic. To say that someone is a responsible individual means that he makes choices, typically, on the basis of reasons, arguments, or beliefs—and that he remains open to the claims of reason, so that further rational argument might lead him to change his mind. It is to say that a person is capable of making and carrying through a life-plan—that he is prepared to act on the basis of his choices. It is to say that a person is capable of living with his life-plan; he can live with the consequences of his choices, he *takes responsibility* for his choices.[10] Of course, none of these are absolutes: all responsible people are at times pigheaded, at times short-sighted, at times flighty. That is to say, all responsible men at times act irresponsibly. Should the lack of responsibility persist, of course, to an extreme degree, we may say that the person has left the community of responsible folk.

Voluntarism and Reward

The other requirement of valid consent is that it be given voluntarily. The choice which the consent expresses must be freely made.

We all know some conditions which, if satisfied, make us say that a consent has been given involuntarily. The case which immediately springs to mind occurs when an individual succumbs under a threat: we call this duress or coercion. But the threat need not be overt; and perhaps there need not be a threat at all to render consent involuntary.

Hence, the major problem currently engendered by the requirement of voluntariness. It is typified by the prisoner who "volunteers" for an experiment in the hope or expectation of a reward: significantly higher wages, an opportunity for job training, better health care while involved in the experiment, a favorable report to his parole board. Is the consent which the prisoner offers a voluntary consent? The problem may be stated more generally thus: At what point does reward render consent involuntary?

The problem of reward is particularly difficult, since it involves questions of degree. Is a prisoner's consent involuntary if the reward for his participation in the experiment is a three-month reduction of sentence? Is it relevant here that the prisoner is serving a twenty-year sentence, rather than a one-to-five-year sentence? Does a possible increase in wages from twenty-five cents per hour to one dollar per hour constitute duress? Should we consider the percentage increase, or the increase in absolute value, or the increase in actual value which the seventy-five cent disparity represents in the prison environment?

To some, of course, questions like these have little meaning. They have little meaning to those who are indifferent to the demands of justice and autonomy which the consent doctrine represents, to those who are willing to buy guinea pigs, rather than to reward human beings. And they have little meaning for those who are convinced that prisoners are inherently unfree, and who thus would call for a total cessation of prison experimentation. Each of these positions denies, in an *a priori* fashion, freedom to prisoners; each must be rejected. A recognition of the fact that decisions about consent may be over- as well as under-protective forces us to deal with this sort of question, complex though it may be.

As is so often the case, posing the question in a different way may facilitate response. We have been considering the question of how much reward nullifies the validity of consent, how much reward renders the subject unfree. But is it in fact the case that *reward* is the disruptive factor here?

This problem may be clarified by the following examples. Imagine an upper-middle-class individual, who can provide for his family all of their needs and most of the amenities of civilized life. Let us say that this person is offered one hundred dollars to cross the street—if you like, make it one thousand or ten thousand dollars? He chooses to cross the street. Is his choice *involuntary*? Despite the substantial reward, I think most of us would agree that the consent was freely offered (and would that we should have such problems!).

Consider a person who deeply wants to be an astronaut. He is told that as part of the program he must participate in experiments to determine resistance to high-G conditions. Is his consent to this invalid, involuntary? I think not. We would say, this is part of his job; he should have expected it; and if he can't stand the heat, he should get out of the kitchen. In this vein, consider Evel Knievel, a financially prosperous man, who is offered millions of dollars to perform daredevil stunts. His choice may be bizarre, even crazy: but has his reward rendered it unfree?

Finally, consider a man who is informed by his doctor that he will most likely die unless he has open-heart surgery. His "reward" for consenting is his life; the penalty for not consenting is death. Does this mean this man cannot give the doctor valid consent—morally valid consent—to proceed?

There are two distinctions which, I think, go a long way towards dispelling these problems. First, I think it must be granted that natural contingencies ("acts of God," things which come to pass naturally, those contingencies which we cannot hold anyone responsible for) do not render a person unfree, nor do they render unfree the choices which a person makes in light of those contingencies.[11]

That natural contingencies do not render a man unfree is a point which is apt to be forgotten in the present context. I am not—in the morally relevant sense—lacking in freedom because I cannot, unaided, fly through the air, or live on grass. Nor am I unfree because my heart is about to give out. Nor am I unfree when, recognizing that my heart may give out, I choose to undergo surgery. I may, of course, be so crazed by knowing that I am near death's door that I am in a state of general impotence, and hence must have the choice made for me; but general incompetence is not in question here. The distinction between choices forced by man, and choices forced by nature, is, then, of importance.

The second distinction is between those pressures which are, and those which are not, in Daube's words, "consonant with the dignity and responsibility of free life."[12] I would explain this as follows: there are certain basic freedoms and rights which we possess which *entitle* us (morally) to certain things (or states of affairs). We would all, no doubt, draw up different lists of these rights and freedoms; but included in them would be safety of person, freedom of conscience and religion, a right to a certain level of education, and, for some of us, a right to some level of health care. When the "reward" is such as only to give us the necessary conditions of these rights and freedoms—when all that the reward does is to bring us up to a level of living to which we are entitled, and of which we have been deprived by man—then the "reward," I think, constitutes duress. A reward which accrues to one who has achieved this level, or who can easily achieve it (other than by taking the reward-option), and which hence serves only to grant us "luxury" items, does not constitute duress, and hence does not render choice unfree, no matter how great this reward may be.

The rewards above the moral subsistence level are true rewards. In contrast, we may say (with some touch of metaphor) that the "rewards" which only bring us up to the level to which we were in any event entitled are properly viewed as functioning as *threats:* "Do this, or stay where you are:"—when you should not have been "where you are" in the first place.

The astronaut, Evel Knievel, and the upper-middle-class street-crosser are being granted "luxury" items, and hence are capable of giving free consent. But consider a man who will not be admitted to the hospital for treatment unless he agrees to be a subject in an experiment (unrelated to his treatment). Those who feel, as I do, that we are, here and now, morally entitled to medical treatment would agree, I trust, that this illegitimate option coerces the man into agreeing. Or consider a man who has religious scruples against donating blood, who takes his daughter to a hospital for treatment. He is told that the doctors will not treat her unless the family donates a certain amount of blood. His freedom has been nullified: his "consent" to donating blood is morally invalid. Similarly, the college student whose grade is contingent upon his participation in the instructor's psychological experiments is not validly consenting to serve. He is entitled to have his grade based upon his classroom work.

It yet remains to apply this distinction to our original problem, prison experimentation. The application will not be attempted here, for we would first need to be clear in our minds what rights and freedoms a prisoner is entitled to. I would not hesitate to say, though, that when a situation is created whereby a prisoner can only receive decent health care by participating in an experiment, he is being coerced into that experiment. I would have little hesitation in claiming that if subjecting himself to experimentation is the only way in which a prisoner could learn a trade which may be used "outside," then that prisoner is being coerced, his consent is not free. When we take into account the condition of our society, these would seem to be reasonable entitlements for the prisoner. Other rewards—for example, higher pay—

may or may not constitute rewards above the moral subsistence level; if they are, then consent in light of these rewards could be freely offered. Perhaps too much has been said already; judgments like these must be made in an individualized fashion, one which is sensitive to the realities of prison life.

II. Consent and the Incompetent

In this section will be discussed, first, the question of how the age of majority and minority with reference to valid consent ought to be set; and secondly, the problems associated with the concept of proxy consent.

The Age of Consent

It has been argued that the requirements for obtaining valid consent are that the patient/subject must have consented freely and that he must be a responsible individual. The requirement of voluntariness does not raise any novel problems when applied to minors. Rather, what we usually have in mind when restricting the power of the minor to consent is that he is not, in the sense required, a responsible individual.

I have claimed that to be a responsible individual one must be capable of rationally adopting, following through, and accepting the consequences of a life-plan. The age, therefore, at which society indicates a presumption that individuals can satisfy these conditions can be said to be the age at which society ought to grant the right to give valid consent to serious medical procedures. The examples which spring to mind are the age of conscription and the age of marriageability. At these ages society has indicated that one is capable of acting, in a complex society, as an individual.

This is not an argument like that which says "If you are old enough to fight, then you are old enough to vote." The requirements necessary for being a soldier may be wholly unrelated to the requirements necessary before the franchise may be properly exercised. In contrast, the responsibility which we assume to be possessed by those capable of soldiering and contracting marriage is the same responsibility which is required to make consent valid: the ability to work through and with a life-plan.

The first thing which needs to be said, then, is

that the age of consent should be lowered from 21 to 18 in those jurisdictions which have not yet done so. This should not entail merely that an 18-year-old may consent in the absence of parental disapproval; it should be a full power to consent, irrespective of what others might say.

But the setting of an age of consent indicates only a presumption and nothing more. The fact that someone has passed the age of consent is not conclusive proof that he is responsible (in the sense required); the fact that someone is below the age of consent is not conclusive proof of irresponsibility. The presumption may be defeated in either direction.

It is clear, for example, that an adult is not, *ipso facto*, responsible. The adult may be insane.

It is equally clear that a minor need not be irresponsible. People mature at different rates. If evidence of responsibility may be supplied on behalf of one below the age of consent, the presumption of irresponsibility should be defeated. The sort of evidence which would be necessary is that which indicates that the person can work through a life-plan. It may be said that this notion is being approached by the law in the special provisions sometimes made for the "emancipated minor." Marriage or economic self-sufficiency are among the common requirements for being considered an emancipated minor. One of the special prerogatives of the emancipated minor is that he may consent on his own behalf to medical care. I would argue that this should be extended to cover participation in experimentation as well.

Proxy Consent

Proxy consent is consent given on behalf of an individual who is himself incapable of granting consent. The major category of those who require proxy consent are minors, but proxy consent may need to be obtained for the insane or the unconscious as well. My comments will nevertheless be restricted to the case of minors, leaving the other cases to be dealt with by implication. In minors, proxy consent is ordinarily granted by the child's parent or guardian; exceptionally, it may be given by another close relative or by an individual appointed by the court for the specific purpose of granting consent to some procedure.

I have argued that the function of informed consent is to respect the autonomy and dignity of the individual. This cannot be the function of proxy consent. The minor patient/subject cannot fully express autonomy and dignity through choices. It may be said that the function of proxy consent is to protect the right of the parents to raise their child as they see fit, to do with the child as they like. But the child is not the property of the parents; parents do not have an absolute right of disposal over the child. In law we recognize constraints upon the parental power, and common morality affirms the justice in this. What then is the function of proxy consent?

I think it would be best to turn this question on its head. By virtue of what right which the child possesses do we require the granting of proxy consent before a medical procedure may be initiated? What *could* be the source of such an obligation? We ordinarily recognize that there is only one fundamental right possessed by minors, a right to be protected and aided in development. " . . . A child, unlike an adult, has a right 'not to liberty but to custody.' "[13] All other rights which a child possesses, all other duties which we have towards children, are derivative from this single right, and are void when inconsistent with it. Broadly speaking, in consequence of this right, we must do what we may to promote the welfare of the child; we must abstain from doing what will injure the child, physically or otherwise; and, as far as this right goes, we are at liberty to deal with the child in ways which neither help nor hurt.

That proxy consent is ordinarily to be obtained from the parent or guardian of the child is understandable. We feel that the parent has the best interests of the child at heart, and knows how best to seek the child's welfare. It also follows from this right, however, that, when the parent does not have the best interests of the child in mind, the power of proxy consent should be transferred to another. It is on such a basis that society feels justified in removing a child from his parent's custody, and in appointing another to act *in parens patriae*. If this system is to be effective, society must, by and large, act on the basis of shared common views about what the welfare of the child consists of. We cannot allow anything which a parent considers to be a benefit to the child—being boiled in oil to save his eternal soul—to count as action in the child's best interests. This does not preclude a certain amount of leeway in a liberal society as to permitted views of welfare: if most feel that it is better, when the money is available, to send the child to a private school, we yet will not fault an affluent parent who decides to send his child to a public school.

The consequences of these propositions for cases when proxy consent is being sought for the purpose of giving therapy to a child accord well with the way the law handles this subject. The problem situation which arises concerns parents who, because of religious scruples, refuse to consent to needed medical treatment for their child. Jehovah's Witnesses, for example, who believe that blood transfusions are forbidden by the law of God, will not consent on behalf of their child to blood transfusions. Society feels that the benefit of the child is to be found in allowing the procedure. Because of this, the hospital will often turn to a judge, who appoints someone to act *in parens patriae* for the purpose of consenting to the specific procedure. I suggest that if it were clearly the view of society that it is to the mongoloid infant's benefit to survive, should a parent refuse to consent to a life-saving procedure for that infant, a similar course would be followed: the consent of a court-appointed guardian would be substituted.

Proxy consent to experimentation on children is a more complicated matter. In law, there are two kinds of intervention in the person of another which are actionable in the absence of consent: those interventions where harm does, and where harm does not, result. The latter are termed "wrongful" or "harmful touchings" (though no harm has occurred). In other words, the mere *doing* of something to a person without his consent is, in itself, an actionable wrong.

We may say that, corresponding to this division, there are two sorts of experiments: those which do, and those which do not, injure the subject appreciably. Beecher has noted, for example, that "Many thousands of psychomotor tests and sociological studies have been carried out in children during the child's development and have revealed much information of value. . . . Sound nutritional studies without risk have been carried out. So have certain blood studies."[14] It must be added that many studies of value cannot, due to metabolic and other differences, be carried out in adults with results which will be valid for children.

It is clear, on the basis of the principle of ben-

efit, that proxy consent to dangerous or harmful experiments on children cannot be valid. What about those experiments which carry no appreciable risk—the "wrongful touchings" sort? In an adult, it would seem, the right to autonomy, the right "to be let alone," is sufficient basis for the action of wrongful touching. But the child does not have a right to autonomy, except insofar as some measure of autonomy is necessary to promote the child's development and well-being.

Harmless experiments on children, therefore, which satisfy the other canons of medical ethics—good design, well-trained experimenters, and so forth—could be performed. Parents would not be derelict in their duty should they consent, on behalf of their child, to experiments of this sort. Participation in these experiments does not infringe the child's right to welfare, unless they would result in a *harmful* (and not just any) restriction of autonomy.

As I see it, the fundamental problem with those who would forbid *all* experimentation upon children[15] is that they confuse consent in adults with proxy consent for children. These two are fundamentally different requirements. Children are not small adults; our relations with children must not be made to approach as nearly as possible to our relations with adults. There are things which you ought to grant to children which need not be granted to adults: if a child is thirsty you provide him with drink. And there are things which may licitly be done to children which could not be done with adults: if my parents annoy me I may not send them to their room. A child is (morally) a different sort of thing than is an adult; we must adjust our relations with them according to their claims upon us.

Conclusion

This paper represents an attempt to formulate what I call a "moral theory" of the requirement of consent to serious medical procedures. The method used involves an interplay between cases and principles, such that each influences the other. Well-established moral intuitions about cases suggested some principles and called for the rejection of others. These principles in turn, once established, enabled the clarification of a proper approach to other, borderline cases.

Under the influence of situation ethics, much of the work on medical ethics has stressed the respects in which cases differ. This has resulted in the development of an *ad hoc* literature on cases which pose difficulty for the doctrine of informed consent. As the cases accumulated, the doctrine began to seem more and more amorphous.

In contrast, this paper has sought to unify the doctrine of consent. Principles which are developed through considering the problems raised by prison experimentation in turn suggested solutions to other situations; rather than stressing the differences between the experimental and the therapeutic contexts, their similarities were emphasized. There is, I think, a need for such efforts at unification, as there is a need for a literature which is committed to the unique aspects of different cases.

Notes

The research for this paper was begun during an internship at the Institute of Society, Ethics and the Life Sciences in the month of June, 1973. I gratefully acknowledge the help of Drs. Daniel Callahan, Marc Lappé, Peter Steinfels, and Robert Veatch, of the Institute, who helped make my internship profitable and enjoyable. My wife Barbara read the manuscript and suggested a number of needed changes.

1. For examples of a similar method applied to different problems, see Thomas I. Emerson, *Toward A General Theory of the First Amendment* (New York: Vintage Books, 1967).

2. "Brain Surgery in Aggressive Epileptics," in *Hastings Center Report*, February 1973.

3. See the insert to Alexander M. Capron's call for a moratorium on prison experimentation, "Medical Research in Prisons," *Hastings Center Report*, June 1973. The insert is a report from the New York *Times*, April 15, 1973, and reads in part: "Ninety-six of the 175 inmates at Lancaster County prison have written to a newspaper here protesting a recent decision by the state to halt all medical experiments on state prisoners. In their letter to the *Lancaster New Era*, they urged that state to allow the research

[which] did not harm them and enabled them to pay off their fines and court costs."

4. See Henry K. Beecher, *Research and the Individual: Human Studies* (Boston: Little, Brown, 1970), p. 56. Professor Beecher notes a study of prison inmates, who, for participation in an experiment involving malaria, received pay but no reduction of sentence. Half of the volunteers cited "altruism" rather than money as their motive for volunteering. Those inmates who did not volunteer "expressed or implied respect for those who did volunteer."

5. *Cobbs* v. *Grant*, 502 P. 2d 1, 11.

6. Alexander M. Capron, "Legal Rights and Moral Rights," in Hilton, *et al.*, eds., *Ethical Issues in Human Genetics* (Plenum Press, 1973), 228.

7. If this sort of explanation were given as a matter of course in *all* experiments, this might still further reduce the problem of artifacts. The remarks, it should be noted, are directed towards medical experiments. By and large, they are inapplicable to, say, experiments in social psychology.

8. The counter-suggestion may be made that children cannot *really* make choices. This would, I think, put too great a weight upon the requirement of voluntarism. We would be recruiting the concepts of choice and volition to do a job which they have not been designed for.

9. I am speaking of course in the moral, not the legal, context. It may be that in an emergency a child may, in the absence of his parents, give legally valid consent.

10. This gives us the link between "responsible" in the dispositional sense explained here, and "responsible" in the blame-sense of the word ("I'll hold you responsible for that.").

11. The *caveat* must be added: natural contingencies do not have, as their *sole* result, the rendering of a person unfree, in the sense which vitiates consent: a man's brain tumor can make the man an idiot, schizophrenia can make a man insane, but these do not so much affect a person's volition as they do disturb his entire psychic structure.

12. David Daube, quoted in Beecher, p. 146.

13. *In re Gault*, 387 U.S. 1 (1967).

14. Beecher, p. 67.

15. See, for example, Paul Ramsey, "Consent as a Canon of Loyalty With Special Reference to Children in Medical Investigations," in *The Patient as Person* (New Haven: Yale University Press, 1970).

The Willowbrook Letters: Criticism and Defense _____

Stephen Goldby, Saul Krugman, M. H. Pappworth, and Geoffrey Edsall

SIR.—You have referred to the work of Krugman and his colleagues at the Willowbrook State School in three editorials. In the first article the work was cited as a notable study of hepatitis and a model for this type of investigation. No comment was made on the rightness of attempting to infect mentally retarded children with hepatitis for experimental purposes, in an institution where the disease was already endemic.

The second editorial again did not remark on the ethics of the study, but the third sounded a note of doubt as to the justification for extending these experiments. The reason given was that some children might have been made more susceptible to serious hepatitis as the result of the administration of previously heated icterogenic material.

I believe that not only this last experiment, but the whole of Krugman's study, is quite unjustifiable, whatever the aims, and however academically or therapeutically important are the results. I am amazed that the work was published and that it has been actively supported editorially by the *Journal of the American Medical Association* and by Ingelfinger in the 1967–68 *Year Book of Medicine*. To my knowledge only the *British Journal of Hospital Medicine* has clearly stated the ethical position on these experiments and shown that it was indefensible to give potentially dangerous infected material to children, particularly those who were mentally retarded, with or without parental consent, when no benefit to the child could conceivably result.

Krugman and Giles have continued to publish the results of their study, and in a recent paper go to some length to describe their method of obtaining parental consent and list a number of influential medical boards and committees that have approved the study. They point out again that, in their opinion, their work conforms to the World Medical Association Draft Code of Ethics on Human Experimentation. They also say that hepatitis is still highly endemic in the school.

This attempted defence is irrelevant to the central issue. Is it right to perform an experiment on a normal or mentally retarded child when no benefit can result to that individual? I think that the answer is no, and that the question of parental consent is irrelevant. In my view the studies of Krugman serve only to show that there is a serious loophole in the Draft Code, which under General Principles and Definitions puts the onus of consent for experimentation on children on the parent or guardian. It is this section that is quoted by Krugman. I would class his work as "experiments conducted solely for the acquisition of knowledge," under which heading the code states that "persons retained in mental hospital or hospitals for mental defectives should not be used for human experiment." Krugman may believe that his experiments were for the benefit of his patients, meaning the individual patients used in the study. If this is his belief he has a difficult case to defend. The duty of a pediatrician in a situation such as exists at Willowbrook State School is to attempt to improve that situation, not to turn it to his advantage for experimental purposes, however lofty the aims.

Every new reference to the work of Krugman and Giles adds to its apparent ethical respectability, and in my view such references should stop, or at least be heavily qualified. The editorial attitude of *The Lancet* to the work should be reviewed and openly stated. The issue is too important to be ignored.

If Krugman and Giles are keen to continue their experiments I suggest that they invite the parents of the children involved to participate. I wonder what the response would be.

Stephen Goldby

SIR.—Dr. Stephen Goldby's critical comments about our Willowbrook studies and our motives for conducting them were published without extending us the courtesy of replying in the same

Reprinted by permission of the authors and publisher from The Lancet, *April 10, May 8, June 5, and July 10, 1971.*

issue of *The Lancet*. Your acceptance of his criticisms without benefit of our response implies a blackout of all comment related to our studies. This decision is unfortunate because our recent studies on active and passive immunisation for the prevention of viral hepatitis, type B, have clearly demonstrated a "therapeutic effect" for the children involved. These studies have provided us with the first indication and hope that it may be possible to control hepatitis in this institution. If this aim can be achieved, it will benefit not only the children, but also their families and the employees who care for them in the school. It is unnecessary to point out the additional benefit to the world-wide populations which have been plagued by an insoluble hepatitis problem for many generations.

Dr. Joan Giles and I have been actively engaged in studies aimed to solve two infectious-disease problems in the Willowbrook State School—measles and viral hepatitis. These studies were investigated in this institution because they represented major health problems for the 5000 or more mentally retarded children who were residents. Uninformed critics have assumed or implied that we came to Willowbrook to "conduct experiments on mentally retarded children."

The results of our Willowbrook studies with the experimental live attenuated measles vaccine developed by Enders and his colleagues are well documented in the medical literature. As early as 1960 we demonstrated the protective effect of this vaccine during the course of an epidemic. Prior to licensure of the vaccine in 1963 epidemics occurred at two-year intervals in this institution. During the 1960 epidemic there were more than 600 cases of measles and 60 deaths. In the wake of our ongoing measles vaccine programme, measles has been eradicated as a disease in the Willowbrook State School. We have not had a single case of measles since 1963. In this regard the children at the Willowbrook State School have been more fortunate than unimmunised children in Oxford, England, other areas in Great Britain, as well as certain groups of children in the United States and other parts of the world.

The background of our hepatitis studies at Willowbrook has been described in detail in various publications. Viral hepatitis is so prevalent that newly admitted susceptible children become infected within 6 to 12 months after entry in the institution. These children are a source of infection for the personnel who care for them and for their families if they visit with them. We were convinced that the solution of the hepatitis problem in this institution was dependent on the acquisition of new knowledge leading to the development of an effective immunising agent. The achievements with smallpox, diphtheria, poliomyelitis, and more recently measles represent dramatic illustrations of this approach.

It is well known that viral hepatitis in children is milder and more benign than the same disease in adults. Experience has revealed that hepatitis in institutionalised, mentally retarded children is also mild, in contrast with measles, which is a more severe disease when it occurs in institutional epidemics involving the mentally retarded. Our proposal to expose a small number of newly admitted children to the Willowbrook strains of hepatitis virus was justified in our opinion for the following reasons: (1) they were bound to be exposed to the same strains under the natural conditions existing in the institution; (2) they would be admitted to a special, well-equipped, and well-staffed unit where they would be isolated from exposure to other infectious diseases which were prevalent in the institution—namely, shigellosis, parasitic infections, and respiratory infections—thus, their exposure in the hepatitis unit would be associated with less risk than the type of institutional exposure where multiple infections could occur; (3) they were likely to have a subclinical infection followed by immunity to the particular hepatitis virus; and (4) only children with parents who gave informed consent would be included.

The statement by Dr. Goldby accusing us of conducting experiments exclusively for the acquisition of knowledge with no benefit for the children cannot be supported by the true facts.

Saul Krugman

SIR.—The experiments at Willowbrook raise two important issues: What constitutes valid consent, and do ends justify means? English law definitely forbids experimentation on children, even if both parents consent, unless done specifically in the interests of each individual child. Perhaps in the U.S.A the law is not so clear-cut. According to Beecher, the parents of the children at Willowbrook were informed that, because of overcrowding, the institution was to be closed; but only a week or two later they were told that there would be vacancies in the "hepatitis unit" for children whose parents allowed them to form part of the hepatitis research study. Such consent, ethically if not legally, is invalid because of its element of coercion, some parents being desperately anxious to institutionalise their mentally defective children. Moreover, obtaining consent after talking to parents in groups, as described by Krugman, is extremely unsatisfactory because even a single enthusiast can sway the diffident who do not wish to appear churlish in front of their fellow citizens.

Do ends justify the means? Krugman maintains that any newly admitted children would inevitably have contracted infective hepatitis, which was rife in the hospital. But this ignores the statement by the head of the State Department of Mental Hygiene that, during the major part of the 15 years these experiments have been conducted, a gamma-globulin inoculation programme had already resulted in over an 80 percent reduction of that disease in that hospital. Krugman and Pasamanick claim that subsequent therapeutic effects justify these experiments. This attitude is frequently adopted by experimenters and enthusiastic medical writers who wish us to forget completely how results are obtained but instead enjoy any benefits that may accrue. Immunisation was not the purpose of these Willowbrook experiments but merely a by-product that incidentally proved beneficial to the victims. Any experiment is ethical or not at its inception, and does not become so because it achieved some measure of success in extending the frontiers of medicine. I particularly object strongly to the views of Willey, " . . . risk being assumed by the subjects of the experimentation balanced against the potential benefit to the subjects *and* [Willey's italics] to society in general." I believe that experimental physicians never have the right to select martyrs for society. Every human being has the right to be treated with decency, and that right must always supersede every consideration of what may benefit mankind, what may advance medical science, what may contrib-

ute to public welfare. No doctor is ever justified in placing society or science first and his obligation to patients second. Any claim to act for the good of society should be regarded with distaste because it may be merely a highflown expression to cloak outrageous acts.

M. H. Pappworth

Sir.—I am astonished at the unquestioning way in which *The Lancet* has accepted the intemperate position taken by Dr. Stephen Goldby concerning the experimental studies of Krugman and Giles on hepatitis at the Willowbrook State School. These investigators have repeatedly explained—for over a decade—that natural hepatitis infection occurs sooner or later in virtually 100% of the patients admitted to Willowbrook, and that it is better for the patient to have a known, timed, controlled infection than an untimed, uncontrolled one. Moreover, the wisdom and human justification of these studies have been repeatedly and carefully examined and verified by a number of very distinguished, able individuals who are respected leaders in the making of such decisions.

The real issue is: Is it not proper and ethical to carry out experiments in children, which would apparently incur no greater risk than the children were likely to run by nature, in which the children generally receive better medical care when artificially infected than if they had been naturally infected, and in which the parents as well as the physician feel that a significant contribution to the future well-being of similar children is likely to result from the studies? It is true, to be sure, that the W.M.A. code says, "Children in institutions and not under the care of relatives should not be the subjects of human experiments." But this unqualified *obiter dictum* may represent merely the well-known inability of committees to think a problem through. However, it has been thought through by Sir Austin Bradford Hill, who has pointed out the unfortunate effects for these very children that would have resulted, were such a code to have been applied over the years.

Geoffrey Edsall

Judgment on Willowbrook

Paul Ramsey

In 1958 and 1959 the *New England Journal of Medicine* reported a series of experiments performed upon patients and new admittees to the Willowbrook State School, a home for retarded children in Staten Island, New York.[1] These experiments were described as "an attempt to control the high prevalence of infectious hepatitis in an institution for mentally defective patients." The experiments were said to be justified because, under conditions of an existing controlled outbreak of hepatitis in the institution, "knowledge obtained from a series of suitable studies could well lead to its control." In actuality, the experiments were designed to duplicate and confirm the efficacy of gamma globulin in immunization against hepatitis, to develop and improve or improve upon that inoculum, and to learn more about infectious hepatitis in general.

The experiments were justified—doubtless, after a great deal of soul searching—for the following reasons: there was a smoldering epidemic throughout the institution and "it was apparent that most of the patients at Willowbrook were naturally exposed to hepatitis virus"; infectious hepatitis is a much milder disease in children; the strain at Willowbrook was especially mild; only the strain or strains of the virus already disseminated at Willowbrook were used; and only those small and incompetent patients whose parents gave consent were used.

The patient population at Willowbrook was 4478, growing at a rate of one patient a day over a three-year span, or from 10 to 15 new admissions per week. In the first trial the existing population was divided into two groups: one group served as uninoculated controls, and the other group was inoculated with 0.01 ml. of gamma globulin per pound of body weight. Then for a second trial new admittees and those left uninoculated before were again divided: one group served as uninoculated controls and the other was inoculated with 0.06 ml. of gamma globulin per pound of body weight. This proved that Stokes et al. had correctly demonstrated that the larger amount would give significant immunity for up to seven or eight months.[2]

Serious ethical questions may be raised about the trials so far described. No mention is made of any attempt to enlist the adult personnel of the institution, numbering nearly 1,000 including nearly 600 attendants on ward duty, and new additions to the staff, in these studies whose excusing reason was that almost everyone was "naturally" exposed to the Willowbrook virus. Nothing requires that major research into the natural history of hepatitis be first undertaken in children. Experiments have been carried out in the military and with prisoners as subjects. There have been fatalities from the experiments; but surely in all these cases the consent of the volunteers was as valid or better than the proxy consent of these children's "representatives." There would have been no question of the understanding consent that might have been given by the adult personnel at Willowbrook, if significant benefits were expected from studying that virus.

Second, nothing is said that would warrant withholding an inoculation of some degree of known efficacy from part of the population, or for withholding in the first trial less than the full amount of gamma globulin that had served to immunize in previous tests, except the need to test, confirm, and improve the inoculum. That, of course, was a desirable goal; but it does not seem possible to warrant withholding gamma globulin for the reason that is often said to justify controlled trials, namely, that one procedure is *as likely* to succeed as the other.

Third, nothing is said about attempts to control or defeat the low-grade epidemic at Willowbrook by more ordinary, if more costly and less experimental, procedures. Nor is anything said about admitting no more patients until this goal had been accomplished. This was not a massive urban hospital whose teeming population would have to be turned out into the streets, with resulting dangers to themselves and to public health, in order to sanitize the place. Instead, between 200 and 250 patients were housed in each of 18 buildings over approximately 400 acres in a semirural setting of fields, woods, and well-kept, spacious lawns. Clearly it would have been possible to secure other accommodation for new admissions away from the infection, while eradicating the infection at Willowbrook building by building. This might have cost money, and it would certainly have required astute detective work to discover the source of the infection. The doctors determined that the new patients likely were not carrying the infection upon admission, and that it did not arise from the procedures and routine inoculations given them at the time of admission. Why not go further in the search for the source of the epidemic? If this had been an orphanage for normal children or a floor of private patients, instead of a school for mentally defective children, one wonders whether the doctors would so readily have accepted the hepatitis as a "natural" occurrence and even as an opportunity for study.

The next step was to attempt to induce "passive-active immunity" by feeding the virus to patients already protected by gamma globulin. In this attempt to improve the inoculum, permission was obtained from the parents of children from 5 to 10 years of age newly admitted to Willowbrook, who were then isolated from contact with the rest of the institution. All were inoculated with gamma globulin and then divided into two groups: one served as controls while the other group of new patients were fed the Willowbrook virus, obtained from feces, in doses having 50 percent infectivity, i.e., in concentrations estimated to produce hepatitis with jaundice in half the subjects tested. Then twice the 50 percent infectivity was tried. This proved, among other things, that hepatitis has an "alimentary-tract phase" in which it can be transmitted from one person to another while still "inapparent" in the first person. This, doubtless, is exceedingly important information in learning how to control epidemics of infectious hepatitis. The second of the two articles mentioned above describes studies of the incubation period of the virus and of whether pooled serum remained infectious when aged and frozen. Still the small, mentally defective patients who were deliberately fed infectious hepatitis are described as having

suffered mildly in most cases: "The liver became enlarged in the majority, occasionally a week or two before the onset of jaundice. Vomiting and anorexia usually lasted only a few days. Most of the children gained weight during the course of hepatitis."

That mild description of what happened to the children who were fed hepatitis (and who continued to be introduced into the unaltered environment of Willowbrook) is itself alarming, since it is now definitely known that cirrhosis of the liver results from infectious hepatitis more frequently than from excessive consumption of alcohol! Now, or in 1958 and 1959, no one knows what may be other serious consequences of contracting infectious hepatitis. Understanding human volunteers were then and are now needed in the study of this disease, although a South American monkey has now successfully been given a form of hepatitis, and can henceforth serve as our ally in its conquest. But not children who cannot consent knowingly. If Peace Corps workers are regularly given gamma globulin before going abroad as a guard against their contracting hepatitis, and are inoculated at intervals thereafter, it seems that this is the least we should do for mentally defective children before they "go abroad" to Willowbrook or other institutions set up for their care.

Discussions pro and con of the Willowbrook experiments that have come to my attention serve only to reinforce the ethical objections that can be raised against what was done simply from a careful analysis of the original articles reporting the research design and findings. In an address at the 1968 Ross Conference on Pediatric Research, Dr. Saul Krugman raised the question, Should vaccine trials be carried out in adult volunteers before subjecting children to similar tests?[3] He answered this question in the negative. The reason adduced was simply that "a vaccine virus trial may be a more hazardous procedure for adults than for children." Medical researchers, of course, are required to minimize the hazards, but not by moving from consenting to unconsenting subjects. This apology clearly shows that adults and children have become interchangeable in face of the overriding importance of obtaining the research goal. This means that the special moral claims of children for care and protection are forgotten, and especially the claims of children who are most weak and vulnerable. (Krugman's reference to the measles vaccine trials is not to the point.)

The *Medical Tribune* explains that the 16-bed isolation unit set up at Willowbrook served "to protect the study subjects from Willowbrook's other endemic diseases—such as shigellosis, measles, rubella and respiratory and parasitic infections—while exposing them to hepatitis."[4] This presumably compensated for the infection they were given. It is not convincingly shown that the children could by no means, however costly, have been protected from the epidemic of hepatitis. The statement that Willowbrook "had endemic infectious hepatitis and a sufficiently open population so that the disease could never be quieted by exhausting the supply of susceptibles" is at best enigmatic.

Oddly, physicians defending the propriety of the Willowbrook hepatitis project soon begin talking like poorly instructed "natural lawyers"! Dr. Louis Lasagna and Dr. Geoffrey Edsall, for example, find these experiments unobjectionable—both, for the reason stated by Edsall: "the children would apparently incur no greater risk than they were likely to run by nature." In any case, Edsall's examples of parents consenting with a son 17 years of age for him to go to war, and society's agreements with minors that they can drive cars and hurt themselves were entirely beside the point. Dr. David D. Rutstein adheres to a stricter standard in regard to research on infectious hepatitis: "It is not ethical to use human subjects for the growth of a virus for any purpose."[5]

The latter sweeping verdict may depend on knowledge of the effects of viruses on chromasomal difficulties, mongolism, etc., that was not available to the Willowbrook group when their researches were begun thirteen years ago. If so, this is a telling point against appeal to "no discernible risks" as the sole standard applicable to the use of children in medical experimentation. That would lend support to the proposition that we always know that there are unknown and undiscerned risks in the case of an invasion of the fortress of the body—which then can be consented to by an adult in behalf of a child only if it is in the child's behalf medically.

When asked what she told the parents of the subject-children at Willowbrook, Dr. Joan Giles replied, "I explain that there is no vaccine against infectious hepatitis. . . . I also tell them that we can modify the disease with gamma globulin but we can't provide lasting immunity without letting them get the disease."[6] Obviously vaccines giving "lasting immunity" are not the only kinds of vaccine to be used in caring for patients.

Doubtless the studies at Willowbrook resulted in improvement in the vaccine, to the benefit of present and future patients. In September 1966, "a routine program of GG [gamma globulin] administration to every new patient at Willowbrook" was begun. This cut the incidence of icteric hepatitis 80 to 85 percent. Then follows a significant statement in the *Medical Tribune* article: "A similar reduction in the icteric form of the disease has been accomplished among the employees, who began getting routine GG earlier in the study."[7] Not only did the research team (so far as these reports show) fail to consider and adopt the alternative that new admittees to the staff be asked to become volunteers for an investigation that might improve the vaccine against the strain of infectious hepatitis to which they as well as the children were exposed. Instead, the staff was routinely protected earlier than the inmates were! And, as we have seen, there was evidence from the beginning that gamma globulin provided at least some protection. A "modification" of the disease was still an inoculum, even if this provided no lasting immunization and had to be repeated. It is axiomatic to medical ethics that a known remedy or protection—even if not perfect or even if the best exact administration of it has not been proved—should not be withheld from individual patients. It seems to a layman that from the beginning various trials at immunization of all new admittees might have been made, and controlled observation made of their different degrees of effectiveness against "nature" at Willowbrook. This would doubtless have been a longer way round, namely, the "anecdotal" method of investigative treatment that comes off second best in comparison with controlled trials. Yet this seems to be the alternative dictated by our received medical ethics, and the only one expressive of minimal care of the primary patients themselves.

Finally, except for one episode, the obtaining of parental consent (on the premise that this is ethically valid) seems to have been very well handled. Wards of the state were not used, though by law the administrator at Willowbrook could have signed consent for them. Only new admittees whose parents were available were entered by proxy consent into the project. Explanation was made to groups of these parents, and they were given time to think about it and consult with their own family physicians. Then late in 1964 Willowbrook was closed to all new admissions because of overcrowding. What then happened can most impartially be described in the words of an article defending the Willowbrook project on medical and ethical grounds:

> Parents who applied for their children to get in were sent a form letter over Dr. Hammond's signature saying that there was no space for new admissions and that their name was being put on a waiting list.
>
> But the hepatitis program, occupying its own space in the institution, continued to admit new patients as each new study group began. "Where do you find new admissions except by canvassing the people who have applied for admission?" Dr. Hammond asked.
>
> So a new batch of form letters went out, saying that there were a few vacancies in the hepatitis research unit if the parents cared to consider volunteering their child for that. In some instances the second form letter apparently was received as closely as a week after the first letter arrived.[8]

Granting—as I do not—the validity of parental consent to research upon children not in their behalf medically, what sort of consent was that? Surely, the duress upon these parents with children so defective as to require institutionalization was far greater than the duress on prisoners given tobacco or paid or promised parole for their cooperation! I grant that the timing of these events was inadvertent. Since, however, ethics is a matter of criticizing institutions and not only of exculpating or making culprits of individual men, the inadvertence does not matter. This is the strongest possible argument for saying that even if parents have the right to consent to submit the children who are directly and continuously in their care to nonbeneficial medical experimentation, this should not be the rule of practice governing institutions set up for their care.

Such use of captive populations of children for purely experimental purposes ought to be made legally impossible. My view is that this should be stopped by legal acknowledgement of the moral invalidity of parental or legal proxy consent for the child to procedures having no relation to a child's own diagnosis or treatment. If this is not done, canons of loyalty require that the rule of practice (by law, or otherwise) be that children in institutions and not directly under the care of parents or relatives should *never* be used in medical investigations having present pain or discomfort and unknown present and future risks to them, and promising future possible benefits only for others.

Notes

1. Robert Ward, Saul Krugman, Joan P. Giles, A. Milton Jacobs, and Oscar Bodansky, "Infectious Hepatitis: Studies of Its Natural History and Prevention," *New England Journal of Medicine* 258, no. 9 (February 27, 1958): 407–16; Saul Krugman, Robert Ward, Joan P. Giles, Oscar Bodansky, and A. Milton Jacobs, "Infectious Hepatitis: Detection of the Virus during the Incubation Period and in Clinically Inapparent Infection," *New England Journal of Medicine* 261, no. 15 (October 8, 1959): 729–34. The following account and unannotated quotations are taken from these articles.

2. J. Stokes, Jr., et al., "Infectious Hepatitis: Length of Protection by Immune Serum Globulin (Gamma Globulin) during Epidemics," *Journal of the American Medical Association* 147 (1951): 714–19. Since the half-life of gamma globulin is three weeks, no one knows exactly why it immunizes for so long a period. The "highly significant protection against hepatitis obtained by the use of gamma globulin," however, had been confirmed as early as 1945 (see Edward B. Grossman, Sloan G. Stewart, and Joseph Stokes, "Post-Transfusion Hepatitis in Battle Casualties," *Journal of the American Medical Association* 129, no. 15 [December 8, 1945]: 991–94). The inoculation *withheld* in the Willowbrook experiments had, therefore, proved valuable.

3. Saul Krugman, "Reflections on Pediatric Clinical Investigations," in *Problems of Drug Evaluation in Infants and Children*, Report of the Fifty-eighth Ross Conference on Pediatric Research, Dorado Beach, Puerto Rico, May 5–7, 1968 (Columbus: Ross Laboratories), pp. 41–42.

4. "Studies with Children Backed on Medical, Ethical Grounds," *Medical Tribune and Medical News* 8, no. 19 (February 20, 1967): 1, 23.

5. *Daedalus*, Spring 1969, pp. 471–72, 529. See also pp. 458, 470–72. Since it is the proper business of an ethicist to uphold the proposition that only retrogression in civility can result from bad moral reasoning and the use of inept examples, however innocent, it is fair to point out the startling comparison between Edsall's "argument" and the statement of Dr. Karl Brandt, plenipotentiary in charge of all medical activities in the Nazi Reich: "Do you think that one can obtain any worth-while, fundamental results without a definite toll of lives? The same goes for technological development. You cannot build a great bridge, a gigantic building—you cannot establish a speed record without deaths!" (quoted by Leo Alexander, "War Crimes: Their Social-Psychological Aspects," *American Journal of Psychiatry* 105, no. 3 [September 1948]: 172). Casualties to progress, or injuries accepted in setting speed limits, are morally quite different from death or maiming or even only risks, or unknown risks, directly and deliberately imposed upon an unconsenting human being.

6. *Medical Tribune*, February 20, 1967, p. 23.

7. *Medical Tribune*, February 20, 1967, p. 23.

8. *Medical Tribune*, February 20, 1967, p. 23.

Who Benefits from the Artificial Heart?

Thomas A. Preston

The debate over the artificial heart is not just a matter of one physician treating one patient. Nor is it a matter of two, or seven, or a hundred patients dealing in isolation with one medical team.

When Dr. William DeVries replaced first Barney Clark's and then William Schroeder's failing hearts with artificial ones, he initiated a sequence of events that will affect all patients. In time, the artificial heart program will have an indirect but certain influence on levels and types of Medicare expenditures, medical research, mechanisms and limits of insurance, the federal health care budget, and more. How all this works out will determine who gets what and how much medical care, how we apportion our expenditures between medical and nonmedical services, and whether individuals perceive the distribution of services as just.

The central issue is whether our utilization of the artificial heart shall be directed by a small group of medical investigators and their entrepreneurial backers, or by representatives of the society that has developed the technology and will have to live with its consequences. It is a classic conflict between the economic independence of individuals, and the determination of the public good in an increasingly interdependent society.

Tradition, inertia, the peculiarities of medical financing, and the absence of an effective mechanism for public direction of medical policies combine to favor the independent course of Dr. DeVries, his medical team, and Humana, Inc. Time and a rising insistence for public accountability are working against them. In my opinion, resolution of the many political and ethical issues surrounding the artificial heart will not be possible until we come to grips with the central issue of who shall make policy.

The Claim of Therapeutic Benefit

Virtually every statement by the Humana team and its representatives revolves around two arguments: we desperately need a technology by which we can save the lives of the thousands who die from heart disease, our number one killer; and, the present model of the artificial heart can achieve this goal. The first assertion—that we need more effective therapy for patients with end-stage heart disease—is indisputable. But physicians and the public usually assume that what *can* be done through modern technology *must* be done. What is missing is a hard look at whether the new technology is likely to be of net benefit to all of us, and is a better choice than other options. There is almost never a mechanism to do this kind of assessment.

From The Hastings Center Report, *February 1985, Vol. 15, no. 1, pp. 5–7. Reproduced by permission.*
© *The Hastings Center.*

In answering criticism while Barney Clark was still alive, Dr. Chase Peterson defended the artificial heart as a "legitimate idea," and added, "If this country somehow ever got the notion that an idea is dangerous, we would be in the intellectual Dark Ages." Dr. DeVries used the same metaphor a few weeks after the implantation of Mr. Schroeder. But the issue has nothing to do with an *idea* as such, or the freedom to pursue one. The distinction is between the freedom of investigators to ask questions and seek solutions, and the right of society to impose restrictions on the implementation of technology. We might decide that the artificial heart is a good idea, but one that we do not want to implement.

The second assertion—that the present model of the artificial heart is of therapeutic value—edges the advocates onto shakier ethical ground by making dubious claims of clinical success. Virtually the first statement Dr. DeVries made after the first implant was that Barney Clark would have been dead within hours had he not received the artificial heart. Other physicians might argue that life actually was shortened by the procedure. By predicting Barney Clark's imminent demise, the team precluded the most serious objection to the implantation of the artificial heart.

But is the claim correct? Before his operation Barney Clark suffered life-threatening arrhythmias because of drugs he was given, but he had had the same complication, even more sustained and for the same reason, on several occasions during the previous year and a half. And William Schroeder underwent an uncomplicated elective removal of his gall bladder just eight days before swapping hearts. Such an operation is never performed on a patient "hours" from death.

The only patient who can be said to be within hours of death is one who has in fact died already and been resuscitated. Even then, as volumes of medical evidence attest, one cannot be sure of when death might recur. We'll never know how long Clark or Schroeder would have lived without an artificial heart.

The team also has made general claims of therapeutic benefit for the artificial heart. DeVries, in explaining his move from Salt Lake City to Louisville, said, "I don't like to see people die while I wait for the red tape." The claim has locked the team into producing a patina of therapeutic success (or denial of setback) covering each clinical development. This framework foreclosed the far more legitimate option of proceeding strictly as a research project, with quiet approval of the medical community and relative indifference to the media. Instead, the team's primary goal is a substantiation of their claim; to be "vindicated," as Dr. DeVries put it. Good research needs no vindication.

The need to show benefit led to a publicity barrage. Barney Clark was set up as a media event, and then cancelled. Two video-taped interviews in which Clark had nothing positive to say were not released; finally, a short clip was culled from an extensive interview in which, encouraged by Dr. DeVries, Clark issued a semblance of a positive statement. The same thing with Schroeder. After "prolonging his life," the team was "astounded" by his fast recovery. Schroeder recovered "brilliantly"—how is this done?—from his stroke. This is not medical research. What a tangled web they weave, when first they practice to achieve.

The confusion between research and therapy runs afoul of national medical policy as established by the National Institutes of Health (NIH) and the Food and Drug Administration (FDA). For more than a decade, the NIH has favored the development of left ventricular assist devices (partial artificial hearts) rather than total artificial hearts. Moreover, NIH officials vigorously opposed FDA approval of Utah's request for permission to use the Jarvik-7 heart. The FDA did not approve the artificial heart as a device capable of achieving therapeutic benefit, but rather gave its users an *exemption* from the need to show therapeutic benefit, so that it might be used strictly on an experimental basis. In allowing claims of therapeutic benefit without demonstration of such, the FDA is exceeding its mandate from Congress and condoning a violation of its own rules.

As things now stand, the Humana team will slow down only if the clinical outcome of Mr. Schroeder and those who may follow him is poor enough to alarm the public, which has been primed to expect miraculous outcomes. This unwise and unscientific approach is a consequence of the team's unnecessary claim of therapeutic benefit. In the startup phase of any medical technology, and especially the artificial heart, adverse clinical results are expected, and the team may ironically abort its mission because of failure to achieve what seems unrealistic to most other investigators.

A Corporate Marketing Strategy

The National Institutes of Health (NIH) have been the primary source of approximately $250 million of federal expenditures for development of the artificial heart over the last twenty years, including work done on the model now being used. But the Humana team and Symbion, Inc., the manufacturer of the artificial heart, have used the quirks of our legal system to become free of the public agencies that nurtured them. By shifting patent rights from the University of Utah to Symbion, Inc., Jarvik and his co-workers became free of any NIH control.

The surgical team became impatient with the Utah Institutional Review Board (IRB), which moved cautiously and insisted on a review after each case. Humana offered DeVries freedom, funding for his artificial heart patients, plus a tripling of salary, and he left for Louisville. The Humana IRB approved the team's application shortly after its arrival. There is now no assurance of an independent mechanism to protect the rights of patients, as the Utah IRB attempted to do.

Humana, Inc. answers to its stockholders, not to the community or to a university, as do non-profit research centers. To be sure, universities also seek publicity, do not want to lose money, and have to answer to trustees: but there is in my view a fundamental difference between the broader goals of universities and enterprises whose existence depends on making a profit. Humana's interest in research is to create an "enhanced reputation," according to its chairman, David Jones. For this company with 1983 profits of $193 million, a few million dollars spent over a year or more to achieve this status should be an extremely good investment. But the artificial heart program as it now exists will fail as research because it is a corporate marketing strategy, not research.

Nevertheless, the Humana team holds that they can implant the artificial heart better than anyone else; therefore they should push on and find its value. They reiterate that we must first find out how well it works, or else we will never know and may lose a life-saving technology. Then, if it is of value, we can work out the social and economic problems attending it. DeVries, who thinks the debate is premature, said, "We have to find out if it works and then (debate) what it costs."

This argument is entirely within medical precedent, and that is what bothers most critics. A medical practice, once established, and especially if it is compensable through insurers and is popular with the public, is almost impossible to reduce or eliminate so long as it is not patently of no value. Therefore, in our medical system in which rationing exists indirectly (a lot of medical services lack forceful advocates and so never become available), what physicians establish is what we get, with indifference to relative social or medical value.

Once the artificial heart is established as workable—and it need not be even demonstrably of real benefit for the public to clamor for it—and especially if channels of public funding are established, it will be on the slippery slope from which it can not be withdrawn. Dr. DeVries expressed this to a *Washington Post* reporter with another metaphor: "I think the snowball's started and I don't think anybody can stop it now." But when everyone who might benefit from the artificial heart will want it, will Humana pay? The federal government will be asked to pay, and then it will be too late to say no. The only alternative would be to make the heart accessible only to those who can afford it, an ethically unacceptable policy in an egalitarian society.

Assessing Technologies

In thinking about whether we want the artificial heart we must consider first its technologic capabilities, and then our priorities for expending our resources. Dr. Robert Jarvik, in a 1981 *Scientific American* article, said "Neither the Jarvik-7 nor any of the several other total artificial hearts being developed is yet ready to permanently replace a human heart, even on a trial basis. . . ." I suspect that this statement, written before the decision to push ahead, is still correct.

The artificial pacemaker provides a good analogy of development during which there were repeated failures due to a number of causes, most of which were not anticipated by medical and engineering investigators. Pacemakers are an order of magnitude simpler than artificial hearts, having only one moving part and requiring one-millionth the power to run. Furthermore, when a pacemaker stops suddenly, as they still do, the consequences are seldom serious and deaths are extremely rare.

Sudden failure of an artificial heart could result in death or irreversible brain damage within ten to fifteen seconds. If and when we get to the point when artificial heart patients leave the protective environment of a hospital, we will undoubtedly encounter disasters due to unanticipated failures at times and places where patients cannot receive immediate emergency treatment. It will take a decade or more for investigators to learn what the problems are and how to deal with them, and artificial hearts will always run the risk of sudden failure. We must give serious thought to whether we want to promote this sort of existence.

Setting Priorities

Finally, we must decide whether the artificial heart is a high-priority item. The cost, if it is some day successful enough to be used for all who could benefit from it, would be great. By best estimates, approximately 50,000 persons a year are candidates for a reliable new heart. At an average cost of $125,000 apiece (half the cost for Barney Clark), the annual bill would be $6.25 billion by today's prices. The $2 billion a year now spent on end-stage kidney disease is seriously straining the Medicare budget, which is already threatened with cuts. By the most optimistic estimates the artificial heart will extend the life expectancy of the recipient by one to two years and of the total population by an average of a few days. Is the cost worth the limited gain?

If the goal is to save lives, that can be done more quickly, more broadly, and more surely by other means. Let us spend our resources instead on reducing our infant mortality rate, or treating hypertension in the inner cities, or taking care of the twenty-five million Americans who are without insurance or means of attaining adequate medical care. Let us work on prevention of heart disease, an approach that is preferable to a crude

method of altering the lives of a few who already have the disease. Recent studies suggest that a reduction of fat in the average American's diet would prolong lives far in excess of what could be achieved with any high technology.

All medical expenses ultimately are paid for by the public through individual insurance, which is shared by the public-at-large, employers, or the government. The public already is paying for these experiments. Medicare and private insurance paid about $60,000 of Barney Clark's bill at Utah, and Humana has applied to a private insurance company for partial payment of Schroeder's expenses. We must decide whether we want to spend our money on what will be at best a troublesome stopgap device, or adequate nutrition for school children, or better schools, or more parks.

In the tug for our minds and our money, all too often we place drama above reason. It is easy to empathize with a Barney Clark, or a William Schroeder, media heroes. It's much harder to send our well-wishes to someone dying in anonymity who must base his hope not on a sensational technological breakthrough but on our love and support. When President Reagan telephoned Mr. Schroeder he chose not to call the tens of thousands of others who were dying at that moment, many for lack of care from us, and some for lack of adequate medical attention. Who will call these people and offer them the help they need?

What is happening now is not good medicine, is not good science, and is not in the public interest. The artificial heart team should proceed under the public purview of an impartial commission, such as could be formed under the aegis of the National Academy of Sciences. The FDA has jurisdiction over medical devices, and it alone can represent the public in this matter. I believe that the FDA should refuse allowance of further implants because they do not represent good science, and because the claims of therapeutic efficacy are unwarranted and exceed the terms of FDA approval.

The artificial heart is still crude. Whether within two decades we can achieve a device that can predictably add two years of life without serious complications is questionable. Meanwhile, the existence of the artificial heart, with its potential for benefit, forces decisions that are for the most part not medical, but ethical and political. The stakes are too high, and the consequences too great, to exclude the public from these decisions.

When Well-Meaning Science Goes Too Far

Alexander Morgan Capron

Baby Fae has joined such figures as Barney Clark and Karen Ann Quinlan in the vocabulary of popular bioethics. Her transformation from tiny baby to larger-than-life symbol is not without problems, however, partly because of the way in which it occurred and partly because of ambiguities about the role she played in the whole drama.

There was a time when the public learned of biomedical developments after they had been reviewed by, and generally reported to, the researchers' scientific and medical peers. This method not only preserved the dignity of all involved—from scientists to patients—but also meant that the public learned about genuine "advances" rather than merely being titillated by bizarre cases of as-yet unproven import.

Today, it seems that *People* magazine has replaced *The New England Journal of Medicine* as the preferred forum for reporting events on the medical frontiers. This occurs not only in instances where a court (and, hence, usually public records, as in the *Quinlan* case) is involved, but also when the hospital actively courts the media or lamely asserts its inability to prevent media coverage. (Would we accept as readily a hospital's inability to prevent the spread of an infection into the community?)

As a result, the public receives a distorted view about the process by which scientific knowledge and useful technology actually unfold. Moreover, it may be misled about the usefulness of techniques like the baboon-heart transplant technique used on Baby Fae. Even when the press is able to obtain opinions on such an experimental procedure from members of the biomedical community, the latter are typically unable to offer the sorts of careful, well-informed evaluations that require the full data from a completed experiment (usually including matched or randomized controls or at least a series of cases).

And the research process itself may be distorted by the drive for publicity. As Ellen Goodman asked recently in questioning the way Humana Hospital was handling the William Schroeder artificial-heart implant, "Must every research project now come complete with a press kit and an attractive, articulate patient available perhaps for talk shows and certainly evening-news programs?" How can research in epidemiology or preventive care possibly compete?

One final concern about the manner in which Baby Fae was transformed into a familiar though fleeting part of our lives: this episode illustrates the unseemly way that traditional medical privacy is now frequently invaded by media spotlights merely because a patient is participating in unusual research. Some people may regard this concern as pure paternalism. After all, it might be argued, if a patient consents to the publicity (perhaps out of a desire for fame or to reward a researcher to whom the patient feels indebted), who am I to complain that his hematocrit level or urinary output is reported on the evening news?

But it is precisely here that the Baby Fae case becomes so sticky. Whatever difficulties attend the process of negotiation between a researcher and his or her subject—fraught as it is with barriers to understanding, with transferences and countertransferences, as Jay Katz has recently reminded us in *The Silent World of Doctor and Patient*—they are insignificant compared to those that arise when someone else (such as a parent) must consent on behalf of the patient-subject. Reading over the documents in the Barney Clark case, I have my doubts about the "informed consent" he gave to many aspects of what occurred, but at least some possibility of genuine communication and choice existed. Obviously, for Baby Fae, it was impossible.

This leads to the second, and more important, set of issues, which grow out of the role little Fae played in the drama that brought all that attention to Loma Linda University Medical Center. What was she: hero, victim, or patient?

The ancient dictum *primum non nocere* is simply inadequate guidance for those who treat very sick and dying patients. For them, the greatest kindness may not always to be avoid doing any

From The Hastings Center Report, *February 1985, Vol. 15, no. 1, pp. 8–9. Reproduced by permission.*
© *The Hastings Center.*

harm, if they wish to risk harm for a chance at improvement. Indeed, some patients decide to join with physician-investigators in path-breaking research—almost as collaborators, as Renée Fox observed in *Experiment Perilous*. On such medical frontiers, they are rightly regarded as heroes.

A child who is "volunteered" for research is not in the same position, however. For this reason, some ethicists have opposed research involving children. Others have suggested that allowing children into experiments (on their parents' consent, for example) serves to teach a moral lesson, that people in a community owe it to one another to behave altruistically, as by contributing to the discovery of new, useful knowledge.

Such arguments may be persuasive for low-risk studies, but certainly not for innovative therapy of the baboon-heart transplant sort. Here the choice to use a child must rest on the firmest scientific and ethical grounds. Regarding the first, I argued some years ago for a "model of successive approximations," by which one would try to get down to the least vulnerable child-subjects for procedures designed and tested to involve the least possible risk (for example, only those that had first been proven on older subjects).

When a procedure cannot be tested first on other subjects because it is intended especially for infants (as is said to be the case for babies with Fae's heart problems), there should be no ambiguity about the obligations of all involved toward the child as patient. For the physicians this means never advancing their research at the expense of the child by foregoing an alternative treatment that offers a better chance. Did Dr. Leonard Bailey and his colleagues seek a human heart for Baby Fae? Apparently not. Was one available? So a transplant expert in Los Angeles has said.

Hence the concern that Baby Fae may have ended up—like the children in the Willowbrook hepatitis research—as a victim of well-meaning science. And like them, doubts linger not only about the adequacy of the information supplied to Baby Fae's parents but about whether their personal difficulties made it possible for them to choose freely, and whether the realization that their child was dying may have left them with the erroneous conclusion that consenting to the transplant was the only "right" thing to do.

More will have to be known about this case before these doubts can be answered. Until then, Baby Fae's short life will remain with us as a reminder that certain good things—like biomedical research—sometimes go too far, and that others— like the publicity that so often now attends such experiments-in-process—need a very critical reexamination.

Principles of the Nuremberg Code

1. The voluntary consent of the human subject is absolutely essential.

2. The experiment should be such as to yield fruitful results for the good of society, unprocurable by other methods or means of study, and not random and unnecessary in nature.

3. The experiment should be so designed and based on the results of animal experimentation and a knowledge of the natural history of the disease or other problem under study that the anticipated results will justify the performance of the experiment.

4. The experiment should be so conducted as to avoid all unnecessary physical and mental suffering and injury.

5. No experiment should be conducted where there is an a priori reason to believe that death or disabling injury will occur; except, perhaps, in those experiments where the experimental physicians also serve as subjects.

6. The degree of risk to be taken should never exceed that determined by the humanitarian importance of the problem to be solved by the experiment.

From Trials of War Criminals before the Nuremberg Military Tribunals under Control Council Law No. 10, *vol. 2, pp. 181–182. Washington, D.C.: United States Government Printing Office, 1949.*

7. Proper preparations should be made and adequate facilities provided to protect the experimental subject against even remote possibilities of injury, disability, or death.

8. The experiment should be conducted only by scientifically qualified persons. The highest degree of skill and care should be required through all stages of the experiment of those who conduct or engage in the experiment.

9. During the course of the experiment the human subject should be at liberty to bring the experiment to an end if he has reached the physical or mental state where continuation of the experiment seems to him to be impossible.

10. During the course of the experiment the scientist in charge must be prepared to terminate the experiment at any stage, if he has probable cause to believe, in the exercise of good faith, superior skill and careful judgment required of him that a continuation of the experiment is likely to result in injury, disability, or death to the experimental subject.

Principles of the Declaration of Helsinki

World Medical Association

I. Basic Principles

1. Biomedical research involving human subjects must conform to generally accepted scientific principles and should be based on adequately performed laboratory and animal experimentation and on a thorough knowledge of the scientific literature.

2. The design and performance of each experimental procedure involving human subjects should be clearly formulated in an experimental protocol which should be transmitted to a specially appointed independent committee for consideration, comment, and guidance.

3. Biomedical research involving human subjects should be conducted only by scientifically qualified persons and under the supervision of a clinically competent medical person. The responsibility for the human subject must always rest with a medically qualified person and never rest on the subject of research, even though the subject has given his or her consent.

4. Biomedical research involving human subjects cannot legitimately be carried out unless the importance of the objective is in proportion to the inherent risk to the subject.

5. Every biomedical research project involving human subjects should be preceded by careful assessment of predictable risks in comparison with foreseeable benefits to the subject or to others. Concern for the interests of the subject must always prevail over the interests of science and society.

6. The right of the research subject to safeguard his or her integrity must always be respected. Every precaution should be taken to respect the privacy of the subject and to minimize the impact of the study on the subject's physical and mental integrity and on the personality of the subject.

7. Doctors should abstain from engaging in research projects involving human subjects unless they are satisfied that the hazards involved are believed to be predictable. Doctors should cease any investigation if the hazards are found to outweigh the potential benefits.

8. In publication of the results of his or her research, the doctor is obliged to preserve the accuracy of the results. Reports of experimentation not in accordance with the principles laid down in this Declaration should not be accepted for publication.

9. In any research on human beings, each potential subject must be adequately informed of the aims, methods, anticipated benefits and potential hazards of the study and the discomfort it may entail. He or she should be informed that he or she is at liberty to abstain from participation in the study and that he or she is free to withdraw his

Adopted by the 18th World Medical Assembly, Helsinki, Finland, 1964, and revised by the 29th World Medical Assembly, Tokyo, Japan, October 1975. Reprinted with permission of the World Medical Association, Inc. from the "Declaration of Helsinki," revised edition.

or her consent to participation at any time. The doctor should then obtain the subject's freely given informed consent, preferably in writing.

10. When obtaining informed consent for the research project the doctor should be particularly cautious if the subject is in a dependent relationship to him or her or may consent under duress. In that case the informed consent should be obtained by a doctor who is not engaged in the investigation and who is completely independent of this official relationship.

11. In case of legal incompetence, informed consent should be obtained from the legal guardian in accordance with national legislation. Where physical or mental incapacity makes it impossible to obtain informed consent, or when the subject is a minor, permission from the responsible relative replaces that of the subject in accordance with national legislation.

12. The research protocol should always contain a statement of the ethical consideration involved and should indicate that the principles enunciated in the present Declaration are complied with.

II. Medical Research Combined with Professional Care (Clinical Research)

1. In the treatment of the sick person, the doctor must be free to use a new diagnostic and therapeutic measure, if in his or her judgment it offers hope of saving life, reestablishing health or alleviating suffering.

2. The potential benefits, hazards and discomfort of a new method should be weighed against the advantages of the best current diagnostic and therapeutic methods.

3. In any medical study, every patient—including those of a control group, if any—should be assured of the best proven diagnostic and therapeutic method.

4. The refusal of the patient to participate in a study must never interfere with the doctor-patient relationship.

5. If the doctor considers it essential not to obtain informed consent, the specific reasons for this proposal should be stated in the experimental protocol for transmission to the independent committee (I, 2).

6. The doctor can combine medical research with professional care, the objective being the acquisition of new medical knowledge, only to the extent that medical research is justified by its potential diagnostic or therapeutic value for the patient.

III. Non-therapeutic Biomedical Research Involving Human Subjects (Non-clinical Biomedical Research)

1. In any purely scientific application of medical research carried out on a human being, it is the duty of the doctor to remain the protector of the life and health of that person on whom biomedical research is being carried out.

2. The subjects should be volunteers—either healthy persons or patients for whom the experimental design is not related to the patient's illness.

3. The investigator or the investigating team should discontinue the research if in his/her or their judgment it may, if continued, be harmful to the individual.

4. In research on man, the interest of science and society should never take precedence over considerations related to the well-being of the subject.

Decision Scenario 1 ....

You are an agent of the Ethics Committee of the National Association of Physicians. You have been sent to Laural, Mississippi, to look into the experimental work of Dr. Joseph Camwell at the Laural State Hospital.

"Our basic concern," Dr. Camwell tells you, "was to test the effectiveness of a hormone-based substance in controlling conception by the regulation of ovulation."

"A birth control pill."

"Exactly," says Dr. Camwell. "We ran a double-blind test with HB-4, the test substance, and a sucrose-based compound flavored and shaped to be phenomenologically indistinguishable from the tablets of HB-4."

"So that neither the experimenter nor the subjects knew who was getting HB-4 and who was getting the sugar pills. But who were your test subjects?"

"Patients who presented themselves at our state-sponsored outpatient clinic and requested contraceptive medication formed our candidate population. We drew from them subjects with a good medical history, and no present major illnesses, who seemed reliable enough to take their medications on schedule."

"What were the racial percentages?"

"We didn't consider that to be a relevant factor in the experiment. It just happened that about 90 percent of our subjects were black, although race was not a criterion for selection."

"Did you secure from these women their informed consent to be subjects in this experiment?"

"Of course," Dr. Camwell says. "I personally explained to each of them that they were going to participate in an experiment but that it wouldn't hurt them any. I told them they would be given birth control pills that we were testing for effectiveness. 'You might get pregnant while you're taking these pills,' I said."

"But you didn't tell them that at least half of them would be receiving sugar pills that would do absolutely nothing to prevent pregnancy?"

"I think that I warned them sufficiently," says Dr. Camwell. "I told them they might get pregnant. None of these women is able to understand medical sophistications. If I tried to tell them about the experiment, they wouldn't understand me. They knew they might get pregnant, and I figured that was enough."

"Did they all agree to participate?"

"Every last person we approached agreed to participate," Dr. Camwell says. "People always want to help out doctors, and they'll do it if you just put it to them in the right way. I never have any trouble getting subjects for my work."

Would you recommend to the ethics committee that Dr. Camwell's consent procedures be condemned? If so, on what grounds?

Camwell apparently endorses Ingelfinger's view that informed consent is impossible. Evaluate this claim.

What sort of information would have to be provided to the potential subjects to satisfy the principles of informed consent argued for by Freedman?

Decision Scenario 2 ···

"In effect," said Dr. Sanchez, "the drug is a powerful tranquilizer. We are not sure how it works, but we know that it has a great calming effect on people diagnosed as schizophrenics. It's much like thorazine, which you may have heard of."

"Does it have any side effects?" Monica Jones asked.

"If taken over a period of a couple of weeks, it produces a palsied condition—muscular tremors, difficulty in walking and in controlling the face muscles, and so on. These don't seem to be permanent."

"That's in schizophrenics," Monica said.

"That's right. We don't know the likely effects in other people. Perhaps you will notice no change whatsoever, and perhaps you will never develop the muscular tremors. But perhaps you'll develop them sooner or more severely. That's part of what we need to find out."

"I'm not in danger of death, then?"

"Not to any great extent. That is, all medication has associated with it some risk. But we don't believe the risk here to be great. There is some possibility of long-term nerve or brain damage. We simply don't know the risks here."

"And you need so-called normal people like me to act as subjects so that you can compare the effects of the drug on us with its effects on schizophrenics?"

"Exactly right," said Dr. Sanchez. "But I should tell you that you may not get the drug. None of us involved in the experiment as patients or experimenters will know who is getting the tranquilizer and who is getting a placebo."

"So maybe I'm not running any risk at all," said Monica.

"Maybe not. But your participation is still important. This drug may do much to relieve the symptoms of a great number of schizophrenics."

"Now if I understand correctly," said Monica Jones, "I will be paid for my participation."

"That's right. You will be paid a flat fee for participation—half at the beginning of the study and the rest at the end. I want you to be clear on one thing, however. You must waive your right to claim compensation due to any injury or ill-effects you may suffer as a result of the medication."

"I understand that. I've got to take a risk. I'm not too happy about that, but I can't get a job and I need the money so I can go back to school next semester."

"Fine," said Dr. Sanchez. "I have the consent forms right here."

Is a society in which risking one's health for financial gain one compatible with Rawls's principles of justice?

Do Kant's principles allow one to take such a risk?

Does the natural law doctrine of Catholicism?

Would the view of human experimentation advocated by Jonas regard such an experiment as legitimate? Would the view of Lasagna? Would Freedman's theory allow such a financial transaction?

Do you think it is possible for Sanchez to give Jones good reasons for participating that do not involve some form of pressure or duress?

Decision Scenario 3 ···

The drug DES—diethylstilbestrol—was once believed to be effective in preventing miscarriages. But in 1971 sufficient evidence was available to establish a link between DES and vaginal cancer and cervical cell abnormalities in the daughters of women given the drug. About one million women were given DES in the first trimester of pregnancy, and over 120 daughters of these women have been shown to have cancer. Sons, apparently, do not develop cancer, but the group shows a higher than average proportion of genital abnormalities and sterility.

In late 1951 and early 1952, women receiving prenatal care at the University of Chicago's Lying-In Hospital were given unmarked tablets of DES as part of a study conducted by Dr. William Dieckmann. One of those receiving the tablets was Ms. Patsy T. Mink, who later became an Assistant Secretary of State.

"I remember quite clearly the doctor giving me those pills and telling me they were vitamins," Ms. Mink says.

Ms. Mink's daughter Gwendolyn was born in the hospital in 1952. Ms. Mink was not notified that she had been given DES until twenty-four years later. She rushed her daughter to a medical examination, and it was discovered that Gwendo-

lyn had abnormal cell changes in the cervix—a condition known as adenosis and thought to be a precursor of cancer.

Ms. Mink is outraged by the experiment in which she was an unwitting subject. She feels that she was not given the drug for a legitimate medical reason and that she was deceived by her doctor. "There's no way we could know," she says. "If they had given me a choice, if they had said, 'We think you are a risk case and this drug may help you.' That's different. That's the choice we should have been presented with. But I wasn't a risk case, and I wasn't told anything."

Did those who gave her DES act immorally? After all, at the time she was given the drug there was no reason to believe that it might be harmful effects.

If Ms. Mink's informed consent had been obtained, the outcome would have been exactly the same because she could not have been warned of dangers that no one knew existed. Doesn't this show that the whole notion of informed consent is pointless and that one simply must trust in the integrity and best judgment of a physician, as Ingelfinger suggests?

Decision Scenario 4 ....

"You realize," Dr. Thorne said, "that you may not be in the group that receives medication? You may be in the placebo group for at least part of the time."

"Right," Ms. Ross said. "You're just going to give me some medicine."

"And do you understand the aims of the experiment?"

"You want to help me get better," Ms. Ross suggested hesitantly.

"We hope you get better, of course. But that's not what we're trying to accomplish here. We're trying to find out if this particular medication will help other people in your condition if we can treat them earlier than we were able to treat you."

"You want to help people," Ms. Ross said.

"That's right. Now, do you understand that we may not be helping you in this experiment?"

"But you're going to try?"

"Not exactly. I mean, we aren't going to try to harm you. But we aren't necessarily going to be giving you the preferred treatment for your complaint either. Do you know the difference between research and therapy?"

"Research is when you're trying to find something out. You're searching around."

"That's right. And we're asking you to be part of a research effort. As I told you, there are some risks. Besides the possibility of not getting treatment that you need, the drug may produce some limited hepatic portal damage. We're not sure how much."

"I think I understand," Ms. Ross said.

"I hope so," said Dr. Thorne. "Now I understand that you are freely volunteering to participate in this research."

"Yes, sir. Mrs. Woolerd, she told me if I volunteered I'd get a letter put in my file and I could get early release."

"Mrs. Woolerd told you the Review Board would take your volunteering into account when they considered whether you should be put on work-release."

"Yes, sir. And I'm awfully anxious to get out of here. I've got two children staying with my aunt, and I need to get out of this place as quick as I can."

"I understand. We can't promise you release, of course. But your participation will look good on your record. Now I have some papers here I want you to sign."

Discuss some of the difficulties involved in explaining research procedures to nonexperts and determining whether they are aware of the nature and risks of their participation.

What reasons are there for believing that Ms. Ross does not understand what she is volunteering for?

Also discuss the problems involved in securing free and voluntary consent from a person involuntarily confined to an institution (a prisoner, for example).

Is there a reason to believe that Ms. Ross is not giving free consent?

What conditions does Freedman require satisfied before a prisoner's consent can be regarded as legitimate?

Decision Scenario 5 ....

The ad in the newspapers was simple and uninformative:

> Subjects (male and female) wanted to participate in scientific study. Must be 21 or over. $2.00 per hour.

Karen Barty wrote down the address. She could use the money, and in 1962 $2.00 an hour wasn't bad pay for what was sure to be very little work. Besides, the hours were probably flexible, and she could fit the time into her class schedule.

Next Tuesday morning at ten o'clock, Karen and nine other people reported to room 711 of the Basic Sciences Building in the Western Medical Center. A man who introduced himself as Dr. Carlo Raphael explained what would be required of them as research subjects.

"First of all, you must all sign consent forms," he said. "These state that you are voluntary participants in this study and that for your assistance you will receive a financial reward. If you are not willing to sign the forms, then we cannot accept you as a subject."

He interrupted himself to pass out badly mimeographed sheets of paper that had "Voluntary Consent of Research Subjects" printed at the top. Karen signed hers at once, without bothering to read it. The others in her group, she noticed, did the same thing.

"Very good," Dr. Raphael said, after collecting the forms. "We are going to ask that you provide us with the answers to a series of questions. Some of you may think of these as 'tests,' but I want to assure you that they are not tests in the way you ordinarily think of them. You can neither pass or fail. Just give us your immediate and truthful responses."

With the help of two assistants, Dr. Raphael distributed test booklets with coded answer sheets tucked inside. Everyone was then supplied with a black IBM pencil with soft, black lead.

Karen listened, half bored, as Dr. Raphael explained how the answer sheets were to be filled in. She had heard the same kind of explanation a dozen times before, but she guessed that the same thing always had to be said as part of the test procedure. Despite herself, she felt a twinge of anxiety. It was all well and good to say these weren't tests they were taking, but they were enough like every other test she had taken to make her adrenalin flow.

At noon, they handed in their test booklets and took a break for lunch. When they reported back, it was to another room in the same building. It was not a classroom this time, but a lounge. Steel-framed chairs and sofas covered in grey and orange plastic were set about the room, and the floor was covered with beige carpet, its industrial finish looking flat and somewhat dirty.

A long table at the front was draped with white crepe paper, and pitchers of water surrounded by glasses were set at one end. At the opposite end, a red cafeteria tray with small paper cups was watched over by a woman Karen hadn't seen before.

The cups looked like the sort that are usually filled with nuts or hard candies. When Karen got close enough, she saw that each cup contained only what looked like a single cube of sugar.

That's what it tasted like when Karen got hers. Dr. Raphael lined up the ten subjects, and as each one reached the table, the woman handed over one of the cups.

"Let the cube dissolve in your mouth," Dr. Raphael told them. "Then have some water, if you like, but don't eat or drink anything else. Then you may just sit around in this room and talk to each other."

It was pretty disgusting, just eating plain sugar. But within twenty minutes, Karen knew that it wasn't just plain sugar. She was sitting on one of the sofas talking to another woman about an English group called the Beatles. The woman had never heard of them, and Karen spelled the name for her.

But as she started to spell it, she suddenly found it very hard to concentrate. She knew where she was and what she was doing, but the woman in front of her began to look strange. She seemed to be surrounded by a halo of brightly colored light. The features of her face lost their outlines and became twisted and distorted.

In a few minutes, Karen gave up trying to talk. Somewhere at the back of her mind, she felt fear and confusion. But what was happening to her wasn't unpleasant. It was interesting, really, and she surrendered herself to the fantastic images that seemed to take over her mind without her being able to control them.

Somewhere in that time, Karen fell asleep or at least she thought she did. She vaguely remembered one of Dr. Raphael's assistants holding her by the arm and leading her back to the classroom. She tried to talk to him, but she wasn't sure what she said. When she was handed another test booklet, she was surprised to find how easy it was to fill out the answer sheet. This time there was no anxiety at all.

By five o'clock that afternoon, Karen was herself again. It was not until seventeen years later that she realized she had been an unwitting participant in a research project sponsored by the army to determine psychological effects of LSD.

What kind of information would Karen Barty have had to be given to satisfy Freedman's principles of informed consent?

On what grounds would Jonas disapprove of the way in which Karen was employed as a subject?

This was clearly a case of nontherapeutic research. Can a case be made for it on utilitarian grounds?

Does Karen have any grounds for claiming compensation if in years after the research she suffers

from effects that may reasonably be attributed to her participation as a subject?

Suppose that Dr. Raphael had fully informed the group about the nature and aims of the research and warned them about potential dangers. Given that very little was known in 1962 about the possible effects of LSD, would any person be justified in risking life or health by participating in the experiment?

Decision Scenario 6 ·······································

"That is truly absurd," Dr. Kuhmwar Raita said. "The mother wanted to get rid of the fetus. That's why she elected to have the abortion in the first place. The fetus has no status. It's just a lump of tissue."

Dr. Allan Smith shook his head in disagreement. "It is not, Kuhmwar. That's just the point. The fetus is not viable, but it's out of the uterus and alive at this very instant."

"Well, it will be dead in a short while, then it will be of no use to me. If I'm going to find out anything about cerebral glucose uptake, I've got to have a functioning system."

"But we can't just kill this child."

"The child, as you call it, is as good as dead. And if we can ever gain an understanding of the fundamental processes involved here, we may actually be able to save the lives of countless babies."

"I can't believe you would resort to such a crude argument."

"Call it whatever you want to, but I think it's right."

Is it possible to construct a utilitarian argument to support the position taken by Dr. Raita?

In what way is the status of the fetus relevant to this issue of fetal experimentation?

Are the issues of fetal experimentation exactly analogous to the arguments about abortion? Or are they more closely analogous to the arguments about human experimentation?

What view might a Kantian take on this question?

Decision Scenario 7 ·······································

In April of 1979, a suit was filed in Illinois by the Cook County Public Guardian against the Illinois Department of Mental Health. The suit alleged that during the 1950s and 1960s between twenty-five and one hundred patients underwent "unauthorized and secret" surgery at a state mental health center.

The suit charged that the patients, without their consent, were subjected to experimental surgery to remove their adrenal glands. A memo from a psychiatrist was cited that described the health center as "virtually a human dog lab."

A spokesman for the mental health department publicly denied the charges in the suit. He

claimed that an internal investigation showed that consent from the patients had been obtained and each had been informed of the possible risks and of the short- and long-term effects.

Moreover, the surgery was said to have a therapeutic aim, as well as an experimental one. A theory at the time suggested that the removal of the adrenal gland might correct a hormonal imbalance that some research psychiatrists believed to be a cause of schizophrenia. Furthermore, it was claimed that only four schizophrenic patients were involved.

As a matter of fact, the surgery did not lead to improvement in any of the patients, and the theory which suggested that it might is no longer held. Those who had their adrenal glands removed required injections of cortisone for the rest of their lives to compensate for the loss of natural secretions from the gland.

> *Suppose that the charge made by the Public Guardian is correct. What utilitarian argument might be offered to support the use of mental patients as subjects in the experimental surgery?*

> *Clearly the only proper candidates for an experimental procedure aimed at treating schizophrenia are people who are schizophrenics. Is it reasonable*

> *to believe that people who suffer from a psychosis are capable of giving informed consent?*

> *On Freedman's view, would proxy consent obtained for such people be legitimate?*

> *Is it possible to argue that the principle of autonomy requires that patients diagnosed as psychotic ought to be allowed to consent to any procedure that may help their condition? If not, why not?*

> *How relevant to the moral issue of consent is the nonmoral question of the degree of confirmation of a theory which is the basis of an experimental procedure with a therapeutic aim?*

Decision Scenario 8 ···

At six A.M. on Wednesday, March 6, 1985, Dr. Kevin Cheng of Phoenix got a call from cardiac surgeon Dr. Cecil Vaughn. "Is your heart ready to be implanted?" Dr. Vaughn asked.

Dr. Cheng thought the question was about implanting the artificial heart he had invented into a calf, an experiment he and Dr. Vaughn had done once before and were planning to do again. When he learned that the intended recipient was a human, he hesitated. "Wait a minute," Dr. Cheng said. "It's designed for a calf and not ready for a human yet."

"Think about it, decide, and I'll call back in ten minutes," Dr. Vaughn told him.

The heart was needed because Thomas Creighton, a thirty-three-year-old automobile mechanic and divorced father of two, had rejected the heart he had received from an accident victim. Dr. Jack Copeland and the transplant team at University Medical Center in Tucson immediately began a search for another donor heart, and Mr. Creighton was placed on the heart–lung machine. Dr. Copeland had also called Utah and requested that the Jarvik-7 heart be flown in.

"I knelt and prayed," Dr. Cheng recalled later. When Dr. Vaughn called him back, he said, "The pump is sterile and ready to go."

Around noon of the same day, Dr. Vaughn implanted the device in Mr. Creighton. Mr. Creighton's physicians had decided that it would be dangerous to leave him on the heart–lung machine any longer, and the Jarvik-7 heart had not yet arrived. The Phoenix heart maintained Mr.

Creighton's circulation until a donor heart was located.

At eleven that night, the device was turned off, and Mr. Creighton was put back on the heart–lung machine. At three A.M. on Thursday, Dr. Copeland transplanted the second donor heart. However, despite all efforts, Mr. Creighton died the following day. The Phoenix heart had had nothing to do with causing his death.

However, in deciding to use the Phoenix heart, Dr. Vaughn and Dr. Copeland had apparently violated FDA regulations by employing a device that had not been approved for experimental use in humans. They and their defenders justified their action by claiming that their use of the device was an emergency measure. They were not performing an experiment with Mr. Creighton, but attempting to save his life. The only other option was just to let him die. "We had nothing to lose" by using the heart, Dr. Copeland said.

> *Would the line of reasoning taken by Dr. Copeland lead to the conclusion that anything at all can be done to a patient, if it can be justified as an effort to save the patient's life?*

> *What response can be given to the charge that Mr. Creighton's condition was not a true medical emergency, because transplant rejection is one of the anticipated risks of that kind of surgery?*

> *Although Mr. Creighton gave consent to the original surgery, he was in no condition to give consent to the use of the artificial heart. (Consent was*

given by his mother and sister.) Because of the risks known to be associated with artificial hearts (strokes and consequent brain damage, for example), the fact that he consented to a heart transplant does not mean that he would have consented

to even the temporary use of an artificial heart. So far as he knew, the matter would never arise. Does this mean that Mr. Creighton was illegitimately denied the opportunity to decide what sort of risks he was willing to take?

Decision Scenario 9 ·····································

The first human heart was transplanted in 1967 in South Africa by Dr. Christiaan Barnard. However, this was not the first heart transplant on a human being. In January of 1964, Dr. James D. Hardy of the University of Mississippi transplanted a chimpanzee heart into Boyd Rush.

Boyd Rush was a deaf-mute who was brought to the University of Mississippi Medical Center unconscious and on the verge of dying. A stepsister, the only relative who could be located, signed a consent form permitting, if necessary, "the insertion of a suitable heart transplant." The form made no reference to the sort of heart that might be employed. Mr. Rush lived for two hours after the transplant.

Dr. Hardy justified his use of the chimpanzee heart on the ground that it was impossible to obtain a human heart. Also, he was encouraged to think the transplant might be successful because of the limited success obtained by Dr. Keith Reemtsma in transplanting chimpanzee kidneys into a man dying of glomerulonephritis. The kidney recipient lived for two months.

Dr. Leonard Bailey, the surgeon who trans-

planted the baboon heart into the child known as Baby Fae, expressed his view of Dr. Hardy in an interview: "He's an idol of mine because he followed through and did what he should have done . . . he took a gamble to try to save a human life."

Evaluate the quality of the consent that was secured for transplant surgery in this case.

Suppose that Mr. Rush's stepsister did know that it was possible that a chimpanzee heart might be used. Should anyone be permitted to give consent to such a transplant on behalf of someone else?

If the only way to save the life of Mr. Rush was to transplant a chimpanzee heart, was the surgery justified?

If the transplant could have been expected to postpone Mr. Rush's death for only a relatively short time, was the surgery justifiable?

Evaluate the criticism that Dr. Hardy was doing no more than performing a medical experiment in which Mr. Rush was the unknowing and unconsenting subject.

PART III

CONTROLS

CHAPTER 6

GENETICS: INTERVENTION, CONTROL, AND RESEARCH

CASE PRESENTATION
Huntington's Disease: The Search for a Marker

Huntington's disease is a particularly cruel and frightening genetic disorder. Those diagnosed as having the disease soon become aware of the facts that the disease is invariably fatal and that there is no effective treatment for it. What is more, each of their children has a fifty percent chance of developing the disease.

The disease typically makes its appearance between the ages of thirty-five and forty-five in men and women who have shown no previous symptoms. The signs of its onset may be quite subtle—a certain clumsiness in performing small tasks, a slight slurring of speech, a few facial twitches. But the disease is progressive. Eventually the small, subtle signs develop into massive physical and mental changes. Walking becomes jerky and unsteady, the face contorts into wild grimaces, the hands repeatedly clench and relax, and the whole body writhes with involuntary muscle spasms. The victim eventually loses the power of speech, becomes disoriented, and gives way to irrational emotional outbursts. Before mental deterioration becomes too advanced, HD victims often kill themselves out of sheer hopelessness and despair. Death may occur naturally from fifteen to twenty years after the beginning of the

symptoms. Usually it results from massive infection and malnutrition, for as the disease progresses, the victim loses the ability to swallow normally.

In the United States, at any given time, some 20,000 people are diagnosed as having the disease. It has been estimated that as many as 100,000 more may have the gene responsible for the disease. The incidence of the disease is only 1 in 10,000, but for the child of a victim of the disease, the chances are 1 out of 2.

The disease is transmitted from generation to generation in a hereditary pattern that indicates that it is caused by a single gene. However, since the disease makes its appearance relatively late in life, an unsuspecting victim may already have passed on the gene to a child before he or she shows any sign of the disease. In the absence of a genetic test to detect the presence of the gene, there is no way for an individual to know whether he or she is a carrier of the gene.

In 1983 a major step toward the development of a genetic test for determining the presence of the HD gene was announced by Dr. James F. Gusella and his group at Massachusetts General Hospital. The team did not locate the gene itself, but a ''genetic marker'' that appears to indicate that it is present.

The group began by studying the DNA taken from members of a large American family with a history of Huntington's disease. They then employed recombinant-DNA techniques to attempt to locate a genetic marker for the HD gene. The techniques involve using a group of proteins known as restriction enzymes. A particular enzyme, when mixed with a single strand of DNA, cuts the strand at specific locations known as recognition sites. After the DNA strand has been cut up by restriction enzymes, short sections of radioactive, single-stranded DNA are added to serve as probes. The probes bind to particular segments of the DNA. Because the probes are radioactive, the segments of DNA to which they are attached can be identified on photographic film.

The number and location of recognition sites vary among individuals and appear to be inherited. The various fragments of DNA produced by the restriction enzymes and identified by probes form a pattern that is typical of individuals. A mutation of a normal gene may change the point at which an enzyme makes a cut. This produces a DNA fragment that is not the usual length and alters the pattern of that person. Thus, if the pattern of someone who does not have the disease is compared with the pattern of a family member who does, the fragments that include the faulty gene can be identified, even though the gene itself is unknown. The abnormal pattern serves as a *marker* for the presence of the gene.

Dr. Gusella's group faced the problem of attempting to find a marker that was consistently inherited by those with Huntington's disease but not inherited by those free of the disease. This meant identifying perhaps as many as eight hundred markers and determining whether one could serve as the marker for the HD gene. Fortunately, after only eleven attempts the team identified a good candidate. It was a marker found in all members of the family they were studying. All those with the disease had the same form of the marker, and those free of the disease had some other form.

In collaboration with the Hereditary Disease Foundation, plans were made to test this finding in a larger population. It was known that a large family with a high incidence of HD lived along the shores of Lake Maracaibo in Venezuela. Nancy Wexler led a team to this remote location to collect the family history and to obtain blood and skin samples for analysis. The lake-dwelling family included some one hundred people with the disease and 1,100 children with the risk of developing it.

Analysis of the samples showed that those with the disease also carried the same form of the marker as their American counterparts. Gusella estimated that the odds are 100 million to one that the marker is linked to the HD gene. Subsequent work by Susan Naylor located the marker on chromosome number four. The gene itself still has not been identified, and it is still not known whether the gene is located on chromosome four of all who carry the HD gene. Also, the mechanisms through which the gene acts to cause the disease are not yet known.

A standard genetic test for the presence of the HD marker has yet to be developed. It is reasonably certain that one will be soon. The current test is elaborate and expensive and can be used only with those who have large enough families to detect a linkage with the marker. The identification of the gene should permit a blood test and the use of a DNA probe to search for the presence of the gene.

A study conducted in Wales in the 1970s revealed that more than half of those whose parents or relatives were victims of Huntington's disease would not want to have a test that would tell them whether they had the HD gene, even if such a test were available. Considering that the disease is virtually untreatable and invariably fatal, this is perhaps not a surprising finding. It is difficult to imagine the dread and horror that would be suffered by someone who knows that eventually the disease will announce itself and who must wait for that moment.

But what about obligations to others? If a test is available, is it fair to a potential marriage partner to marry without finding out whether one is a carrier of the HD gene and informing the potential partner of the result? Perhaps he or she may be willing to take the chance that the offspring of an HD victim will not have the disease. Yet because of the tremendous burden the disease places on the other spouse, the possibility of being tested for the presence of the gene deserves serious consideration.

The decision about whether to have children

might also be affected by the knowledge that one partner is a carrier of the HD gene so there is a 50 percent chance any child will also inherit the gene and develop the disease. Should a potential carrier of the gene impose the risk of having a child who will inherit the disease on the other partner? Should such a risk be imposed on a potential child? A genetic test could determine whether there is any risk at all. If the risk is present, then the couple could at least make a decision with a knowledge of the relevant facts.

The present test can also be used in conjunction with amniocentesis to determine whether a developing fetus has the marker for the HD gene, and any subsequent test will also have this capability. Possessing such information adds a particular difficulty to making an abortion decision, for those who do not oppose abortion in principle. A child born with the HD gene will inevitably develop the disease but may not do so for three, four, or even five or more decades. Is the fact that the child will eventually succumb to the disease reason enough to make an abortion morally obligatory?

The development of a standard, inexpensive test for the HD gene is sure to raise other moral and social issues as well. For example, it is possible that insurance companies may refuse to provide life or health insurance to those from families with Huntington's disease, unless they prove that they are not carriers of the gene. Employers may refuse to provide health benefits to family members unless they are tested and found to lack the gene.

Informing someone that he or she carries the marker or the gene also has problems associated with it. Such news can be devastating, both to the person and to the person's family. About 10 to 12 percent of HD victims kill themselves, and 30 percent of those at risk say that this is what they will do if they learn they have the disease. Thus, the mere act of conveying the information that someone will later develop the signs of a fatal disease can itself constitute a threat to life.

In the best of all worlds, an effective means of avoiding or treating the disease would be available. Then the moral and social issues associated with a genetic test for it would disappear without having to be resolved. Regrettably, that world still lies in the future.

CASE PRESENTATION
Gene Therapy

In 1980 Dr. Martin J. Cline of UCLA treated two patients suffering from an incurable blood disorder called beta-zero thalassemia with an entirely new therapeutic technique. The disease is one in which the gene for beta globulin, one of the constituents of the hemoglobin in red blood cells, is either missing or unexpressed. Those with the disease usually die very early, and frequently they suffer from anemia, cirrhosis of the liver, and serious heart problems because of the inability of their blood to transport sufficient oxygen to their tissues.

The aim of Dr. Cline's treatment was to provide the patients with the gene required to produce normal hemoglobin. The technique he employed, called *transformation*, is one that had been developed through research with animals. The basic idea behind the technique is simple.

Copies of a normal gene are inserted into the cells of a patient who lacks the gene or who possesses it only in a malfunctioning form. The DNA of the cells is induced to incorporate the new gene so that, when the cells reproduce themselves, copies of the new gene are made along with copies of the other genes encoded by the cellular DNA. In this way, the patient acquires a population of normal cells. The problem that was caused by the missing or defective gene is thus corrected. The technique as applied by Cline in this particular situation depended on the chemical properties of DNA and on the fact that cells take in calcium from their environment. Under proper conditions, the cells will take up DNA fragments, which include new genes, along with the calcium. Cells in the bone marrow (stem cells) are among those responsible for the production of red blood cells.

Accordingly, Cline and his associates took bone marrow from the patients and added the appropriate DNA segments to a cell culture of that material. The hope was that the DNA would be incorporated into the genetic code of the cells—that the cells would be transformed. Afterward, the treated cells would then multiply, and their copies would include the new genes. The patients would thus be supplied with the cells necessary to produce beta globulin.

The plan was not successful. Transformation is a very ineffective process, and very few cells in a culture actually incorporate the foreign DNA. Perhaps the material injected into the patients did not contain enough transformed cells to make a difference. Or perhaps the transformed cells did not multiply sufficiently or otherwise perform as expected. In any case, the patients were not helped by the attempt at therapy, although there was no indication they were harmed, either.

Cline was reprimanded by the National Institutes of Health for engaging in medical experiments without securing the approval of the appropriate UCLA committees. In his own view, the experiments were both scientifically and morally justifiable.

The techniques developed in recombinant-DNA research are crucial to the procedures of gene therapy. It must be possible to identify the defective gene and manipulate the cell's DNA so that a new DNA segment containing a functioning gene is included in it. What is more, these tasks must be accomplished without damaging the cell or destroying its ability to reproduce normally. Although Cline made use of transformation as a technique, the more common technique in animal research is to employ a genetically engineered retrovirus to introduce the new gene into the cellular DNA. Unmodified retroviruses frequently cause diseases in humans, such as AIDS and certain forms of cancer. Consequently, one of the aims of recent gene-therapy research has been to modify retroviruses so that they will insert a desired gene into the DNA of a human cell but will not cause a dangerous infection. (See the Introduction for more information about recombinant-DNA.)

So far gene therapy has not been successfully used with humans. However, animal research suggests that it will be only a very short time before genetic modifications in human cells can also

be made with the assurance that the genes will function as they are supposed to. The promise that an effective gene therapy holds for those who suffer from a variety of genetic disorders is enormous.

In the view of many researchers, the first diseases to receive attention should be those that are both life-threatening and hold out the possibility of successful treatment. Prime candidates meeting these criteria are deficiency diseases in which a crucial enzyme is missing because of a single defective gene, such as adenosine deaminase (ADA) deficiency and purine nucleoside phosphorylase (PNP) deficiency. Both diseases are invariably fatal, and both are caused by the lack of a single effective gene. Replacing the gene in a victim's cells would allow them to produce the missing enzyme. In principle, people suffering from such diseases could be completely cured by genetic modification.

Another disease that is widely considered a major candidate for gene therapy is Lesch-Nyhan disease. Those suffering from the disease show signs of dwarfism, palsy, bone deformities, and a peculiar compulsion of self-mutilation. Children who are untended may literally chew off their lips and tear at their fingers with their teeth. The disease is known to be the result of a single defective gene, one that fails to produce an adequate amount of the enzyme HPRT. However, exactly what role the lack of the enzyme plays in causing the disease is not yet known. The symptoms may be the result of the buildup of some biochemical in the brain that is ordinarily broken down when the enzyme is present.

Copies of the normal gene that produces HPRT have been grown in the laboratory and transplanted into cell cultures. However, unlike deficiency diseases such as ADA and PNP, the enzyme in Lesch-Nyhan may be needed in the brain. Some researchers are of the opinion that this may involve a difficulty not easily overcome. Other single-gene deficiency diseases can be treated by taking cells from the bone marrow, modifying them into the bloodstream. The modified cells then migrate back to the bone marrow. In Lesch-Nyhan the modified cells may have to be injected directly into the brain, and whether they will then reproduce normally and produce the HPRT enzyme remains to be seen.

In the future, it may be possible to treat such

relatively common diseases as cystic fibrosis, hemophilia, phenylketonuria, and sickle-cell anemia by gene therapy. Current strategy is to concentrate on diseases with causes that are comparatively simple. Initial success seems certain to spur research to make it possible to treat more complicated diseases, including genetic disorders that are the result of a more than one malfunctioning gene.

Paralleling the development of gene therapy are other treatment strategies also based on the technology of recombinant-DNA. One of the most promising is the use of drugs to alter the function of genes that are not behaving normally. The drugs in effect "turn on" a malfunctioning gene so that it plays the role it is supposed to. Some promising results in the treatment of thalassemia and sickle-cell anemia have been reported.

Another technique involves transplanting cells into the brain, and it has been used experimentally in the treatment of Parkinson's disease. The disease appears to result from the destruction of brain cells in the substantia nigra and the consequent reduction in dopamine production. Dopamine is a neurotransmitter involved in the movement of voluntary muscles. Its absence results in loss of control and shaky, involuntary movements. Researchers in Sweden in 1982 reported some success in transplanting cells from a patient's adrenal glands into the substantia nigra tissue of his brain. Recent work transplanting cells into animal brains supports the idea that transplant therapy for diseases such as Parkinson's and Alzheimer's will be effective in the not-too-distant future.

The gene therapy in humans that is currently under development is somatic-cell therapy. That is, the modifications are in the body cells of patients, not in the sex cells. This means that even if the therapy can eliminate the disease produced in an individual who has inherited a defective gene, the therapy will do nothing to alter the probability that a child of that person will inherit the same defective gene. To change this circumstance, so-called germ-line cells would have to be altered. That is, the defective gene in an ovum or sperm cell would have to be replaced.

If this were possible, then certain genetic diseases could be eliminated from families. Germ-line therapy would make it unnecessary to perform somatic-cell therapy for each generation of af-

fected individuals. As appealing as this prospect is, at the present germ-line therapy has many more technical difficulties associated with it than does somatic-cell therapy. Uniformly encouraging results have not so far been produced in animal research, and somatic-cell therapy in humans remains a distant prospect.

Most of the moral issues discussed in connection with gene therapy have centered around germ-line therapy. It holds out the prospect of genetically engineering sex cells to produce offspring with virtually any set of characteristics desired. This possibility has led many critics to warn that "genetic surgery" may be leading us into a sort of Brave New World in which we practice eugenics and manufacture our children to order. (See the Introduction for a fuller discussion.) However, any dangers posed by germ-line therapy are far from immediate.

Somatic-cell therapy in humans is likely to become an established form of treatment within the next two to five years. It will for some time remain an experimental treatment, and as such it raises the same sorts of moral questions typical of any experimental procedure—ones of informed consent, benefit, and risk. The basic issue raised by researchers themselves is the question of when it is legitimate to move from laboratory experiments to the actual treatment of humans. The generally accepted answer has been that gene therapy is ready to employ when it has been demonstrated to be safe and effective. However, such an answer is helpful only when specific criteria are formulated to determine safety and effectiveness.

INTRODUCTION

The two great triumphs of nineteenth-century biology were Darwin's formulation of the theory of organic evolution and Mendel's statement of the laws of transmission genetics. One of the twentieth century's outstanding accomplishments has been the development of an understanding of the molecular structures and processes that are involved in genetic inheritance. All three great achievements give rise to moral and social issues of considerable complexity. The theories are abstract, but the problems they generate are concrete and immediate.

Major problems are associated with our increased knowledge of inheritance and genetic change. One class of problems concerns the use we make of the knowledge we possess in dealing with individuals. We know a great deal about the ways in which genetic diseases are transmitted and about the sorts of errors that can occur in human development. We have the means to make reliable predictions about the chances of the occurrence of a disease in a particular case, and we have the medical technology to detect some disorders before birth.

To what extent should we employ this knowledge? One possibility is that we might use it to detect, treat, or prevent genetic disorders. Thus, we might require that everyone submit to screening and counseling before having children. Or we might require that children be tested either prenatally or immediately after birth. We might recommend or require selective abortions. In this way, it might be possible to bring many genetic diseases under control in much the same way that we have brought contagious diseases under control.

Requiring screening and testing suggests another possibility, one that involves taking a broader view of human genetics. Eliminating genetic disease might simply become part of a much more ambitious plan for deliberately improving the entire species. Shall we attempt to control human evolution by formulating policies and practices designed to alter the genetic composition of the human population? Shall we make use of "gene surgery" and recombinant-DNA technology to shape physical and mental attributes of our species? That is, shall we practice some form of eugenics?

Another class of problems has to do with the wider social and environmental consequences of genetic research and technology. Research in molecular genetics that is concerned with recombinant-DNA has already revealed to us ways in which the machinery of cells can be altered in beneficial ways. We are able to make bacteria synthesize such important biological products as human insulin, and we are able to alter bacteria to serve as vaccines against some diseases. In effect, recombinant-DNA technology produces life forms that have never existed before. Should biotech industries be allowed to patent such forms, in exactly the same way as new inventions are patented? Or do organisms belong to us all?

Also, what are we to say about the deliberate release of genetically altered organisms into the environment? Is the threat that such organisms pose greater than the benefits they are likely to produce? We have already witnessed the great damage that can be done by pesticides and chemical pollution. Is there any way that we can avoid the potential damage that might be caused by genetically engineered organisms?

In the following three sections, we shall focus attention on the issues that are raised by the actual and potential use of genetic information. Our topics are these: genetic intervention (screening, counseling, and prenatal diagnosis), eugenics, and genetic research (therapy, technology, and biohazards).

GENETIC INTERVENTION: SCREENING, COUNSELING, AND DIAGNOSIS

Our genes play a major role in making us what we are. Biological programs of genetic information work amazingly well to produce normal, healthy individuals. But sometimes things can go wrong, and when they do, the results can be tragic.

Almost two thousand human diseases have been identified as involving genetic factors. Some of the diseases are quite rare, while others are relatively common. Some are invariably fatal, while others are comparatively minor. Some respond well to treatment, while others do not.

The use of genetic information in predicting and diagnosing diseases has significantly increased during the last two decades. New scientific information, new medical techniques, and new social programs have all contributed to this increase.

Three approaches in particular have been adopted by the medical community as means of acquiring and employing genetic information related to diseases: genetic screening, genetic counseling, and prenatal genetic diagnosis. Each approach has been the source of significant ethical and social issues, but before examining the approaches and the problems they present, we need to consider what is usually meant in talking about genetic disease.

Genetic Disease

The concept of a "genetic" disease is far from being clear. Generally speaking, a genetic disease is one in which genes or the ways in which they are expressed are causally responsible for particular biochemical, cellular, or physiological defects. Rather than rely upon such a general definition, it is more useful for the purpose of understanding genetic diagnosis to consider some of the ways in which genes may play a role in producing diseases.

Gene defects. The program of information that is coded into DNA (the genetic material) may in some way be abnormal because of the occurrence of a mutation at some time or other. (That is, a particular gene may have been lost or damaged, or a new gene added.) Consequently, when the DNA blueprint is "read" and its instructions followed, the child that develops will have defects.

For example, a number of diseases (such as PKU and Tauri's disease) are the result of so-called "inborn errors of metabolism." The diseases are produced by the lack of a particular enzyme necessary for ordinary metabolic functioning. In each case, the genetic information required in coding for the production of the enzyme is simply not present. The gene for the enzyme is missing.

A missing or defective gene may be due to a new mutation, but more often the condition has been inherited. It has been transmitted to the offspring through the genetic material contributed by its parents. Because defective genes can be passed on in this way, the diseases that they produce are themselves described as heritable. (Thus, PKU is a genetically transmissible disease.) The diseases follow regular patterns through generations, and tracing out those patterns has been one of the great accomplishments of modern biology and medicine.

Developmental defects. The biological development of a human being from a fertilized egg to a newborn child is an immensely complicated process. It involves an interplay among both genetic and environmental factors, and the possibility of the occurrence of errors is quite real.

Mistakes that result as part of the developmental process are ordinarily called "congenital." Such defects are not in the original blueprint (genes) but result either from genetic damage or from the reading of the blueprint. When either happens, the manufacture and assembly of materials required for normal fetal development are affected.

Radiation, drugs, chemicals, and nutritional deficiencies can all cause changes in an otherwise normal process. Also, biological disease agents, such as certain viruses, may intervene in development. They may alter the machinery of the cells, interfere with the formation of tissues, and defeat the carefully programmed processes that lead to a normal child.

Finally, factors internal to fetal development may also alter the process and lead to defects. The most common form of Down's syndrome, for example, is known to be caused by a failure of chromosomes to separate normally. (However, the cause of this failure is presently unknown.) The result is a child that has failed to develop properly and displays physical anomalies and some degree of mental retardation.

Defects that occur during the developmental process are not themselves the results of inheritance, and they cannot be passed on to the next generation.

Genetic carriers. Some diseases are produced only when an individual inherits both genes (alleles) for the disease from his or her parents. The parents themselves possess only one gene for the disease, and generally show none of its symptoms. However, sometimes a parent may have symptoms of the same kind as are associated with the disease, although to a much lesser degree of severity.

In the metabolic disease PKU, for example, individuals who have inherited only one of the genes (that is, the offspring are heterozygous, rather than homozygous) may show a greater than normal level of phenylalanine in their blood. Such people are somewhat deficient in the enzyme required to metabolize this substance. The level of the substance may not be high enough to have caused any damage to them. Yet they are the carriers of a gene which, when passed on with the same gene from the other parent, can cause the disease PKU in their offspring. (As we will see later, the same is also true for those who are carriers of sickle-cell trait.) The individual who receives both genes for PKU obviously has the disease, but what about the parents? Clearly, the point at which a condition becomes a disease is often a matter of degree.

Genetic predisposition. It has been suggested that virtually every disease involves a genetic component in some way or other. Whether or not this is true, there is good evidence that hypertension, heart disease, various forms of cancer, and differential responses to environmental agents (such as sunlight, molds, or chemical pollutants) run in families, and it has been established in a number of cases that the genetic makeup of particular individuals may predispose them to specific diseases.

At present, it is not generally possible to say just what genetic factor might be partly responsible for a particular disease, just what role it plays, or through what mechanism it expresses itself. It is important to keep in mind that predispositions are not themselves diseases. At best, they can be regarded only as causal conditions which, in conjunction with other conditions, can produce disease.

The action of genes in disease processes is much more complicated than we have been able to discuss here. Nevertheless, our general categories are adequate to allow us to talk about the use made of information in genetic diagnosis.

Genetic Screening

In 1962 Dr. Robert Guthrie of the State University of New York developed an automated procedure for testing the blood of newborn children for the disease PKU. Although a diagnostic test for PKU had been available since 1934, it was time-consuming and labor-intensive. The Guthrie test made it practical to diagnose a large number of infants at a relatively low price.

PKU (phenylketonuria) is a serious metabolic disorder. Infants affected are deficient in the enzyme phenylalanine hydroxylase. Since the enzyme is necessary to convert the amino acid phenylalanine into tyrosine, as part of the normal metabolic process, a deficiency of the enzyme leads to a high concentration of phenylalanine in the infant's blood. The almost invariable result is severe mental retardation.

However, if the high level of phenylalanine in an infant's blood is detected very early, the infant can be put on a diet that is very low in that particular amino acid. Keeping children on the diet until they are around the age of six significantly reduces the severity of the retardation that is otherwise inescapable.

The availability of the Guthrie test and the prospects of saving newborn children from irreparable damage encouraged state legislatures to pass mandatory screening laws. Massachusetts passed the first such law in 1963, and by 1967 similar legislation had been adopted by forty-one states.

The term "genetic screening" is sometimes used to refer to any activity having to do with locating or advising people with genetically connected diseases. In our discussion, we will restrict the term's application and use it to refer only to public health programs which survey or test target populations with the aim of detecting individuals who are at risk of disease for genetic reasons.

The Massachusetts PKU law pointed the way for the development of public screening programs. PKU was the first disease tested for, but before long others were added to the list. For example, New York state law requires that an infant be tested for seven diseases. A number of public health programs now screen particular populations for such conditions as sickle-cell anemia, sickle-cell trait, metabolic disorders, hypothyroidism, and chromosome anomalies.

Although genetic screening is relatively new as a social program, the concept is historically connected with public health measures for the detection of communicable diseases like tuberculosis and syphilis. If an individual with such a disease is identified, then he or she can receive treatment. Furthermore, the diseased individual can be prevented from spreading the disease to other members of the population.

Similarly, it is possible to think of diseases with a genetic basis as resembling contagious diseases. Individuals are affected, and they can pass on the disease. But with genetic diseases, the potential spread is not horizontal through the population, but vertical through the generations.

In terms of this model, public health measures similar to the ones that continue to be so effective in the control of contagious diseases might be used to help bring genetic diseases under control. When screening locates an individual with a genetic disorder, then steps can be taken to ensure that he receives appropriate therapy. Furthermore, when carriers of genes that produce diseases are identified, then they can be warned about their chances of having children that are genetically defective. Thus, at least a limited amount of control over the spread of genetic disease can be exercised, and the suffering of at least some individuals can be reduced or eliminated.

The justification of laws mandating screening programs can be sought in the power and responsibility of government to see to the welfare of its citizens. Here again, the public health measures employed to control contagion might be looked to as a model. We do not permit the parents of a child to decide on their own whether the child should be vaccinated against smallpox. We believe that the society, operating through its government, has a duty to protect the child. Similarly, it can be argued that the society owes it to the child with PKU to see to it that the condition is discovered as quickly as possible so that appropriate treatment can be instituted.

Critics of screening programs have not been convinced that the contagious-disease model is at all appropriate in dealing with genetic diseases. Because the way in which genetic diseases are spread is so different, only a very small part of the population can be said to suffer any risk at all. By contrast, an epidemic of smallpox may threaten millions of people. Furthermore, some genetic screening programs do not have follow-up or counseling services attached to them so often nothing is done that benefits participants. By being told that they are the carriers of a genetic disease, people may be more harmed than helped by the programs.

In general, there are serious questions about whether the benefits of screening programs are sufficient to outweigh the liabilities. In particular, are screening programs so worthwhile that they justify the denial of individual choice entailed by required participation?

These issues and others related to them are easier to appreciate when they are considered in the context of particular kinds of screening programs. We will discuss briefly two programs that have been both important and controversial.

PKU screening. As we pointed out earlier, screening for PKU was the first mass testing program to be mandated by state laws. It is generally agreed that it has also been the most successful program.

PKU is a relatively rare disease. It accounts for only about 0.8 percent of mentally retarded people who are institutionalized, and among the infants screened during a year in a state like Massachusetts, only about three of four cases of PKU may be discovered. (The incidence is 5.4 per 100,000 infants.) Given this relatively low incidence of the disease, some critics have argued that the abrogation of the freedom of choice required by a mandatory program does not make the results worthwhile.

This is particularly true, they suggest, because of the difficulties with the testing procedure itself. The level of phenylalanine in the blood may fluctuate so that not all infants with a higher than normal level at the time of the test actually have PKU. If they are put on the restricted diet, then they may suffer consequences from the diet that are harmful to their health. Thus, in attempting to protect the health of some infants, a mandatory pro-

gram may unintentionally injure the health of other infants.

Tests more refined than the Guthrie one are possible. However, their use increases considerably the cost of the screening program, even if they are employed only when the Guthrie test is positive for PKU. In social terms, then, the financial cost of preventing a few cases of PKU may be much greater than allowing the cases to remain undetected and untreated.

Furthermore, there are additional hidden social costs. Female infants who are successfully treated for PKU may grow into adults and have children of their own. Their children run a very high risk of being born with brain damage. The reason for this is not genetic but developmental. The uterine environment of PKU mothers is one high in phenylalanine, and in high concentrations it causes damage to the infant. Thus, one generation may be saved from mental retardation by screening only to cause mental retardation in the next.

Sickle-cell. Sickle-cell disease is a disorder of the hemoglobin in red blood cells. The cells assume a characteristic sickle shape and do not transport oxygen as well as normal red cells. They are also fragile and break apart more frequently. The result is anemia and, often, the blocking of blood vessels by fragments of ruptured cells.

The disease occurs only in those who have inherited both genes for the disease from their parents. (That is, the gene for the disease is recessive, and those who are homozygous for the gene are the ones who develop the disease.) Those with only one gene for the disease (that is, are heterozygous) are said to have sickle-cell trait.

Sickle-cell disease may develop at infancy, or it may manifest itself later in life in painful and debilitating symptoms. Those with sickle-cell trait rarely show any of the clinical symptoms.

In the United States, the disease is most common among blacks and those of Mediterranean ancestry. The trait is carried by about 7–9 percent of the black population, and the disease occurs in about 0.3 percent of the population. Many people with the disease are not severely affected and can live relatively normal lives. However, the disease may also be fatal, and at the present there is no adequate therapy for it. There is no cure, although there is now a means of diagnosing the disease prenatally.

In 1970 a relatively inexpensive and accurate test for sickle-cell hemoglobin was developed, making it possible to identify the carriers of sickle-cell trait. This technological development combined with political pressures generated by rising consciousness in the black population was to lead to the passage of state laws mandating sickle-cell screening. During 1971 and 1972, twelve states enacted sickle-cell legislation.

The results were socially disastrous. Some laws required blacks who applied for a marriage license to undergo screening. Since the only way to reduce the incidence of the disease is for two carriers to avoid having children, many blacks charged that the mandatory screening laws were a manifestation of a plan for genocide.

Medical reports that carriers of sickle-cell trait sometimes suffered from the pain and disability of sickling crises came to serve as a new basis of discrimination. Some employers and insurance companies began to require tests of black employees, and as a result some job possibilities were closed off to blacks with sickle-cell trait.

In 1972, Congress passed the National Sickle-Cell Anemia Control Act. In order to qualify for federal grants under the act, states were required to make sickle-cell screening voluntary, provide genetic counseling, and take steps to protect the confidentiality of participants. The most significant impact of the act was to force states to modify their laws to bring them into conformity with the act's requirements. In response, the seventeen states with sickle-cell screening laws now require only voluntary programs.

The National Genetic Diseases Act, passed in 1976 and funded annually since then, provides testing and counseling for the diagnosis and treatment of a number of genetic diseases. The act further strengthens the commitment to voluntary participation and to guarantees of confidentiality.

The lesson learned from the public controversy over the first sickle-cell screening programs is that genetic information can be used in ways that are harmful to the interests of individuals. Furthermore, the information can be used as a basis for systematic discrimination.

Genetic Counseling

Much is known about the ways in which a number of genetic diseases are inherited. Ones like PKU, sickle-cell, and Tay-Sachs follow the laws of Mendelian transmission genetics. Accordingly, given the appropriate information, it is often possible to determine how likely it is that a particular couple will have a child with a certain disease.

Suppose, for example, that a black couple is concerned about the possibility of having a child with sickle-cell disease. They will be tested to discover whether either or both of them is a carrier of sickle-cell trait.

Sickle-cell disease occurs only when two recessive genes are both present—one inherited from the mother, one from the father. If only one of the parents is a carrier of the trait (is heterozygous), then no child will have the disease. However, if both parents are carriers of the trait, then the chances are one out of four that their child will have the disease. (This is determined simply by considering which combinations of the two genes belonging to each parent will produce a combination that is a homozygous recessive. The combination of Ss and Ss will produce ss in only 25 percent of the possible cases.)

Such information can be used to explain to potential parents the risks they might run in having children. But, as the case of sickle-cell disease illustrates quite well, it is often very difficult for individuals to know what to do with such information.

Is a 25 percent risk of having a child with sickle-cell disease sufficiently high that a couple ought to decide to have no children at all? Since the prenatal test for the disease is not easily available to everyone, this question is one that is best considered in advance of a pregnancy. If the couple is opposed to abortion, the question becomes especially crucial. Answering it is made more difficult by the fact that sickle-cell disease varies greatly in severity. A child with the disease may be virtually normal, or doomed to a short life filled with suffering. No one can say in advance of its birth which possibility is more likely.

It is generally agreed that the question of whether to have a child when a serious risk is involved is a decision that must be made by the couple. The counselor may provide information about the risk, and just as important, the counselor may provide information about medical therapies that are available for a child born with a hereditary disease.

In diseases in which prenatal diagnosis is possible, the option of abortion may be open to potential parents. Here, too, the object of counseling is to see to it that the couple is educated in ways relevant to their needs.

Prenatal Genetic Diagnosis

A variety of new technological developments now make it possible to secure a great amount of information about the developing fetus while it is still in the uterus. Ultrasound, radiography, and fiber optics allow examination of soft-tissue and skeletal development. Anatomical abnormalities can be detected early enough to permit an abortion to be safely performed, if that is the decision of the woman carrying the fetus.

Yet the most common method of prenatal diagnosis continues to be amniocentesis. The amnion (the membrane surrounding the fetus) is filled with a fluid that contains fetal cells, urine, and metabolic products. By means of a needle puncture through the woman's abdomen, some of the amniotic fluid can be removed for study.

The procedure cannot be usefully performed until fourteen to sixteen weeks into the pregnancy. Until that time, there is an inadequate amount of fluid. The risk to the woman and to the fetus from the procedure is relatively small, something less than 1 percent. (Still undergoing clinical trials is the new procedure of chorion villi sampling that employs cells taken from the developing fetus. The advantage of the test is that it can be employed eight to ten weeks after conception.)

Amniocentesis came into wide use only in the early 1960s. At first, it was mostly restricted to testing fetuses in cases in which there was a risk of Rh incompatibility. When the mother lacks a group of blood proteins called the Rh (or Rhesus) factor, and the fetus has it, then the immune system of the mother may produce antibodies against the fetus. The result for the fetus may be anemia, brain damage, and even death.

It was soon realized that additional information about the fetus could be gained from further analysis of the amniotic fluid and the fetal cells in it. The fluid can be chemically assayed, and the cells can be grown in cultures for study. An examination of the chromosomes from the cells will show whether there are any known abnormalities that are likely to cause serious physical or mental defects. The presence or absence of the Y chromosome will also show the sex of the fetus. (Only males have a Y chromosome, so it is impossible to examine the chromosomes without discovering the sex of the fetus.)

Some metabolic disorders (such as Tay-Sachs disease) can be detected by chemical analysis of the amniotic fluid. However, some of the more common ones, such as PKU and cystic fibrosis, cannot be diagnosed in this way.

Amniocentesis does have some hazard attached to it. Accordingly, it is not at all regarded as a routine procedure to be performed in every pregnancy. There must be some indication that the fetus is at risk from a genetic or developmental disorder.

One indication is the age of the mother. Down's syndrome is much more likely to occur in fetuses conceived in women over the age of thirty-five. Since the syndrome is produced by a chromosome abnormality, an examination of the chromosomes in the cells of the fetus can reveal the defect. (See the introduction to Chapter 2 for a fuller discussion.)

Genetic screening can also provide an indication of a need to perform amniocentesis. For example, Tay-Sachs disease is a metabolic disorder that occurs ten times as often among Jews originating in central and eastern Europe (the Ashkenazy) as in the general population. (The disease is invariably fatal and follows a sad course. An apparently normal child progressively develops blindness and brain damage, then dies at an early age.) Carriers of the Tay-Sachs gene can be identified by a blood test, and couples who are both carriers of the trait run a 25 percent risk of having a child with the disease. In such a case, there would be a good reason to perform amniocentesis.

Until recently, there was no way to use amniocentesis to determine whether a fetus was affected with a neural-tube defect. (See Chapter 2 for a discussion of such defects as spina bifida.) The situation has now changed quite dramatically.

The cause of neural-tube defects is unknown, and they occur in about one out of every 500 births in the United States. They follow no known family patterns, have no known genetic basis, and cannot be predicted by genetic screening. They are also considered to be among the worst of all birth defects.

However, a test is available to indicate the presence of a neural-tube defect in a developing fetus. In 1972 David H. Brock of Edinburgh discovered that there is an unusually large amount of the substance alpha-fetoprotein (AFP) in the amniotic fluid taken from women who give birth to children with neural-tube defects.

The reason for this, Brock decided, is that the open spine or skull of the fetus allows the AFP it normally contains to leak into the amniotic fluid. Through additional research, Brock determined that there is also a greater level of AFP in the blood of women carrying a fetus with the defect than in that of women with normal fetuses. The AFP enters the mother's circulatory system by passing through the umbilical cord and the placenta.

The blood test is not wholly reliable. Because the level of AFP varies in all women, the test produces many false positives. Also, women with twins or triplets have a level of AFP that is higher than that of women carrying a single fetus. Consequently, the blood test must be supplemented by ultrasound examination to determine whether only one fetus is present. If so, then amniocentesis is performed to get a more accurate measurement of the AFP present.

Selective Abortion

In most cases in which prenatal diagnosis indicates that the fetus suffers from a genetic disorder or developmental defect, the only means of avoiding the birth of an impaired child is abortion.

Because those who go through the tests required to determine the condition of the fetus are concerned with having a child, abortion performed under such circumstances is called *selective*. That is, the woman decides to have an abortion to avoid producing a child with birth defects, not just to avoid having a child.

Those who oppose abortion in principle (see Chapter 1) also oppose selective abortion. In the view of some, the fact that a child will be born impaired is in no way a justification for terminating the life of the fetus.

Those who are prepared to endorse abortion at all typically approve of selective abortion as an acceptable way of avoiding suffering. In their view, it is better that the potential person that is the fetus not become an actual person, full of pain, disease, and disability.

At this time, there is some hope that the painful decision between having an abortion or giving birth to a defective child may someday be avoided. In the last few years, techniques of fetal surgery have been employed to correct certain abnormal physical conditions.

Repairs to the heart, the insertion of shunts to drain off excess brain fluids, and the placement of tubes to inflate collapsed lungs are some of the intrauterine surgical procedures now being performed. It is believed that it may be possible to expose the fetus within the uterus, perform surgery, then close up the amnion again. This would make possible more extensive surgery for a greater variety of conditions.

The present hope is that as new surgical techniques for the treatment of fetuses are perfected and expanded, the need to rely on abortion to avoid the birth of defective children will significantly decline. Of course, surgery cannot, even in principle, provide a remedy for a large number of hereditary disorders. Surgery can do nothing for a child with Tay-Sachs disease or PKU.

Helplessness in this regard is matched by another hope. Perhaps in future years pharmaceutical and biochemical therapies will be available to employ in cases involving missing enzymes. Or perhaps "gene surgery" will make it possible to insert the proper gene for manufacturing a needed biochemical into the DNA of the cells of a fetus.

Hopeful though we may be, the painful present reality is that for most children born with genetic diseases or defects very little can be done. Selective abortion continues to be the primary means to avoid the birth of a child known to be genetically impaired.

Difficulties with Genetic Intervention

Genetic screening, counseling, and prenatal diagnosis present bright possibilities for those who believe in the importance of exercising control through rational planning and decision making. The prospect of avoiding the birth of children with crippling impairments is seen by them as one of the triumphs of contemporary medicine.

Furthermore, the additional prospect of wholly eliminating some genetic diseases by counseling and control holds the promise of an even better future. For example, if people who are carriers of diseases caused by a dominant gene (such as Huntington's) produced no children with the disease, the disease would soon disappear entirely. The gene causing the disease would simply not be passed on to the next generation.

A vision of a world without the misery caused by genetic defects is a motivating factor among those who are strong advocates of programs of genetic intervention. (See the section on eugenics in this chapter for more details.) The vision must have its appeal to all who are moved by compassion in the face of suffering. Yet whether or not one shares this vision and is prepared to use it as a basis for social action, there are serious ethical questions about genetic intervention that must be faced.

We have already mentioned some of the issues in connection with particular programs and procedures. We can now add some more general questions to that list, but it should be kept in mind that our discussion cannot be complete. The moral and social issues connected with genetic intervention are woven into a complicated fabric of personal and social considerations. We can merely sketch the main outline of the pattern.

1. Is there a right to have children who are likely to be impaired? Suppose that a woman is informed, after the AFP test and amniocentesis, that the child she is carrying will be born with a neural-tube defect. Does she have the right to refuse an abortion and have the child anyway?

Those who are opposed to all abortion on the grounds of natural law would favor the woman's having the child. By contrast, a utilitarian might well argue that the decision would be wrong. The amount of suffering the potential child might be expected to undergo outweighs any parental loss. For different reasons, a Kantian might endorse this same point of view. Even if we assume the fetus is a person, a Kantian might argue that we are obliged to prevent its suffering. (For more details of these and similar arguments, see Chapters 1 and 2.)

Suppose we decide that a woman does have a right to have a child that is almost certain to be impaired. If so, then is the society obligated to bear the expense of caring for such a child? On the natural law view, the answer is almost certainly yes. The child, impaired or not, is a human person, and, as such, is entitled to the support and protection of the society. If we agree that the impaired child is a person, then he or she is also a disadvantaged person. Thus, an argument based on Rawls's principles of justice would support the view that the child is entitled to social support. (Again, see Chapter 2 for more detail.)

2. Is the society justified in requiring that people submit to genetic screening, counseling, and prenatal diagnosis? Children born with genetic diseases and defects require the expenditure of large amounts of public funds. Mandatory diagnosis need not be coupled with mandatory abortion or abstention from bearing children. (A related question is whether society ought to make available genetic testing to all who wish it, regardless of their ability to pay.)

On utilitarian grounds, it might be argued that society has a legitimate interest in seeing to it that, no matter what people ultimately decide, they should at least have the information about the likelihood that they will produce an impaired child.

If this view is adopted, then a number of specific medically related questions become relevant. For example, who should be screened? It is impractical and unnecessary to screen everyone. Why should we screen schoolchildren or prisoners, those who are sterile, or those past the age of childbearing?

This is closely connected with a second question: What should people be screened for? Should everyone be screened for Tay-Sachs disease, even though it is the Jewish population that is most at risk? Should everyone be screened for sickle-cell trait, even though it is primarily the black population that is at risk?

Those who accept the contagious-disease model of genetic screening frequently defend it on the utilitarian grounds that screening promotes the general social welfare. However, one might argue that screening can also be justified on deontological grounds. It could be claimed that we owe it to developing fetuses, regarded as persons, to see to it that they receive the opportunity for the most effective treatment. For example, it might be said that we have an obligation to provide a PKU child with the immediate therapy required to save him or her from severe mental retardation. The restriction of the autonomy of individuals by requiring screening might be regarded as justified by this obligation. If screening is voluntary, then the welfare of the child is made to depend on ignorance and accidental opportunity.

3. Do physicians have an obligation to inform their patients who are prospective parents about the kinds of genetic tests that are available? A study of one population of women screened for Tay-Sachs disease showed that none had sought testing on the recommendation of her physician.

If the autonomy of the individual is to be preserved, then it seems clear that it is the duty of a physician to inform patients about genetic testing. A physician who disapproves of abortion might be reluctant to inform patients about tests that might encourage them to seek an abortion. Nevertheless, to the extent that abortion is a moral decision, it is a decision properly made by the individual, not by someone acting paternalistically in her behalf.

The duty of a physician to inform patients about the possibility of genetic tests seems quite straightforward. Yet the issue becomes more complicated in light of the next question about truth telling.

4. Do patients have a right to be informed of all of the results of a genetic test? Ethical theories that are based on respect for the autonomy of the individual (such as Kant's and Ross's) suggest that patients are entitled to know what has been learned from the tests.

But what if the test reveals that the fetus has only a quite minor genetically transmissible disease? Should the physician run the risk of the patient's deciding to have an abortion merely because she is committed to the ideal of a "perfect" baby? Is such a decision really one for the physician to make?

Furthermore, what about the matter of sex determination? Screening tests that involve chromosome examination also reveal the sex of the fetus. Are prospective parents entitled to know this information? When abortion is elective, it is quite possible for the woman to decide to have an abortion to avoid giving birth to a child of a particular sex.

It might be argued on both utilitarian and deontological grounds that the sex of the fetus is information that is not relevant to the health of the fetus. Accordingly, the physician is under no obligation to reveal the sex of the fetus. Indeed, the physician may be under an obligation *not* to reveal the sex of the fetus in order to avoid the possibility of its destruction for a basically trivial reason. But, again, is this really a decision for the physician?

5. Should public funds be used to pay for genetic tests when an individual is unable to pay? This is a question that holders of various ethical theories may not be prepared to answer in a simple yes or no fashion. Those who oppose abortion on natural law grounds might advocate providing funds only for genetic screening and counseling. That is, they might favor providing prospective parents with information that they might then use to decide whether to refrain from having children. Yet opponents of abortion might be against spending public money on tests that might encourage the use of abortion to prevent the birth of a defective child.

The views of Rawls and of utilitarianism might well support the use of public funds for genetic testing as part of a more general program of providing for health-care needs. Whether genetic testing programs are funded and the level of funding would then depend on judgments about their expected value in comparison with other health-care programs.

A present ethical and social difficulty is caused by the fact that federal funds may be employed to pay for genetic screening and testing, yet federal money cannot legally be used to pay for abortions. Consequently, it is possible for a woman to discover that she is carrying a fetus with a serious genetic disease, wish to have an abortion, yet lack the financial means to pay for it.

Issues about the confidentiality of test results, informed consent, the use of genetic testing to gather epidemiological information, and a variety of other matters might be mentioned here in connection with genetic intervention. Those that have been discussed are sufficient to indicate that the difficulties presented by genetic intervention are at least as numerous as the benefits it promises.

EUGENICS

Like other organisms, we are the products of millions of years of evolutionary development. This process has taken place through the operation of natural selection on randomly produced genetic mutations. Individual organisms are successful in an evolutionary sense when they contribute a number of genes to the gene pool of their species proportionately greater than the number of contributed by others. Most often, this means that the evolutionarily successful individuals are those with the largest number of offspring. These are the individuals favored by natural selection. That is, they possess the genes for certain properties that are favored by existing environmental factors. (This favoring of properties is natural selection.) The genes of "favored" individuals will occur with greater frequency than the genes of others in the next generation. If the same environmental factors continue to operate, these genes will spread through the entire population.

Thanks to Darwin and the evolutionary biologists who have come after him, we now have a sound understanding of the evolutionary process and the mechanisms by which it operates. This understanding puts us in a position to intervene in the process. That is, we no longer have to consider ourselves subject to the blind working of natural selection. If we choose to do so, we can modify the course of human evolution. As the evolutionary biologist Theodosius Dobzhansky expressed the point: "Evolution need no longer be a destiny imposed from without; it may conceivably be controlled by man, in accordance with his wisdom and values.

Those who advocate eugenics accept just this point of view. They favor social policies and practices which, over time, offer the possibility of increasing the number of genes in the human population responsible for producing or improving traits (for example, intelligence) that we value.

The aim of increasing the number of favorable genes in the human population is called *positive eugenics*. By contrast, *negative eugenics* aims at decreasing the number of undesirable or harmful genes. Those who advocate negative eugenics are generally most interested in eliminating or reducing the number of those genes that are responsible for various kinds of birth defects and genetic diseases.

Both positive and negative eugenics require instituting some sort of control over human reproduction. Several kinds of policies and procedures have been advocated, and we will discuss a few of the possibilities below.

Genetic Intervention

The discussion in the preceding section of genetic screening, counseling, and prenatal genetic diagnosis makes it unnecessary to repeat here information about the possibilities and procedures we currently possess for predicting and diagnosing genetic diseases. It is enough to recall that, given information about the genetic makeup and background of potential parents, a number of genetic diseases can be predicted with a certain degree of probability as likely to occur in a child of such parents. This is true of such diseases as PKU, sickle-cell anemia, hemophilia, Huntington's disease, and Tay-Sachs disease.

When genetic information is not adequate to serve as a basis for a reliable prediction, then information about the developing fetus can often be obtained by employing one of several procedures of prenatal diagnosis. Even when genetic information is adequate for a statistical prediction, whether the fetus has a certain disease can be determined by prenatal testing. Thus, in addition to the disorders named above, prenatal tests can be performed for such other defects as neuraltube anomalies and Down's syndrome.

A proponent of negative eugenics might advocate that a screening process for all or some currently detectable genetic diseases be required by law. When the probability of the occurrence of a disease is high (whatever figure that might be taken to be), then the potential parents might be encouraged to have no children. Indeed, the law might *require* that such a couple abstain from having children and prescribe a penalty for going against the decision of the screening board. If those carrying the genes for some genetic diseases could be prevented from having children, then over time the incidence of the diseases in the population would decrease. In some cases, when the disease is the result of a dominant gene (as it is in Huntington's disease), the disease would eventually disappear.

When the disease is a kind that can be detected only after a child is conceived, then if the results of a prenatal diagnosis show that the developing fetus has a heritable disease, an abortion might be encouraged. Short of a law requiring abortion, a variety of social policies might be adopted to make abortion an attractive option. (For example, the cost of an abortion might be paid for by government funds, or women choosing abortion might be financially rewarded.) The aborting of a fetus found to have a transmissible genetic disease would not only prevent the birth of an impaired infant, it would eliminate a potential carrier of the genes responsible for the disease.

Similarly, the sterilization of people identified as having genes that are responsible for certain kinds of physical or mental impairments would prevent them from passing on these defective genes. (See Chapter 7 for a discussion of sterilization.) In this way, the number of such genes in the population would be proportionately reduced.

Currently, there are no state or federal laws that make it a crime for couples who are genetically a bad risk to have children. Yet there may be developing a tendency toward more genetic regulation. As we mentioned earlier, several states now require the screening of newborn infants in order to detect the presence of certain genetic diseases that respond well to early treatment. Also, genetic screening programs are frequently offered in communities to encourage people to seek information about particular diseases.

At present, genetic screening (for adults) and genetic counseling are voluntary. They aim at providing information and then leave reproductive decisions up to the individuals concerned. Most often, they are directed toward the immediate goal of decreasing the number of children suffering from birth defects and genetic diseases. Yet genetic screening and counseling might also be viewed as a part of negative eugenics. To the extent that they discourage the birth of children carrying deleterious genes, they also discourage the spread of those genes in the human population.

Obviously, screening programs and genetic counseling might also be used to promote *positive* eugenics. Individuals possessing genes for traits that society values might be encouraged to have large numbers of children. In this way, genes for traits that are considered worthwhile would increase in relative frequency within the population.

There are no programs of positive eugenics. Yet is is easy to imagine a variety of social and economic incentives (for example, government bonuses) that might be introduced as part of a plan to promote the spread of certain genes by rewarding favored groups of people for having children.

Use of Desirable Germ Cells

Artificial insemination by the use of stored sperm is already a reality. The implantation of a donor ovum in the wall of the uterus is also possible, and we have developed a biotechnology that permits the long-term storage of ova. Thus, a man or woman might choose to have a child by selecting stored germ cells contributed by individuals possessing traits that they admire. Sperm banks and ova banks would then provide a way for the human population to improve itself—that is, to increase the number of genes for desirable traits in the population. (See Chapter 7.)

Difficulties with Eugenics

Critics have been quick to point out that the proposals we have discussed suffer from serious drawbacks. First, negative eugenics is not likely to make much of a change in the species as a whole. Most hereditary diseases are genetically recessive and so occur only when both parents possess the same defective gene. Even though a particular couple might be counseled (or required) not to have children, the gene will still be widespread in the population among people we would consider wholly normal. For a similar reason, sterilization would have few long-range effects. Also, there is the uncomfortable fact that geneticists have estimated that, on the average, everyone carries recessive genes for five genetic defects or diseases. Genetic counseling may help individuals, but negative eugenics does not promise much for the population as a whole.

Positive eugenics can promise little more. It is difficult to imagine that we would all agree on what traits we would like to see increased in the human species. But even if we could, it is not clear that we would be able to increase them in any simple way. For one thing, we have little understanding of the genetic basis of traits such as "intelligence," "honesty," "musical ability," and so on. It is clear, however, that there is not just a single gene for them, and the chances are that they are the result of a complicated interplay between genetic endowment and social and environmental factors. Consequently, the task of increasing their frequency is quite different from that of, say, increasing the frequency of short-horned cattle. Furthermore, the desirable traits may well be accompanied by less desirable traits, and we may not be able to increase the first without also increasing the second.

Quite apart from biological objections, eugenics also raises questions of a moral kind. Have we indeed become the "business manager of evolution" as Julian Huxley once claimed? If so, then do we have a responsibility to future generations to improve the human race? Would this responsibility justify our requiring genetic screening? Would it justify our establishing a program of positive eugenics? Affirmative answers to these questions may generate conflicts with notions of individual dignity and self-determination.

Of the ethical theories we have discussed, it seems likely that only utilitarianism might be construed as favoring a program of positive eugenics. The possibility of increasing the frequency of desirable traits in the human species might, in terms of the principle of utility, justify present restrictions on reproduction. It is not clear that this is so, however. The goal of an improved society or human race might well be regarded as too distant and uncertain to warrant the imposition of restrictions that would increase current human unhappiness.

So far as negative eugenics is concerned, the principle of utility could certainly be appealed to in order to justify social policies that would discourage or prohibit parents who are serious genetic risks from having children. The aim here need not be the remote one of improving the human population but the more immediate one of preventing the increase in sorrows and pains that would be caused by an impaired child.

Natural law doctrines of Roman Catholicism forbid abortion (see the introduction to Chapter 1 and the introductory chapter) and sterilization. Thus, these means of practicing negative eugenics are ruled out. Also the natural law view that reproduction is a natural function of sexual intercourse seems, at least prima facie, to rule out negative eugenics as a deliberate policy altogether. It could be argued, however, that voluntary abstinence from sexual intercourse or some other acceptable form of birth control would be a legitimate means of practicing negative eugenics.

Ross's prima facie duty of causing no harm might be invoked to justify negative eugenics. If there is good reason to believe that a child is going to suffer from a genetic disease, then we may have a duty to prevent the child from being born. Similarly, Rawls's theory might permit a policy that would require the practice of some form of negative eugenics for the benefit of its immediate effects of preventing suffering and sparing all the cost of supporting those with genetic diseases.

It is difficult to determine what sort of answer to the question of negative eugenics might be offered in terms of Kant's ethical principles. Laws regulating conception or forced abortion or sterilization might well be considered to violate the dignity and autonomy of individuals. Yet moral agents as rational decision makers require information on which to base their decisions. Thus, programs of genetic screening and counseling might be considered to be legitimate.

GENETIC RESEARCH, THERAPY, AND TECHNOLOGY

By replacing natural selection with artificial selection that is directly under our control, we can, over time, alter the genetic composition of populations of organisms. This has been done for thousands of years by animal and plant breeders, and our improved understanding of genetics allows us to do it today with more effectiveness and certainty of results. Yet such alterations require long periods of time. Molecular genetics holds out the possibility of immediate changes. Bacteria continue to be the major organisms of research, but genetic technology is already being applied to plants and animals. The same technology is now on the verge of being applied to humans.

Recombinant DNA

The information required for genetic inheritance is coded in the two intertwined strands of DNA (deoxyribonucleic acid) found in plant and animal cells—the double helix. The strands are made up of four kinds of chemical units called nucleotides, and the genetic message is determined by the particular sequence of nucleotides. Three nucleotides in sequence form a triplet codon. Each codon directs the synthesis of a particular amino acid and determines the place that it will occupy in making up a protein molecule. Since virtually all properties of organisms (enzymes, organs, eye color, and so on) depend on proteins, the processes directed by DNA are fundamental.

Alterations in the nucleotide sequence in DNA occur naturally as mutations—random changes introduced as "copying errors" when DNA replicates (reproduces) itself. These alterations result in changes in the properties of organisms since the properties are under the control of DNA. Much research in current molecular genetics is directed toward bringing about desired changes by deliberately manipulating the nucleotide sequences in DNA. The major steps toward this goal have involved the development of techniques for recombining DNA from different sources.

The recombinant process begins by taking proteins known as restriction enzymes from bacteria and mixing them with DNA that has been removed from cells. These enzymes cut open the DNA strands at particular nucleotide locations. DNA nucleotide sequences from another source can then be added, and certain of these will attach to the cut ends. Thus, DNA from distinct sources can be recombined to form a single molecule.

This recombinant DNA can then be made to enter a host cell. The organism almost universally employed as a host is the one-celled bacterium *E. coli* that inhabits the human intestine by the billions. In addition to the DNA that makes up the chromosome of the cell, *E. coli* also possesses small circular strands of DNA known as plasmids. The DNA of a plasmid can be recombined with the DNA of a foreign source and returned to the cell. There the plasmid will start replicating again. It will make copies of the original nucleotides *plus* copies of the added segments. Thus, a strain of bacteria can be produced that will make limitless numbers of copies of the foreign DNA.

The obvious question is, what benefits might this recombinant technique produce? It might lead to the understanding and control of the molecular processes involved in such diseases as cancer, diabetes, and hemophilia. It might provide more effective treatment for metabolic diseases like PKU and Tay-Sachs.

From the more commercial standpoint, recombinant DNA technology might lead to the development of new breeds of plants that are able to utilize nitrogen from the air and thus require no fertilizer. Specially engineered bacteria might be used to clean up the environment by breaking down currently nonbiodegradable compounds like DDT and Agent Orange. Other bacteria might be used to convert petroleum into other useful chemical compounds, including plastics.

The most immediate benefits of recombinant DNA are likely to be the use of modified bacteria as chemical factories to produce biological materials of medical importance. In addition, the transplanting of human genes into nonhuman embryos promises to lead to an understanding of the ways in which genes can be made to reproduce themselves and be passed on to succeeding generations.

Just a glance at a few of the many recent research developments is enough to gain an appreciation of the powerful potential of genetic technology:

Hypopituitary dwarfism is a condition caused by a deficiency in growth hormone. The hormone itself consists of molecules that are too large and structurally complex to synthesize in the laboratory. In 1979 researchers in California employed recombinant-DNA technology to induce bacteria to produce the hormone. It is now available in quantities large enough to be used in medical therapy.

In 1982 Dr. John D. Baxter and his associates developed a bacterial strain capable of producing endorphin. Because endorphin is a natural opiate, the hope is that it can be used as an effective substitute for such addictive drugs as morphine.

Modified bacteria now produce human insulin in quantities large enough to meet the need of diabetics who are allergic to swine or bovine insulin.

Genetically engineered bacteria have also been used to produce a vaccine against hepatitis B and against a strain of genital herpes. The clotting factor employed in the treatment of hemophilia has been similarly produced.

In 1985 the Cetus Corporation was awarded the first patent for an altered form of the protein interleukin-2. Il-2 activates the immune system and shows promise in the treatment of some forms of cancer. It occurs naturally in such small amounts that it was not possible to test its effectiveness until it was produced in quantity by genetically altered bacteria.

In 1986 two research teams reported the development of a genetically engineered modification of the virus used as a vaccine against smallpox for use as a vaccine against AIDS. The altered *vaccinia* virus has been used experimentally, and it is reported that it evokes antibody production against the AIDS virus in both mice and monkeys.

Gene Therapy

The rapid advancement in genetic knowledge during the last few years makes it seem likely to most experts that the use of recombinant DNA techniques as part of a program of medical therapy is now virtually at hand. In particular, the possibility of performing some sort of gene surgery, in which a defective gene is cut out or a needed gene is inserted, is likely to be employed in an experimental way within the next few years. (See the Case Presentation for more details.)

The ability to alter the basic machinery of life to correct its malfunctioning is surely the most powerful form of therapy imaginable. The immediate prospects for gene therapy are most likely to involve the relatively modest, but very dramatic, task of splicing into the DNA of body cells a gene that controls the production of a specific substance. Diseases such as PKU that are caused by the absence of a particular enzyme might then be corrected by inducing the patient's cells to manufacture that enzyme. Some genetic diseases involve dozens or even hundreds of genes, and often the mechanism by which the genes produce the disease is not understood. Consequently, it is likely to be a long while before most genetic diseases can be treated by gene therapy. However, the treatment of single-gene disorders is a most promising possibility.

Few special moral or social issues are raised by the use of gene therapy so long as the cells modified are somatic (body) cells. However, the issues change significantly with the prospect of modifying human germ-line (sex) cells. Somatic-cell changes cannot be inherited, but germ-line cell changes can be. This possibility holds out the benign prospect of eliminating forever a number of sex-linked diseases. However, it also points toward the more frightening outcome of "engineering" human beings to produce people that meet our predetermined specifications. We will discuss this possibility further below. Here it is relevant only to note that the technology that would be required to alter the sex cells of human beings does not exist at present.

Commercial Applications

Commercial uses of recombinant-DNA technology are a present reality, and an entire industry of biotechnology has emerged. Large-scale production of many drugs, hormones, and enzymes is already underway, and more than a hundred diagnostic and therapeutic products based on biotechnology are currently waiting for Food and Drug Administration approval. Some financial analysts have estimated that by 1995 the market for such biological goods will amount to tens of billions of dollars. In the view of many, during the coming decade biotechnology is likely to develop with the same explosive force that characterized the development of the computer-chip industry during the 1970s.

The great commercial expansion has brought with it a number of legal, moral, and social problems. In 1981, the Supreme Court ruled that new organisms created by recombinant techniques can be patented in the same way as other commercial products or processes. Many members of the scientific community have been critical of this decision. Some object that it is simply wrong to grant exclusive rights to life forms that should belong to all.

Others have argued that the information used to create new forms is the result of scientific research paid for through public grants to universities and research establishments. Consequently, the fruits of that research ought be belong to everyone.

This issue is clearly seen in a case involving Genentech, one of the first and largest of the biotechnology companies. Genentech obtained cells from the National Cancer Institute. From those cells, Genentech workers were able to extract the gene responsible for the production of interferon and splice it into bacterial genes. Scientists at UCLA who had identified the cells as ones producing interferon and sent samples of them to the NCI objected to Genentech's being given the cells. They claimed that the commercial organization had no right to use the cell line they had identified for the purposes of profit.

The traditional character of universities has also been challenged by the prospect of being directly involved with the development of commercially valuable organisms and organic products. For example, Stanford is one of the holders of a patent which it has licensed on the condition of royalty payments by users. Some have questioned whether universities, which have traditionally been committed to the pursuit of knowledge for its own sake, ought to be permitted to profit from research done by faculty members. The suggestion is that universities ought to be functioning for the benefit of society and humanity, not for their own welfare.

In addition, new commercial alliances call into question the impartiality of universities and their faculties. In 1981, MIT accepted one hundred million dollars from a commercial concern to establish an independent research institute in molecular biology. Although a variety of safeguards have been built into the agreement, some critics are still of the opinion that there is substantial risk that academic values (such as independent research and the transmission of free information) run a high risk of being compromised.

Similarly, a number of scientists on the faculties of universities have become personally involved with biotechnology companies. In the view of some, such personal and financial interests may result in scientists' losing their credibility with the public and with the government. Such a loss of trust may mean that we will no longer be able to rely on the impartiality of scientific experts in attempting to decide matters affecting public interest and policy.

Screening and Industry

The enzyme AHH (amyl hydrocarbon hydroxylase) acts to break down hydrocarbons in smoke and other industrial pollutants. About 10 percent of the population possess variant forms of the genes that produce the enzyme, and their bodies produce it in an excessive amount. The excess enzyme reacts with hydrocarbons and turns them into carcinogenic substances. People with the variant genes are thus some 26 times more likely to get lung cancer from breathing air polluted with hydrocarbons.

This is just one example of the way in which genetic factors may predispose individuals to certain kinds of diseases. Researchers are well on the way to identifying an entire catalog of such factors and their associated diseases. Such information offers the opportunity for individuals who are screened and found to be particularly susceptible to a certain environmental pollutant or manufacturing substance to avoid contact with that agent. For example, people who are prone to develop an acute form of anemia after exposure to naphthalene should avoid jobs in which that chemical is employed.

In principle, susceptible workers could be assigned to jobs that would allow them to avoid being exposed to the chemicals particularly harmful to them. With such an end in view, in 1982 some 59 percent of large companies surveyed indicated that they either had a genetic screening program or intended to institute one. Their motivation was partly based on economic self-interest, for the costs of damage suits and insurance premiums could be lowered by keeping susceptible workers out of danger.

By 1986 most plans to screen workers had been abandoned by corporations that had initially favored them. This was mostly in response to criticisms from civil rights groups, women's organizations, and labor unions. The critics pointed out that the results of the genetic screening could be used to discriminate against the hiring of entire classes of workers. Because blacks are more susceptible to environmentally induced anemia, they would be effectively shut out of jobs in which the risk to them was greater than to other workers. Similarly, because fetuses are likely to be affected by a number of chemicals used in manufacturing, pregnant women would not be hired for a wide variety of jobs. Indeed, the possibility that a woman might be or might become pregnant might result in the exclusion of women as a group.

As Morton Hunt points out in the essay included here, the possibility of genetic screening in connection with employment presents us with a number of dilemmas of a moral and social kind. We wish to promote equal opportunity for workers, yet we also wish to protect their health and safety. If those genetically predisposed to certain diseases are allowed to compete for jobs that place them at risk, then we are not seeing to their health and safety. Yet if we see to their health, we are not allowing them equal opportunity. Similarly, we wish to promote individual freedom in the society, but at what point do we decide that an individual is taking an unacceptable risk? If we allow someone to risk her health, are we willing to bear the social cost associated with her falling ill?

A worker found to be susceptible to a common manufacturing chemical would be at a clear disadvantage in attempting to get a job and might claim that an employer who required him to take a screening test as a condition of employment was violating his right to privacy. Yet should employers be allowed no protection from the added costs of damage suits and higher insurance premiums caused by a higher rate of illness among susceptible workers?

These are some of the difficulties that are raised by the new possibilities of screening for genetic predisposition to diseases. The promise of being able to prevent the occurrence of disease in many individuals is a genuine one, but we have yet to make an adequate effort to resolve the social and moral issues that fulfilling the promise presents. Until we resolve them, a powerful technology will remain unutilized.

Biohazards

The issues connected with gene therapy and the commercial use of genetic technology may be overshadowed in significance by questions concerning the dangers that are inherent in the development of the technology and in the release of its products into the natural environment.

The question of whether recombinant-DNA research ought to be halted is no longer a serious social issue. However, this has not always been so. In 1974 a group of scientists active in such research issued a report in which they recommended that scientists should be asked to suspend work voluntarily on recombinant experiments involving tumor viruses, increase in drug resistance in harmful bacteria, and increase in toxicity in bacteria. The discussion that ensued resulted in the formulation of guidelines by the National Institutes of Health to regulate research.

The major concern initially was that recombinant techniques might be employed to produce essentially new organisms that would threaten human health. Suppose that the nucleotide sequence for manufacturing a lethal toxin were combined with the DNA of *E. coli*. This currently harmless inhabitant of the intestine might be transformed into a deadly organism that would threaten the existence of the entire human population. Or perhaps a nucleotide sequence that transforms normal cells into cancerous ones might trigger an epidemic of cancer. Without a thorough knowledge of the molecular mechanisms involved, little could be done to halt the outbreak. Indeed, it is not clear what would happen if an insulin-producing strain of bacteria spread through the human population.

These and similar dangers prompted some critics to call for an end to all genetic engineering research. However, over a decade of recombinant-DNA research has passed without the occurrence of any biological catastrophes. Most observers regard this as sufficient proof of the essential safety of the research. Yet in the view of others, the fact that no catastrophes have yet occurred must not be allowed to give us a false sense of security. Almost no one advocates that the research be abandoned, but several molecular geneticists have argued that the very fact that we still do not know enough to estimate the risks involved with a high degree of certainty is a good reason for continuing to control it severely.

The release of genetically altered organisms into the environment still remains a focus of concern, more so than does research itself. In October 1985, a transformed virus designed to serve as a vaccine to inoculate pigs against a disease caused by the pseudorabies virus was used to inoculate 250 piglets on a farm in Bradford, Illinois. This was the first time that an organism created by the techniques of genetic engineering was used in the field.

In April 1986 the Department of Agriculture suspended the license of the Biologics Corporation, manufacturers of the vaccine.

The department's Animal and Plant Health Inspection Service, which had approved the license, had failed to present evidence concerning the virus's impact on the environment to the department's own Recombinant DNA Research Committee. Critics have pointed to this as an example of the way in which a government bureaucracy might bypass regulatory controls and public awareness and take actions that could have disastrous consequences.

The concern is based on the possibility that genetically altered organisms may multiply, mutate, and cause unforeseeable damage. Most animal viruses do not infect people, although some, such as the AIDS virus, may. Furthermore, an altered virus might behave differently, and it almost certainly could spread to other animals, both domestic and wild. The virus might act in ways that would cause disease in other animals or make them more susceptible to other diseases.

The swine-vaccine case has led to a tightening of standards governing environmental testing of genetically altered organisms by the Environmental Protection Agency. Very few critics are calling for abandoning the possibility of employing such organisms, for they hold too much promise as vaccines, growth enhancers, and pesticides. However, within the scientific community there is a widespread attitude of caution and a demand for rigorous testing.

Quite apart from the possible hazards associated with genetic engineering, many people continue to be uneasy about the direction of research. A number of biotechnological possibilities are on the horizon, some of which might have far-reaching consequences. As we noticed earlier, gene surgery offers more possibilities than just medical therapy. If undesirable DNA segments can be sliced out of the genetic code and replaced by others, then this would permit the "engineering" of human beings to an extent and to a degree of precision never before imagined. The eugenic dream of producing people to match an ideal model would be a reality. What would happen then to such traditional and moral values as autonomy, diversity, and the inherent worth of the individual?

The same techniques employed to manufacture the ideal person might also be used to design others to fit special needs. It is not difficult to imagine using genetic surgery to engineer a subhuman race to serve as a slave class for the society. The scenarios of cautionary science fiction might be acted out in our own future.

In addition, the biological technique of asexual reproduction known as cloning might be employed to produce individuals that are exact genetic copies of the DNA donor. These "Xeroxed" organisms—including human beings—are within the scope of technological imagination.

To mention just one last possibility, virtually new organisms might be produced by splicing together DNA from two or more sources. Thus, the world might be faced with creatures of an unknown and unpredictable nature that are not the product of the natural processes of evolution.

It is little wonder that molecular biologists have become concerned about the nature and direction of their research. As Robert Sinsheimer of the California Institute of Technology says, "Biologists have become, without wanting it, custodians of great and terrible power." Such power in the hands of a tyrannical government could be used with irresistible effectiveness to control its subjects. Societies might create a race of semihuman slaves or armies of genetically engineered soldiers. The possibilities are both fantastic and unlimited.

Difficulties with Genetic Research, Therapy, and Technology

The risks involved in gene therapy are not unique ones. In most respects, they ex-

actly parallel those involved in any new medical treatment. Accordingly, it seems reasonable to believe that the same standards of safety and the same consideration for the welfare of the patient that are relevant to the use of other forms of therapy should be regarded as relevant to gene therapy.

The principles of Kant and Ross would suggest that the autonomy of the individual be respected and preserved. In particular, the individual ought not be viewed as an experimental case for testing out a procedure that may later prove helpful. If the person is well enough to be adequately informed and to give consent, and if there is no alternative therapy likely to be effective, it would be morally legitimate for the patient to be given the opportunity to benefit from the therapy. However, if the hazards are great or if they are completely unknown, then it is doubtful whether the patient would be justified in risking his or her life.

By contrast, on utilitarian principles, if the outcome of gene therapy can be reasonably expected to produce more benefit than harm, then the use of the therapy might be considered justifiable. If we assume that a person is likely to die anyway, then that in itself might be enough to warrant the use of the therapy. In addition, since each case treated is likely to contribute to increased understanding and to benefit others, this tends to support the use of gene therapy, even in cases in which it is of doubtful help to the individual. (See Chapter 5 for a fuller discussion.)

Genetic research and its associated technology present issues that are much greater in scope than those raised by gene therapy. They are issues that require us to decide what sort of society we want to live in.

Very few responsible people currently believe that we should call a halt to research in molecular genetics and forgo the increase in power and understanding that it is likely to bring. However, the possibilities of genetic engineering include ones that are frightening and threatening, ones that could wholly alter our society and destroy some of our most cherished values. These are the possibilities that require that we make decisions about whether or to what extent we want to see them realized.

The natural law view of ethics would not, in general, support any policy of restricting scientific inquiry in the area of molecular genetics. For on this view, there is a natural inclination (and hence a natural duty) to seek knowledge. Yet certain types of experiments and gene engineering would be ruled out. Those that aim at altering human beings or creating new species from mixed DNA are most likely to be considered to violate the natural order. On the Roman Catholic view, such a violation of nature would run counter to God's plan and purpose and so be immoral.

The principle of utility might be invoked to justify limiting, directing, or even ending research in molecular genetics. If research or its results are more likely to bring about more harm than benefit, then regulation would be called for. Yet if the promise of relieving misery or increasing well-being is great, then some risks that we might also acquire dangerous knowledge in the process might be acceptable. On the utilitarian view, knowledge may be recognized as a good, but it is only one good among others. Possessing the knowledge to alter human beings in accordance with a eugenic ideal or to create new species means that we have to make a decision about whether doing so would result in an overall benefit. That judgment will then be reflected in our social policies and practices. Such an analysis also seems to be consistent with Rawls's principles. There is not, for Rawls, an absolute right to seek knowledge, nor is there any obligation to employ knowledge that is available. Restriction might well be imposed on scientific research and on the technological possibilities it presents if the good of society seems to demand it.

THE SELECTIONS

In the first selection, L. M. Purdy claims that it is wrong to reproduce when we know there is a high risk of transmitting a serious genetic disease to an offspring. In support of this claim, Purdy presents three interconnected arguments: (1) we have a duty to provide every child with a normal opportunity for a good life, (2) we do not harm possible children by preventing them from existing, (3) the duty to provide a normal opportunity for a good life takes precedence over a potential parent's right to reproduce.

Purdy uses Huntington's disease (chorea) as an example in her argument. The recent identification of a genetic marker (see the Case Presentation) has opened up new possibilities for early detection of the disease in some cases. However, this fact does not substantially affect Purdy's argument. Also, the line of reasoning she develops is applicable to a wide variety of genetic diseases, such as thallasemia and cystic fibrosis, and is not uniquely tied to Huntington's disease.

Leon R. Kass, in "Implications of Prenatal Diagnosis for the Human Right to Life," expresses concern that the practice of "genetic abortion" will strongly affect our attitudes towards all who are "defective" or abnormal. Those who escape the net of selective abortion might receive less care and might even come to think of themselves as second-class specimens. Furthermore, on Kass's view, genetic abortion might encourage us to accept the general principle that defectives of any kind ought not be born. This, in turn, would threaten our commitment to the basic moral principle that each person, despite any physical or mental handicap, is the inherent equal of every other person.

Kass presents six criteria that he suggests ought to be satisfied to justify the abortion of a fetus for genetic reasons. In the remainder of his paper, he focuses on the question raised by the last criterion: According to what standards should we judge a fetus with genetic abnormalities unfit to live? As candidates for such standards, Kass examines the concepts of social good, family good, and the "healthy and sound" fetus. He finds difficulty with all, and in the end, he professes himself unable to provide a satisfactory justification for genetic abortion. Kass's difficulty with the "healthy and sound" fetus as a standard puts his general position in conflict with that taken by Purdy. What Purdy regards as a relatively clear-cut criterion, Kass views as a relatively vague and arbitrary social standard.

Critics of genetic screening and selective abortion have often charged that it is only a small social step from such programs to the practice of eugenics. In the selection included here, Ruth Macklin reviews four arguments against any proposal to establish a eugenics program. Macklin holds that if we accept these arguments as sound, then there is no justification for restricting individual decision making in matters of reproduction for eugenic considerations. Eugenics programs are likely to be misguided or dangerous, and decisions about genetic screening, selective abortion, and the like are best left to the individuals concerned.

W. F. Anderson and J. C. Fletcher, in "Gene Therapy in Human Beings," address the question of when it is legitimate to make the transition from experimental investigation to medical therapy. Before humans are made the subjects of gene therapy, they argue, evidence from animal experiments must show that patients are likely to benefit from it and that the level of risk to them is acceptably low. In particular, animal studies should demonstrate that a new gene can be put into target cells, remain in them, and do no harm to those cells. In their view, this is the minimum required to justify gene alteration as a form of therapy. (Their concern is restricted to alterations in the somatic cells, as distinct from the sex cells. See the Case Presentation for some of the issues connected with sex-cell changes.)

In "The Total Gene Screen," Morton Hunt summarizes the current state of screening to detect genetic predispositions to certain diseases. Hunt focuses on the screening of workers by employers and points out how the existence and use of the technology of screening give rise to five "profoundly troublesome" moral dilemmas. As he makes clear, whether we decide to use the technology or not to use it, the decision itself causes a conflict between values that we generally acknowledge and promote. Hunt suggests that the most socially practical and beneficial response to the possibility of genetic screening for predispositions to diseases would be to work out compromises that allow us to gain as much benefit as we can, while preserving, to the extent we are able, such values as privacy and autonomy.

Genetic Diseases: Can Having Children Be Immoral?

L. M. Purdy

I. Introduction

Suppose you know that there is a fifty percent chance you have Huntington's chorea, even though you are still free of symptoms, and that if you do have it, each of your children has a fifty percent chance of having it also.

Should you now have children?

There is always some possibility that a preg-

Reprinted with permission of the author.

nancy will result in a diseased or handicapped child. But certain persons run a higher than average risk of producing such a child. Genetic counselors are increasingly able to calculate the probability that certain problems will occur; this means that more people can find out whether they are in danger of creating unhealthy offspring *before* the birth of a child.

Since this kind of knowledge is available, we ought to use it wisely. I want in this paper to defend the thesis that it is wrong to reproduce when we know there is a high risk of transmitting a serious disease or defect. My argument for this claim is in three parts. The first is that we should try to provide every child with a normal opportunity for health; the second is that in the course of doing this it is not wrong to prevent possible children from existing. The third is that this duty may require us to refrain from childbearing.[1]

One methodological point must be made. I am investigating a problem in biomedical ethics: this is a philosophical enterprise. But the conclusion has practical importance since individuals do face the choice I examine. This raises a question: what relation ought the outcome of this inquiry bear to social policy?[2] It may be held that a person's reproductive life should not be interfered with. Perhaps this is a reasonable position, but it does not follow from it that it is never wrong for an individual to have children or that we should not try to determine when this is the case. All that does follow is that we may not coerce persons with regard to childbearing. Evaluation of this last claim is a separate issue which cannot be handled here.

I want to deal with this issue concretely. The reason for this is that, otherwise, discussion is apt to be vague and inconclusive. An additional reason is that it will serve to make us appreciate the magnitude of the difficulties faced by diseased or handicapped individuals. Thus it will be helpful to consider a specific disease. For this purpose I have chosen Huntington's chorea.[3]

II. Huntington's Chorea: Course and Risk

Let us now look at Huntington's chorea. First we will consider the course of the disease, then its inheritance pattern.

The symptoms of Huntington's chorea usually begin between the ages of thirty and fifty, but young children can also be affected. It happens this way:

> Onset is insidious. Personality changes (obstinacy, moodiness, lack of initiative) frequently antedate or accompany the involuntary choreic movements. These usually appear first in the face, neck, and arms, and are jerky, irregular, and stretching in character. Contractions of the facial muscles result in grimaces; those of the respiratory muscles, lips, and tongue lead to hesitating, explosive speech. Irregular movements of the trunk are present; the gait is shuffling and dancing. Tendon reflexes are increased . . . Some patients display a fatuous euphoria; others are spiteful, irascible, destructive, and violent. Paranoid reactions are common. Poverty of thought and impairment of attention, memory, and judgment occur. As the disease progresses, walking becomes impossible, swallowing difficult, and dementia profound. Suicide is not uncommon.[4]

The illness lasts about fifteen years, terminating in death.

Who gets Huntington's chorea? It is an autosomal dominant disease; this means it is caused by a single mutant gene located on a non-sex chromosome. It is passed from one generation to the next via affected individuals. When one has the disease, whether one has symptoms and thus knows one has it or not, there is a fifty percent chance that each child will have it also. If one has escaped it then there is no risk to one's children.[5]

How serious is this risk? For geneticists, a ten percent risk is high.[6] But not every high risk is unacceptable: this depends on what is at stake.

There are two separate evaluations in any judgment about a given risk. The first measures the gravity of the worst possible result; the second perceives a given risk as great or small. As for the first, in medicine as elsewhere, people may regard the same result differently:

> . . . The subjective attitude to the disease or lesion itself may be quite at variance with what informed medical opinion may regard as a realistic appraisal. Relatively minor limb defects with cosmetic overtones are examples here. On the other hand, some patients regard with equanimity genetic lesions which are of major medical importance.[7]

For devastating diseases like Huntington's chorea, this part of the judgment should be unproblematic: no one could want a loved one to suffer so.

There may be considerable disagreement, however, about whether a given probability is big or little. Individuals vary a good deal in their attitude toward this aspect of risk.[8] This suggests that it would be difficult to define the "right" attitude to a particular risk in many circumstances. Nevertheless, there are good grounds for arguing in favor of a conservative approach here. For it is reasonable to take special precautions to avoid very bad consequences, even if the risk is small. But the possible consequences here *are* very bad: a child who may inherit Huntington's chorea is a child with a much larger than average chance of being subjected to severe and prolonged suffering. Even if the child does not have the disease, it may anticipate and fear it, and anticipating an evil, as we all know, may be worse than experiencing it. In addition, if a parent loses the gamble, his child will suffer the consequences. But it is one thing to take a high risk for oneself; to submit someone else to it without his consent is another.

I think that these points indicate that the morality of procreation in situations like this demands further study. I propose to do this by looking first at the position of the possible child, then at that of the potential parent.[9]

III. Reproduction: The Possible Child's Position

The first task in treating the problem from the child's point of view is to find a way of referring to possible future offspring without seeming to confer some sort of morally significant existence upon them. I will call children who might be born in the future but who are not now conceived "possible" children, offspring, individuals, or persons. I stipulate that this term implies nothing about their moral standing.

The second task is to decide what claims about children or possible children are relevant to the morality of childbearing in the circumstances being considered. There are, I think, two such claims. One is that we ought to provide every child with at least a normal opportunity for a good life. The other is that we do not harm possible children if we prevent them from existing. Let us consider both these matters in turn.

A. Opportunity for a Good Life

Accepting the claim that we ought to try to provide for every child a normal opportunity for a good life involves two basic problems: justification and practical application.

Justification of the claim could be derived fairly straightforwardly from either utilitarian or contractarian theories of justice, I think, although a proper discussion would be too lengthy to include here. Of prime importance in any such discussion would be the judgment that to neglect this duty would be to create unnecessary unhappiness or unfair disadvantage for some persons.

The attempt to apply the claim that we should try to provide a normal opportunity for a good life leads to a couple of difficulties. One is knowing what it requires of us. Another is defining "normal opportunity." Let us tackle the latter problem first.

Conceptions of "normal opportunity" vary among societies and also within them: *de rigueur* in some circles are private music lessons and trips to Europe, while in others providing eight years of schooling is a major sacrifice. But there is no need to consider this complication since we are here concerned only with health as a prerequisite for normal opportunity. Thus we can retreat to the more limited claim that every parent should try to ensure normal health for his child. It might be thought that even this moderate claim is unsatisfactory since in some places debilitating conditions are the norm. One could circumvent this objection by saying that parents ought to try to provide for their children health normal for that culture, even though it may be inadequate if measured by some outside standard. This conservative position would still justify efforts to avoid the birth of children at risk for Huntington's chorea and other serious genetic diseases.

But then what does this stand require of us: is sacrifice entailed by the duty to try to provide normal health for our children? The most plausible answer seems to be that as the danger of serious disability increases, the greater the sacrifice demanded of the potential parent. This means it would be more justifiable to recommend that an individual refrain from childbearing if he risks passing on spina bifida than if he risks passing on webbed feet. Working out all the details of such a schema would clearly be a difficult matter: I do not think it would be impossible to set up workable guidelines, though.

Assuming a rough theoretical framework of this sort, the next question we must ask is whether Huntington's chorea substantially impairs an individual's opportunity for a good life.

People appear to have different opinions about the plight of such persons. Optimists argue that a child born into a family afflicted with Huntington's chorea has a reasonable chance of living a satisfactory life. After all, there is a fifty percent chance it will escape the disease even if a parent has already manifested it, and a still greater chance if this is not so. Even if it does have the illness, it will probably enjoy thirty years of healthy life before symptoms appear; and, perhaps, it may not find the disease destructive. Optimists can list diseased or handicapped persons who have lived fruitful lives. They can also find individuals who seem genuinely glad to be alive. One is Rick Donohue, a sufferer from the Joseph family disease: "You know, if my mom hadn't had me, I wouldn't be here for the life I have had. So there is a good possibility I will have children."[10] Optimists therefore conclude that it would be a shame if these persons had not lived.

Pessimists concede these truths, but they take a less sanguine view of them. They think a fifty percent risk of serious disease like Huntington's chorea appallingly high. They suspect that a child born into an afflicted family is liable to spend its youth in dreadful anticipation and fear of the disease. They expect that the disease, if it appears, will be perceived as a tragic and painful end to a blighted life. They point out that Rick Donohue is still young and has not yet experienced the full horror of his sickness.

Empirical research is clearly needed to resolve this dispute: we need much more information about the psychology and life history of sufferers and potential sufferers. Until we have it we cannot know whether the optimist or the pessimist has a better case: definitive judgment must therefore be suspended. In the meantime, however, common sense suggests that the pessimist has the edge.

If some diseased persons do turn out to have a worse than average life there appears to be a case against further childbearing in afflicted families. To support this claim two more judgments are necessary, however. The first is that it is not wrong to refrain from childbearing. The second is that asking individuals to so refrain is less of a sacrifice than might be thought.[11] I will examine each of these judgments.

B. The Morality of Preventing the Birth of Possible Persons

Before going on to look at reasons why it would not be wrong to prevent the birth of possible persons, let me try to clarify the picture a bit. To understand the claim it must be kept in mind that we are considering a prospective situation here, not a retrospective one: we are trying to rank the desirability of various alternative future states of affairs. One possible future state is this: a world where nobody is at risk for Huntington's chorea except as a result of random mutation. This state has been achieved by sons and daughters of persons afflicted with Huntington's chorea ceasing to reproduce. This means that an indeterminate number of children who might have been born were not born. These possible children can be divided into two categories: those who would have been miserable and those who would have lived good lives. To prevent the existence of members of the first category it was necessary to prevent the existence of all. Whether or not this is a good state of affairs depends on the morality of the means and the end. The end, preventing the existence of miserable beings, is surely good; I will argue that preventing the birth of possible persons is not intrinsically wrong. Hence this state of affairs is a morally good one.

Why then is it not in itself wrong to prevent the birth of possible persons? It is not wrong because there seems to be no reason to believe that possible individuals are either deprived or injured if they do not exist. They are not deprived because to be deprived in a morally significant sense one must be able to have experiences. But possible persons do not exist. Since they do not exist, they cannot have experiences. Another way to make this point is to say that each of us might not have been born, although most of us are glad we were. But this does not mean that it makes sense to say that we would have been deprived of something had we not been born. For if we had not been born, we would not exist, and there would be nobody to be deprived of anything. To assert the contrary is to imagine that we are looking at a world in which we do not exist. But this is not the way it would be: there would be nobody to look.

The contention that it is wrong to prevent possible persons from existing because they have a right to exist appears to be equally baseless. The most fundamental objection to this view is that there is no reason to ascribe rights to entities which do not exist. It is one thing to say that as-yet-nonexistent persons will have certain rights if and when they exist: this claim is plausible if made with an eye toward preserving social and environmental goods.[12] But what justification could there be for the claim that nonexistent beings have a right to exist?

Even if one conceded that there was a presumption in favor of letting some nonexistent beings exist, stronger claims could surely override it.[13] For one thing, it would be unfair not to recognize the prior claim of already existing children who are not being properly cared for. One might also argue that it is simply wrong to prevent persons who might have existed from doing so. But this implies that contraception and population control are also wrong.

It is therefore reasonable to maintain that because possible persons have no right to exist, they are not injured if not created. Even if they had that right, it could rather easily be overridden by counterclaims. Hence, since possible persons are neither deprived nor injured if not conceived, it is not wrong to prevent their existence.

C. Conclusion to Part III

At the beginning of Part III I said that two claims are relevant to the morality of childbearing in the circumstances being considered. The first is that we ought to provide every child with at least a normal opportunity for a good life. The second is that we do not deprive or injure possible persons if we prevent their existence.

I suggested that the first claim could be derived from currently accepted theories of justice: a healthy body is generally necessary for happiness and it is also a prerequisite for a fair chance at a good life in our competitive world. Thus it is right to try to ensure that each child is healthy.

I argued, with regard to the second claim, that we do not deprive or injure possible persons if we fail to create them. They cannot be deprived of anything because they do not exist and hence cannot have experiences. They cannot be injured because only an entity with a right to exist could be injured if prevented from existing: but there are no good grounds for believing that they are such entities.

From the conjunction of these two claims I conclude that it is right to try to ensure that a child is healthy even if by doing so we preclude the existence of certain possible persons. Thus it is right for individuals to prevent the birth of children at risk for Huntington's chorea by avoiding parenthood. The next question is whether it is seriously wrong *not* to avoid parenthood.

IV. Reproduction: The Potential Parent's Situation

I have so far argued that if choreics live substantially worse lives than average, then it is right for afflicted families to cease reproduction. But this conflicts with the generally recognized freedom to procreate and so it does not automatically follow that family members ought not to have children. How can we decide whether the duty to try to provide normal health for one's child should take precedence over the right to reproduce?

This is essentially the same question I asked earlier: how much must one sacrifice to try to ensure that one's offspring is healthy? In answer to this I suggested that the greater the danger of serious disability, the more justifiable considerable sacrifice is.

Now asking someone who wants a child to refrain from procreation seems to be asking for a large sacrifice. It may, in fact, appear to be too large to demand of anyone. Yet I think it can be shown that it is not as great as it initially seems.

Why do people want children? There are probably many reasons, but I suspect that the following include some of the most common. One set of reasons has to do with the gratification to be derived from a happy family life—love, companionship, watching a child grow, helping mold it into a good person, sharing its pains and triumphs. Another set of reasons centers about the parents as individuals—validation of their place within a genetically continuous family line, the conception of children as a source of immortality, being surrounded by replicas of themselves.

Are there alternative ways of satisfying these desires? Adoption or technological means provide ways to satisfy most of the desires pertaining to family life without passing on specific genetic defects. Artificial insemination by donor is already available; implantation of donor ova is likely within a few years. Still another option will exist if cloning becomes a reality. In the meantime, we might permit women to conceive and bear babies for those who do not want to do so themselves.[14] But the desire to extend the genetic line, the desire for immortality, and the desire for children that physically resemble one cannot be met by these methods.

Many individuals probably feel these latter desires strongly. This creates a genuine conflict for persons at risk for transmitting serious genetic diseases like Huntington's chorea. The situation seems especially unfair because, unlike normal people, through no fault of their own, doing something they badly want to do may greatly harm others.

But if my common sense assumption that they are in grave danger of harming others is true, then it is imperative to scrutinize their options carefully. On the one hand, they can have children: they satisfy their desires but risk eventual crippling illness and death for their offspring. On the other, they can remain childless or seek nonstandard ways of creating a family: they have some unfulfilled desires, but they avoid risking harm to their children.

I think it is clear which of these two alternatives is best. For the desires which must remain unsatisfied if they forgo normal procreation are less than admirable. To see the genetic line continued entails a sinister legacy of illness and death; the desire for immortality cannot really be satisfied by reproduction anyway; and the desire for children that physically resemble one is narcissistic and its fulfillment cannot be guaranteed even by normal reproduction. Hence the only defence of these desires is that people do in fact feel them.

Now, I am inclined to accept William James' dictum regarding desires: "Take any demand, however slight, which any creature, however weak, may make. Ought it not, for its own sole sake be satisfied? If not, prove why not."[15] Thus I judge a world where more desires are satisfied to be better than one in which fewer are. But not all desires should be regarded as legitimate, since, as James suggests, there may be good reasons why these ought to be disregarded. The fact that their

fulfillment will seriously harm others is surely such a reason. And I believe that the circumstances I have described are a clear example of the sort of case where a desire must be judged illegitimate, at least until it can be shown that sufferers from serious genetic diseases like Huntington's chorea do not live considerably worse than average lives. Therefore, I think it is wrong for individuals in this predicament to reproduce.

V. Conclusion

Let me recapitulate. At the beginning of this paper I asked whether it is wrong for those who risk transmitting severe genetic disease like Huntington's chorea to have "blood" children. Some despair of reaching an answer to this question.[16] But I think such pessimism is not wholly warranted, and that if generally accepted would lead to much unnecessary harm. It is true that in many cases it is difficult to know what ought to be done. But this does not mean that we should throw up our hands and espouse a completely laissez-faire approach: philosophers can help by probing the central issues and trying to find guidelines for action.

Naturally there is no way to derive an answer to this kind of problem by deductive argument from self-evident premises, for it must depend on a complicated interplay of facts and moral judgments. My preliminary exploration of Huntington's chorea is of this nature. In the course of discussion I suggested that, if it is true that sufferers live substantially worse lives than do normal persons, those who might transmit it should not have children. This conclusion is supported by the judgments that we ought to try to provide for every child a normal opportunity for a good life, that possible individuals are not harmed if not conceived, and that it is sometimes less justifiable for persons to exercise their right to procreate than one might think.

I want to stress, in conclusion, that my argument is incomplete. To investigate fully even a single disease, like Huntington's chorea, empirical research on the lives of members of afflicted families is necessary. Then, after developing further the themes touched upon here, evaluation of the probable consequences of different policies on society and on future generations is needed. Until the results of a complete study are available, my argument could serve best as a reason for persons at risk for transmitting Huntington's chorea and similar diseases to put off having children. Perhaps this paper will stimulate such inquiry.

Notes

1. There are a series of cases ranging from low risk of mild disease or handicap to high risk of serious disease or handicap. It would be difficult to decide where the duty to refrain from procreation becomes compelling. My point here is that there are some clear cases.

   I'd like to thank Lawrence Davis and Sidney Siskin for their helpful comments on an earlier version of this paper.

2. This issue is one which must be faced most urgently by genetic counselors. The proper role of the genetic counselor with regard to such decisions has been the subject of much debate. The dominant view seems to be that espoused by Lytt Gardner who maintains that it is unethical for a counselor to make ethical judgments about what his clients ought to do. ("Counseling in Genetics." *Early Diagnosis of Human Genetic Defects: Scientific & Ethical Considerations,* ed. Maureen Harris, [H.E.W. Publication No. (NIH) 72–25; Fogarty Center Proceedings No. 6]; p. 192.) Typically this view is unsupported by an argument. For other views see Bentley Glass "Human Heredity and Ethical Problems" *Perspectives in Biology & Medicine,* Vol. 15 (winter '72) 237–53, esp. 242–52; Marc Lappé, "The Genetic Counselor Responsible to Whom? *Hastings Center Report,* Vol. 1, No. 2 (Sept. '71) 6–8; E. C. Fraser, "Genetic Counseling" *Am. J. of Human Genetics* 26: 636–659, 1974.

3. I have chosen Huntington's chorea because it seems to me to be one of the clearest cases of high risk serious genetic disease known to the public, despite the fact that it does not usually manifest itself until the prime of life. The latter entails two further facts. First an individual of reproductive age may not know whether he has the disease; he therefore does not know the risk of passing on the disease. Secondly, an affected person may have a substantial number of years of healthy life before it shows itself. I do not think that this factor materially changes my case, however. Even if an individual does not in fact risk passing the disease to his children, *he cannot know that this is true.* And even thirty years of healthy life may well be seriously shadowed by anticipation and fear of the disease. Thus the fact that the disease develops late does not diminish its horror.

If it could be shown that these factors could be adequately circumvented, my claim that there is a *class* of genetic disease of such severity that it would be wrong to risk passing them on would not be undermined.

It might also be thought that Huntington's chorea is insufficiently common to merit such attention. But, depending on reproductive patterns, the disease could become a good deal more widespread. Consider the fact that in 1916 nine hundred and sixty-two cases could be traced from six seventeenth-century arrivals in America. (Gordon Rattray Taylor, *The Biological Time Bomb,* [New York, 1968], p. 176.) But more importantly, even if the disease did not spread, it would still be seriously wrong. I think, to inflict it unnecessarily on *any* members of new generations. Finally, it should be kept in mind that I am using Huntington's chorea as an example of the sort of disease we should try to eradicate. Thus the arguments presented here would be relevant to a wide range of genetic diseases.

4. *The Merck Manual,* (Rahway, N.J.: Merck, 1972). p. 1346.

5. Hymie Gordon, "Genetic Counseling," JAMA, Vol. 217 No. 9 (August 30, 1971), 1217.

6. Charles Smith, Susan Holloway, and Alan E. H. Emery, "Individuals at Risk in Families—Genetic Disease," *J. of Medical Genetics,* 8 (1971), 453. See also Townes in *Genetic Counseling* ed. Daniel Bergsma, *Birth Defects Original Article Series,* Vol. VL No. 1 (May 1970).

7. J. H. Pearn, "Patients' Subjective Interpretation of Risks offered in Genetic Counseling," *Journal of Medical Genetics,* 10 (1973) 131.

8. Pearn, p. 132.

9. There are many important and interesting points that might be raised with respect to future generations and present society. There is no space to deal with them here, although I strongly suspect that conclusions regarding them would support my judgment that it is wrong for those who risk transmitting certain diseases to reproduce—for some discussion of future generations, see Gerald Leach, *The Biocrats,* (Middlesex, England: Penguin Books, 1972), p. 150; M. P. Golding, "Obligations to Future Generations," *Monist* 56 (Jan. 1972) 84–99; Gordon Rattray Taylor, *The Biological Time Bomb* (New York, 1968), esp. p. 176. For some discussions of society, see Daniel Callahan, "The Meaning and Significance of Genetic Disease: Philosophical Perspectives," *Ethical Issues in Human Genetics,* ed. Bruce Hilton et al., (New York, 1973), p. 87ff.; John Fletcher, "The Brink: The

Parent-Child Bond in the Genetic Revolution," *Theological Studies* 33 (Sept. '72) 457–486; Glass (supra 2ª); Marc Lappé, "Human Genetics," Annals of the *New York Academy of Sciences*, Vol. 26 (May 18, 1973) 152–59; Marc Lappé, "Moral Obligations and the Fallacies of Genetic Control," *Theological Studies* Vol. 33, No. 3 (Sept. '72) 411–427; Martin P. Golding. "Ethical Issues in Biological Engineering," *UCLA Law Review* Vol. 15: 267 (1968) 443–479; L. C. Dunn, *Heredity and Evolution in Human Populations*, (Cambridge, Mass., 1959), p. 145; Robert S. Morison in *Ethical Issues in Human Genetics*, ed. Bruce Hilton et al., (New York, 1973), p. 208.

10. *The New York Times*, September 30, 1975, p. 1. col. 6. The Joseph family disease is similar to Huntington's chorea except that symptoms start appearing in the twenties. Rick Donohue is in his early twenties.

11. There may be a price for the individuals who refrain from having children. We will be looking at the situation from their point of view shortly.

12. This is in fact the basis for certain parental duties. An example is the maternal duty to obtain proper nutrition before and during pregnancy, for this is necessary if the child is to have normal health when it is born.

13. One might argue that as many persons as possible should exist so that they may enjoy life.

14. Some thinkers have qualms about the use of some or all of these methods. They have so far failed to show why they are immoral, although, naturally, much careful study will be required before they could be unqualifiedly recommended. See, for example, Richard Hull, "Genetic Engineering: Comment on Headings," *The Humanist*, Vol. 32 (Sept./Oct. 1972). 13.

15. *Essays in Pragmatism*, ed. A. Castell (New York, 1948), p. 73.

16. For example, see Leach, p. 138. One of the ways the dilemma described by Leach could be lessened would be if society emphasized those aspects of family life not dependent on "blood" relationships and downplayed those that are.

Implications of Prenatal Diagnosis for the Human Right to Life

Leon R. Kass

Any discussion of the ethical issues of genetic counseling and prenatal diagnosis is unavoidably haunted by a ghost called the morality of abortion. This ghost I shall not vex. More precisely, I shall not vex the reader by telling ghost stories. However, I would be neither surprised nor disappointed if my discussion of an admittedly related matter, the ethics of aborting the genetically defective, summons that hovering spirit to the reader's mind. For the morality of abortion is a matter not easily laid to rest, recent efforts to do so notwithstanding. . . .

Yet before leaving the general question of abortion, let me pause to drop some anchors for the discussion that follows. Despite great differences of opinion both as to what to think and how to reason about abortion, nearly everyone agrees that abortion is a moral issue.[1] What does this mean? Formally, it means that a woman seeking or refusing an abortion can expect to be asked to justify her action. And we can expect that she should be able to give reasons for her choice other than "I like it" or "I don't like it." Substantively, it means that, in the absence of good reasons for intervention, there is some presumption in favor of allowing the pregnancy to continue once it has begun. A common way of expressing this presumption is to say that "the fetus has a right to continued life."[2] In this context, disagreement concerning the moral permissibility of abortion concerns what rights (or interests or needs), and whose, override (take precedence over, or outweigh) this fetal

Reprinted from Ethical Issues in Human Genetics: Genetic Counseling and the Use of Genetic Knowledge, *edited by Bruce Hilton, Daniel Callahan, Maureen Harris, Peter Condliffe, and Burton Berkley (New York: Plenum Press, 1973), pp. 185–199. A revised version of this essay ("Perfect Babies: Prenatal Diagnosis and the Equal Right to Life") appears in Dr. Kass's book,* Toward a More Natural Science: Biology and Human Affairs *(New York: The Free Press, 1985).*

"right." Even most of the "opponents" of abortion agree that the mother's right to live takes precedence, and that abortion to save her life is permissible, perhaps obligatory. Some believe that a woman's right to determine the number and spacing of her children takes precedence, while yet others argue that the need to curb population growth is, at least at this time, overriding.

Hopefully, this brief analysis of what it means to say that abortion is a moral issue is sufficient to establish two points. First, that the fetus is a living thing with some moral claim on us not to do it violence, and therefore, second, that justification must be given for destroying it.

Turning now from the general questions of the ethics of abortion, I wish to focus on the special ethical issues raised by the abortion of "defective" fetuses (so-called "abortion for fetal indications"). I shall consider only the cleanest cases, those cases where well-characterized genetic diseases are diagnosed with a high degree of certainty by means of amniocentesis, in order to sidestep the added moral dilemmas posed when the diagnosis is suspected or possible, but unconfirmed. However, many of the questions I shall discuss could also be raised about cases where genetic analysis gives only a statistical prediction about the genotype of the fetus, and also about cases where the defect has an infectious or chemical rather than a genetic cause (e.g., rubella, thalidomide).

My first and possibly most difficult task is to show that there is anything left to discuss once we have agreed not to discuss the morality of abortion in general. There is a sense in which abortion for genetic defect is, after abortion to save the life of the mother, perhaps the most defensible kind of abortion. Certainly, it is a serious and not a frivolous reason for abortion, defended by its proponents in sober and rational speech—unlike justifications based upon the false notion that a fetus is a mere part of a woman's body, to be used and abused at her pleasure. Standing behind genetic abortion are serious and well-intentioned people, with reasonable ends in view: the prevention of genetic diseases, the elimination of suffering in families, the preservation of precious financial and medical resources, the protection of our genetic heritage. No profiteers, no sex-ploiters, no racists. No arguments about the connection of abortion with promiscuity and licentiousness, no perjured testimony about the mental health of the mother, no arguments about the seriousness of the population problem. In short, clear objective data, a worthy cause, decent men and women. If abortion, what better reason for it?

Yet if genetic abortion is but a happily wagging tail on the dog of abortion, it is simultaneously the nose of a camel protruding under a rather different tent. Precisely because the quality of the fetus is central to the decision to abort, the practice of genetic abortion has implications which go beyond those raised by abortion in general. What may be at stake here is the belief in the radical moral equality of all human beings, the belief that all human beings possess equally and independent of merit certain fundamental rights, one among which is, of course, the right to life.

To be sure, the belief that fundamental human rights belong equally to all human beings has been but an ideal, never realized, often ignored, sometimes shamelessly. Yet it has been perhaps the most powerful moral idea at work in the world for at least two centuries. It is this idea and ideal that animates most of the current political and social criticism around the globe. It is ironic that we should acquire the power to detect and eliminate the genetically unequal at a time when we have finally succeeded in removing much of the stigma and disgrace previously attached to victims of congenital illness, in providing them with improved care and support, and in preventing, by means of education, feelings of guilt on the part of their parents. One might even wonder whether the development of amniocentesis and prenatal diagnosis may represent a backlash against these same humanitarian and egalitarian tendencies in the practice of medicine, which, by helping to sustain to the age of reproduction persons with genetic disease has itself contributed to the increasing incidence of genetic disease, and with it, to increased pressures for genetic screening, genetic counseling, and genetic abortion.

No doubt our humanitarian and egalitarian principles and practices have caused us some new difficulties, but if we mean to weaken or turn our backs on them, we should do so consciously and thoughtfully. If, as I believe, the idea and practice of genetic abortion points in that direction, we should make ourselves aware of it. And if, as I believe, the way in which genetic abortion is described, discussed, and justified is perhaps of even greater consequence than its practice for our notions of human rights and of their equal possession by all human beings, we should pay special attention to questions of language and in particular, to the question of justification. . . .

Genetic Abortion and the Living Defective

The practice of abortion of the genetically defective will no doubt affect our view of and our behavior toward those abnormals who escape the net of detection and abortion. A child with Down's syndrome or with hemophilia or with muscular dystrophy born at a time when most of his (potential) fellow sufferers were destroyed prenatally is liable to be looked upon by the community as one unfit to be alive, as a second-class (or even lower) human type. He may be seen as a person who need not have been, and who would not have been, if only someone had gotten to him in time.

The parents of such children are also likely to treat them differently, especially if the mother would have wished but failed to get an amniocentesis because of ignorance, poverty, or distance from the testing station, or if the prenatal diagnosis was in error. In such cases, parents are especially likely to resent the child. They may be disinclined to give it the kind of care they might have before the advent of amniocentesis and genetic abortion, rationalizing that a second-class specimen is not entitled to first-class treatment. If pressed to do so, say by physicians, the parents might refuse, and the courts may become involved. This has already begun to happen.

In Maryland, parents of a child with Down's syndrome refused permission to have the child operated on for an intestinal obstruction present at birth. The physicians and the hospital sought an injunction to require the parents to allow surgery. The judge ruled in favor of the parents, despite what I understand to be the weight of precedent to the contrary, on the grounds that the child was Mongoloid, that is, had the child been "normal," the decision would have gone the other way. Although the decision was not appealed to and hence not affirmed by a higher court, we can see through the prism of this case the possibility that the new powers of human genetics will strip the blindfold from the lady of justice and will make official the dangerous doctrine that some men are more equal than others.

The abnormal child may also feel resentful. A child with Down's syndrome or Tay-Sachs disease will probably never know or care, but what about a child with hemophilia or with Turner's syndrome? In the past decade, with medical knowledge and power over the prenatal child increasing and with parental authority over the postnatal child decreasing, we have seen the appearance of a new type of legal action, suits for wrongful life. Children have brought suit against their parents (and others) seeking to recover damages for physical and social handicaps inextricably tied to their birth (e.g., congenital deformities, congenital syphilis, illegitimacy). In some of the American cases, the courts have recognized the justice of the child's claim (that he was injured due to parental negligence), although they have so far refused to award damages, due to policy considerations. In other countries, e.g., in Germany, judgments with compensation have gone for the plaintiffs. With the spread of amniocentesis and genetic abortion, we can only expect such cases to increase. And here it will be the soft-hearted rather than the hard-hearted judges who will establish the doctrine of second-class human beings, out of compassion for the mutants who escaped the traps set out for them.

It may be argued that I am dealing with a problem which, even if it is real, will affect very few people. It may be suggested that very few will escape the traps once we have set them properly and widely, once people are informed about amniocentesis, once the power to detect prenatally grows to its full capacity, and once our "superstitious" opposition to abortion dies out or is extirpated. But in order even to come close to this vision of success, amniocentesis will have to become part of every pregnancy—either by making it mandatory, like the test for syphilis, or by making it "routine medical practice," like the Pap smear. Leaving aside the other problems with universal amniocentesis, we could expect that the problem for the few who escape is likely to be even worse precisely because they will be few.

The point, however, should be generalized. How will we come to view and act toward the many "abnormals" that will remain among us—the retarded, the crippled, the senile, the deformed, and the true mutants—once we embark on a program to root out genetic abnormality? For it must be remembered that we shall always have abnormals—some who escape detection or whose disease is undetectable *in utero*, others as a result of new mutations, birth injuries, accidents, maltreatment, or disease—who will require our care and protection. The existence of "defectives" cannot be fully prevented, not even by totalitarian breeding and weeding programs. Is it not likely that our principle with respect to these people will change from "We try harder" to "Why accept second best?" The idea of "the unwanted because abnormal child" may become a self-fulfilling prophecy, whose consequences may be worse than those of the abnormality itself.

Genetic and Other Defectives

The mention of other abnormals points to a second danger of the practice of genetic abortion. Genetic abortion may come to be seen not so much as the prevention of genetic disease, but as the prevention of birth of defective or abnormal children—and, in a way, understandably so. For in the case of what other diseases does preventive medicine consist in the elimination of the patient-at-risk? Moreover, the very language used to discuss genetic disease leads us to the easy but wrong conclusion that the afflicted fetus or person is rather than has a disease. True, one is partly defined by his genotype, but only partly. A person is more than his disease. And yet we slide easily from the language of possession to the language of identity, from "He has hemophilia" to "He is a hemophiliac," from "She has diabetes" through "She is diabetic" to "She is a diabetic," from "The fetus has Down's syndrome" to "The fetus is a Down's." This way of speaking supports the belief that it is defective persons (or potential persons) that are being eliminated, rather than diseases.

If this is so, then it becomes simply accidental that the defect has a genetic cause. Surely, it is only because of the high regard for medicine and science, and for the accuracy of genetic diagnosis, that genotypic defectives are likely to be the first to go. But once the principle, "Defectives should not be born," is established, grounds other than cyto-logical and biochemical may very well be sought. Even ignoring racialists and others equally misguided—of course, they cannot be ignored—we should know that there are social scientists, for example, who believe that one can predict with a high degree of accuracy how a child will turn out from a careful, systematic study of the socioeconomic and psychodynamic environment into which he is born and in which he grows up. They might press for the prevention of socio-psychological disease, even of "criminality," by means of prenatal environmental diagnosis and abortion. I have heard rumor that a crude, unscientific form of eliminating potential "phenotypic defectives" is already being practiced in some cities, in that submission to abortion is allegedly being made a condition for the receipt of welfare payments. "Defectives should not be born" is a principle without limits. We can ill-afford to have it established.

Up to this point, I have been discussing the possible implications of the practice of genetic abortion for our belief in and adherence to the idea that, at least in fundamental human matters such as life and liberty, all men are to be considered as equals, that for these matters we should ignore as irrelevant the real qualitative differences amongst men, however important these differences may be for other purposes. Those who are concerned about abortion fear that the permissible time of eliminating the unwanted will be moved forward along the time continuum, against newborns, infants, and children. Similarly, I suggest that we should be concerned lest the attack on gross genetic inequality in fetuses be advanced along the continuum of quality and into the later stages of life.

I am not engaged in predicting the future; I am not saying that amniocentesis and genetic abortion will lead down the road to Nazi Germany. Rather, I am suggesting that the principles underlying genetic abortion simultaneously justify many further steps down that road. The point was very well made by Abraham Lincoln (1854):

> If A can prove, however conclusively, that he may, of right, enslave B—Why may not B snatch the same argument and prove equally, that he may enslave A?
>
> You say A is white, and B is black. It is color, then; the lighter having the right to enslave the darker? Take care. By this rule,

you are to be slave to the first man you meet with a fairer skin than your own.

You do not mean color exactly? You mean the whites are intellectually the superiors of the blacks, and, therefore have the right to enslave them? Take care again. By this rule, you are to be slave to the first man you meet with an intellect superior to your own.

But, say you, it is a question of interest; and, if you can make it your interest, you have the right to enslave another. Very well. And if he can make it his interest, he has the right to enslave you.

Perhaps I have exaggerated the dangers; perhaps we will not abandon our inexplicable preference for generous humanitarianism over consistency. But we should indeed be cautious and move slowly as we give serious consideration to the question "What price the perfect baby?"[3]

Standards for Justifying Genetic Abortion

The rest of this paper deals with the problem of justification. What would constitute an adequate justification of the decision to abort a genetically defective fetus? Let me suggest the following formal characteristics, each of which still begs many questions. (1) The reasons given should be logically consistent, and should lead to relatively unambiguous guidelines—note that I do not say "rules"—for action in most cases. (2) The justification should make evident to a reasonable person that the interest or need or right being served by abortion is sufficient to override the otherwise presumptive claim on us to protect and preserve the life of the fetus. (3) Hopefully, the justification would be such as to help provide intellectual support for drawing distinctions between acceptable and unacceptable kinds of genetic abortion and between genetic abortion itself and the further practices we would all find abhorrent. (4) The justification ought to be capable of generalization to all persons in identical circumstances. (5) The justification should not lead to different actions from month to month or from year to year. (6) The justification should be grounded on standards that can, both in principle and in fact, sustain and support our actions in the case of genetic abortion and our notions of human rights in general.

Though I would ask the reader to consider all these criteria, I shall focus primarily on the last. According to what standards can and should we judge a fetus with genetic abnormalities unfit to live, i.e., abortable? It seems to me that there are at least three dominant standards to which we are likely to repair.

The first is societal good. The needs and interests of society are often invoked to justify the practices of prenatal diagnosis and abortion of the genetically abnormal. The argument, full blown, runs something like this. Society has an interest in the genetic fitness of its members. It is foolish for society to squander its precious resources ministering to and caring for the unfit, especially for those who will never become "productive," or who will never in any way "benefit" society. Therefore, the interests of society are best served by the elimination of the genetically defective prior to their birth.

The societal standard is all-too-often reduced to its lowest common denominator: money. Thus one physician, claiming that he has "made a cost-benefit analysis of Tay-Sachs disease," notes that "the total cost of carrier detection, prenatal diagnosis and termination of at-risk pregnancies for all Jewish individuals in the United States under 30 who will marry is $5,730,281. If the program is set up to screen only one married partner, the cost is $3,122,695. The hospital costs for the 990 cases of Tay-Sachs disease these individuals would produce over a thirty-year period in the United States is $34,650,000."[4] Another physician, apparently less interested or able to make such a precise audit has written: "Cost-benefit analyses have been made for the total prospective detection and monitoring of Tay-Sachs disease, cystic fibrosis (when prenatal detection becomes available for cystic fibrosis) and other disorders,and in most cases, the expenditures for hospitalization and medical care far exceed the cost of prenatal detection in properly selected risk populations, followed by selective abortion." Yet a third physician has calculated that the costs to the state of caring for children with Down's syndrome is more than three times that of detecting and aborting them. (These authors all acknowledge the additional nonsocietal "costs" of personal suffering, but insofar as they consider society, the costs are purely economic.)

There are many questions that can be raised

about this approach. First, there are the questions about the accuracy of the calculations. Not all the costs have been reckoned. The aborted defective child will be "replaced" by a "normal" child. In keeping the ledger, the "costs" to society of his care and maintenance cannot be ignored—costs of educating him, or removing his wastes and pollutions, not to mention the "costs" in nonreplaceable natural resources that he consumes. Who is a greater drain on society's precious resources, the average inmate of a home for the retarded or the average graduate of Harvard College? I am not sure we know or can even find out. Then there are the costs of training the physician, and genetic counselors, equipping their laboratories, supporting their research, and sending them and us to conferences to worry about what they are doing. An accurate economic analysis seems to me to be impossible, even in principle. And even if it were possible, one could fall back on the words of the ordinary language philosopher, Andy Capp, who, when his wife said that she was getting really worried about the cost of living, replied: "Sweet'eart, name me one person who wants t'stop livin' on account of the cost."

A second defect of the economic analysis is that there are matters of social importance that are not reducible to financial costs, and others that may not be quantifiable at all. How does one quantitate the costs of real and potential social conflict, either between children and parents, or between the community and the "deviants" who refuse amniocentesis and continue to bear abnormal children? Can one measure the effect on racial tensions of attempting to screen for and prevent the birth of children homozygous (or heterozygous) for sickle-cell anemia? What numbers does one attach to any decreased willingness or ability to take care of the less fortunate, or to cope with difficult problems? And what about the "costs" of rising expectations? Will we become increasingly dissatisfied with anything short of the "optimum baby"? How does one quantify anxiety? Humiliation? Guilt? Finally, might not the medical profession pay an unmeasurable price if genetic abortion and other revolutionary activities bring about changes in medical ethics and medical practice that lead to the further erosion of trust in the physician?

An appeal to social worthiness or usefulness is a less vulgar form of the standard of societal good. It is true that great social contributions are unlikely to be forthcoming from persons who suffer from most serious genetic diseases, especially since many of them die in childhood. Yet consider the following remarks of Pearl Buck (1968) on the subject of being a mother of a child retarded from phenylketonuria:

> My child's life has not been meaningless. She has indeed brought comfort and practical help to many people who are parents of retarded children or are themselves handicapped. True, she has done it through me, yet without her I would not have had the means of learning how to accept the inevitable sorrow, and how to make that acceptance useful to others. Would I be so heartless as to say that it has been worthwhile for my child to be born retarded? Certainly not, but I am saying that even though gravely retarded it has been worthwile for her to have lived.
>
> It can be summed up, perhaps, by saying that in this world, where cruelty prevails in so many aspects of our life, I would not add the weight of choice to kill rather than to let live. A retarded child, a handicapped person, brings its own gift to life, even to the life of normal human beings. That gift is comprehended in the lessons of patience, understanding, and mercy, lessons which we all need to receive and to practice with one another, whatever we are.

The standard of potential social worthiness is little better in deciding about abortion in particular cases than is the standard of economic cost. To drive the point home, each of us might consider retrospectively whether he would have been willing to stand trial for his life while a fetus, pleading only his worth to society as he now can evaluate it. How many of us are not socially "defective" and with none of the excuses possible for a child with phenylketonuria? If there is to be human life at all, potential social worthiness cannot be its entitlement.

Finally, we should take note of the ambiguities in the very notion of societal good. Some use the term "society" to mean their own particular political community, others to mean the whole human race, and still others speak as if they mean both simultaneously, following that all-too-human belief that what is good for me and mine is good for mankind. Who knows what is genetically best for mankind, even with respect to Down's syndrome? I would submit that the genetic heritage of the human species is largely in the care of persons who do not live along the amniocentesis frontier. If we in the industrialized West wish to be really serious about the genetic future of the species, we would concentrate our attack on mutagenesis, and especially on our large contribution to the pool of environmental mutagens.

But even the more narrow use of society is ambiguous. Do we mean our "society" as it is today? Or do we mean our "society" as it ought to be? If the former, our standards will be ephemeral, for ours is a faddish "society." (By far the most worrisome feature of the changing attitudes on abortion is the suddenness with which they changed.) Any such socially determined standards are likely to provide too precarious a foundation for decisions about genetic abortion, let alone for our notions of human rights. If we mean the latter, then we have transcended the societal standard, since the "good society" is not to be found in "society" itself, nor is it likely to be discovered by taking a vote. In sum, societal good as a standard for justifying genetic abortion seems to be unsatisfactory. It is hard to define in general, difficult to apply clearly to particular cases, susceptible to overreaching and abuse (hence, very dangerous), and not sufficient unto itself if considerations of the good community are held to be automatically implied.

A second major alternative is the standard of parental or familial good. Here the argument of justification might run as follows. Parents have a right to determine, according to their own wishes and based upon their own notions of what is good for them, the qualitative as well as the quantitative character of their families. If they believe that the birth of a seriously deformed child will be the cause of great sorrow and suffering to themselves and to their other children and a drain on their time and resources, then they may ethically decide to prevent the birth of such a child, even by abortion.

This argument I would expect to be more attractive to most people than the argument appealing to the good of society. For one thing, we are more likely to trust a person's conception of what is good for him than his notion of what is good for society. Also, the number of persons involved is small, making it seem less impossible to weigh all the relevant factors in determining the good of the family. Most powerfully, one can see and appreciate the possible harm done to healthy children if the parents are obliged to devote most of their energies to caring for the afflicted child.

Yet there are ambiguities and difficulties perhaps as great as with the standard of societal good. In the first place, it is not entirely clear what would be good for the other children. In a strong family, the experience with a suffering and dying child might help the healthy siblings learn to face and cope with adversity. Some have even speculated that the lack of experience with death and serious illness in our affluent young people is an important element in their difficulty in trying to find a way of life and in responding patiently yet steadily to the serious problems of our society (Cassell, 1969). I suspect that one cannot generalize. In some children and in some families, experience with suffering may be strengthening, and in others, disabling. My point here is that the matter is uncertain, and that parents deciding on this basis are as likely as not to be mistaken.

The family or parental standard, like the societal standard, is unavoidably elastic because "suffering" does not come in discontinuous units, and because parental wishes and desires know no limits. Both are utterly subjective, relative, and notoriously subject to change. Some parents claim that they could not tolerate having to raise a child of the undesired sex; I know of one case where the woman in the delivery room, on being informed that her child was a son, told the physician that she did not even wish to see it and that he should get rid of it. We may judge her attitude to be pathological, but even pathological suffering is suffering. Would such suffering justify aborting her normal male fetus?

Or take the converse case of two parents, who for their own very peculiar reasons, wish to have an abnormal child, say, a child who will suffer from the same disease as grandfather or a child whose arrested development would preclude the threat of adolescent rebellion and separation. Are these acceptable grounds for the abortion of "normals"?

Granted, such cases will be rare. But they

serve to show the dangers inherent in talking about the parental right to determine, according to their wishes, the quality of their children. Indeed, the whole idea of parental rights with respect to children strikes me as problematic. It suggests that children are like property, that they exist for the parents. One need only look around to see some of the results of this notion of parenthood. The language of duties to children would be more in keeping with the heavy responsibility we bear in affirming the continuity of life with life and in trying to transmit what wisdom we have acquired to the next generation. Our children are not our children. Hopefully, reflection on these matters could lead to a greater appreciation of why it is people do and should have children. No better consequence can be hoped for from the advent of amniocentesis and other technologies for controlling human reproduction.

If one speaks of familial good in terms of parental duty, one could argue that parents have an obligation to do what they can to insure that their children are born healthy and sound. But this formulation transcends the limitation of parental wishes and desires. As in the case of the good society, the idea of "healthy and sound" requires an objective standard, a standard in reality. Hard as it may be to uncover it, this is what we are seeking. Nature as a standard is the third alternative.

The justification according to the natural standard might run like this. As a result of our knowledge of genetic diseases, we know that persons afflicted with certain diseases will never be capable of living the full life of a human being. Just as a no-necked giraffe could never live a giraffe's life, or a needleless porcupine would not attain true "porcupine-hood," so a child or fetus with Tay-Sachs disease or Down's syndrome, for example, will never be truly human. They will never be able to care for themselves, nor have they even the potential for developing the distinctively human capacities for thought or self-consciousness. Nature herself has aborted many similar cases, and has provided for the early death of many who happen to get born. There is no reason to keep them alive; instead, we should prevent their birth by contraception or sterilization if possible, and abortion if necessary.

The advantages of this approach are clear.

The standards are objective and in the fetus itself, thus avoiding the relativity and ambiguity in societal and parental good. The standard can be easily generalized to cover all such cases and will be resistant to the shifting sands of public opinion.

This standard, I would suggest, is the one which most physicians and genetic counselors appeal to in their heart of hearts, no matter what they say or do about letting the parents choose. Why else would they have developed genetic counseling and amniocentesis? Indeed, the notions of disease, of abnormal, of defective, make no sense at all in the absence of a natural norm of health. This norm is the foundation of the art of the physician and of the inquiry of the health scientist. Yet, as Motulsky and others in this volume have pointed out, the standard is elusive. Ironically, we are gaining increasing power to manipulate and control our own nature at a time in which we are increasingly confused about what is normal, healthy, and fit.

Although possibly acceptable in principle, the natural standard runs into problems in application when attempts are made to fix the boundary between potentially human and potentially not human. Professor Lejeune (1970) has clearly demonstrated the difficulty, if not the impossibility, of setting clear molecular, cytological, or developmental signposts for this boundary. Attempts to induce signposts by considering the phenotypes of the worst cases is equally difficult. Which features would we take to be the most relevant in, say, Tay-Sachs disease, Lesch-Nyhan syndrome, Cri du chat, Down's syndrome? Certainly, severe mental retardation. But how "severe" is "severe"? As Abraham Lincoln and I argued earlier, mental retardation admits of degree. It too is relative. Moreover, it is not clear that certain other defects and deformities might not equally foreclose the possibility of a truly or fully human life. What about blindness or deafness? Quadriplegia? Aphasia? Several of these in combination? Not only does each kind of defect admit of a continuous scale of severity, but it also merges with other defects on a continuous scale of defectiveness. Where on this scale is the line to be drawn: after mental retardation? blindness? muscular dystrophy? cystic fibrosis? hemophilia? diabetes? galactosemia? Turner's syndrome? XYY? club foot? Moreover, the identical two continuous scales—

kind and severity—are found also among the living. In fact, it is the natural standard which may be the most dangerous one in that it leads most directly to the idea that there are second-class human beings and subhuman human beings.

But the story is not complete. The very idea of nature is ambiguous. According to one view, the one I have been using, nature points to or implies a peak, a perfection. According to this view, human rights depend upon attaining the status of humanness. The fetus is only potential; it has no rights, according to this view. But all kinds of people fall short of the norm: children, idiots, some adults. This understanding of nature has been used to justify not only abortion and infanticide, but also slavery.

There is another notion of nature, less splendid, more humane and, though less able to sustain a notion of health, more acceptable to the findings of modern science. Animal nature is characterized by impulses of self-preservation and by the capacity to feel pleasure and to suffer pain. Man and other animals are alike on this understanding of nature. And the right to life is ascribed to all such self-preserving and suffering creatures. Yet on this understanding of nature, the fetus—even a defective fetus—is not potential, but actual. The right to life belongs to him. But for this reason, this understanding of nature does not provide and may even deny what it is we are seeking, namely a justification for genetic abortion, adequate unto itself, which does not simultaneously justify infanticide, homicide, and enslavement of the genetically abnormal.

There is a third understanding of nature, akin to the second, nature as sacrosanct, nature as created by a Creator. Indeed, to speak about this reminds us that there is a fourth possible standard for judgments about genetic abortion: the religious standard. I shall leave the discussion of this standard to those who are able to speak of it in better faith.

Now that I am at the end, the reader can better share my sense of frustration. I have failed to provide myself with a satisfactory intellectual and moral justification for the practice of genetic abortion. Perhaps others more able than I can supply one. Perhaps the pragmatists can persuade me that we should abandon the search for principled justification, that if we just trust people's situational decisions or their gut reactions, everything will turn out fine. Maybe they are right. But we should not forget the sage observation of Bertrand Russell: "Pragmatism is like a warm bath that heats up so imperceptibly that you don't know when to scream." I would add that before we submerge ourselves irrevocably in amniotic fluid, we take note of the connection to our own baths, into which we have started the hot water running.

Notes

1. This strikes me as by far the most important inference to be drawn from the fact that men in different times and cultures have answered the abortion question differently. Seen in this light, the differing and changing answers themselves suggest that it is a question not easily put under, at least not for very long.

2. Other ways include: one should not do violence to living or growing things; life is sacred; respect nature; fetal life has value; refrain from taking innocent life; protect and preserve life. As some have pointed out, the terms chosen are of different weight, and would require reasons of different weight to tip the balance in favor of abortion. My choice of the "rights" terminology is not meant to beg the questions of whether such rights really exist, or of where they come from. However, the notion of a "fetal right to life" presents only a little more difficulty in this regard than does the notion of a "human right to life," since the former does not depend on a claim that the human fetus is already "human." In my sense of the terms "right" and "life," we might even say that a dog or a fetal dog has a "right to life," and that it would be cruel and immoral for a man to go around performing abortions even on dogs for no good reason.

3. For a discussion of the possible biological rather than moral price of attempts to prevent the birth of defective children see Neel (1970) and Motulsky, Fraser, and Felsenstein (1971).

4. I assume this calculation ignores the possibilities of inflation, devaluation, and revolution.

References

Buck, P. S. (1968). Foreward to *The Terrible Choice: The Abortion Dilemma*. New York, Bantam Books, pp. ix–xi.

Cassell, E. (1969). "Death and the Physician," Commentary (June), pp. 73–79.

Lejeune, J. (1970). *American Journal of Human Genetics*, 22, p. 121.

Lincoln, A. (1854). In *The Collected Works of Abraham Lincoln*, R. P. Basler, editor. New Brunswick, New Jersey, Rutgers University Press, Vol. II, p. 222.

Motulsky, A. G., G. R. Fraser, and J. Felsenstein

(1971). In Symposium on Intrauterine Diagnosis, D. Bergsma, editor. *Birth Defects: Original Article Series*, Vol. 7, No. 5.

Neel, J. (1972). In *Early Diagnosis of Human Genetic Defects: Scientific and Ethical Considerations*, M. Harris, editor. Washington, D.C. U.S. Government Printing Office, pp. 366–380.

Moral Issues in Human Genetics: Counseling or Control?

Ruth Macklin

The notion of genetic engineering appears to have a narrower and a broader definition. The narrow conception refers to approaches involving laboratory manipulation of genes or cells: somatic cell alteration and germ cell alteration.[1] When this meaning is assigned to genetic engineering, the term 'eugenics' is used to refer to selection of parents or of their germ cells.[2] But sometimes the term 'genetic engineering' is used in a fully general sense, to refer to any manipulation of the reproductive acts or capacities of persons or their parts. It is this latter sense that will be used in the remainder of this account.

At least the idea behind eugenics—if not the practice itself in some form—is ancient. Positive eugenics was promoted in Plato's *Republic*, long before the science of genetics provided the theoretical basis and systematic data that today's proponents of genetic engineering have to work with. The lack of personal freedoms allowed the citizens in the *Republic* is well known to those familiar with Plato's work, and is evident in the following passage discussing regulation of unions between the sexes:

> It is for you, then, as their lawgiver, who have already selected the men, to select for association with them women who are so far as possible of the same natural capacity. . . . [A]nything like unregulated unions would be a profanation in a state whose citizens lead the good life. The Rulers will not allow such

a thing. . . . [I]f we are to keep our flock at the highest pitch of excellence, there should be as many unions of the best of both sexes, and as few of the inferior, as possible, and . . . only the offspring of the better unions should be kept. . . . Moreover, young men who acquit themselves well in war and other duties, should be given, among other rewards and privileges, more liberal opportunities to sleep with a wife, for the further purpose that, with good excuse, as many as possible of the children may be begotten of such fathers.[3]

But lest we conclude that a eugenics movement can only be promoted or gain adherents in a rigidly controlled society like Plato's *Republic* or a totalitarian regime such as Nazi Germany, let us consider the view of a 20th century Nobel Prize winning geneticist. The late Hermann Muller was an arch proponent of positive eugenics, based on his belief that the human gene pool is deteriorating. Muller argued for voluntary programmes of positive eugenics, rejecting any form of state-imposed regulations. He claimed that "democratic control . . . implies an upgrading of the people in general in both their intellectual and social faculties, together with a maintenance or, preferably, an improvement in their bodily condition."[4] Muller was one of a number of contemporary geneticists who have made gloomy prophecies about the increasing load of mutations in the human gene pool. The particular brand of positive eugenics

Reprinted by permission from Dialogue, *Vol. XVI, no. 3 (1977), pp. 386–396. [Editor's note. In the first part of this article, which is omitted here, Macklin discusses genetic counseling and argues that individuals "should have final decision-making authority" in matters of reproduction when "the reasons for these decisions refer to genetic factors."]*

that he advocated was a voluntary artificial insemination programme using donor semen (AID). He envisaged preserving the semen of outstanding men for future use in artificial insemination, choosing such greats as Einstein, Pasteur, Descartes, Leonardo and Lincoln as men whose child no woman would refuse to bear.[5]

Muller's method of freezing the semen of intellectual and creative men is only one of several proposals favouring some form of *positive* eugenics—a programme for improving the species, breeding a better race, or trying to prevent further deterioration by taking active countermeasures. Greater attention has been directed to the question of whether *negative* eugenics should be practiced on carriers or those afflicted with heritable diseases, in the form of enforced or encouraged abortions, sterilization, or less repressive but nonetheless coercive measures. The dilemma of choosing between preserving the individual freedom to marry and procreate as one chooses, and preventing further pollution of the gene pool would, indeed, pose an agonizing moral choice if the facts were as clear-cut as the eugenicists take them to be. There seems, however, to be enough uncertainty about the possible and probable outcomes of any attempts at eugenics to warrant extreme caution in mounting such grandiose schemes for genetic improvement. Many scientists agree that trying to reduce the load of mutations in the human gene pool through negative eugenics would be ineffective, at best. And the arguments against positive eugenics point to a number of potentially infelicitous outcomes. There are at least five separate arguments against the feasibility or desirability of any large-scale attempt at genetic engineering for eugenic purposes—arguments which, if taken together, give strong support to my conclusion that genetic engineering with this aim is misguided or dangerous or both. A sixth argument is the religious one that creating or modifying the human species is a task not for man, but for God.[6] For those to whom this sort of argument is compelling, it may lend added strength to the other five. I shall confine my discussion to four of the five considerations that do not require belief in a supernatural deity. Each of the following arguments against a systematic effort to mount any sort of eugenics programme will be discussed in turn below:

1. We're too ignorant to do it right;

2. In any case, we are likely to alter the gene pool for ill;

3. Negative eugenics can't possibly work unless carriers are eliminated, but this would soon eliminate the entire species;

4. Some methods of genetic engineering carry grave moral risks of mishap.

The fifth argument is essentially that most—if not all—methods of genetic engineering are dehumanizing in basic ways.[7] While I think this attack contains some interesting points and raises questions of the value that generally deserve important consideration, it is a gratuitous argument in this context. If the first four arguments are sound, they obviate the necessity for the fifth, since the scientific and practical objections to eugenic programmes would rule them out before the value issues need be brought into consideration. So I shall treat only the first four arguments in what follows.

(1) The claim that we are too ignorant to do the job right has several variants, each with significant implications. The first consideration points to our general ignorance about the value of a gene to a given race to the species. As one prominent geneticist notes:

> We know only about its value to the individual carrying it and then only in instances where the effect is severe. In the light of such ignorance, it seems to me that the best procedure is to avoid all changes in the environment which are likely to change the mutation rate. . . . The quality of a gene or genotype may be determined only by the reaction of the associated phenotype in the environment in which it exists. A phenotype may be disadvantageous in some environments, essentially neutral in others, and advantageous in others. In the face of a rapidly changing and entirely new environment (new in an evolutionary sense), I do not believe that we can determine the value of specific genotypes to the species.[8]

This brand of ignorance constitutes our lack of knowledge of what to select for—a form of ignorance that some may argue is confined to the present state of development of the science of genetics. But a second variant of the "we're too ignorant" argument notes that "if we alter the gene pool, independent of environment, we are acting on the basis of present environmental criteria to select a gene pool for the future. Since the environment is changing a thousandfold times faster than our gene pool, it would be a disastrous approach.[9] But the difficulty here is not simply one of our inability to predict accurately what the future will be like. Questions of value enter in—questions that invariably resurrect the memory of attempts at positive eugenics among the Nazis. One writer asks:

> Who will be the judges and where will be the separation between good and bad? The most difficult decisions will come in defining the borderline cases. Will we breed against tallness because space requirements become more critical? Will we breed against near-sightedness because people with glasses may not make good astronauts? Will we forbid intellectually inferior individuals from procreating despite their proved ability to produce a number of superior individuals?[10]

The last variant on the "we're too ignorant" theme that we shall consider here requires us to recall Hermann Muller's proposal for positive eugenics. Muller would not be alone in including Abraham Lincoln on a list of men whose child no woman would refuse to bear. Yet there is now considerable evidence that Lincoln was afflicted with Marfan's syndrome, a heritable disease of the connective tissue that is transmitted by a dominant gene. The evidence is based on a number of factors. Lincoln's bodily characteristics and facial features—the very qualities we term "Lincoln-esque"—are typical features of bone deformities common to Marfan's syndrome. The disease was first named in 1896, some thirty years after Lincoln's death. It was believed for some time that Lincoln had Marfan's disease, on the basis of physical defects he was known to have had, as well as the early death of one of his children. One sign of the disease was Lincoln's abnormally long limbs. Also, casts made of Lincoln's body in the year of his inauguration reveal that his left hand was much longer than his right hand, and his left middle finger was elongated. He is also known to have suffered from severe farsightedness, in addition to having difficulty with his eyesight that stemmed from distortions in his facial bone struc-

ture. These bodily asymmetries are common to Marfan's syndrome, as is cardiac disease. It is believed that Lincoln inherited the disease from his father's side. His father was blind in one eye, his son Robert had difficulties with his eyes, and his son Tad had a speech defect and died at the age of eighteen, probably from cardiac trouble. The likelihood that Lincoln himself suffered from Marfan's syndrome was further confirmed in 1959, when a California physician named Harold Schwartz recognized the disease in a boy of seven who was known to share an ancestor with Lincoln.[11] Since the gene for Marfan's disease is dominant, those who have it and reach child-bearing age stand a fifty percent chance of having an afflicted child.

Now consider the consequences for the gene pool if Lincoln's frozen sperm were to be disseminated widely in the population. At least until the facts became evident, the result would be exactly the opposite of what Muller intended by his proposal. And if the mistake went beyond the case of Lincoln and Marfan's syndrome, including other individuals who, despite their outstanding achievements might be afflicted with or be carriers of other little known or as yet undiagnosed genetic diseases, the results would be dysgenic in the extreme. This last consideration leads directly to the second argument against eugenics programmes to which we turn next.

(2) This argument holds that in any event, we are likely to alter the gene pool for ill. Leaving aside the less likely incidence of this occurrence as exemplified just now in the Abraham Lincoln story, we may look at another prominent consideration noted by some geneticists.

This consideration is often referred to as "heterozygote advantage." One geneticist explains as follows:

> There is . . . good evidence that individuals who carry two different forms of the same gene, that is, are heterozygous, appear to have an advantage. This is true even if that gene in double dose, that is, in the homozygous state, produces a severe disease. For example, individuals homozygous for the gene coding for sickle-cell hemoglobin invariably develop sickle-cell anemia which is generally fatal before the reproductive years. Heterozygotes for the gene are, however, protected more than normals from the effects of the most malignant form of malaria. It has

been shown that women who carry the gene in single dose have a higher fertility in malarial areas than do normals.[12]

Here again, it is not only in the cases where there is known heterozygote advantage that the likelihood exists of altering the gene pool for ill by trying to eliminate genes for heritable diseases. There are, in addition, all of the cases where heterozygote advantage may exist but is at present unknown. If one uses risk-benefit ratios or something like a utilitarian schema for deciding moral issues in biomedical contexts, the evidence seems clearly to indicate a greater risk of dysgenic consequences than a possibility of beneficial results from attempts to alter the human gene pool by means of negative eugenics. A successful effort to eliminate carriers for heritable diseases would result at the same time in eliminating heterozygote advantage, which is believed to be beneficial to the species or to sub-populations within the species. While little is known at the present stage of inquiry in genetics about all of the particular advantages that exist, it is an inference made by many experts in the field on the basis of present data and well-confirmed genetic theory. One biologist asks us to:

> Consider the gene leading to cystic fibrosis (C.F.). Until quite recently homozygotes for this gene died in infancy. Yet the gene causing C.F. is very common among all Caucasoid populations thus far studied. . . . It is too widespread in the race to be accounted for by genetic drift. The gene is also too frequent for it to be likely to be maintained by mutation pressure. Hence, we are driven to assume heterozygote advantage.[13]

It would seem, then, that what is gained by the elimination of homozygotes may well be lost by the elimination of heterozygotes, resulting in no clear benefits and possibly some significant disadvantages in populations that suffer from genetic diseases. But the argument just given assumes that it would in fact be possible to eliminate genes for heritable diseases by preventing carriers from reproducing and thereby passing on such genes to future generations. The next argument against genetic engineering questions such a possibility.

(3) This argument maintains, in sum, that negative eugenics can't possibly work unless carriers are eliminated as well as diseased individuals;

but a successful attempt to prevent all carriers of potentially lethal genes from reproducing would effectively eliminate the entire species. The effects of negative eugenics on the general population are assessed by one geneticist as follows:

> With a few exceptions, dominant diseases are rare and interfere severely with reproductive ability. They are generally maintained in the population by new mutations. Therefore, there is either no need or essentially no need for discouraging these individuals from reproduction . . . The story is quite different for recessive conditions. . . .[A]ny attempt to decrease the gene frequency of these common genetic disorders in the population by prevention of fertility of all carriers would be doomed to failure. First, we all carry between three and eight of these genes in a single dose. Secondly, for many of these conditions, the frequency of carriers in the population is about 1 in 50 or even greater. Prevention of fertility for even one of these disorders would stop a sizable proportion of the population from reproducing. . . .[14]

If this assessment is sound, it has significant implications for the prospects of favourably altering the human gene pool by negative eugenics. Such an argument is persuasive if the purpose of negative eugenics is viewed as that of improving the human gene pool for the sake of future generations. But if the purpose of negative eugenics is seen as improving the quality of life for those in the present and next generation, then the argument just given is beside the point. We should recall the dual purpose for which proposals for genetic engineering are put forth. The one we have been discussing here is the proposed improvement or prevention of deterioration of the gene pool for the sake of future generations of humans. The other purpose, tied to voluntary genetic screening programmes and the activity of genetic counseling, is to present options to individuals or couples that will help them avoid the birth of a defective child whose quality of life will be poor and who will most likely be a burden on both parents and society. For this latter purpose, the practice of negative eugenics through voluntary screening and sensitive genetic counseling can serve to improve the quality of life of persons in this and the next generation. But when transformed into a programme designed to control the reproductive acts or capacities of people for the sake of future generations, then the practice of negative eugenics seems to be scientifically and practically misguided. Indeed, taking this argument and the previous one together, the conclusion may be put succinctly in the words of one writer:

> Neither positive nor negative eugenics can ever significantly improve the gene pool of the population and simultaneously allow for adequate evolutionary improvement of the human race. The only useful aspect of negative eugenics is in individual counseling of specific families in order to prevent some of the births of abnormal individuals.[15]

(4) The fourth argument against genetic engineering focuses specifically on those practices involving manipulation of genetic material itself. This argument raises questions about the grave risks involved in any such manipulation, especially since mishaps that may arise are likely to be far worse than what happens when nature takes its course. One geneticist sees the prospects as follows:

> The problem of altering an individual's genes by direct chemical change of his DNA presents technically an enormously difficult task. Even if it became possible to do this, the chance of error would be high. Such an error, of course, would have the diametrically opposite effect to that desired and would be irreversible; in other words, the individual would become even more abnormal.[16]

Some observers fear the creation of hapless monsters as a result of various manipulations on genetic material. Whether or not the laboratory techniques are sufficiently refined at present to enable researchers to develop procedures for widespread use, it is likely that these techniques will be available soon enough to deserve careful reflection now. We need to ask, once again, whether the purpose served by laboratory methods of genetic engineering is helping those who are at risk for bearing defective children to prevent such occurrences, or instead, breeding a genetically improved species for the future. If such techniques are perfected and become available for use in spite of the attendant risks of mishap, they would then be offered to couples on a voluntary basis in the same way that current methods of genetic intervention are employed. Where a practice is aimed at the genetic improvement of a couple's own progeny, there are no grounds for methods that involve coercion. What is needed in such cases is counseling and education, not coercion and control.

At the outset, I said I would argue for two separate but related theses. First, the individual or couple should have final decision-making authority in matters of his or her own reproductive acts and capacities, as well as continuation or termination of pregnancy where the reasons for these decisions refer to genetic factors. Second, attempts at government-based or scientist-directed eugenic programmes are bound to be misguided or dangerous or both. The four arguments at the end were offered in support of the second thesis. If those arguments are sound, they demonstrate that there is no warrant for those in power to take final decision-making authority away from the individual where the reasons for such actions refer to eugenic considerations. Recall also our earlier conclusion that final decision-making should be left to the individual or couple in the context of genetic counseling, except in cases where the decision requires medical expertise that a patient is unlikely to have. Now if genetic screening should be practiced on a voluntary basis; and if decisions arising out of counseling should be left to the individual; and if in addition, positive and negative eugenics aimed at future generations is basically misguided; then there sems to be only one consideration remaining that might argue in favour of limiting individual rights for the sake of social benefits. That consideration points to the burden placed on society for treating and maintaining defective infants and others who might have been aborted or never even conceived by dint of state policy. Time does not permit an examination of this last issue, but is worth making a final observation in closing. If the notion of social benefit is understood largely in terms of increased financial resources that would otherwise be allocated to caring for those afflicted with heritable diseases, then something crucial is being left out of the balance between individual rights and social benefits. What is socially beneficial must be viewed not only in terms of increases in financial and other tangible resources, but also in terms of a range of freedom and autonomy that members of a society can reasonably expect to enjoy. It is important to preserve that freedom and autonomy through insuring the individual's right to decide about his or her own reproductive acts and capacities. With increased availability of voluntary genetic screening programmes and widespread education of the public, it is hard to imagine that most people will choose to burden themselves and society with defective children when other options are open to them. Even if there are some who refuse screening or abortion, society as a whole would be better off to accommodate their freely chosen reproductive acts than to impose compulsory genetic screening, abortion, or sterilization on its members.

Notes

1. Bernard D. Davis. "Threat and Promise in Genetic Engineering," ed. by Preston Williams in *Ethical Issues in Biology and Medicine* (Cambridge, Mass.: Schenkman Publishing Company, 1973), pp. 17–24.

2. *Ibid.*

3. Francis MacDonald Cornford (tr.). *The Republic of Plato* (New York: Oxford University Press), pp. 157–60.

4. Hermann J. Muller, "Genetic Progress by Voluntarily Conducted Germinal Choice," ed. by Gordon Wolstenholme, in *Man and His Future* (Boston: Little, Brown and Co., 1963), p. 256.

5. Theodosius Dobzhansky, *Mankind Evolving* (New Haven: Yale University Press, 1962), p. 328.

6. Such arguments are offered by Paul Ramsey in *Fabricated Man* (New Haven: Yale University Press, 1970).

7. This argument is given by Ramsey, *op. cit.*, and also by Leon R. Kass, "Making Babies—The New Biology and the 'Old' Morality," *The Public Interest*, Vol. 26, Winter, 1972.

8. Arthur Steinberg, "The Genetic Pool. Its Evolution and Significance—'Desirable' and 'Undesirable' Genetic Traits," in C.I.O.M.S. *Recent Progress in Biology and Medicine*, pp. 83–93.

9. Kurt Hirschhorn, "Symposium: Ethics of Genetic Counseling," *Contemporary OB/GYN*," Vol. 2, no. 4, p. 128.

10. Kurt Hirschhorn, "Practical and Ethical Problems in Human Genetics," *Birth Defects*, Vol. VIII, July, 1972, p. 28.

11. *Ibid.* p. 23.

12. Steinberg, *op. cit.*

13. Rene Dubos and Maya Pines, *Health and Disease* (New York: Time, Inc., 1965), pp. 123–24.

14. Kurt Hirschhorn, "Practical and Ethical Problems in Human Genetics," pp. 22–23.

15. *Ibid*, p. 25.

16. *Ibid*, p. 27.

Gene Therapy in Human Beings: When Is It Ethical to Begin?

W. French Anderson and John C. Fletcher

The recent rapid expansion of research in the area of molecular genetics, resulting in large part from the application of recombinant-DNA technology, has produced uncertainty in the minds of some physicians about how much has been accomplished in the area of genetic engineering. Successful introduction of genes into intact mice[1,2] and into mouse embryos[3] indicates that the transfer of certain genes into human beings may now be technically feasible. Indeed, the *Los Angeles Times* reported on October 8 that an attempt at gene therapy in human beings was conducted this summer.[4] Is it ethical to carry out such a new therapeutic procedure, aimed at alleviating a serious or lethal disease in a patient, before the probable benefits and risks of the procedure have been determined in animals? The ethical arguments that have guided therapy-oriented medical research in the recent past have indicated overwhelmingly that the answer is no (although exceptions may be permissible for critically ill subjects). At what point, then, is it ethical to begin a revolutionary new treatment procedure? In this paper, we briefly summarize some of the relevant ethical ar-

Reprinted by permission from The New England Journal of Medicine, *vol. 303 (November 27, 1980), pp. 1293–1297. Copyright 1980 Massachusetts Medical Society.*

guments and the current state of the art of gene therapy; we then attempt to explain what still needs to be learned from animal studies before experiments with human beings should begin.

Ethical Background

One of the cornerstones of the ethics of clinical investigation is the rule governing when to start experimental therapy in human beings. A persistent problem is embodied in the question, "When is it ethical to begin the experiment?" Beginning with the Nuremberg Code,[5] a body of ethical guidelines for investigators and peer-review groups has accumulated. As stated by Rule 3 of the Nuremberg Code:

> The experiment should be so designed and based on the results of animal experimentation and a knowledge of the natural history of the disease or other problems under study that the anticipated results will justify the performance of the experiment.[5]

This rule is repeated or paraphrased in every major code of ethics governing clinical investigation and developed by international groups,[6] medical associations,[7] and single institutions.[8] Henry Beecher summarized the ethical considerations involved in preparing to begin experiments with human beings by stating: "A study is ethical or not at its inception; it does not become ethical because it succeeds in producing valuable data. . . ."[9] The fundamental principle is that it should be determined in advance that the probable benefits outweigh the probable risks.

These statements were made in an era when the first (and only) line of defense in clinical research was the conscience of the individual investigator. Two additional procedures intended for the protection of subjects have been broadly accepted: prior review of research protocols by a local Institutional Review Board (IRB), and procurement of the written consent of the subject or proxy. The Belmont Report,[10] the most definitive recent statement of the ethical guidelines that should govern IRB review, stressed that the adequacy of preparation for research in human beings is vitally related to answering the paramount question of the review process: Are the benefits and risks in a favorable ratio? A systematic analysis of risks and benefits requires an examination of information about all aspects of the proposed research, including consideration of whether additional animal research might be more appropriate than subjecting human beings to the possible risks, given the existing state of knowledge. The investigators are obliged to explain how they know that the presuppositions of the research have probable validity and whether the information can be obtained in any safer way than by trials in human beings. Such considerations are inherent in the requirements of the Food and Drug Administration for treatment of a patient with a new drug. In short, the moral justification for initiating therapeutic research in human beings rests on an assessment of the validity of the hope of success. This assessment is usually based on results of experiments with animals or other studies in human beings that suggest, on balance, that the proposed research question may be answered with acceptable risk to the subject.

The definition of acceptable risk is complex and depends in part on the severity of the patient's illness. Current standards for medical research in the area of cancer therapy, for example, permit experimental use of highly dangerous therapeutic agents in patients with fatal illnesses for which no effective conventional therapy is known. These agents include toxic mutagens that are capable of killing or altering the genetic composition of somatic and germ cells. The use of such treatments obviously requires very thoughtful prior assessment. Similarly, considerable caution should be exercised before giving a patient genetic material in an attempt at therapy. The severity of the illness, despite existing therapy, would have to be so great that a potentially considerable risk from the new therapy might be justified. There are a number of genetic diseases that fall into this "severe-illness" category. Two of them, β-thalassemia and sickle-cell anemia, have been extensively studied at the molecular level and are known to result from an abnormality in the amount (in β-thalassemia) or type (sickle-cell anemia) of beta-globin chains. In theory, these two seriously debilitating genetic anemias could be treated by insertion of a beta-globin gene into the patient's bone marrow; this approach would direct the erythroid cells to produce normal amounts of normal beta globin.

Although IRB's have faced questions of benefit versus risk in new and potentially dangerous therapeutic regimens before, they have never had to evaluate treatment procedures designed to influence the genotype of human cells. Correction of the germ line of the patient so that future offspring will be phenotypically normal may even be possible. Such new therapy may involve substantial risks, as we shall discuss, although gene therapy may turn out to be far safer and more effective than existing treatments for some disorders, including these lethal anemias.

In summary, the conclusion drawn from consideration of these ethical codes[5-10] is that before any gene is administered to a human being, animal studies must ensure that the new gene has a reasonable chance of producing the desired result and that there is a reasonable expectation that it will not produce a harmful result.

Present State of the Art of Gene Therapy

Our present concept of a gene is that it is a specific sequence of nucleotides in the DNA of a cell. A gene is recognized by the product that it makes. Any gene coding for a molecule can, in theory, be identified in total cellular DNA. The gene can then be isolated, purified, modified, and attached to other DNA sequences—for example, to other genes isolated from other sources. This final DNA fragment, perhaps containing several genes, can then be inserted into living mammalian cells in a number of ways: genes can be injected directly into an individual cell with a micropipette[11]; they can be introduced into a population of cells in a culture dish by exposing the cells to a precipitate of DNA containing the desired genes[12]; or they can be inserted into a viral particle (modified so that it will no longer be pathogenic), with the recombinant virus then used to infect a population of cells.[13,14] A number of genes have been inserted into living cells with these techniques. In summary, a gene can be isolated from normal cells, attached to other selected DNA sequences, and inserted into other cells in which, in some cases, the inserted gene will function.

With use of these techniques, experiments with genetic material inserted into intact animals have begun. It has been possible to introduce a gene that confers resistance to the toxic drug methotrexate into the bone-marrow cells of mice.[1,2] The treated mice were more resistant to the drug as the result of the gene therapy. In another experiment, a viral gene was injected into mouse embryos, and a small number of newborn mice retained the viral DNA sequences in their cells.[3] Clearly, research in the area of mammalian genetic engineering has progressed dramatically in recent years. Some workers may believe that the progress is so great that gene therapy in human beings should begin. Let us examine what we think should still be accomplished before experiments with human beings are justified.

Animal Studies Needed before Attempting Gene Therapy in Human Beings

Successful experimentation with genetic material inserted into laboratory animals needs to be accomplished before that material is introduced into human subjects. At least three requirements should be met for each gene introduced: First of all, the new gene should be put into the proper target cells and should remain there. If, however, the gene also enters other cells, it should be shown that the presence of the gene or its product does not damage the non-target cells.

Secondly, the new gene should be regulated appropriately in the target cells. In other words, the gene's product should be made in amounts that are sufficient to correct the genetic defect but not so large as to have a detrimental effect.

Thirdly, the presence of the new gene (and all other DNA sequences associated with it) should not harm the cell. Specifically, the inserted genetic material should not produce mutagenic events in the organism, interfere with regulatory pathways within the cell, or otherwise adversely affect critical cell functions.

We submit that these three criteria should be satisfied to a considerable degree in animals before gene therapy is attempted in human beings. Although advances may shorten the time or effort needed to meet these criteria, no advance can eliminate the necessity that all three requirements be met. However, we think that once all three are satisfied, attempts to cure human genetic diseases by treatment with gene therapy will be ethical.

The goal of biomedical research is, and has always been, to alleviate human suffering. Gene therapy is a proper and logical part of that effort.

What Knowledge Is Necessary to Meet the Three Requirements?

The New Gene Should Be Put into the Target Cells and Remain in Them

As yet, little is known about the cell's recognition signals. Ultimately, it may be possible to add nucleotide sequences to a gene that will allow that gene to enter or function only in a particular type of cell, but this is not feasible at present. Inserting a gene into the proper target cells may not be difficult in a few cases, however. Experiments in mice have shown that bone-marrow cells can be removed, given a drug-resistance gene (see above), and replaced in the animal, with successful function of the gene.[1,2] Similarly, bone-marrow cells could be removed from a patient with β-thalassemia or sickle-cell anemia and given the normal beta-globin gene; the genetically altered marrow could then be introduced into the patient (nonerythroid marrow cells would also be exposed to the gene in this case). If animal studies were successful, liver cells could be obtained by biopsy from patients with phenylketonuria, the normal phenylalanine hydroxylase gene could be inserted into the liver cells, and then the cells could be reimplanted under conditions (such as partial liver resection) that encourage multiplication of the implanted cells. For other diseases, skin fibroblasts could be used.

Will the new gene get out of the target cells and spread to other cells and tissues? Recent evidence indicates that genes inserted into cells in the form of gene-containing plasmids (plasmids are bacterial extrachromosomal DNA molecules used as molecular vehicles to carry genetic material in experiments on gene transfer) may exist not only as integrated genes but also as free extrachromosomal elements within the cell.[11] It is not known whether or to what extent these gene-containing plasmids may move between cells. Furthermore, it is not known whether the new gene will persist unchanged inside the cell. A plasmid now being commonly used for gene transfer (known as pBR322) appears to manifest recombination and

deletion events with itself (including any inserted genes) when placed in mammalian cells, thus leading to replication of mutant genes with the host cell.[11]

These unsettling questions concerning the stability of new genes transferred into target cells can probably be answered in experiments with animals. The presence of gene-containing plasmids or the genes themselves can be monitored in various animal tissues after administration of the gene to a specific target organ. However, such experiments will take time to complete, and they are just now being initiated. If the new genes are found in non-target tissues, their level of function must be assessed together with the resulting effects, if any, on the non-target cell.

The New Gene Should Be Regulated Appropriately

Appropriate regulation (the ability of the gene to correct or ameliorate the genetic defect) does not necessarily mean normal regulation. For example, it may take many years to understand normal regulation of the hemoglobin genes (i.e., the proper switching on and off of the genes for the embryonic, fetal, and adult globin chains).[15] At present, although globin genes have been inserted into animal cells, it has not been possible to make them function except at ineffectively low levels. Correction of the defect in β-thalassemia and alleviation of the defect in sickle-cell anemia may be accomplished by linking a "naked" beta-globin gene (i.e., one without any normal regulatory sequences) to a known regulatory region that will cause the beta-globin gene to express at the right level (i.e., to produce enough normal beta globin to equal the amount of alpha globin produced in β-thalassemia or to dilute the sickle hemoglobin in sickle-cell anemia). This latter approach is now under active investigation. However, to find the most effective regulatory region and to fine tune it to ensure the beta-globin gene will make the right amount of product will undoubtedly require considerable experimentation in animal cells. Fortunately, there are strains of mice that have a disease analogous to thalassemia.[16,17] Experimental studies with these animals should be helpful.

On the other hand, enzymes such as thymidine kinase or hypoxanthine phosphoribosyl transferase (HPRT) that are required in every cell may be regulated efficiently in whatever cell they are located. The evidence appears to indicate that a viral thymidine kinase gene functions effectively when inserted into any of a number of different mammalian cells.[18] The human HPRT gene might, therefore, be regulated appropriately if inserted into the cells of a patient with Lesch-Nyhan disease.

The Presence of the New Gene Should Not Harm the Cell

This requirement will be the most difficult to study since it will require determining what problems may develop years or generations after gene therapy. Treated animals (e.g., mice) and their offspring should be studied carefully throughout their lifetimes to determine whether any pathologic process is detectable. It is possible that the introduction of a new gene into a cell would interfere with the normal regulatory system of that cell and cause, for example, slow growth, organ-system dysfunction, reduced fertility, increased incidence of cancer, or early death. Fortunately, the short life span of mice should allow meaningful data to be obtained fairly rapidly. The extent of studies in larger animals and primates that should be completed before studies in human beings begin is difficult to estimate. The decision about how much is adequate should be based on the realization that results in larger animals will take a long time to obtain, that human beings may react differently from other animals and, therefore, may respond better or have fewer side effects, and that we are attempting to treat tragic and lethal human diseases. It would be just as inappropriate to delay treatment of patients while we are awaiting long-term results in primates as it would be to rush into experimentation with patients before studies of small animals have been completed.

What Can and Cannot Be Expected from Research on Gene Therapy in Human Beings

Many fear where research on gene therapy may be leading us. Despite the enormous amount of information obtained on DNA in recent years, our basic understanding of cells and how they function is still exceedingly elementary. At this point we can purify only genes whose products are known and can be isolated. We can transfer such a gene into animal cells, in which, in a few cases, it will function. But we are dealing only with single genes. We are currently attempting to influence in a known way only single-gene defects. Intelligence, personality, fertility, organ structure, and physical, mental, and emotional characteristics are all presumably controlled or influenced by vast arrays of genes about which we know little or nothing. There are dozens (hundreds?) of genes within every cell that make regulatory substances used by the cell in unknown ways. We do not know what the substances are, how they work, or what genes are involved. Any planned alteration of multigenic traits will not be accomplished by gene therapy for many decades to come, if ever.

Conclusions

We argue that gene therapy for some genetic disorders will be possible in the foreseeable future. Ethical codes[5-10] emphasize that before any experiments are performed in human beings, there should be reasonable evidence from studies in animals that the patient will benefit (or that knowledge that may benefit future patients will be acquired), and there should be a reasonable expectation of minimal, or at least acceptable, risk. It is our view that knowledge in several areas should be obtained from studies in animals before gene transfer in human beings is ethically justified. Specifically, experiments in animals should demonstrate that the new gene can be put into the target cells and remain in them, that the new gene can be regulated appropriately, and that the presence of the new gene does not harm the cell.

We must await a full scientific report of the facts of the recently reported attempt to treat β-thalassemia with gene therapy before judgment can be made about this experiment.

We recognize that the urgent desire to treat patients having lethal or extremely serious genetic diseases may lead the attending physician to attempt promising, though not fully tested, new regimens. In this sense, treatment of a critical illness by gene therapy differs little from treatment of cancer with a new chemotherapeutic agent or treatment of a congenital malformation with a complex and dangerous new surgical procedure.

In each case, the ethical principles governing experimentation in human beings apply. The successful application of gene therapy in human beings offers the strong possibility of enormous good by reducing the suffering and death caused by genetic diseases. We hope that this laudable goal will not be jeopardized by premature experiments that could prove needlessly ineffective or hazardous.

References

1. Cline MJ, Stang H, Mercola K, et al. Gene transfer in intact animals. Nature. 1980: 284:422–5.

2. Mercola KE, Stang HD, Browne J, Salser W, Cline MJ. Insertion of a new gene of viral origin into bone marrow cells of mice. Science. 1980. 208:1033–5.

3. Gordon JW, Scangos GA, Plotkin DJ, Barbosa JA, Ruddle FH. Genetic transformation of mouse embryos by microinjection of purified DNA. Proc Natl Acad Sci USA. (in press).

4. Jacobs P. Pioneer genetic implants revealed. Los Angeles Times. 1980; October 8:1.

5. Nuremberg Military Tribunal: United States versus Karl Brandt, et al. ("The Medical Case"). In: Trials of war criminals, Vol. 2. Washington, D.C.: Government Printing Office, 1947:181–4.

6. Declaration of Helsinki. (Adopted by the 18th World Medical Assembly, 1964, revised 1975.)

7. Ethical guidelines for clinical investigation. (Adopted by the House of Delegates, American Medical Association, November 30, 1966.)

8. Research investigations involving human beings: code and methods of procedure. Houston, Tex.: M.D. Anderson Hospital, 1965.

9. Beecher HK. Some guiding principles for clinical investigation. JAMA. 1966; 195:1135–6.

10. The National Commission for the Protection of Human Subjects of Biomedical and Behavioral Research. The Belmont Report. Ethical principles and guidelines for the protection of human subjects in research. Washington, D.C.: Government Printing Office, 1978:16–7. (DHEW publication no. [OS]78–0012).

11. Anderson WF, Killos L, Sanders-Haigh L, Kretschmer PJ, Diacumakos EG. Replication and expression of thymidine kinase and human globin genes microinjected into mouse fibroblasts. Proc Natl Acad Sci USA. 1980; 77:5399–403.

12. Pellicer A, Wigler M, Axel R, Silverstein S. The transfer and stable integration of the HSV thymidine kinase gene into mouse cells. Cell. 1978; 14:133–41.

13. Mulligan RC, Howard BH, Berg P. Synthesis of rabbit β-globin in cultured monkey kidney cells following infection with a SV40 β-globin recombinant genome. Nature. 1979; 277:108–14.

14. Hamer DH, Smith KD, Boyer SH, Leder P. SV40 recombinants carrying rabbit β-globin gene coding sequences. Cell. 1979; 17:725–35.

15. Proudfoot NJ, Shander MHM, Manley JL, Gefter ML, Maniatis T. Structure and in vitro transcription of human globin genes. Science. 1980; 209:1329–36.

16. Popp RA, Stratton LP, Hawley DK, Effron K. Hemoglobin of mice with radiation-induced mutations at the hemoglobin loci. J Mol Biol. 1979; 127:141–8.

17. Whitney JB III, Russell ES. Linkage of genes for adult α-globin and embryonic α-like globin chains. Proc Natl Acad Sci USA. 1980; 77:1087–90.

18. Pellicer A, Robins D, Wold B, et al. Altering genotype and phenotype by DNA-mediated gene transfer. Science. 1980; 209:1414–22.

The Total Gene Screen

Morton Hunt

Jogging down a New Jersey park trail one morning, Ed Morgan felt wonderfully content. A tall man of 62, lean and fit, he particularly enjoyed running on such a day; his business, selling insulation supplies, was doing better than ever and his children and grandchildren were all thriving.

As always, nearing home he broke into a sprint, but that day, to his surprise, he ended up gasping desperately for air. Alarmed, he went to his doctor and got bad news: an X-ray showed a large tumor on his right lung. A few weeks later, he was operated on. The tumor proved to be a pleural mesothelioma, a type of cancer; the surgeon removed as much as he could. Chemotherapy and radiation would buy Ed Morgan (not his real name) a little time, but the end was predictable.

Why me, he wondered bitterly, his world in ruins. Before starting his own business, he'd been an insulation installer for 20 years, working mainly with asbestos. Dangerous stuff, to be sure—yet many men he'd worked with, side by side, had spent as long or longer doing the same thing and were still healthy. In fact, only one asbestos worker in 15 dies of asbestos-related cancer. So why me? He never learned why; he lived two years, then became that one in 15.

The likely answer: Ed Morgan was hereditarily more susceptible to asbestos than the other 14. The problem was in his genes.

Of the billions of units called nucleotides strung together in the DNA molecules of each person's genes, it takes only one or two, altered or misplaced at some biochemically critical site, to cause serious disease. This is the general explanation, now emerging from biomedical research, of one of the long-impenetrable mysteries of human illness—why, other things being equal, some people are harmed by various substances in the environment while others are not.

Clearly, it would be a major boon to humankind, more plagued than ever by noxious substances, if each of us could have our entire set of genes searched—or screened—for abnormalities that create vulnerability to chemicals in the environment. With that information, we would then know what jobs, locales and habits to avoid so we could improve our chances of a long and healthy life.

Although genetic screening has been talked about in the past in connection with hereditary conditions such as sickle-cell anemia and Tay-Sachs disease, there recently have been a number of new developments, some with far wider applications and greater potential benefits for all. Elaborate genetic screening—a method of examining a person's complete genetic makeup, or genome, for variations that might lead to diseases, including cancer—is now thought to be on the horizon. Some researchers contend it will be with us in a very few years. The field of ecogenetics, which includes the study of genetic variations in suscep-tibility to disease, is rapidly growing. And, ironically, even as science is perfecting genetic screening, industry is conducting less of it.

Each year, 390,000 employees of American industries contract disabling occupational illnesses, including lung, bladder, and other cancers; anemias; dermatitis; asthma, and emphysema, and 100,000 die annually of some of these diseases. Yet their co-workers remain unaffected. Many of those made ill by materials in the workplace are, as geneticists now believe, "hypersusceptible" to them. It isn't chance that makes some fall prey to these illnesses; it's unseen variations in their genetic equipment.

For example, one person in every 10 has, among his or her 100,000 genes, a pair of variant genes that produces an excess of the enzyme aryl hydrocarbon hydroxylase, or AHH. Normally, AHH rids the body's cells of hydrocarbons containing benzopyrene, such as those in the air in many industrial plants. But when the enzyme is made in excess amounts, it turns some of the hydrocarbon molecules into carcinogens. People with this genetic variant are more than 26 times as apt to get lung cancer from inhaling such vapors as most other people.

What is true in the workplace is true everywhere. Many of the numerous serious diseases induced by certain pesticides, exhaust fumes and other pollutants, by drugs, cosmetics, charcoal-broiled and fatty foods and by radiation occur in those who are hereditarily vulnerable. Government agencies advise us of the "safe limits" of exposure to many environmental agents, but these limits are based on averages; individually, we may be less susceptible—or several to 100 times more so—to particular chemicals than are most people. Hence such anomalies as these:

Naphthalene and many widely used amino and nitro compounds have no effect on most people. But 2 percent to 5 percent of Chinese, 11 percent of Mediterranean Jews and 13 percent to 16 percent of black males in the United States exposed to them will develop an acute and highly dangerous form of anemia.

A number of important drugs—the sulfas, hydralazine (an antihypertensive) and many others—are well tolerated by most patients but in a minority produce dangerous toxic reactions.

One out of five men who are heavy smokers develops lung cancer; the rest do not.

Genetic screening for such variations is very likely to become commonplace, and it could be the greatest advance in disease prevention since Edward Jenner's work on vaccination in the late 18th century. Or so it would seem. But in several respects this giant step for humankind will conflict with our notions of equality and fairness and with the laws that embody them. Already, genetic screening has been—and it will continue to be—strenuously opposed by unions, women's groups, civil liberties groups and others who see it as anti-egalitarian, antilabor, racist, invasive of privacy and, in general, a grave threat to democratic ideals. Genetic screening is certain to call forth a major national debate on social policy, compared to which the present shouting match about the ethics of blood testing for drug use and the AIDS antibody is a disagreement couched in polite murmurs.

Undeterred by the unresolved problems and despite the inevitability of the debate that lies ahead, scientists are pressing on in their research, investigating genetic variation at the molecular level. As Dr. Philip Leder, head of the department of genetics at the Harvard University Medical School, puts it, "We need to reach in and lay our hands on the gene." Geneticists and biomedical researchers working in scores of university, hospital and government laboratories in this country and abroad are swiftly gathering the basic knowledge that, many feel, will make comprehensive genetic screening practical soon, perhaps within a decade. Listening to these scientists, one gets a sense of great excitement and imminent breakthrough.

A couple of examples will serve. Dr. Harry V. Gelboin, chief of the laboratory of molecular carcinogenesis at the National Cancer Institute in Bethesda, Md., is a tall, gray-haired man whose long sober face lights up with enthusiasm as he talks and scribbles on the blackboard in his cluttered little office.

"In my laboratory, we're working out how the body metabolizes benzopyrene, or BP, the most common carcinogen in our environment," he explains. "It occurs in tobacco smoke, auto exhausts, heating emissions and so on. Our cells get rid of BP—and virtually all other harmful foreign compounds—by enzymatically converting them to water-soluble form and excreting them in the urine. The body's key detoxifier is the enzyme cytochrome P-450—or, actually, the P-450's, because we produce 15 to 20 variant forms of it and maybe many more.

"The P-450's perform the first step in converting BP into more than 40 harmless compounds. And sometimes, depending on the particular P-450's present, one or two active carcinogens are formed that aren't excreted but bind to DNA, starting the cell on the way to cancer. So the array of P-450's you make determines whether you're more or less susceptible to foreign substances and more or less resistant to cancer. Right now, we're identifying the genes that produce each of the P-450's and soon we'll be able to determine the individual's P-450 profile—and how he handles carcinogens and many other environmental agents. We're very excited by our results."

One can actually see hypersusceptibility operating at the genetic level. At Columbia University's College of Physicians and Surgeons, Dr. I. Bernard Weinstein showed me an electron microscope photograph of pale threads of DNA marked by black spots that indicated the presence of antibodies.

"Each spot," he explained, "is an antibody tagged by an iron molecule that shows up dark. Each antibody has found a carcinogen molecule bound to the DNA." The carcinogen would not have been able to bind to the DNA—the first step in the cancerous transformation of the cell—unless, as Dr. Weinstein explained, "it had been converted to a highly reactive chemical. It appears that individuals differ in the ability to activate this chemical to bind to DNA. They would therefore vary in their susceptibility to the hazardous effects of this carcinogen in their environment."

When genetic screening becomes a reality, one or a very few tests may suffice for pre-employment screening at any given plant; whoever might be damaged by the materials present in the milieu could be spared the consequences of exposure to them.

But genetic researchers have a grander dream of using screening to benefit anyone, anywhere. Dr. Paul A. Marks, president of New York's Memorial Sloan-Kettering Cancer Center, believes that screening the entire genome of a human may be possible by means of about 100 "DNA probes" or tests. A recent report by a Presidential commission predicted that such a repertory, capable of yielding all relevant information about a person's abnormal genes and chromosomes, will exist by the end of the century. Many biomedical researchers agree and expect the total gene screen in 10 to 15 years.

Enthusiasts like Dr. Gelboin at the National Cancer Institute believe the dream will be realized far sooner and in automated form: a programmed machine will divide up a blood sample, process the portions through a battery of tests and produce a printout of the results. "Automated screening for susceptibility to certain drugs may be only months away," says Dr. Gelboin, "and an automated genetic profile of the whole individual may be only several years away."

The liberation from the ills that flesh is heir to, so exciting in concept to the scientists, is now being strenuously opposed on the grounds that it conflicts with American ideals and laws concerning equality and fairness. Such alarms were not sounded when hypersusceptibility research began in the 1950's. At that time, a number of researchers reported that certain chemicals and foods could produce acute hemolytic anemia in a number of black, Asiatic and Mediterranean males, but in very few white males of Northern European origin. Dr. Marks of Memorial Sloan-Kettering, who did some of the early research, says: "Nobody in the late 1950's or early 1960's saw this as anything but an important contribution to the health of a substantial segment of the population." It was not thought of as a racist finding.

Likewise seeing no evil, Dr. Herbert E. Stokinger, a now-retired Government toxicologist, began enthusiastically advocating genetic screening of workers as early as 1963. By 1970, he had listed 92 occupational illnesses, including anemias, leukemia and diseases of the skin, lungs and bladder, that seemed to be the result of enzyme deficiencies due to genetic variations—and that could be avoided by assigning hypersusceptible workers to jobs elsewhere. In 1973, Dr. Stokinger complained that few companies were trying to minimize occupational illness by using such tests as existed.

But more were doing so than he knew and keeping it quiet to avoid confrontations with unions and government agencies. A survey was later conducted by the National Opinion Research Center, commissioned by Representative (now Senator) Albert Gore Jr. for his subcommittee of the House Committee on Science and Technology. It found that between 1970 and 1982, at least 18 of the country's largest companies and private utilities used one or more of these tests. As of 1982, 59 intended to, or thought they might, do so within the next five years. The real figures were surely higher, since one-third of the 561 organizations in the sample did not reply. The survey was confidential, but among the companies that have spoken of their interest in such testing were Du Pont, Dow Chemical and Johns-Manville.

All these companies had good reason to be keenly interested. Workers' compensation and damage suit awards were rising steeply and insurance premiums, accordingly, were soaring. Moreover, if companies could exclude hypersusceptibles, they could come closer to meeting the formidable requirement of the Occupational Safety and Health Act of 1970 that workplaces be safe for all employees. But the fair employment rules of the Civil Rights Act of 1964 made any form of discrimination illegal unless justified by business necessity. To avoid hiring people with a special vulnerability, such as the anemia far more common among blacks than whites, employers had to show that hypersusceptibility and its extra costs, not race, was the reason.

Unions, perceiving a threat to their interests, began to attack the idea of genetic screening vociferously. So did women's groups, since women were being barred from many jobs on the ground that fetuses were highly susceptible to certain workplace chemicals. Though this was not genetic screening, it seemed akin to it. They were joined by the Hastings Center and the Kennedy Institute of Ethics at Georgetown University—both centers of bioethical studies—and by civil rights groups, legal theorists and others who saw genetic screening as endangering privacy, equality and freedom of choice.

These views were increasingly voiced in management-labor bargaining sessions, biomedical research conferences, the lobbies of the Capitol and the news media. Representative Gore conducted hearings on the matter in 1981 and 1982; the resulting rash of articles in the press gave opponents of genetic screening ample chance to get their message across to the public. Genetic researchers and industry spokesmen countered with the arguments in favor of screening, but the hostile view made splashier copy and captured public attention, since it played on the fear of science that is endemic in our time.

"Genetic screening has a potential for unjust application," said Sheldon W. Samuels, health director of the Industrial Union Department, A.F.L.-C.I.O. "Who would employ these susceptibles, who would protect their dignity and place in the community? Here is the stuff by which war and revolution have been made and by which human progress has been destroyed."

"The emphasis on the susceptible worker is a manifestation of social policy and not of science," said Dr. Jeanne Stellman, executive director of the Women's Occupational Health Resource Center at Columbia University. "I am the child of a survivor of the Holocaust," she continued, saying she "and many millions of others suffered very directly and convincingly the results of policies based on dubious genetic traits . . . While I don't see gas ovens being built in the United States, I do see that many of the premises which led to that terrible time are again beginning to surface here."

No wonder most companies either quickly lost or hid their interest in genetic screening. By 1983, after Representative Gore's survey made headlines, only five big companies admitted they were still testing; today, virtually none do. Gordon D. Strickland of the Chemical Manufacturers Association, for instance, says, "As far as we know, only one or two of our companies are doing genetic screening—and only for the benefit of doctor and patient, not job selection."

Although industry is generally silent on the subject, its reasons for being interested in genetic screening are as strong as ever and perhaps stronger, given the example of the multibillion-dollar mass of lawsuits against Johns-Manville, many of them filed on the part of employees who developed asbestosis and other diseases. Citing the cost of the suits, the company filed for bankruptcy in 1982.

Major chemical and pharmaceutical companies are sending representatives to the growing stream of conferences on genetic screening and ecogenetics. A number of large companies sup-

port laboratories doing ecogenetic research. In 1983, Dow, Exxon, Du Pont, I.B.M., Eli Lilly and other corporations sponsored a major international ecogenetics conference at Cold Spring Harbor, N.Y. And the opposition to genetic screening has had no effect on the pace of research, which has steadily increased.

Ecogenetic research seems sure to continue to provoke a major national debate—or, if one takes seriously the warnings of Sheldon Samuels of the A.F.L.-C.I.O., it may lead to war and revolution. Even if the conflict remains nonviolent, it will be prolonged and bitter, for it involves cherished values that genetic screening puts at odds. We face a number of moral dilemmas. Five will be profoundly troublesome.

1. Equal opportunity versus health protection.

Most Americans believe that job discrimination based on sex, race or ethnic origin is morally wrong; the Civil Rights Act of 1964 makes it illegal. Most of us also believe that employers and government should protect workers from health hazards in the workplace; the Occupational Safety and Health Act makes that the law of the land. But when genetic screening is perfected, it will make the two beliefs and laws incompatible, since using screening to protect hypersusceptibles from working at jobs dangerous to them would disproportionately exclude members of certain ethnic and racial groups.

Union leaders, ethicists and some legal authorities believe both goals are desirable but consider equality of job opportunity the more important one. Judith C. Areen, associate dean of the Georgetown University Law School, is typical of those who hold this view: "People should have equal opportunity in the job market, regardless of race, sex or genetic makeup. But genetic screening, even when there is no intent to discriminate, will create de facto discrimination."

To most biogeneticists, however, the preservation of life and health is the controlling moral value. When the question of de facto discrimination is raised, Dr. Leon E. Rosenberg, research geneticist and dean of the Yale University School of Medicine, testily says: "That's the *wrong* question! The *right* one is, how much can genetic screening benefit humanity?" The argument that genetic testing will increase inequality seems to him to ignore reality. "The whole notion of genetics is that we're *not* all the same," he says. "The whole notion of risk factors is that they *aren't* equally distributed."

2. *Equal opportunity versus free enterprise.*

A solution often proposed by union leaders and ethicists to the preceding dilemma is that workers at special risk should be given no-risk jobs with comparable pay and benefits. But this fails to resolve a second dilemma: the conflict between the worker's right to equal employment opportunity and the employer's right to run a business. It seems as unfair to require companies in a competitive market to create alternate safe jobs as it is to deny jobs to workers for genetic traits they cannot control.

For now, the dilemma is being resolved on the side of equal employment. Most employers make no effort to screen or exclude the genetically susceptible. But as genetic screening becomes better known and more feasible, their failure to use it might enable employees who became ill to sue for massive damages over and above workers' compensation. A jury, told by a gaunt, dying man that his employer failed to use available tests and so allowed him to contract his fatal disease, might well find the company grossly negligent and award the dying man generous damages. Even one such award could weaken many a company.

3. *Fairness to the handicapped versus "the greatest happiness of the greatest number."*

The Federal Rehabilitation Act of 1973 and similar laws in 45 states and the District of Columbia embody the moral principle that burdens should be shared; society is held to have an obligation to help the handicapped lead a full life. One way is to ban job discrimination against them whenever "reasonable accommodation" to their needs—ramps, modified work schedules and so on—is economically feasible.

But these laws conflict with the common sense assumption that the ethically soundest guide to social policy is the greatest happiness (or greatest good) of the greatest number. According to this dictum, the most efficient, lowest-cost production of goods and services, benefiting the largest number of people, is the best course.

Americans have tended to assign greater weight to the first principle than to the second, giving special protections and privileges to the handicapped. So far, this has not cost us dearly,

but if the courts should decide that genetic susceptibility is a protected handicap, the cost will expand explosively. Employers required to hire hypersusceptibles would have to make the workplace safe for them. But industry officials and many neutral observers say that in most cases a workplace so clean as to be safe for every hypersusceptible is technically impossible. Even when it is not, experts say, it would be extremely costly—and the costs would have to be passed along to the consumer. This would not be a "reasonable accommodation" or conducive to the greatest happiness of the greatest number.

4. *Individual freedom versus social control.*

Do people have a right to risk their own health, or does society have an obligation to restrain them for their own good and to prevent them from becoming a burden on the rest of us? Both values exist in our culture. We permit people to smoke and climb mountains, yet we make it a crime to ride a motorcycle without a helmet or to use heroin.

The same clash of values exists in regard to taking risks on the job. We require employers to make jobs as nearly risk-free as possible, yet it is not unusual for employees to fight for the right to hold high-paying jobs even though they are at far greater risk than others. They even fight for the right to further risk their health. A few years ago, Johns-Manville prohibited smoking in its asbestos plants because smoking greatly increases the health hazards of working with asbestos. The International Association of Machinists local at the Denison, Tex., plant, filed a grievance; the arbitrator, and later the court, agreeing with the union, struck down the no-smoking rule in that plant on the grounds that "the danger . . . is to the smoker who willingly courts it."

By that reasoning, hypersusceptibles should be free to take jobs where they are in greater danger than other people. But it can be argued that this is unfair to their employers and to the rest of us, for workers who accept special risks will not bear all or even most of the cost of their risk-taking. Under workers' compensation and similar laws, employers cannot defend themselves against injury claims by arguing that the employees knowingly assumed the risk. So the employer will pay—and we all will, because products will cost more and because many hypersusceptibles, felled by chronic illness, will eventually turn to Medicaid.

5. *Knowledge versus privacy; paternalism versus autonomy.*

Government, most of us believe, has a right to gather some information about individuals and establishments and to use its knowledge for the general good. Schoolchildren and restaurant kitchens, for instance, are subject to examination. Yet every such intervention diminishes the privacy and freedom that are part of our tradition; we and our courts fiercely guard what remains, considering it a crucial part of our constitutional endowment. Genetic screening would be a new battleground for the conflict between these values.

On the one hand, most biomedical researchers feel that the knowledge provided by genetic screening will enable us to make more rational decisions about work and health. On the other, ethicists and legal scholars fear that genetic screening and the knowledge it yields will rob us of some of our essential rights. Political scientist Ronald Bayer of the Hastings Center says that the legal right of employers to insist that some job applicants and employees—airline pilots and bus drivers, for instance—submit to medical tests is a "stunning exception" to the right of individuals to refuse medical interventions and "involves bodily intrusions and invasions of privacy."

Even more serious is the potential of genetic screening to disclose defects we would prefer to keep secret. To be known as a cancer risk in any workplace contaminated with the ubiquitous BP is to be stigmatized; in a town with a single industry, it could mean unemployability. Socially, moreover, the hypersusceptible person may be perceived as defective, and shunned.

Given the choice between knowledge or ignorance of their own genetic defects, some people may opt for ignorance. Many Hasidic Jews have refused to take part in mass screening for Tay-Sachs disease, the hereditary condition affecting descendants of Eastern European Jews, because when it comes to marriage, known carriers would be at a severe disadvantage. More generally, even if genetic information is kept confidential, a susceptible individual might find the knowledge hard to live with. Dr. Stuart H. Yuspa, who heads a research team at the National Cancer Institute, says: "We shouldn't rush genetic screening. What happens to you if you're identified at age 20 as high risk? Ask a young person with Huntington's chorea, which develops later in life; he's living with a death warrant. That's how a cancer-prone individual might feel."

Many of us, considering these dilemmas, will take one side or the other. But the most socially practical and beneficial option would be a set of compromise regulations worked out by lawmakers after careful consultation with all factions. Now, before the crisis is upon us, is the right time to do so, but the present Administration, strongly oriented toward deregulation, is hardly likely to initiate such legislation.

When lawmakers finally have to act, will they listen to the scientists or to the opponents of genetic screening and impose such strict controls on it as to deprive us of much of its benefit? Perhaps at first they will do the latter; in the long run, probably not, if we can judge from how such dilemmas have been resolved in the past. In the 1960's, when Congress and government agencies sought to protect human subjects of biomedical and behavioral research, they nearly strangled some lines of valuable scientific inquiry; later, compromises made it possible to protect both the rights of human subjects and those of researchers to seek knowledge—and of all of us to benefit from it. Similarly, if genetic screening is overcontrolled at first, adjustments will probably be made later.

Such solutions to dilemmas please no one—but they work. As Edmund Burke told the British Parliament, "All government—indeed, every human benefit and enjoyment, every virtue and every prudent act—is founded on compromise and barter." Parliament ignored him, but would have done better to pay heed; he was urging compromise with America, in 1775.

Decision Scenario 1 ••

"My mother was fifty when she died," Lauri Ross said. "From the time the first symptoms of Hungtington's appeared until the time she died was about twelve years. It was terribly sad to watch. I would hate to think that I was going to put a child through the ordeal my sister and I suffered."

"Do you ever worry about yourself?" Dr. Haskins asked.

"About whether I'm going to develop Huntington's? Yes, I do. I know that there is a fifty-fifty chance that I will. I'm twenty-five now, and I can't keep from thinking about what the next ten or fifteen years may bring." Lauri smiled and shrugged. "But life has been pretty good to me in a lot of ways. We all have to go some way so I guess I'm prepared for it."

"You don't seem to have let the possibility affect your life too much. You've gone to college, established yourself in a career, gotten married. You've done all the things others do, and I think that's a tribute to your courage."

"I haven't done quite everything," Lauri said. "Bob and I would like to have children. Quite frankly, I don't know whether we should. That's connected with what I wanted to ask you. Is there any prenatal test that can be used to determine whether a child is going to have Huntington's? Or is there any test I can take that will show whether I'm going to have it?"

"Without going into detail, the answer is: not yet. If we had a lot of family history and we had blood samples from you and a large number of family members, it would be possible to use a genetic probe technique to see whether you are carrying the gene. But all of that is still in the experimental stage, and for the moment it doesn't offer any practical solution."

"So Bob and I just have to decide for ourselves whether we're willing to take the risk."

"Fundamentally, that is correct."

Lauri nodded. "What bothers me most, I guess, is that we also have to decide the fate of the potential child. I don't know whether it's right to saddle a child with our decision."

Dr. Haskins shrugged. "If you decide not to have a child, then you're deciding not to let that potential child live at all. Maybe it's better to allow the child at least some years of a normal life, rather than no life at all."

According to Purdy, would it be wrong for Lauri and Bob to decide to have no children?

On what grounds can it be argued that we have an obligation to provide every child with at least a normal opportunity for a good life?

Is there a right to reproduce? If so, does it override the duty to provide a child with a normal life?

Decision Scenario 2 ••

Sara Straus was frightened. She sat in the counselor's office with her hands folded in her lap, trying to look calm.

"Mrs. Straus," the counselor said, "I have the results back on your AFP test. I'm sorry to tell you that the level of alpha protein in your blood is quite high."

"What does that mean?" Mrs. Straus asked.

"It means," said the counselor, "that your chances of having a baby with what we call neural tube defect are quite high. Your child might be born with an open spine or with part of its brain missing."

"Oh, my God. Is there anything I can do?"

The counselor shook her head. "If you mean can you do anything to make the baby normal, the answer is no. This test is about 90 percent accurate. The only reasonable course is to have an abortion and begin another child when you feel ready."

"But I don't believe in abortion," said Mrs. Straus.

"There's no way we can force you to have one. But according to the law if you have been informed of the chances of a defect and do not have an abortion, then you and your husband must accept full financial responsibility for the care of the impaired child."

"How much would that cost?"

"Probably around fifty thousand dollars a year."

"We can't afford that," said Mrs. Straus. "Nobody could afford to pay money like that."

"I'm just telling you the law," said the counselor.

"What if we have the child and then can't pay?"

"The law requires that you and your husband declare yourselves bankrupt. The child will then be placed in a public institution, and a fixed percentage of your future earnings will go to pay for its upkeep. Even after its death you must continue to pay until the accumulated costs to the state have been repaid."

"That's unfair," said Mrs. Straus. "We're being forced to go against what we think is right."

At this time, there is no such law as that mentioned by the counselor. Should there be such a law? After all, don't we generally believe that people should accept responsibility for their actions and decisions?

Is it ever right for society to force people to act in ways they consider to be morally wrong?

Does involuntary prenatal or genetic screening necessarily involve a violation of the autonomy of individuals?

Should screening programs be voluntary and advisory, or should they be backed up by laws that aim to protect society by requiring that individuals acts in certain ways as the results of the screening?

Following Purdy's line of argument, might one claim that when there is a reason to believe that a child may suffer from a serious genetic disease, the parents have a duty to undergo genetic screening?

Decision Scenario 3 ••

"I'm sorry I wasn't able to bring you better news," Dr. Valery Mendez said. "I hope our first consultation helped prepare you for it."

Timothy Schwartz shook his head. "We gambled and lost," he said. "We can't say we didn't know what we were doing."

"That doesn't make it much easier," Judith Schwartz said. "When you said we were both Tay-Sachs carriers, I thought, 'Well, it won't happen to us.' But I was wrong."

"The odds were in our favor," Mr. Schwartz said. "I still think we did the right thing."

"Maybe we shouldn't even have had ourselves tested," Mrs. Schwartz said. "Then we wouldn't even know we've got a problem."

"But we'd have one anyway," her husband said. "Ignorance is bliss only when it's folly to be wise. Now we at least know what we're up against."

"What about this new test?" Mrs. Schwartz asked. "Can we really trust the results?"

"I'm afraid so," said Dr. Mendez. "The fetal cells taken during amniocentesis were cultured, and the chromosome study showed that the child you're carrying will have Tay-Sachs."

"What do you recommend?" Mr. Schwartz asked.

"It's not for me to recommend. I can give you some information—tell you the options—but you've got to make your own decision."

"Is abortion the only solution?" Mrs. Schwartz asked.

"If you call it a solution," Mr. Schwartz said.

"The disease is almost invariably fatal," Dr. Mendez said. "And there is really no effective treatment for it. A lot of people think there may be in the future, but that doesn't help right now."

"So what does it involve?" Mr. Schwartz asked.

"At first your child will seem quite normal, but that's only because it takes time for a particular chemical to build up in the brain. After the first year or so, the child will start to show signs of deterioration. He'll start losing his sight. Then as brain damage progresses, he'll lose control over his muscles, and eventually he will die."

"And we just have to stand by and watch that happen?" Mrs. Schwartz asked.

"Nothing can be done to stop it," Dr. Mendez said. "It's a terrible and sad disease."

"We certainly do want to have a child," Mr. Schwartz said. "But we don't want to have one that is going to suffer all his life. I don't think I could stand that."

How persuasive is Kass's argument that genetic abortion constitutes a threat to the principle that all persons are of equal worth?

Can Purdy's argument that every child deserves a normal opportunity for a good life be used to justify requiring abortion in a case such as this?

Kass contends that none of the three standards he examines can allow us to justify selective abortion. State and evaluate his arguments.

How unfavorable must the odds be against having a normal child before (according to Purdy) parents have a duty not to reproduce? In what way is the seriousness of the disease at issue relevant to the odds?

Decision Scenario 4 ....

"The concept behind the bill is very simple, Senator," said Mrs. Laude. "We want to improve the human race, and we know exactly how to do it. The principles of genetics can be used to guide changes in the population."

"You mean," said the Senator, "you can make people smarter?"

"Not as individuals. But we can increase the level of intelligence in society. We can do this by seeing to it that intelligent people have more children than the less intelligent. Over time, the statistical balance will shift towards intelligence."

"And does your draft of the bill make that possible?"

"By a system of financial incentives and disincentives," said Mrs. Laude. "Those above a certain level of intelligence will be offered a yearly stipend to pay part of the expenses for each of their children. Those below that level will receive nothing, and, having to bear the full cost themselves, they are likely to limit the number of children they have. We will also make use of genetic counseling programs to encourage or discourage children, whatever is appropriate in each case."

"These genetic counseling programs will be government run and supported?" the Senator asked.

"That's right. The law will require that everyone be screened and classified before his or her fifteenth birthday."

"Is intelligence all that you'll screen for?"

"It's the only positive trait we will try to increase. We will also screen against genetic diseases, like Tay-Sachs and sickle-cell anemia."

"This will be very controversial, you know," said the Senator.

"We know," Mrs. Laude said. "It will take a person of courage to introduce such a bill into the Senate. But we think it's the most important piece of legislation imaginable. The improvement of our society and of the whole human race will be the end result."

What problems and dangers are inherent in Mrs. Laude's proposal for a program of positive and negative eugenics?

What can be said in defense of such a program?

Would a utilitarian be likely to favor such a program?

Could such a program be defended as compatible with Rawls's principles of justice?

What arguments against any such program does Macklin present?

Decision Scenario 5 ....

"Here's the theory," said Dr. Larry Torland. "Homocystinuria is produced because cystahionine synthetase is not available to catalyze the condensation of homocystine to form cystahionine."

"Another inborn error of metabolism," Cynthia Pruett said. "What are the clinical signs?"

"Renal hypertension, arterial thrombosis, myocardial infarction, and stroke are some of the outcomes. Usually there are skeletal abnormalities, variable mental retardation, progressive arterial thrombosis, and mental confusion that's easily confused with schizophrenia if you don't know what you're looking at. And of course there's a lot of homocystine excreted in the urine."

"Okay," Cynthia said. "Now get back to the theory."

"The enzyme we're talking about is produced in several places. In the kidney, the liver, and the brain primarily. Now one possibility is that it's not produced because there is a missing precursor. If that's the case, there's not much we can do."

"But there's another possibility?"

"Right. It may be that we're dealing with a missing or dysfunctioning gene the way we are in PKU or Tay-Sachs. So if we could get some cells in place that manufacture cystahionine synthetase, get them to multiply, they might produce enough CS to do some good."

"I assume there's no good therapy for this disease."

"None. It can be treated symptomatically by medical means, but there's no way to really bring it under control."

"So what are you going to try to do?" Cynthia asked.

"I've got a cell line already that will produce CS. It's one I developed from mouse tumor cells. I want to inject some into the kidney of a patient and just see if we can get some CS production."

"You're not going to use whole cells, are you?"

"Of course not," Larry said. "Just the DNA. I'm going to try for transformation."

"Do you have any animal data?" Cynthia asked.

"Not yet. I'm going to do a large-scale trial if I get a grant. But right now, I'm just going to go on the basis of the likelihood that the procedure might do some good."

"I think you're making a big mistake," Cynthia said.

According to Anderson and Fletcher, what standards must be met before the direct use of recombinant DNA in gene therapy can be considered morally acceptable?

Explain the relevance of animal experiments to the standards. What, according to Anderson and Fletcher, must such experiments show?

If the gene therapy is not likely to do any harm, and if it holds the promise of doing some good, and if the patient is fully informed, then what reason can there be for not employing the therapy?

What advantages are there to having review boards or committees decide when a proposed therapy can be employed? Is there any merit in the charge made by some researchers that review boards stand in the way of progress and that the only relevant consideration is whether the physician and patient agree to initiate the therapy?

Decision Scenario 6 ....

"The screening program is for the *benefit* of our employees," Carl Larski said. "Amchem production involves radiologic agents and potentially harmful chemical substances. It is absolute madness not to monitor people for overexposure to radiation. I'm sure you agree with that. And it's ridiculous to expose women who are pregnant to a radiation hazard, because that could cause serious impairments in the child. Of course sometimes women are pregnant for a while before they realize it so it makes sense to keep all women of childbearing age away from radiation."

Susan Spencer shook her head to show that she disagreed. "You're using company policy to make decisions that people ought to make for themselves," she said. "If a woman wants to take a risk, she should be allowed to. After all, radiation can make men sterile, as well as causing them direct harm. Amchem's practices are inherently discriminatory. And they don't stop with radiation and they don't stop with women. The company excludes blacks from jobs that put them into contact with naphthalene."

"That's correct," Larski said. "That's because they are much more likely to develop a serious form of anemia than most other workers. And we also keep women away from most of the chemicals we work with. We're concerned about them, of course, but no more so than we are concerned about the men who work with them. We are, once again, worried about the effects on their children."

"Mostly you are worried about insurance claims and lawsuits."

"That's a factor," Larski admitted. "If some people are more prone to develop serious illnesses than others and we can detect it in advance, then we have a corporate duty to keep them out of harm's way. It's true that we help control our insurance cost by doing that, but we also help people avoid getting ill."

"We are impressed with Amchem's humane concerns," Spencer said. "But the Committee Against Screening is much more interested in protecting the individual's right to seek employment of her or his choice. Also, CAS believes that the data used to exclude people from jobs may also be used to exclude them from other benefits. For example, insurance companies are likely to refuse health insurance to someone who runs a greater than average risk of developing a serious disease. The result is that people are penalized because of their genetic makeup, and that's an accident of birth. Our society has a duty to protect individuals from just that sort of discrimination, and CAS intends to do all it can to make sure that society lives up to that duty."

"That's very eloquent," Larski said. "But you're trying to force equality where none exists. People are different, and the society can't alter that fact."

What are the "dilemmas" that Hunt identifies as produced by the conflict in values that genetic screening presents?

Is it a legitimate function of society to protect individuals from hazards in the workplace? Is there a limit to steps that can be taken to provide protection?

If certain jobs present greater hazards to women and blacks than to others, then excluding women and blacks is discriminatory. Are all forms of discrimination that are not directly related to job performance unjustifiable?

"We value individual autonomy, and it may seem enough to warn people of the hazards they may face in accepting a particular job. However, the need to earn a living may force some to accept jobs that put them at a greater than average risk. Consequently, it is misleading to think that we are preserving autonomy by allowing individuals to decide for themselves whether they wish to accept a job that is more than normally hazardous to them. Economic necessity makes a mockery out of the notion that people are free to choose." Evaluate this argument.

Decision Scenario 7 ....

"The trick," said Martin Anders, "is to make use of the virus as part of our production system."

"How's that?" Hilda Presti asked.

"The DNA of the virus contains a segment of DNA that we introduced into it. When the virus attacks a bacterial cell, it injects the DNA into it. The viral DNA then takes over the cell machinery enough to get the cell to make copies of the DNA and get it to synthesize the proteins coded for by the DNA segment we spliced in."

"That means that if the proteins are something that are useful—like a hormone—then you've got a chemical factory working to produce it."

"That's the idea," Anders said. "We can har-

ness the power of literally billions of bacteria to make what we want."

"Isn't that dangerous, though?" Presti asked. "Isn't it at least possible that the viruses might contain some DNA segments that would make the bacteria resistant to antibiotics?"

"That's the sort of Andromeda Strain scenario people used to worry about in the seventies, but we realize today that that's just not something that's going to happen."

"Can you really be sure of that?" Presti asked.

"Reasonably certain," Anders said. "Nothing serious has happened so far. Besides, we've taken a lot of steps to avoid the danger. Even when genetically altered bacteria are released directly into the environment or when altered viruses have been used as vaccines, everything reasonable has been done to make them safe. The bacteria are harmless ones, and the viruses are always weakened strains."

"Probably you're right," Presti said. "But the risks seem to me genuine. Why can't we do without genetically altered organisms? What is there to be gained?"

"The most immediate gain is that we can exploit an entirely new form of technology. We can grow better crops, manufacture better and more effective drugs. There is really no end to what we might be able to do in the future."

"If there is one," Presti said.

What are the potential dangers of genetically altered organisms? What are the potential benefits?

Why do some scientists believe that the so-called Andromeda Strain scenario is not one that we need to take seriously?

What considerations suggest that we ought to proceed with caution in exploiting the promises of genetic engineering?

CHAPTER 7

REPRODUCTIVE CONTROL: [⎯⎯⎯⎯⎯⎯⎯]
IN VITRO FERTILIZATION,
ARTIFICIAL INSEMINATION,
SURROGATE PREGNANCY,
AND STERILIZATION

CASE PRESENTATION [⎯⎯⎯⎯⎯⎯⎯]
Louise Brown

Under other circumstances, the birth announcement might have been perfectly ordinary, the sort that appears in newspapers every day: *Born to John and Lesley Brown: a baby girl, Louise, 5 lbs. 12 ozs., 11:47 p.m., July 25, 1978, Oldham General Hospital (Oldham, England).*

But the birth of Louise Brown was far from being an ordinary event, and the announcement of its occurrence appeared in headlines throughout the world. For the first time in history, a child was born who was conceived outside the mother's body under controlled laboratory conditions.

Louise Brown was the world's first "test-tube baby."

For John and Lesley Brown, the birth of Louise was a truly marvelous event. "She's so small, so beautiful, so perfect," her mother told a reporter. "It was like a dream. I couldn't believe it," her father said.

The joy of the Browns was understandable, for, from the time of their marriage in 1969, they had both very much wanted to have a child. Then they discovered that Mrs. Brown was unable to conceive because of blocked fallopian tubes—the ova would not descend so fertilization could not occur. In 1970, she underwent an operation in an attempt to correct the condition, but the procedure was unsuccessful.

The Browns decided they would adopt a child, since they couldn't have one of their own. After two years on a waiting list, they gave up that

plan. But the idea of having their own child was rekindled when a nurse familiar with the work of embryologist Robert Edwards and gynecologist Patrick Steptoe referred the Browns to them.

For the previous twelve years, Steptoe and Edwards had been working on the medical and biochemical techniques required for embryo transfer. Steptoe developed techniques for removing a ripened ovum from a woman's ovaries, then reimplanting it in the uterus after it has been fertilized. Edwards improved the chemical solutions needed to keep ova functioning and healthy outside the body and perfected a method of external fertilization with sperm.

Using their techniques, Steptoe and Edwards had successfully produced a pregnancy in one of their patients in 1975, but it had resulted in a miscarriage. They continued to refine their procedures and were confident that their techniques could produce a normal pregnancy that would result in a healthy baby.

They considered Lesley Brown an excellent candidate for an embryo transfer. She was in excellent general health, at thirty-one she was not too old for pregnancy, and she was highly fertile. In 1976, Steptoe did an exploratory operation and found that Mrs. Brown's fallopian tubes were not functional and could not be surgically repaired. He removed them so that he would have clear access to the ovaries.

In November of 1977, Mrs. Brown was given

injections of a hormone to increase the maturation rate of her egg cells. Then in a small private hospital in Oldham, Dr. Steptoe performed a minor surgical procedure. Using a laparoscope to guide him—a tube with a built-in eyepiece and light source that is inserted through a tiny slit in the abdomen—he extracted an ovum with a suction needle from a ripened follicle.

The ovum was then placed in a small glass vessel containing biochemical nutrients and sperm that had been secured from John Brown. Once the egg was fertilized, it was transferred to another nutrient solution. More than fifty hours later, the ovum had reached the eight-cell stage of division. Guided by their previous experience and research, Steptoe and Edwards had decided that it was at this stage that an ovum should be returned to the womb. Although in normal human development, the ovum has divided to produce sixty-four or more cells before it completes its descent down the fallopian tube and becomes attached to the uterine wall, they had learned that attachment is possible at an earlier stage. The stupendous difficulties in creating and maintaining the proper biochemical environment for a multiplying cell made it reasonable to reduce the time outside the body as much as possible.

Mrs. Brown had been given another series of hormone injections to prepare her uterus. Two and a half days after the ovum was removed, the fertilized egg—an embryo—was reimplanted. Using a laparoscope and a hollow plastic tube (a cannula), Dr. Steptoe introduced the small sphere of cells into Mrs. Brown's uterus. It successfully attached itself to the uterine wall.

Mrs. Brown's pregnancy proceeded normally, but because of the special nature of her case, seven weeks before the baby was due, she entered the Oldham Hospital maternity ward so that she could be continuously monitored. About a week before the birth was expected, the baby was delivered by caesarean section. Mrs. Brown had developed toxemia, a condition associated with high blood pressure that can lead to stillbirth.

The baby was normal, and all concerned were jubilant. "The last time I saw the baby it was just eight cells in a test tube," Dr. Edwards said. "It was beautiful then, and it's still beautiful now." After the delivery, Dr. Steptoe said, "She came out crying her head off, a beautiful normal baby."

Mr. Brown almost missed the great event, because no one on the hospital staff had bothered to tell him that his wife was scheduled for the operation. Only when he had been gone for about two hours and called back to talk to his wife did he find out what was about to happen.

He rushed back and waited anxiously until a nurse came out and told him, "You're the father of a wonderful little girl." As he later told a reporter, "Almost before I knew it, there I was holding our daughter in my arms."

Like many ordinary fathers, he ran down the halls of the hospital telling people he passed, "It's a girl! I've got a baby daughter."

To calm down, he went outside and stood in the rain. It was there that a reporter from a London newspaper captured Mr. Brown's view of the event. "The man who deserves all the praise is Mr. Steptoe," he said. "What a man to be able to do such a wonderful thing."

CASE PRESENTATION
The Orphaned Embryos of Mario and Elsa Rios

In 1983 Mario and Elsa Rios died in a plane crash. Their deaths left others to face some unique moral and legal issues.

The Los Angeles couple had been trying to have a child. Ova from Mrs. Rios and sperm from an anonymous donor were combined, and the embryos that developed were frozen and stored at the Queen Victoria Medical Center in Melbourne,

Australia. The aim of freezing the embryos was to allow other attempts at pregnancy without subjecting Mrs. Rios to additional surgery.

A scholarly committee that was asked to study the question of what should be done with the embryos recommended that they be destroyed. However, the Parliament of the State of Victoria rejected the recommendation and passed a bill with an amendment that required the embryos to be put up for adoption and implanted in surrogate mothers. (The amendment was intended to cover only the Rios's embryos, not to establish a general policy. In the future, couples participating in in vitro fertilization programs will be required to indicate what should be done with frozen embryos in the event of death or separation.)

The Rios estate was valued at about one million dollars, and what claim, if any, the embryos might have on it is a complicating factor. According to Victoria law, the embryo implants would be considered the children only of their surrogate/adoptive parents. However, this would not necessarily affect legal actions taken in California.

CASE PRESENTATION
The Unclaimed Infant

In January 1983, Judy Stiver of Lansing, Michigan, gave birth to a child nine months after she was artificially inseminated with sperm from Alexander Malahoff of Queens, New York. Mr. Malahoff had agreed to pay Mrs. Stiver ten thousand dollars for her services as a surrogate mother.

Mrs. Stiver had a long and difficult labor, and trouble started as soon as the child was born. The child, a boy, was microcephalic and suffered from a severe infection. Mr. Malahoff, as the presumed father, refused to authorize the treatment necessary to sustain the life of the infant. However, the hospital obtained a court order, and the infant was successfully treated.

Before Mrs. Stiver and her husband could cash the check given to her by Mr. Malahoff, Mr. Malahoff informed them that there was a problem. The baby's blood type was O-positive, while Mr. Malahoff's was AB-positive. Thus, the child could not be his, and he refused to accept responsibility for it. Before that time, according to Mr. Stiver, Mr. Malahoff had accepted the baby's impairment, had the child baptized, and planned to place him in an institution.

"We don't feel the baby is ours," Mr. Stiver said. "We feel no maternal or paternal relationship. We feel sorry for it, but we don't want it." Mrs. Stiver reported that she felt "some affection" for the baby but "there is no bond."

Mrs. Stiver said that she had a thorough medical examination to guarantee that she was not pregnant before she was inseminated with Mr. Malahoff's sperm. She and her husband then avoided sexual intercourse for thirty days. Mr.

Malahoff, who later separated from his wife, is suing the Stivers for thirty thousand dollars, alleging that they violated the terms of the contract by having intercourse during the insemination period. The Stivers are considering suing the physician who performed the insemination.

A month after the child's birth, his fate was still not determined. His medical condition continued to require hospitalization, and it was not certain whether he would go to the Stiver home or spend his life in a state institution for the brain-damaged.

"It's just that I've always thought this baby was for someone else," Mrs. Stiver said. "Whenever we talked about it, it was never 'my baby,' it was the baby for someone else—their baby—so I never developed a maternal feeling about him. But I'm sure the feeling will come real fast when I hold him, because I love all babies."

INTRODUCTION

"Oh, brave new world that has such people in it!" exclaims Miranda in Shakespeare's *The Tempest*.

It is a phrase from this line that provided Aldous Huxley with the title for his dystopian novel *Brave New World*. A dystopia is the opposite of a utopia, and the future society depicted by Huxley is one which we are invited to view with shock and disapproval.

In this society, "pregnancy" is a dirty

word, sex is purely recreational, and children are produced according to explicit genetic standards in the artificial wombs of state "hatcheries." Furthermore, an individual's genetic endowment determines the social position and obligations that he or she has within the society. Of course, everyone is conditioned to believe that the role he finds himself in is the best one to have.

In significant ways, that future is now. The new and still developing medical technologies of human reproduction have now reached a stage in which the technical innovations imagined by Huxley in 1932 to make such a society possible are well within the limits of feasibility.

We have no state hatcheries and no artificial uteruses. But we do have sperm banks and surrogate mothers. We have it within our power to remove an ovum from a woman's body, fertilize it, then return it so that it may develop into a child. By relatively simple surgical procedures, we can end forever the reproductive potentialities of otherwise fertile men or women.

The new technology associated with human reproduction is so powerful that it differs only in degree from that of Huxley's dystopian world. What we have yet to do is to employ the technology as part of a deliberate social policy to restructure our world along the lines imagined by Huxley.

Yet the potentiality is there. Perhaps more than anything else, it is the bleak vision of such a mechanistic and dehumanized future that has motivated much of the criticism of current reproductive technology. The "brave new world" of Huxley is one in which traditional values associated with reproduction and family life, values based on individual autonomy, have been replaced by values of a purely social kind. In such a society, it is the good of the society or of the species, not the good of individuals, that is the touchstone of justification.

The possible loss of personal values is a legitimate and serious concern. The technologies of human reproduction are sometimes viewed as machines that may be employed to pave the road leading to a world of bleakness and loss. Yet it is important to remember that those same technologies also promise to enhance the lives of those presently living and to prevent potential suffering and despair.

Some women who are unable to bear children may now find it possible to do so through the use of in vitro fertilization techniques. Artificial insemination offers a means of impregnation when biological dysfunction makes the normal means impossible. Further, those women who would be at risk from becoming pregnant may now be protected by choosing surgical sterilization.

These are all potentialities that have become actualities; in vitro fertilization, artificial insemination, and sterilization are all procedures currently being performed. In the view of some, these procedures merely mark a beginning, and the possibilities inherent in reproductive technology still remain relatively unrealized. If we wish, we can employ the technology to change the very fabric and pattern of our society.

Should we do that? Or will the use of the technology necessarily promote the development of a dystopia? One way of thinking about these general questions is to turn once more to Huxley.

It is frequently overlooked that in 1962 Huxley published a utopian novel. Like the society in *Brave New World*, Huxley's ideal society also relies upon the principles of science, but in the ideal society they are used to promote autonomy and personal development.

Island portrays a society on the island of Pala that for over a hundred years has developed itself in accordance with the principles of reason and science. Living is communal, sexual repression is nonexistent, children are cared for by both their biological parents and other adults, drugs are used to enhance perceptual awareness, and social obligations are assigned on the basis of personal interest and ability.

More to the present point, the society makes use of reproductive technology to achieve its ends. It practices contraception, eugenics, and artificial insemination. Negative eugenics to eliminate genetic diseases is considered only rational. But more than this, by the use of "DF" and "AI" (Deep Freeze and Artificial Insemination), sperm from donors with superior genetic endowments is available for the use of couples who wish to improve their chances of having a child with special talents or with higher than usual intelligence.

Huxley's ideal society is not above criticism, even from those who are sympathetic toward the values he endorses. Yet *Brave New World* is such a powerful cautionary tale of what might happen if science were pressed into the service of repressive political goals that it makes it difficult to imagine other possible futures in which some of the same technology plays a more benign role. Since *Island* is an attempt to present such an alternate future, in thinking about the possibilities inherent in reproductive technology, fairness demands that we also consider Palinese society and not restrict our attention to the world of soma and state hatcheries.

IN VITRO FERTILIZATION

The birth of Louise Brown in 1978 (see the Case Presentation) was treated as a major media event. Photographs, television coverage, interviews, and news stories presented the world with minute details of the lives of the people involved and with close accounts of the technical procedures that had led to Louise's conception.

Despite the unprecedented character of the event, few people seemed surprised by it. The idea of a "test-tube baby" was one already familiar from fiction and folklore. The medieval alchemist was thought capable of generating life within his retorts, and hundreds of science fiction stories depicted a future in which the creation of life within the laboratory was an ordinary occurrence. In some ways, then, the birth of Louise Brown was seen as merely a matter of science and medicine catching up with imagination. (Indeed, they didn't quite catch up, for the "test tube" contained sperm and an egg, not just a mixture of chemicals.)

Although it is doubtful whether the public appreciated the magnitude of the achievement that resulted in the birth of Louise Brown, it was one of considerable significance. The first embryo transfer was performed in rabbits in 1890, but it was not until the role of hormones in reproduction, the nutritional requirements of developing cells, and the reproductive process itself were better understood that it became possible to consider seriously the idea of fertilizing an egg outside the mother's body and then returning it for ordinary development.

"In vitro" is a Latin phrase that means "in glass," and in embryology, it is used in contrast with "in utero" or "in the uterus." Ordinary human fertilization takes place in utero (strictly speaking, in the fallopian tubes) when a sperm cell unites with an ovum. In vitro fertilization, then, is fertilization that is artificially performed outside the woman's body—in a test tube, so to speak.

The ovum that produced Louise Brown was fertilized in vitro. But the entire process involved *embryo transfer*. That is, an ovum had to be taken from her mother's body. Then, after it was fertilized and had become an embryo, it was returned for in utero development.

Robert Edwards and Patrick Steptoe were the individuals responsible for developing and performing the techniques of in vitro fertilization and embryo transfer that led to the birth of Louise Brown. Basically, they followed a four-step process that has now become almost standard.

1. The patient is given a reproductive hormone in order to cause ova to ripen. A few hours before ovulation can be expected to occur, a small incision is made in the abdomen just below the navel. A laparoscope is inserted through the incision, and the ovaries are examined directly. When mature eggs are found that are about to break free from the thin walls of the ovarian follicle, the walls are punctured and the contents are removed by a vacuum aspirator (a hollow suction needle). Several eggs may be removed.

2. The eggs are transferred to a nutrient solution that is biochemically similar to that found in the fallopian tubes. Sperm is then added to the solution. As soon as a single sperm cell penetrates the ovum, the ovum is fertilized.

3. The fertilized egg is transferred to another nutrient solution where, after about a day, it begins to undergo cell division. When the ovum reaches the eight-cell stage, it is ready to be returned to the uterus. The patient is given injections of hormones to prepare her uterus to receive the fertilized egg.

4. The small ball of cells is placed in the uterus through the cervix (the opening that leads to the vagina) by means of a hollow plastic tube called a cannula. The fertilized egg continues to divide, and somewhere between the thirty-two- and sixty-four-cell stage, it attaches itself to the uterine wall.

If the attachment is successful, from this point on, development should proceed as though fertilization had taken place in the ordinary fashion.

On December 28, 1981, Elizabeth Jordan Carr was born at Norfolk General Hospital, Norfolk, Virginia. She has the distinction of being the first baby conceived in vitro born in the United States. Like Louise Brown, she also weighed five pounds, twelve ounces, was born ahead of schedule, and was perfectly healthy.

As of 1986, over one thousand births have resulted from using in vitro techniques, and in the United States alone from fifty to one hundred clinics performing the procedure have been opened since the Norfolk program was initiated. (Some estimates place the number of programs worldwide at around two hundred.) Success rates vary, but in the best programs, the chance of a woman's becoming pregnant is about 23 to 25 percent, roughly the same odds as those of a normal, healthy couple attempting conception during the woman's regular monthly cycle. Each fertilization and transplantation attempt costs around five thousand dollars, and in most cases, such expenses are not covered by insurance.

The technical procedures are still fundamentally the same as those pioneered by Steptoe and Edwards. However, modifications and extensions have been introduced. One of the more important ones is the development of a nonsurgical procedure for securing ova. After hormones are used to stimulate the ovarian follicles, ultrasound is employed to locate the follicles, and a hollow needle is inserted through the vaginal wall and into a follicle. Fluid is withdrawn, and egg cells are identified under the microscope. The egg cells are then fertilized with the sperm, cultured, and reimplanted.

An additional modification is to attempt to implant two, three, or even more fertilized ova at a time. This increases the chances that at least one of them will attach to the uterine wall and develop normally. Of course, the procedure also increases the chances of multiple births, and clinics that use this technique have patients that produce a higher than average percentage of twins and triplets.

Another important development is the perfection of techniques for freezing embryos. Evidence to date indicates that embryos can be stored in a frozen condition and then unfrozen and implanted without any damage to the chromosomes. The advantage of the procedure is that it eliminates the need for a woman to undergo the surgery and the lengthy and uncomfortable process required to secure additional ova. If a woman fails to become pregnant at a first attempt, an embryo saved from the initial fertilization can be employed in another effort. Furthermore, the technique makes it possible to delay an embryo transplant until the potential mother has reached the most favorable time in her menstrual cycle.

By virtue of being first, Louise Brown continues to be a symbol of what it is possible to achieve by means of the techniques developed by Steptoe and Edwards. But in the future it is likely she will quietly take her place among the ranks of the literally thousands of others whose conception occurred in a glass bottle.

Benefits

Obviously, the processes involved in in vitro fertilization and embryo transfer are complicated and require a great amount of skill and knowledge. An obvious question to ask about the whole procedure is, what is to be gained by it? That is, what are the benefits of such a technically difficult and expensive medical procedure?

The most direct and perhaps the most persuasive answer is that in vitro fertilization makes it possible for many couples to conceive children who would not otherwise be able to do so. At a time when problems with fertility seem to be on the increase, this is a particularly important consideration. Research shows that 10 percent of married couples in the United States are infertile— that they have attempted to conceive a child for a year or longer without success. During

the period 1981–1982, physicians reported a record two million visits for infertility problems, twice as many as for comparable two-year periods. Also, infertility among younger women seems to be on the increase. In 1965 infertility in women aged 20 to 26 was estimated to be 4 percent; in 1982 the figure was 11 percent.

In vitro fertilization is obviously not a solution to all problems of fertility. However, it is the only solution possible in a large number of cases. Figures show that as much as 45 percent of all cases of female infertility are caused by abnormal or obstructed fallopian tubes. In such cases, although normal ova are produced, they cannot move down the tubes to be fertilized. In some cases, tissue blocking the tubes may be removed, or the tubes reconstructed. In other cases, however, the tubes may be impossible to repair or may be entirely absent. (Only 40 to 50 percent of infertile women can be helped through surgery.) This means that the only way in which the woman can expect to have a child of her own is by means of in vitro fertilization. Thus, the procedure offers a realistic possibility of becoming parents to many people who once had no hope at all of having a child.

Despite some early doubts, the public acceptance of in vitro fertilization has been overwhelmingly positive. A public opinion poll conducted in 1978 showed that by a margin of more than two to one Americans favored making in vitro fertilization an option available to childless couples. Furthermore, there can be little doubt that the great majority of eligible couples who want a child are in favor of the procedure. The Norfolk clinic is reported to have a waiting list of some eight thousand names—a backlog of sixteen years.

A second, and quite ironic, benefit of research into improving in vitro fertilization and embryo transfer is that it may lead to better and more effective contraceptives. This almost paradoxical result is due to the fact that the sort of knowledge required to make fertilization and reimplantation of the embryo successful is also knowledge that can be employed to prevent pregnancy. For example, a knowledge of the biochemical mechanism by which a sperm penetrates an ovum and renders the ovum impenetrable to all other sperm cells can be turned in the direction either of promoting fertilization or of preventing it. Similarly, understanding how the embryo attaches itself to the wall of the uterus may lead to methods for either decreasing or increasing the likelihood of an embryo's becoming attached.

Third, research with animals using the techniques of in vitro fertilization and embryo transfer can be employed to determine the ways in which various environmental toxins and drugs affect the developing fetus. At present, research groups are exposing fertilized monkey ova to chemicals, then reimplanting them. The aim is to discover the means by which specific chemicals alter development and result in defective offspring.

Such information is of obvious value. If we are to be successful in eliminating or reducing human birth defects that are caused by chemical agents, then we must know what the chemicals do. Only in such ways can safe levels of exposure be determined and steps taken to avoid or prevent the presence of environmental toxins and harmful ingredients in drugs.

These are just three of the more direct advantages associated with in vitro fertilization. Other possibilities inherent in the procedure might make up a substantial list. Here are merely two of them.

Gene Repair. The way in which the genetic code contained in the DNA of a fertilized egg directs the development of the egg into a baby is far from being understood. Nonetheless, fragments of the total picture are now emerging. The technology of recombinant DNA (see the introduction to Chapter 6) has made it possible to isolate single genes and to identify their products. It is a long way

from this stage to being able, for example, to outline all of the steps by which the heart develops. Yet such work is promising enough to fuel the hope that we shall eventually understand the way in which DNA controls the entire developmental process.

This kind of detailed knowledge might make it possible to locate defects in genes that, when uncorrected, lead to faulty development of the fetus. At present, to avoid the birth of a child with birth defects associated with damaged or missing genes, abortion is the only recourse.

Additional knowledge might allow faulty genes to be replaced or repaired. Thus, developmental failures like Down's syndrome and spinal bifida or heritable genetic defects like Tay-Sachs disease might be treated at the level of the genes. An entirely new chapter of fetal medicine would then be opened.

Surrogate Mothers. This is perhaps the most dramatic possibility opened up by in vitro fertilization and embryo transfer. It has already been demonstrated in animal experiments that embryos from one female can be removed and transferred to another female to undergo the process of development and birth. Thus a cow that is considered genetically superior (in terms of milk production or resistance to disease, for example) can be artificially inseminated, and as many as sixteen embryos removed. After, the embryos can be implanted in the uteruses of less valuable cows. In this way, a desirable strain of cattle can be developed much more quickly than by ordinary breeding techniques.

Although a few people have advocated using "genetically superior" women as a source of ova and "less superior" women as surrogate mothers, it is highly unlikely that such a program will ever be endorsed by society. (See the introduction to Chapter 6 for the difficulties in determining genetic "superiority.")

Nevertheless, the basic procedure might

well be employed with human beings. A woman with an abnormal uterus who is not capable of a normal pregnancy might contribute an ovum that, after being fertilized in vitro, is implanted in the uterus of a second woman whose uterus has been prepared to receive it. The "host" or surrogate mother then carries the baby to term.

Surrogate mothers of a certain kind are already a fact of contemporary life. However, these cases involve artificial insemination, rather than in vitro fertilization and embryo transfer. But the practice of employing a surrogate mother has already become established to a limited degree. Furthermore, the wives of the couples using the services of a surrogate mother were themselves unable to bear children. However, it is only a short step from being unable to bear children to being *unwilling* to bear children, though physically able.

Thus, it is easy to imagine that some women might choose to free themselves from the rigors of pregnancy by hiring a surrogate mother. The employer would be the source of the ovum, which would then be fertilized in vitro and implanted as an embryo in the uterus of the surrogate. Women who could afford to do so could have their own natural children without ever having to be pregnant.

An additional possibility is what has been called "prenatal adoption." A woman unable to ovulate normally, but otherwise capable of pregnancy, might choose to "adopt" an embryo carried by another woman. The embryo would be transferred to the first woman's uterus (after she had been prepared by appropriate hormone injections), and there it would develop into a child. This procedure is not one that has been performed yet.

The possibilities inherent in in vitro fertilization and embryo transfer that have been mentioned here as sources of immediate or future benefits are all ones considered to be quite realistic by most researchers. By contrast, although it is possible to imagine such a thing, the development of "baby factories" or "hatcheries" similar to those described in *Brave New World* are technologically unlikely, judged in terms of current science and medicine. Machines would have to serve the function now served by the uterus, and designing such machines would require knowing enough about the needs of the developing fetus to reproduce that function. At the present, it is not possible even to state all the problems that would have to be solved.

Difficulties

This is not the place to discuss the ethical and social issues connected with the possibilities of in vitro fertilization mentioned above. There are aspects of the procedure itself and the current way in which it is being employed that some people find troublesome. Very briefly, we shall consider just five.

1. The ova that are removed for fertilization are not all used. Although they may all be mixed with sperm and several may be fertilized, only a single fertilized ovum is selected for implantation. The others are simply discarded.

For those who believe that human life begins at the moment of conception, the destruction of fertilized ova may be viewed as tantamount to abortion. Thus, for some people, the destruction may be regarded as destroying innocent human life.

Others, who are not prepared to ascribe the status of being a person to a fertilized ovum, may still be troubled by its pointless destruction. They may believe that its potentiality to develop, under certain conditions, into a human being at least requires that it be treated with concern and respect. Those who subscribe to such a view might well argue that the only legitimate form of in vitro fertilization is one in which the effort is made to fertilize only a single ovum. A failure in fertilization would then be similar to the failure that occurs naturally, and what would be eliminated would be the necessity of destroying fertilized eggs that cannot be implanted.

2. At present, when human in vitro fertilization is a relatively new procedure, it is impossible to assess the risks to the fetus and to the person it may become. A fetus that is conceived from an ovum that is removed to an alien environment and sustained by a nutrient solution that may not contain some necessary ingredients for development may well be at much greater risk than a fetus conceived in the ordinary way. Not only may the child be more likely to suffer defects evident at birth, but it may suffer some defects that will not show up until years later. (Mrs. Brown is rumored to have signed an agreement stating that she would submit to an abortion if there were signs that the fetus she was carrying was not developing normally.)

Experience has rather much taken the teeth out of this objection. The rate of birth defects in children born of in vitro fertilization is about three percent, virtually the same as that of ordinary births. So far there is no evidence that children conceived in vitro differ in any way from other children.

3. In vitro fertilization may encourage the development of eugenic ideas about improving the species. Rather than having children of their own, would-be parents might be motivated to seek out ova (and sperm) from people who possess physical and intellectual characteristics that are particularly admired. Thus, even without an organized plan of social eugenics (see Chapter 6), individuals might be tempted to follow their own eugenic notions.

4. Similarly, would-be parents might be inclined to exercise the potential for control over the sex of their offspring. Only males contain both an X and a Y chromosome, and their presence is detectable in the cells of the developing embryo. Determination of the sex of the embryo would allow the potential parents to decide whether they wish to have a male or female child. Consequently, a potential human being (the developing fetus) might be destroyed for what is basically a trivial reason.

5. In vitro fertilization is likely to promote a social climate in which having children becomes severed from the family. The procedure places emphasis on the mechanics of fertilization and, in doing so, minimizes the significance of the shared love and commitments of the parents of a child conceived by normal intercourse. Furthermore, the procedure offers the opportunity for an unmarried woman to have a child without having anything at all to do with the biological father of the child.

Obviously, these difficulties are not ones likely to be considered equally serious by everyone. Those who do not believe that life begins at conception will hardly be troubled by the discarding of unimplanted embryos. Additional research and experience will no doubt reduce whatever risks there may be to a fetus conceived in vitro. Sex choice is possible now by the use of amniocentesis so is not a problem unique to in vitro fertilization, and the same is true of the implementation of eugenic ideas. Finally, whether in vitro procedures actually lead to a weakening of the values associated with the family is partly an empirical question that only additional use of the method will show. Even if childbearing does become severed from current family structure, it still must be shown that this is itself something of which we ought to disapprove. It is clearly not impossible that alternative social structures for childbearing and childrearing might be superior to ones currently dominant in Western culture.

Research on in vitro fertilization was effectively halted in the United States when Congress declared a temporary moratorium on fetal research in 1974. Technically, the moratorium ended a year later when the former Department of Health, Education, and Welfare declared that all proposals for research involving federal funding would have to be approved by an Ethics Advisory Board. Although such a board was established, it never approved a single proposal. Before it was dissolved in 1979, the board held hearings and solicited testimony from experts in a variety of fields. In its final report, the board held that research into in vitro fertilization and embryo transfer is ethically acceptable.

Despite the board's conclusion, no secretary of the department has seen fit to lift the de facto moratorium. As a result, most of the research done in the United States has involved little more than observation of patients. Some privately funded work has been done, but for the most part American researchers have been dependent on research conducted in England and Australia.

Understandably frustrated, some researchers worry that the lack of major research efforts will slow our understanding of basic biological processes that are involved in conception and development. In particular, the hope that we might detect and repair defective genes in vitro and generally increase our understanding of genetic diseases may suffer a long delay in being realized.

ARTIFICIAL INSEMINATION

In 1909, an unusual letter appeared in the professional journal *Medical World*. A. D. Hard, the author of the letter, claimed that when he was a student at Jefferson Medical College in Philadelphia, a wealthy businessman and his wife consulted a physician on the faculty about their inability to conceive a child.

A detailed examination of each of the people showed that the man was incapable of producing sperm. The case was presented for discussion in a class of which Hard was a member. According to Hard, the class suggested that semen should be taken from the "best-looking member of the class" and used to inseminate the wife.

The letter claimed that this was done while the woman was anesthetized and that neither the husband nor the wife was told about the process. The patient became pregnant and gave birth to a son. The husband was then told how the pregnancy was produced, and although he was pleased with the result, he asked that his wife not be informed.

The event described by Hard took place in 1884, and there is reason to believe that Hard was "the best-looking member of the class."

The Philadelphia case is generally acknowledged to be the first recorded instance of artificial insemination of donor sperm in a human patient. However, the process of artificial insemination itself has a much longer history. Arab horsemen in the fourteenth century apparently inseminated mares with semen-soaked sponges, and in the eighteenth century the Italian physiologist Spallansani documented experiments in which he fertilized dogs, reptiles, and frogs.

The first recorded case of the artificial insemination of a human being occurred in 1790, when the English physician John Hunter used semen obtained from a husband to inseminate his wife. Sporadic uses of the technique continued to occur in England, France, and the United States, and during the early part of the present century, they became more and more frequent. At present, probably more than two thousand children a year are born in this country who were conceived by artificial insemination.

Artificial insemination has become generally recognized as a legitimate medical procedure. The process is employed by hospitals, fertility clinics, and physicians who specialize in problems involving conception. Before looking at some of the ethical and legal issues involved in artificial insemination, it is useful to consider some relevant factual information about the process.

The Artificial Insemination Procedure

Artificial insemination is a relatively simple procedure. It is initiated when the woman's body temperature indicates that ovulation is to take place in one or two days. It is then repeated one or two more times until her body temperature shows that ovulation is completed. Typically, three inseminations are performed during a monthly cycle.

In the insemination, the patient is usually placed in a position so that her hips are raised. A semen specimen, collected earlier through masturbation or taken from a sperm bank, is placed in a syringe attached to a narrow tube or catheter. The catheter is gently inserted into the cervical canal, and the semen is slowly injected into the uterus. The patient then stays in her position for fifteen or twenty minutes to increase the chances that the sperm will fertilize an ovum.

The overall success rate of artificial insemination is about 85 percent. Success on the first attempt is quite rare, and the highest rate occurs in the third month. In unusual cases, efforts may be made every month for as long as six months or a year. Such efforts are continued, however, only when a detailed examination shows that the woman is not suffering from some unrecognized problem preventing her from becoming pregnant.

When sperm taken from donors is used, the rate of congenital abnormalities is a little lower than that for the general population. There seems to be no evidence to support the fear that manipulating the sperm causes any harm. (Many physicians prefer to employ fresh, rather than frozen, sperm to minimize the amount of environmental change the sperm is subjected to. Other physicians claim that frozen sperm is to be preferred, for it provides a means of screening out defective cells or chromosome abnormalities.)

Reasons for Seeking Artificial Insemination

Artificial insemination may be sought for a variety of reasons. When a couple is involved, the reasons are almost always associated with physiological or physical factors that make it impossible for the couple to conceive a child in the usual sexual way.

About 10 percent of all married couples are infertile, and 40 percent of those cases are due to factors involving the male. In some instances, the male may be unable to produce any sperm at all (a condition called asospermia), or the number of sperm the male produces may be too low to make impregnation of the female likely (a condition called oligospermia). In other cases, adequate numbers of sperm cells may be produced, but they may not function normally. They may not be sufficiently motile to make their way past the vaginal canal and through the opening to the uterus. Hence, their chances of reaching and penetrating an ovum are slight. Finally, the male may suffer from a neurological condition that makes ejaculation impossible or from a disease (such as diabetes) which renders him impotent.

If the female cannot ovulate, or if her fallopian tubes are blocked so that ova cannot descend, then artificial insemination can accomplish nothing. (See the section above on in vitro fertilization.) Yet there are factors affecting the female that artificial insemination can be helpful in overcoming. For example, if the female has a vaginal environment that is biochemically inhospitable to sperm, then artificial insemination may be successful. Because the sperm need not pass through the vagina, they have a better chance of surviving. Also, if the female has a small cervix (the opening to the uterus) or if her uterus is in an abnormal position, then artificial insemination may be used to deliver the sperm to an advantageous position for fertilization, a position they otherwise might not reach.

A couple might also seek artificial insemination for genetic reasons. Both may be carriers of a recessive gene for a genetic disorder (Tay-Sachs disease, for example) or the male may be the carrier of a dominant gene for a genetic disorder (Huntington's chorea, for example). In either case, the couple may not want to run the statistical risk of their child's being born with a genetic disease. To avoid the possibility, they may choose to make use of artificial insemination with sperm secured from a donor.

The traditional recipient of artificial insemination is a married woman who, in consultation with her husband, has decided to have a child. Some physiological or physical difficulty in conceiving leads them to turn to artificial insemination.

But the traditional recipient is no longer the only recipient. Those seeking to have the procedure performed now include single women who wish to have a child but do not wish to have it fathered in the usual fashion. Some estimates place the number of such women at 150 a year. The percentages of such inseminations may increase in the future if the notion of being a single parent continues to be met with acceptance or approval within our society. The increase may be quite rapid if the attitudes of physicians, in particular, change. At present, single women who wish to become mothers are likely to be discouraged, and some physicians will not accept them as candidates for artificial insemination.

Types of Artificial Insemination

Artificial insemination can be divided into types in accordance with the source of the sperm employed in the procedure.

Artificial insemination (homologous) uses sperm obtained from the male partner.

The name of the process is usually abbreviated as AIH, and the H is frequently taken to stand for "husband," While it is true that the male of a couple is most frequently the woman's husband, legal marriage is not necessary for AIH. The male need only be, in some sense, the functional equivalent of a husband.

Artificial insemination (heterologous) uses sperm from a sperm donor. For this reason, the process is usually referred to by the abbreviation AID. The use of semen obtained from a donor is the most frequent of AI procedures, and it is the one that gives rise to most of the social and legal issues surrounding the practice.

Artificial insemination (confused) employs a mixture of sperm from the male partner and sperm obtained from a donor. CAI, as it is commonly called, has no particular biological advantage, but it does offer a couple a degree of psychological support. Because they cannot be sure that it was not sperm from the male partner that resulted in conception, they may be more inclined to accept the child as the product of their union. The role of the third-party sperm donor is thus psychologically minimized.

Sperm Donors

Sperm donors are typically selected from medical-student and hospital-staff volunteers. An effort is made to employ as donors people in excellent health with a high level of intellectual ability. Their family histories are reviewed to reduce the possibility of transmitting a genetic disorder, and their blood type is checked to determine its compatibility with that of the AID recipient.

Such general physical features of the donor as body type, hair and eye color, and complexion are matched in a rough way with those of the potential parents. To be a donor, an individual must also be known to be fertile. This means that he must already be a biological parent or that he must fall within the normal range in several semen analyses.

Donors are typically paid for their services. What is more, their identity is kept secret from the recipient and her husband. A coding system is ordinarily used both to preserve the anonymity of the donor and to ensure that the same donor is used in all inseminations.

Sperm contributed by a donor might be employed in an insemination within one to three hours after the semen is obtained. As mentioned earlier, some physicians prefer to use freshly obtained sperm in the procedure. But sperm may also be maintained in a frozen condition and, after being restored to the proper temperature, used in the same way as fresh sperm. Sperm banks are no more than freezers containing racks of coded plastic tubes holding donated sperm.

The semen stored in sperm banks is not necessarily that of anonymous donors. For a variety of reasons, individuals may wish to have their sperm preserved and pay a fee to a sperm-bank operator for this service. For example, a man planning a vasectomy (see the section on sterilization below) or one expecting to become sterile because of a progressive disease may store his sperm in the event that he may later want to father a child.

Issues in Artificial Insemination

Artificial insemination presents a great variety of moral, legal, and social issues. The truth is, most of those issues have not been addressed in a thorough fashion. Legal scholars have explored some of the consequences that AI has for traditional legal doctrines of paternity, legitimacy, and inheritance. They have also made recommendations for formulating new laws (or reformulating old ones) to take into account the reality of the practice of AI.

Others who have written about AI have mostly focused on its potential for altering the relationship between husbands and wives and for producing undesirable social changes. Many of the objections to in vitro fertilization have also been offered to artificial insemination. For example, it has been argued that AI will take the love out of sexual procreation and make it a purely mechanical process, that AI will promote the practice of eugenics and so denigrate the worth of babies that fall short of some ideal, and that AI is just another step down the road toward the society of *Brave New World.*

While such issues are of great importance, they have usually been discussed in such a general fashion that specific ethical questions about the use of artificial insemination as a medical procedure have rarely been raised. As a result, those questions have not been subjected to the dialectical process of argument and criticism that is important in helping us arrive at reasoned opinions.

Some of the issues that need close attention from philosophers concern individual rights and responsibilities. For example, does a man who has served as a sperm donor have any special moral responsibilities? He certainly must have some responsibilities. For example, it would be wrong for him to lie about any genetic diseases in his family history. But does he have any responsibilities to the child that is produced by AI employing his sperm? If donating sperm is no different from donating blood, then perhaps he does not. But is such a comparison apt?

Can a child born as a result of AI legitimately demand to know the name of his biological father? We need not assume that mere curiosity might motivate such a request. Someone might need to know his family background in order to determine how likely it is that a potential child might have a genetic disorder. After all, it is unreasonable to assume that a donor is fully informed about his own biological background. Perhaps the current practice of maintaining the anonymity of sperm donors is not one that can stand critical scrutiny.

Should a woman be allowed to order sperm donated by someone who approximates her concept of an ideal person? Should she be able to request a donor from a certain ethnic group, with particular eye and hair color, certain minimum or maximum height, physical attractiveness, with evidence of intelligence, and so on? At present, the physician who performs the procedure also makes the choice of the donor. But why should the physician be granted the right to make the selection? One might argue that allowing the physician to exercise such a power violates the autonomy of the AI recipient.

A number of other ethical questions are easily raised about AI: Does any woman (married or single, or any age) have the right to demand AI? Should a physician make AID available to a married woman even if her husband is opposed?

Other questions concerning the proper procedures to follow in the practice of AI are also of considerable significance. For example, how thoroughly must sperm donors be screened for genetic defects? What standards of quality must sperm as a biological material be required to satisfy? What physical, educational, or general social traits (if any) should individual donors possess? Should records be maintained and shared through an established network to prevent the marriage or mating of individuals born from AID with the same biological father?

At present, these questions have been answered only by individual physicians or clinics, if at all. There are no general medical or legal policies that govern the practice of AI. Even if present practices are adequate, most people would agree that there is a need to develop uniform policies to regulate AI.

Obviously, we have touched upon only a few of the ethical and social issues that the practice of artificial insemination generates. Indeed, at the moment, it is not wholly clear even what the more significant issues may be. In this area of medical ethics, in particular, philosophers still have a great deal of work to do.

SURROGATE PREGNANCY

We have already mentioned surrogate mothers in connection with in vitro fertilization. In that connection, a surrogate mother is one who supplies an ovum which may be fertilized and implanted into a host mother or one who serves as the host mother and receives an embryo from the biological parents. These biological possibilities are still under development.

Surrogate mothers in the more usual sense are women who agree to become pregnant by means of artificial insemination with sperm from the male of a married couple. The surrogate mother carries the baby to term, then turns the baby over to the couple for adoption. Surrogate mothers are typically sought by couples who wish to have a child with whom they have some genetic link and who have been unsuccessful in conceiving one themselves.

Various legal complications surround surrogate pregnancy. Although it is not prohibited by state laws, it is not acknowledged as legitimate, either. A number of bills have been introduced into state legislatures either to regulate the arrangements or to forbid them, but none has been passed into law.

A major problem has been finding a legal way to pay women who undertake to be surrogate mothers. Adoption laws forbid the selling of children or even the payment of money to one of the parents in connection with adoption. A Michigan appellate court decision, which the Supreme Court refused to review, held that a couple had the right to the services of a surrogate mother but did not have the right to compensate her for acting in that capacity.

Since a child born to a surrogate mother is legally her child, the child must be adopted by the couple securing her services. How then can the surrogate mother be paid? Some women have simply volunteered to be surrogate mothers so that the issue of payment would not arise. In general the difficulty has been resolved by paying the mother to compensate her for the loss of her time and for her inconvenience. Technically, then, the surrogate mother is not being paid for conceiving and bearing a child, nor is she being paid for the child who is handed over for adoption.

The typical fee paid a surrogate mother is about ten thousand dollars. If the arrangements are made by an attorney or by an organization like the Infertility Center of New York, additional fees must be paid. The couple seeking the service must also pay the medical and hospital-delivery expenses of the surrogate mother. Total costs range from twenty to twenty-five thousand dollars.

Some of the same reasons that can be offered to justify in vitro fertilization and embryo transfer can also be offered for surrogate pregnancy. Fundamentally, those couples who wish to have a child of their own but are unable to do so because of some uncorrectable medical difficulty experienced by the woman view surrogate pregnancy as the only hope remaining to them. Some rule out adoption because of the relative shortage of available infants, and some simply want there to be some genetic connection between them and the child. Some people are simply quite desperate to have a child of their own.

Some critics have charged that surrogate pregnancy is no more than a specialized form of prostitution. A woman, in effect, rents out her body for a period of time and is paid for doing so. Such a criticism rests on the assumption that prostitution is morally wrong, and this is a claim that at least some would

deny is correct. Furthermore, the criticism fails to take into account the differences in aims. Some surrogate mothers have volunteered their services with no expectation of monetary reward, and some women have agreed to be surrogate mothers at the request of their sisters. Even those who are paid mention that part of their motivation is to help those couples who so desperately want a child. Far from condemning surrogate mothers as acting immorally, it is perhaps possible to view at least some of them as acting in a morally heroic way by contributing to the good of others through their actions.

Perhaps the most serious objection to surrogate mothers is that they are likely to be recruited from the ranks of those most in need of money. Women of the upper and middle income groups are not likely to serve as surrogate mothers. Women with low-paying jobs or no jobs at all are obviously the prime candidates for recruiters. It might be charged, then, that women who become surrogate mothers are being exploited by those who have money enough to pay for their services.

However, merely paying someone in need of money to do something does not constitute exploitation. To make such a charge stick, it would be necessary to show that women who become surrogate mothers are under a great deal of social and economic pressure and have no other realistic options. Furthermore, it could be argued that, within limits, individuals have a right to do with their bodies as they choose. If a woman freely decides to earn money by serving as a surrogate mother, then we have no more reason to object to her decision than we would have to object to a man's decision to earn money by working as a construction laborer.

There is good reason to believe that the practice of employing surrogate mothers is likely to increase in the near future. The ethical and social issues are far from being resolved to the general satisfaction of our society. Although surrogate mothers have been featured numerous times in newspapers and magazines, the whole issue of surrogate parenthood has received much less attention than it deserves from philosophers and other ethical theorists.

STERILIZATION

A person is *sterile* when he or she is biologically incapable of reproduction, either because of an inability to produce or supply sex cells (gametes) or because of a more general physiological condition.

Sterility may be the natural result of a variety of causes. In women, for example, undeveloped fallopian tubes may make it impossible for ova to descend to be fertilized. In men, viral diseases such as mumps may impair the capacity of the testes to produce sperm.

Sterility may also be an incidental result of a medical or surgical procedure required for the treatment of an illness. Radiation therapy, for example, may lead to sterility in both men and women. Or the treatment of certain kinds of cancer may require the removal of the ovaries, thus destroying a woman's ability to produce ova.

Finally, sterility may be produced deliberately by surgical intervention. That is, surgery may be performed with the sole aim of rendering the patient incapable of biological reproduction. The most common procedure employed with men is *vasectomy*. This involves the surgical removal of a segment of the vas deferens, the tube that transfers sperm cells to the ejaculatory duct. Although ejaculation remains unimpaired, the ejaculate will no longer contain sperm cells. The surgery involved is relatively minor.

The most frequent sterilization procedure used with women is *tubal ligation*. A surgical incision is made in the abdominal wall to gain access to the fallopian tubes. Then the tubes are simply tied off so that the ova produced by the ovaries cannot descend to the uterus. The surgery has more risk associated with it than does vasectomy, but it is considered a relatively simple and safe procedure. Laparoscopic tubal ligation is even less invasive and has become a relatively common procedure.

The next most common means of female sterilization is *total hysterectomy*. In this procedure, the entire uterus (womb) is removed. After an ovum is fertilized by a sperm cell, during the ordinary course of development, the embryo attaches itself to the wall of the uterus. Thus, removal of the uterus makes it impossible for a woman to have children. (There must be good medical reasons to remove the ovaries when a hysterectomy is performed, for their excision leads to hormonal disturbances. Removing the ovaries just for the purpose of sterilization is not considered good medical practice.) A hysterectomy is regarded as a major surgical procedure, and it involves a much greater risk to the patient than tubal ligation. Today the procedure is not regarded as justifiable if its only purpose is sterilization.

Voluntary Sterilization

Some people choose sterilization voluntarily as a method of contraception. Since it is almost totally reliable as a means of birth control, those who are certain that they want to surrender their option to have children may select sterilization for this reason.

The preferred procedures for contraceptive sterilization are vasectomy and tubal ligation. Although the consequences of both can sometimes be reversed surgically (less often with vasectomy), the results are more reasonably thought of as permanent. In 1983, the last year for which statistics are available, 622,000 women and 455,000 men underwent sterilization for contraceptive reasons. For married women, sterilization has become more favored than birth-control pills. In 1965, only 7 percent of married women were sterilized for contraception, while 24 percent relied on a birth-control pill. By 1983, 26 percent employed sterilization, and 20 percent employed a birth-control pill.

Rates of sterilization have also increased for married men. In 1965, only 5 percent had been sterilized for contraception, while by 1983 the number was up to 15 percent.

Except for those who accept a natural law view of sexual reproduction, voluntary sterilization as a contraceptive measure has not been *in itself* the source of major ethical or social controversy. However, in connection with questions about coercion and individual rights under publicly funded welfare and medical assistance programs, voluntary sterilization has been at the center of a political and ethical storm.

In 1973, it was called to public attention that a clinic in Alabama had sterilized a number of girls under circumstances that suggested either a misunderstanding of what was involved or lack of proper consent. Two of the girls, Minni Relf (age fourteen) and Mary Alice Relf (twelve) were the daughters of Lonni Relf, a poor black man from Montgomery. Mr. Relf was called to testify at a federal hearing in Washington. "I didn't want it done," he told the committee.

Partly as a result of the hearing, federal regulations were issued in 1974 to attempt to guarantee that sterilization would always be voluntary. Despite the regulations, studies by both an independent consumer group and the federal General Accounting Office showed that abuses were not only continuing, but actually seemed to be increasing.

In particular, vulnerable groups such as Indian and Hispanic women, poor blacks, minors, and women just recovering from pregnancy were found to be the targets of a disproportionately large number of sterilizations of doubtful legitimacy. Furthermore, those who agreed to sterilization were often subjected to full hysterectomies, rather than the simpler and safer procedure of tubal ligation. The reason for selecting the more complicated and dangerous procedure seemed to have more to do with the surgeon's desire for challenge than with any legitimate medical reason.

When asked why he chose to perform a hysterectomy to sterilize a patient, one surgeon is reported to have replied: "It's more of a challenge. You know, a well-trained chimpanzee can do a tubal ligation . . . . [A hysterectomy] is good training."

In 1977, the federal government reaffirmed its regulations governing sterilization and proposed to cut off funds to clinics and hospitals if there was evidence that the rules were not being followed. The regulations require that a person be given a "fair" explanation of the sterilization procedure, that the benefits and risks be pointed out, and that the irreversible character of the procedure be made clear. The person must also be informed orally before the question of consent is raised that a refusal to accept sterilization will not be used as a basis for denying welfare benefits. The same information must also appear on a consent form, and a seventy-two-hour waiting period is required between the time the consent form is signed and the surgery is performed.

In addition, in keeping with the 1974 regulations, federal funds cannot be used to sterilize anyone under the age of twenty-one or anyone who is not mentally competent. A federal district court injunction extended these same restrictions to sterilization under state laws.

The federal regulations are clearly aimed at protecting the welfare of those groups that are most vulnerable to pressures to consent to sterilization—the poor, minors, and the mentally incompetent. However, critics of the regulations maintain that they are so strict that they actually deny to women who are dependent on public assistance for their medical care the right to make a decision about their own bodies. While women with money can ordinarily arrange for sterilization without question or delay purely as a result of their own decision, poor women must have their decisions subjected to a government policy and its requirements. Thus, according to the critics, the regulations are no more than a case of unjustifiable paternalism.

Opponents of the regulations object particularly to the mandatory waiting period. They point out that it prevents a woman from being sterilized at the end of a pregnancy while still in the hospital. If she chooses sterilization surgery, she must say that she does, then return to the hospital at additional public and private cost, and once more undergo the risk of anesthesia. Consequently, poor women are more subject to government interference in their private lives than are women with adequate financial resources.

Even the requirement that minors be considered ineligible for sterilization paid for by federal funds is not acceptable to critics of the regulations. They contend that age is not itself an indicator of maturity. In their view, it should be left up to the patient's physician to determine whether she adequately understands the nature and consequences of sterilization—even if the patient is a minor. Like any other medical or surgical procedure, informed consent should be required, and it is the job of the physician to make certain this condition is met. If it is not, then the physician ought to be held liable.

Both defenders and critics of the regulations agree that the sterilization of the mentally incompetent poses special problems.

Involuntary Sterilization and the Mentally Incompetent

Starting at the beginning of this century, a complicated network of federal, state, and even city laws and regulations governing sterilization has developed. Many of the laws were inspired by the eugenics movement of the 1920s and 1930s and were intended to "improve" the human race by preventing the "mentally and morally defective" from reproducing.

The most influential court decision from this period was the 1927 Supreme Court ruling in *Buck* v. *Bell*. Carrie Buck was (in the language of the time) a "feeble-minded" white patient at an institution in Virginia. She was the daughter of a feeble-minded woman confined to the same institution, and she herself was the mother of an illegitimate feeble-minded child.

According to a Virginia law, whenever the superintendent of a state institution considered it in the best interest of the patient and society, a patient "afflicted with hereditary forms of insanity and imbecility" might be considered a candidate for sterilization. A hearing was then held by a special board, and if the board ruled in favor of sterilization, then the patient or her representative might appeal to the courts. Otherwise, the sterilization would take place.

An appeal all the way to the Supreme Court was made on behalf of Carrie Buck, and Justice Oliver Wendell Holmes wrote the majority opinion upholding the Virginia law:

> We have seen more than once that the public welfare may call upon the best citizens for their lives. It would be strange if it could not call upon those who already sap the strength of the state for these lesser sacrifices . . . in order to prevent our being swamped with incompetence. It is better for all the world if, instead of waiting to execute degenerate offspring for crime, or to let them starve for their imbecility, society can prevent those who are manifestly unfit from continuing their kind . . . Three generations of imbeciles are enough.

The Holmes opinion relied on an analogy with laws requiring vaccination. The implicit view was that if we can require vaccination in order to protect the society from the spread of infectious diseases, then we can require sterilization to protect society from the spread of feeble-mindedness.

Holmes's opinion and the sterilization laws themselves rest on assumptions about the nature of mental retardation and mental illness that we now recognize to be both simplistic and fundamentally in error. Mental deficiency varies greatly in severity and can have many causes, many of which are quite unknown. Although some forms of mental impairment involve an indirect genetic component, the most common forms do not. Furthermore, there is no evidence at all to show a causal connection between mental deficiency and crime. So far as "hereditary forms of insanity" are concerned, there is good evidence to show that schizophrenia involves a genetic factor, but the evidence is not conclusive. In addition, the pattern of heritability is not as simple as that assumed in the nineteenth and early twentieth centuries.

The sterilization laws and the Supreme Court decision are an outstanding example of how common beliefs and prejudices can do a great deal of social damage when they are used as a substitute for reliable scientific knowledge. To some extent, we are continuing to pay today for the complacent ignorance of an earlier time.

Some twenty-seven states still have so-called involuntary sterilization laws. Yet medical, legal, and public attitudes toward sterilizing the mentally deficient have undergone a radical change. Today no responsible person advocates the compulsory sterilization of the mentally incompetent. However, most of those who do not oppose sterilization in principle also believe that people who are mentally impaired ought to have the same right to sterilization as those of normal intelligence.

The basic moral and social difficulty consists in providing access to sterilization for the mentally deficient, while protecting them from coercion. The federal regulations discussed earlier forbid the sterilization of minors and those incapable of giving informed consent.

Most professionals who work with the mentally handicapped tend to support these restrictions. At present, there are some five million mentally deficient people in the United States. Most of them can care for themselves, and many hold jobs and have families. There are, however, about three hundred thousand people who are profoundly retarded and require care and supervision.

It is this last group that presents the most difficulty for any policy about sterilization. If they are incapable of giving informed consent, then under the government regulations, they cannot receive sterilization surgery. This has led some people to object that in attempting to protect the mentally deficient, the restrictions deny them a right open to others. Furthermore, the restrictions implicitly force the families of such people to bear all the responsibility for the retarded person's sexual conduct and any resulting pregnancies or births. Families are thus deprived of a means of dealing with the problems that they face.

This is essentially the view taken by three groups of parents in Hartford, Connecticut, who decided to fight a legal battle to have their daughters sterilized. The girls are aged twelve, thirteen, and fifteen; all are blind and severely retarded, and one is deaf.

A hospital in Hartford refused to allow sterilization surgery to be performed, even though the parents requested it and physicians who were consulted agreed that the surgery would be beneficial to the girls. The parents tried several other private hospitals in the area, but they also refused the sterilization request.

The federal regulations do not apply to patients whose expenses are privately paid. Nevertheless, the lawsuits based on the regulations have had a general effect on the medical community and made hospitals and physicians reluctant to perform sterilizations in cases in which consent is at issue. Because the children in the Hartford case were not institutionalized, relevant state laws were not applicable to them either. As a result, the hospitals in Hartford moved in the direction of legal and social pressure and refused to allow the sterilizations. The case dramatically reveals the difficulty of finding a satisfactory way of protecting mentally defective people, while allowing actions to be taken in their interest.

ETHICAL THEORIES AND REPRODUCTIVE CONTROL

One of the themes of Mary Shelley's famous novel *Frankenstein* is that it is both wrong and dangerous to tamper with the natural forces of life. It is wrong because it disturbs the natural order of things, and it is dangerous because it unleashes forces beyond human control. The "monster" that is animated by Dr. Victor Frankenstein stands as a warning and reproach to all who seek to impose their will on the world through the powers of scientific technology.

The fundamental ethical question about the technology of human reproductive control is whether it ought to be employed at all. Is it simply wrong for us to use our knowledge of human biology to exercise power over the processes of human reproduction?

The natural law view, as represented by currently accepted doctrines of the Roman Catholic Church, suggests that all three of the techniques for controlling human reproduction that we have discussed here are fundamentally wrong.

Children may ordinarily be expected as a result of sexual union within marriage. However, if no measures are wrongfully taken to frustrate the possibility of their birth (contraception, for example), then a married couple has no obligation to attempt to conceive children by means such as artificial insemination or in vitro fertilization.

Indeed, those processes themselves are inherently objectionable. Artificial insemination requires male masturbation, which is prima facie wrong, since it is an act that can be considered to be unnatural, given the natural end of sex. Furthermore, AI, even when semen from the husband is used, tends to destroy the values inherent in the married state. It makes conception a mechanical act.

In vitro fertilization is open to the same objections. In addition, the process itself involves the destruction of fertilized ova. On the view that human conception takes place at the moment of fertilization, this means that the discarding of unimplanted embryos amounts to the destruction of human life.

Sterilization, whether voluntary or not, is also inherently wrong, for it involves defeating the natural purpose of the reproductive organs. Furthermore, according to the principle of totality, we have a natural duty to preserve the integrity of our bodies. This means that any procedure that involves "mutilation" or the destruction of the capacity of an organ to function properly is morally wrong. Thus, vasectomies and tubal ligations are both ruled out. (Of course, if sterilization is the unintended consequence of a surgical procedure required to save the patient's life, then it is not wrong. We have a natural duty to preserve our lives, and the principle of double effect justifies such unintended sterilizations.)

On the utilitarian view, no reproductive technology is in itself objectionable. The question that has to be answered is whether the use of any particular procedure, in general or in a certain case, is likely to lead to more good than not. In general, it is reasonable to believe that a utilitarian would be likely to approve of the three sorts of procedures we have discussed here.

However, it is worth mentioning that a

rule utilitarian might well oppose any or all of the procedures. If there is strong evidence to support the view that the use of reproductive technology will lead to a society in which the welfare of its members will not be served, then a rule utilitarian would be on firm ground in arguing that reproductive technology ought to be abandoned.

According to Ross's ethical theory, we have prima facie duties of beneficence. That is, we have an obligation to assist others in bettering their lives. This suggests that the use of reproductive technology may be justified as a means to promote the well-being of others. For example, if a couple desires to have a child but is unable to conceive one, then either in vitro fertilization procedures or artificial insemination might be employed to help them satisfy their shared desire.

Similarly, if someone wishes to be sterilized for the purpose of contraception, then there seems to be no reason why he or she should not be. Of course, there is also a prima facie duty to avoid causing anyone harm. This means that we have an obligation to make certain that a candidate for voluntary sterilization understands the nature and consequences of the procedure. In effect, informed consent is required. Thus, in cases where consent may be in question, sterilization may not be legitimate.

Is the involuntary sterilization of the mentally incompetent ever right on Ross's view? One could argue that it sometimes is. If a person is unable to care for herself, then it may be that we have a duty to promote her interest by removing the possibility that she will be burdened by a child. It may be that by performing a sterilization procedure we are doing her no harm and are, in fact, acting beneficently.

Kantian principles do not seem to supply grounds for objecting either to in vitro fertilization or to artificial insemination as inherently wrong. However, the maxim involved in each action must always be one that satisfies the categorical imperative. Consequently, some instances of in vitro fertilization and artificial insemination would no doubt be morally wrong.

It is not clear whether Kantian principles would make the involuntary sterilization of the mentally retarded an unethical procedure. One could argue that sterilization without consent would violate the autonomy of the person. The act might provide benefits for the person's family or for society, but this would offer no legitimate justification. We would be treating the person as a means to satisfy the wishes of others and not as an end in herself.

However, in contrast, one might argue that in dealing with a severely retarded person who is incapable of giving meaningful consent, we have a duty to treat the person in a way that acknowledges her intrinsic worth. This may mean doing for her what she would do for herself if she were rational and seeking her own welfare. Thus, sterilization might be justifiable if it is done for her sake only.

The technology of reproduction is a reality of ordinary life. So far it has made our society into neither a dystopia nor a utopia. It is just one set of tools among the many others that science and medicine have forged.

Yet the tools are powerful ones, and we should beware of allowing familiarity to produce indifference. The moral and social issues raised by reproductive technology are just as real as the technology. So far we have not treated some of them with the seriousness that they deserve.

THE SELECTIONS

The case for in vitro fertilization, artificial insemination, and surrogate pregnancy is based substantially on the desire of individuals to have children of their own. While not denying the value of overcoming infertility, Leon R. Kass, in " 'Making Babies' Revisited," calls into question our easy endorsement of reproductive technology. He is most concerned over the consequences the technology (particularly in vitro fertilization) will have on the traditional role that lineage and the family play in supplying a basis for a "civilized community" and for a child's self-identity and self-respect. If we continue along the path we have taken, Kass argues, we may, like Oedipus, end by destroying our lives and our families. We too may have to pay "the price of presumption, of overconfidence, of the overweening desire to master and control one's fate."

In "The Case Against Surrogate Parenting," Herbert T. Krimmel argues that it is morally wrong for someone "to create a human life with the intention of giving it up." Thus, Krimmel disapproves both of the role of surrogate mother and of artificial insemination with donor sperm. In both cases, he argues, a child should be desired for its own sake, not as a means for attaining some other end. If surrogate motherhood is permitted, Krimmel claims, there is a risk that we will come to view children as little more than commodities that we can exploit for our own ends. Further, the way is opened for the practice of eugenics. Finally, both surrogate pregnancies and artificial insemination with donor sperm exert pressures upon the family structure. The child of the surrogate mother is taken away from her, the sperm donor never knows his children, and both single females and males can become parents.

Unlike Kass and Krimmel, Gillian Hanscombe sees the possibility of becoming a single parent a major advantage of reproductive technology. In "The Right to Lesbian Parenthood," she argues that homosexual parents are entitled to the same treatment from physicians and institutions as heterosexual ones. The objection that lesbian women should not

be allowed to reproduce by artificial insemination is not one that can be supported by relevant evidence, Hanscombe claims. No studies have demonstrated that lesbian mothering is any different from heterosexual mothering or that children of lesbian mothers "fall victim to negative psychosexual developmental influences." She mentions instances of what she considers to be groundless prejudice against lesbian women by the medical establishment.

In "Artificial Insemination and Donor Responsibility," Ronald Munson argues that there are no morally significant differences between the sperm donor and the blood donor. Prima facie it may seem that there should be, given the fact that sperm may lead to the production of a child. Sperm and blood donors both have some responsibilities by virtue of the fact that both supply a product. However, even though the sperm donor supplies a causal condition for pregnancy, he is not the causal agent of the pregnancy. Lacking causal responsibility, he also lacks moral responsibility for any resulting child.

In the last selection, George J. Annas lists three possible positions that courts can take with respect to the sterilization of the mentally retarded: to refuse approval where consent is not possible, to approve when sterilization is in the best interest of the individual, and to take a "*Quinlan*-type" approach and leave the decision in the hands of the individual's family and physician. Annas reviews the New Jersey case of Lee Ann Grady, in which the state Supreme Court, the same court that made the *Quinlan* decision, took the second approach. Most important, Annas presents the kind of evidence the court considered relevant to establish that sterilization is indeed in the best interest of the individual. Annas suggests that this approach is one that avoids the drawbacks of total prohibition and also provides protection for the person concerned.

"Making Babies" Revisited

Leon R. Kass

I.

Many people rejoiced at the birth of Louise Brown. Some were pleased by the technical accomplishment, many were pleased that she was born apparently in good health. But most of us shared the joy of her parents, who after a long, frustrating, and fruitless period, at last had the pleasure and blessing of a child of their own. The desire to have a child of one's own is acknowledged to be a powerful and deep-seated human desire—some have called it "instinctive"—and the satisfaction of this desire, by the relief of infertility, is said to be one major goal of continuing the work with *in vitro* fertilization and embryo transfer. That this is a worthy goal few, if any, would deny.

Yet let us explore what is meant by *"to have a child of one's own."* First, what is meant by *"to have"*? Is the crucial meaning that of gestating and bearing? Or is it "to have" as a possession? Or is it to nourish and to rear, the child being the embodiment of one's activity as teacher and guide? Or is it rather to provide someone who descends and comes after, someone who will replace oneself in the family line or preserve the family tree by new sproutings and branchings?

More significantly, what is meant by *"one's own"*? What sense of one's own is important? A scientist might define "one's own" in terms of carrying one's own genes. Though in some sense correct, this cannot be humanly decisive. For Mr. Brown or for most of us, it would not be a matter of indifference if the sperm used to fertilize the egg were provided by an identical twin brother—whose genes would be, of course, the same as his. Rather, the humanly crucial sense of "one's own," the sense that leads most people to choose their own, rather than to adopt, is captured in such phrases as "my seed," "flesh of my flesh," "sprung from my loins." More accurately, since "one's own" is not the own of one but of *two*, the desire to have a child of "one's own" is a *couple's desire* to embody, out of the conjugal union of their separate bodies, a child who is flesh of their separate flesh made one. This archaic language may sound quaint, but I would argue that this is precisely what is being celebrated by most people who rejoice at the birth of Louise Brown, whether they would articulate it this way or not. Mr. and Mrs. Brown, by the birth of their daughter, fulfill this aspect of their separate sexual natures and of their married life together, they acquire descendants and a new branch of their joined family tree, and the child Louise is given solid and unambiguous roots from which she has sprung and by which she will be nourished.

If this were to be the *only* use made of embryo transfer, and if providing *in this sense* "a child of one's own" were indeed the sole reason for the clinical use of the techniques, there could be no objection. Yet there will almost certainly be other uses, involving third parties, to satisfy the desire "to have" a child of "one's own" in different senses of "to have" and "one's own." I am not merely speculating about future possibilities. With the technology to effect human *in vitro* fertilization and embryo transfer comes the *immediate* possibility of egg donation (egg from donor, sperm from husband), embryo donation (egg and sperm from outside of the marriage), and foster pregnancy (host surrogate for gestation).

Nearly everyone agrees that these circumstances are morally and perhaps psychologically more complicated than the intra-marital case. Here the meaning of "one's own" is no longer so unambiguous; neither is the meaning of motherhood and the status of pregnancy. On the one hand, it is argued that embryo donation, or "prenatal adoption," would be superior to present adoption, because the woman would have the experience of pregnancy and the child would be born of the "adopting" mother, rendering the maternal tie even more close. On the other hand, the mother-child bond rooted in pregnancy and delivery is held to be of little consequence by those who would endorse the use of surrogate gestational "mothers," say for a woman whose infertility is due to uterine disease rather than ovarian disease or oviduct obstruction. Clearly, the "need" and demand for extra-marital embryo transfer are real and probably large, probably even greater than the intra-marital ones. Already, the Chairman of the Ethics Advisory Board has testified in Congress about the need to define the responsibilities of *the donor* and the recipient "parents." Thus the new techniques will not only serve to ensure and preserve lineage, but will also serve to confound and complicate it. The principle truly at work here is not to provide married couples with a child of *their own*, but to provide anyone who wants one with a child, by whatever possible or convenient means.

"So what?" it will be said. First of all, we already practice and encourage adoption. Second, we have permitted artificial insemination—though we have, after some 40 years of this practice, yet to resolve questions of legitimacy. Third, what with the high rate of divorce and remarriage, identification of "mother," "father," and "child" are already complicated. Fourth, there is a growing rate of illegitimacy and husbandless parentages. Fifth, the use of surrogate mothers for foster pregnancy has already occurred, with the aid of artificial insemination.[1] Finally, our age in its enlightenment is no longer so certain about the virtues of family, lineage, and heterosexuality, or even about the taboos against adultery and incest. Against this background, it will be asked, why all the fuss about some little embryos that stray from the nest?

It is not an easy question to answer. Yet, consider. We practice adoption because there are abandoned children who need a good home. We do not, and would not, encourage people deliberately to generate children for others to adopt; partly we wish to avoid baby markets, partly we think it unfair to the child deliberately to deprive him of his natural ties. Recent years have seen a rise in our concern with roots, against the rootless and increasingly homogeneous background of contemporary American life. Adopted children, in particular, are pressing for information regarding their "real parents," and some states now require that such information be made available (on that typically modern ground of "freedom of information," rather than because of the profound importance of lineage for self-identity). The practice of artificial insemination has yet to be evaluated, the secrecy in which it is practiced being an apparent concession to the dangers of publicity.[2] Indeed, most physicians who practice artificial insemination routinely mix in some semen from the husband, to preserve some doubt about paternity—again, a concession to the importance of lineage and legitimacy. Finally, what about the changing mores of marriage, divorce, single-parent families, and sexual behavior? Do we applaud these changes? Do we want to contribute further to the confusion of thought, identity, and practice?[3]

Properly understood, the largely universal taboos against incest, and also the prohibition against adultery, suggest that clarity about who your parents are, clarity in the lines of generation, clarity about who is whose, are the indispensable foundations of a sound family life, itself the sound foundation of civilized community. Clarity about your origins is crucial for self-identity, itself important for self-respect. It would be, in my view, deplorable public policy further to erode such fundamental beliefs, values, institutions, and practices. This means, concretely, no encouragement of embryo adoption or especially of surrogate pregnancy. While it would be perhaps foolish to try to proscribe or outlaw such practices, it would not be wise for the Federal government to foster them. The Ethics Advisory Board should carefully consider whether it should and can attempt to restrict the use of embryo transfer to the married couple from whom the embryo derives.

The case of surrogate wombs bears a further comment. While expressing no objection to the practice of foster pregnancy itself, some people object that it will be done for pay, largely because of their fear that poor women will be exploited by such a practice. But if there were nothing wrong with foster pregnancy, what would be wrong with making a living at it? Clearly, this objection harbors a *tacit* understanding that to bear another's child for pay is in some sense a degradation of oneself—in the same sense that prostitution is a degradation *primarily* because it entails the loveless surrender of one's body to serve another's lust, and *only derivatively* because the woman is paid. It is to deny the meaning and worth of one's body, to treat it as a mere incubator, divested of its human meaning. It is also to deny the meaning of the bond among sexuality, love, and procreation. The buying and selling of human flesh and the dehumanized uses of the human body ought not to be encouraged. To be sure, the practice of womb donation could be engaged in for love not money, as it apparently has been in the case in Michigan. A woman could bear her sister's child out of sisterly love. But to the degree that one escapes in this way from the degradation and difficulties of the *sale* of human flesh and bodily services, and the treating of the body as stuff (the problem of cannibalism), one approaches instead the difficulties of potential incest and near-incest.

II.

Objections have been raised about the deliberate technological intervention into the so-called natural processes of human reproduction. Some would simply oppose such interventions as ''unnatural,'' and therefore wrong. Others are concerned about the consequences of these interventions, and about their ends and limits. Again, I think it important to explore the meaning and possible significance of such interventions, present and projected, especially as they bear on fundamental beliefs, institutions, and practices. To do so requires that we consider likely future developments in the laboratory study of human reproduction. Indeed, I shall argue that we *must* consider such future developments in reaching a decision in the present case.

What can we expect in the way of new modes of reproduction, as an outgrowth of present studies? To be sure, prediction is difficult. One can never know with certainty what will happen, much less how soon. Yet uncertainty is not the same as simple ignorance. Some things, indeed, seem likely. They seem likely because (1) they are thought necessary or desirable, at least by some researchers and their sponsors, (2) they are probably biologically possible and technically feasible,

and (3) they will be difficult to prevent or control (especially if no one anticipates their development or sees a need to worry about them). One of the things the citizenry, myself included, would expect from an Ethics Advisory Board and our policy makers generally is that they face up to reasonable projections of future accomplishments, consider whether they are cause for social concern, and see whether or not the principles *now* enunciated and the practices *now* established are adequate to deal with any such concerns.

I project at least the following:

1. The growth of human embryos in the laboratory will be extended beyond the blastocyst stage. Such growth must be deemed desirable under all the arguments advanced for developmental research *up to* the blastocyst stage; research on gene action, chromosome segregation, cellular and organic differentiation, fetus-environment interaction, implantation, etc., cannot answer all its questions with the blastocyst. Such *in vitro* post-blastocyst differentiation has apparently been achieved in the mouse, in culture; the use of other mammals as temporary hosts for human embryos is also a possibility. How far such embroys will eventually be perpetuated is anybody's guess, but full-term ectogenesis cannot be excluded. Neither can the existence of laboratories filled with many living human embryos, growing at various stages of development.

2. Experiments will be undertaken to alter the cellular and genetic composition of these embryos, at first without subsequent transfer to a woman for gestation, perhaps later as a prelude to reproductive efforts. Again, scientific reasons now justifying Dr. Soupart's research already justify further embryonic manipulations, including formation of hybrids or chimeras (within species and between species); gene, chromosome, and plasmid insertion, excision, or alteration; nuclear transplantation or cloning, etc. The techniques of DNA recombination, coupled with the new skills of handling embryos, make prospects for some precise genetic manipulation much nearer than anyone would have guessed ten years ago. And embryological and cellular research in mammals is making astounding progress.

On the cover of a recent issue of *Science* is a picture of a hexaparental mouse, born after reaggregation of an early embryo with cells disaggregated from three separate embryos. (Note: That sober journal calls this a "hand-made mouse"—i.e., literally a *manu-factured* mouse—and goes on to say that it was "manufactured by genetic engineering techniques.")[4]

3. Storage and banking of living human embryos (and ova) will be undertaken, perhaps commercially. After all, commercial sperm banks are already well-established and prospering.

Space does not permit me to do more than identify a few kinds of questions that must be considered in relation to such possible coming control over human heredity and reproduction: questions about the wisdom required to engage in such practices; questions about the goals and standards that will guide our interventions; questions about changes in the concepts of being human, including embodiment, gender, love, lineage, identity, parenthood, and sexuality; questions about the responsibility of power over future generations; questions about awe, respect, humility; questions about the kind of society we will have if we follow along our present course.[5]

Though I cannot discuss these questions now, I can and must face a serious objection to considering them at all. Most people would agree that the projected possibilities raise far more serious questions than do simple fertilization of a few embryos, their growth *in vitro* to the blastocyst stage, and their possible transfer to women for gestation. Why burden the present decision with these possibilities? Future "abuses," it is often said, do not disqualify present uses (though these same people also often say that "future benefits justify present questionable uses"). Moreover, there can be no certainty that "A" will lead to "B." This thin-edge-of-the-wedge argument has been open to criticism.

But such criticism misses the point, for two reasons. *First*, critics often misunderstand the wedge argument. The wedge argument is not primarily an argument of prediction, that A *will* lead to B, say on the strength of the empirical analysis of precedent and an appraisal of the likely direction of present research. It is primarily an argument about the *logic* of justification. Do the principles of justification *now* used to justify the current research proposal already justify *in advance* the further developments? Consider some of these principles:

1. It is desirable to learn as much as possible about the processes of fertilization, growth, implantation, and differentiation of human embryos and about human gene expression and its control.

2. It would be desirable to acquire improved techniques for *enhancing* conception and implantation, for *preventing* conception and implantation, for the treatment of genetic and chromosomal abnormalities, etc.

3. In the end, only research using *human* embryos can answer these questions and provide these techniques.

4. There should be no censorship or limitation of scientific inquiry or research.

This logic knows no boundary at the blastocyst stage, or for that matter, at any later stage. For these principles *not* to justify future extensions of current work, some independent additional principles, limiting such justification to particular stages of development, would have to be found. Here, the task is to find such a biologically defensible distinction that could be respected as reasonable and not arbitrary, a difficult—perhaps impossible—task, given the continuity of development after fertilization. The citizenry, myself included, will want to know *precisely* what grounds our policy makers will give for endorsing Soupart's research, and whether their principles have not already sanctioned future developments. If they do give such wedge-opening justifications, let them do so deliberately, candidly, and intentionally.

A better case to illustrate the wedge logic is the principle offered for the embryo-transfer procedures as treatment for infertility. Will we support the use of *in vitro* fertilization and embryo transfer because it provides a "child of *one's own*," in a strict sense of *one's own*, to a married couple? Or will we support the transfer because it is treatment of involuntary infertility, which deserves treatment in or out of marriage, hence endorsing the use of any available technical means (which would produce a healthy and normal child), including surrogate wombs, or even ectogenesis?

Second, logic aside, the opponents of the wedge argument do not counsel well. It would be simply foolish to ignore what might come next, and to fail to make the *best possible* assessment of the implications of present action (or inaction). Let me put the matter very bluntly: the Ethics Advisory Board, in the decision it must now make, may very well be helping to decide whether human beings will eventually be produced in laboratories. I say this not to shock—and I do not mean to beg the question of whether that would be desirable or not. I say this to make sure that they and we face squarely the full import and magnitude of this decision. Once the genies let the babies into the bottle, it may be impossible to get them out again.

An Afterword

This has been for me a long and difficult exposition. Many of the arguments are hard to make. It is hard to get confident people to face unpleasant prospects. It is hard to get many people to take seriously such "soft" matters as lineage, identity, respect, and self-respect when they are in tension with such "hard" matters as a cure for infertility or new methods of contraception. It is hard to talk about the meaning of sexuality and embodiment in a culture that treats sex increasingly as sport and that has trivialized the significance of gender, marriage, and procreation. It is hard to oppose Federal funding of baby-making in a society which increasingly demands that the Federal government supply all demands, and which—contrary to so much evidence of waste, incompetence, and corruption—continues to believe that only Uncle Sam can do it. And, finally, it is hard to speak about restraint in a culture that seems to venerate very little above man's own attempt to master all. Here, I am afraid, is the biggest question and the one we perhaps can no longer ask or deal with: the question about the reasonableness of the desire to become masters and possessors of nature, human nature included.

Here we approach the deepest meaning of *in vitro* fertilization. Those who have likened it to artificial insemination are only partly correct. With *in vitro* fertilization, the human embryo emerges

for the first time from the natural darkness and privacy of its own mother's womb, where it is hidden away in mystery, into the bright light and utter publicity of the scientist's laboratory, where it will be treated with unswerving rationality, before the clever and shameless eye of the mind and beneath the obedient and equally clever touch of the hand. What does it mean to hold the beginning of human life before your eyes, in your hands–even for 5 days (for the meaning does not depend on duration)? Perhaps the meaning is contained in the following story:

Long ago there was a man of great intellect and great courage. He was a remarkable man, a giant, able to answer questions that no other human being could answer, willing boldly to face any challenge or problem. He was a confident man, a masterful man. He saved his city from disaster and ruled it as a father rules his children, revered by all. But something was wrong in his city. A plague had fallen on generation; infertility afflicted plants, animals, and human beings. The man confidently promised to uncover the cause of the plague and to cure the infertility. Resolutely, dauntlessly, he put his sharp mind to work to solve the problem, to bring the dark things to light. No secrets, no reticences, a full public inquiry. He raged against the representatives of caution, moderation, prudence, and piety, who urged him to curtail his inquiry; he accused them of trying to usurp his rightfully earned power, of trying to replace human and masterful control with submissive reverence. The story ends in tragedy: He solved the problem but, in making visible and public the dark and intimate details of his origins, he ruined his life, and that of his family. In the end, too late, he learns about the price of presumption, of overconfidence, of the overweening desire to master and control one's fate. In symbolic rejection of his desire to look into everything, he punishes his eyes with self-inflicted blindness.

Sophocles seems to suggest that such a man is always in principle—albeit unwittingly—a patricide, a regicide, and a practitioner of incest. We men of modern science may have something to learn from our forebear, Oedipus. It appears that Oedipus, being the kind of man an Oedipus is (the chorus calls him a paradigm of man), had no choice but to learn through suffering. Is it really true that we too have no other choice?

Notes

1. An unmarried woman in Dearborn, Michigan, offered to bear a child for her married friend, infertile because of a hysterectomy. She was impregnated by artificial insemination using semen produced by her friend's husband, his wife performing the injection. The threesome lived together all during the pregnancy. The child was delivered at birth by the biological-and-gestational-mother to the wife-and-rearing-mother. The first (pregnancy) mother reports no feelings of attachment to the child she carried and bore. Everyone is reportedly delighted with the event. The trio has publicized its accomplishment and is reported to be considering selling rights to the story for a TV show, a book, and a movie. Their attorney has been swamped with letters requesting similar surrogate "mothers." (*American Medical News*, July 28, 1978, pp. 11–12.)

2. There are today numerous suits pending, throughout the United States, because of artificial insemination with donor semen (AID). Following divorce, the ex-husbands are refusing child support for AID children, claiming, minimally, no paternity, or maximally that the child was the fruit of an adulterous "union." In fact, a few states still treat AID as adultery. The importance of anonymity is revealed in the following bizarre case. A woman wanted to have a child, but abhorred the thought of marriage or of sexual relations with men. She learned a do-it-yourself technique of artificial insemination, and persuaded a male acquaintance to donate his semen. Now some 10 years after this virgin birth, the case has gone to court. The semen donor is suing for visitation privileges, to see his son.

3. To those who point out that the bond between sexuality and procreation has already been effectively and permanently cleaved by "the pill," and that this is therefore an idle worry in the case of *in vitro* fertilization, it must be said that the pill provides only sex without babies. Now the other shoe drops: babies without sex.

4. *Science*, 202:5, October 6, 1978.

5. Some of these questions are addressed, albeit too briefly and polemically, in the latter part of my 1972 "Making Babies" article, to which the reader is referred. It has been pointed out to me by an astute colleague that the tone of the present article is less passionate and more accommodating than the first, which change he regards as an ironic demonstration of the inexorable way in which we get used to, and accept, our technological nightmares. I myself share his concern. I cannot decide whether the decline of my passion is to be welcomed; that is, whether it is due to greater understanding bred of more thought and experience, or to greater callousness and the contempt of familiarity bred from *too much* thought and experience. It does seem to me now that many of the fundamental beliefs and institutions that might be challenged by laboratory growth of human embryos and by laboratory-assisted reproduction are already severely challenged in perhaps more potent and important ways. Here, too, we see the creeping effect of the aggregated powers of modernity and the corrosive power of the familiar. Adaptiveness is our glory and our curse: as Raskolnikov put it, "Man gets used to everything, the beast!"

The Case Against Surrogate Parenting

Herbert T. Krimmel

Is it ethical for someone to create a human life with the intention of giving it up? This seems to be the primary question for both surrogate mother arrangements and artificial insemination by donor (AID), since in both situations a person who is providing germinal material does so only upon the assurance that someone else will assume full responsibility for the child he or she helps to create.

The Ethical Issue

In analyzing the ethics of surrogate mother arrangements, it is helpful to begin by examining the roles the surrogate mother performs. First, she acts as a procreator in providing an ovum to be fertilized. Second, after her ovum has been fertilized by the sperm of the man who wishes to par-

From **The Hastings Center Report**, *October 1983, Vol. 13, no. 5, 35–39. Reproduced by permission.*
© *The Hastings Center.*

ent the child, she acts as host to the fetus, providing nurture and protection while the newly conceived individual develops.

I see no insurmountable moral objections to the functions the mother performs in this second role as host. Her actions are analogous to those of a foster mother or of a wet-nurse who cares for a child when the natural mother cannot or does not do so. Using a surrogate mother as a host for the fetus when the biological mother cannot bear the child is no more morally objectionable than employing others to help educate, train, or otherwise care for a child. Except in extremes, where the parent relinquishes or delegates responsibilities for a child for trivial reasons, the practice would not seem to raise a serious moral issue.

I would argue, however, that the first role that the surrogate mother performs—providing germinal material to be fertilized—does pose a major ethical problem. The surrogate mother provides her ovum, and enters into a surrogate mother arrangement, with the clear understanding that she is to avoid responsibility for the life she creates. Surrogate mother arrangements are designed to separate in the mind of the surrogate mother the decision to create a child from the decision to have and raise that child. The cause of this dissociation is some other benefit she will receive, most often money.[1] In other words, her desire to create a child is born of some motive other than the desire to be a parent. This separation of the decision to create a child from the decision to parent it is ethically suspect. The child is conceived not because he is wanted by his biological mother, but because he can be useful to someone else. He is conceived in order to be given away.

At their deepest level, surrogate mother arrangements involve a change in motive for creating children: from a desire to have them for their own sake, to a desire to have them because they can provide some other benefit. The surrogate mother creates a child with the intention to abdicate parental responsibilities. Can we view this as ethical? My answer is no. I will explain why by analyzing various situations in which surrogate mother arrangements might be used.

Why Motive Matters

Let's begin with the single parent. A single woman might use AID, or a single man might use

a surrogate mother arrangement, if she or he wanted a child but did not want to be burdened with a spouse.[2] Either practice would intentionally deprive the child of a mother or a father. This, I assert, is fundamentally unfair to the child.

Those who disagree might point to divorce or to the death of a parent as situations in which a child is deprived of one parent and must rely solely or primarily upon the other. The comparison, however, is inapt. After divorce or the death of a parent, a child may find herself with a single parent due to circumstances that were unfortunate, unintended, and undesired. But when surrogate mother arrangements are used by a single parent, depriving the child of a second parent is one of the intended and desired effects. It is one thing to ask how to make the best of a bad situation when it is thrust upon a person. It is different altogether to ask whether one may intentionally set out to achieve the same result. The morality of identical results (for example, killings) will oftentimes differ depending upon whether the situation is invited by, or involuntarily thrust upon, the actor. Legal distinctions following and based upon this ethical distinction are abundant. The law of self-defense provides a notable example.[3]

Since a woman can get pregnant if she wishes whether or not she is married, and since there is little that society can do to prevent women from creating children even if their intention is to deprive the children of a father, why should we be so concerned about single men using surrogate mother arrangements if they too want a child but not a spouse? To say that women can intentionally plan to be unwed mothers is not to condone the practice. Besides, society will hold the father liable in a paternity action if he can be found and identified, which indicates some social concern that people should not be able to abdicate the responsibilities that they incur in generating children. Otherwise, why do we condemn the proverbial sailor with a pregnant girlfriend in every port?

In many surrogate mother arrangements, of course, the surrogate mother will not be transferring custody of the child to a single man, but to a couple: the child's biological and a stepmother, his wife. What are the ethics of surrogate mother arrangements when the child is taken into a two-parent family? Again, surrogate mother arrangements and AID pose similar ethical questions: The surrogate mother transfers her parental responsibilities to the wife of the biological father, while with AID the sperm donor relinquishes his interest in the child to the husband of the biological mother. In both cases the child is created with the intention of transferring the responsibility for its care to a new set of parents. The surrogate mother situation is more dramatic than AID since the transfer occurs after the child is born, while in the case of AID the transfer takes place at the time of the insemination. Nevertheless, the ethical point is the same: creating children for the purpose of transferring them. For a surrogate mother the question remains: Is it ethical to create a child for the purpose of transferring it to the wife of the biological father?

At first blush this looks to be little different from the typical adoption, for what is an adoption other than a transfer of responsibility from one set of parents to another? The analogy is misleading, however, for two reasons. First, it is difficult to imagine anyone conceiving children for the purpose of putting them up for adoption. And, if such a bizarre event were to occur, I doubt that we would look upon it with moral approval. Most adoptions arise either because an undesired conception is brought to term, or because the parents wanted to have the child, but find that they are unable to provide for it because of some unfortunate circumstances that develop after conception.

Second, even if surrogate mother arrangements were to be classified as a type of adoption, not all offerings of children for adoption are necessarily moral. For example, would it be moral for parents to offer their three-year-old for adoption because they are bored with the child? Would it be moral for a couple to offer for adoption their newborn female baby because they wanted a boy?

Therefore, even though surrogate mother arrangements may in some superficial ways be likened to adoption, one must still ask whether it is ethical to separate the decision to create children from the desire to have them. I would answer no. The procreator should desire for its own sake, and not as a means to attaining some other end. Even though one of the ends may be stated altruistically as an attempt to bring happiness to an infertile couple, the child is still being used by the surro-

gate. She creates it not because she desires it, but because she desires something from it.

To sanction the use and treatment of human beings as means to the achievement of other goals instead of as ends in themselves is to accept an ethic with a tragic past, and to establish a precedent with a dangerous future. Already the press has reported the decision of one couple to conceive a child for the purpose of using it as a bone marrow donor for its sibling (*Los Angeles Times*, April 17, 1979, p. 1–2). And the bioethics literature contains articles seriously considering whether we should clone human beings to serve as an inventory of spare parts for organ transplants[4] and articles that foresee the use of comatose human beings as self-replenishing blood banks and manufacturing plants for human hormones.[5] How far our society is willing to proceed down this road is uncertain, but it is clear that the first step to all these practices is the acceptance of the same principle that the Nazis attempted to use to justify their medical experiments at the Nuremberg War Crimes Trials: that human beings may be used as means to the achievement of other goals, and need not be treated as ends in themselves.[6]

But why, it might be asked, is it so terrible if the surrogate mother does not desire the child for its own sake, when under the proposed surrogate mother arrangements there will be a couple eagerly desiring to have the child and to be its parents? That this argument may not be entirely accurate will be illustrated in the following section, but the basic reply is that creating a child without desiring it fundamentally changes the way we look at children—instead of viewing them as unique individual personalities to be desired in their own right, we may come to view them as commodities or items of manufacture to be desired because of their utility. A recent newspaper account describes the business of an agency that matches surrogate mothers with barren couples as follows:

> Its first product is due for delivery today. Twelve others are on the way and an additional 20 have been ordered. The "company" is Surrogate Mothering Ltd. and the "product" is babies.[7]

The dangers of this view are best illustrated by examining what might go wrong in a surrogate mother arrangement, and most important, by viewing how the various parties to the contract may react to the disappointment.

What Might Go Wrong

Ninety-nine percent of the surrogate mother arrangements may work out just fine; the child will be born normal, and the adopting parents (that is, the biological father and his wife) will want it. But, what happens when, unforeseeably, the child is born deformed? Since many defects cannot be discovered prenatally by amniocentesis or other means, the situation is bound to arise.[8] Similarly, consider what would happen if the biological father were to die before the birth of the child. Or if the "child" turns out to be twins or triplets. Each of these instances poses an inevitable situation where the adopting parents may be unhappy with the prospect of getting the child or children. Although legislation can mandate that the adopting parents take the child or children in whatever condition they come or whatever the situation, provided the surrogate mother has abided by all the contractual provisions of the surrogate mother arrangement, the important point for our discussion is the attitude that the surrogate mother or the adopting parent might have. Consider the example of the deformed child.

When I participated in the Surrogate Parent Foundation's inaugural symposium in November 1981, I was struck by the attitude of both the surrogate mothers and the adopting parents to these problems. The adopting parents worried, "Do we have to take such a child?" and the surrogate mothers said in response, "Well, we don't want to be stuck with it." Clearly, both groups were anxious not to be responsible for the "undesirable child" born of the surrogate mother arrangement. What does this portend?

It is human nature that when one pays money, one expects value. Things that one pays for have a way of being seen as commodities. Unavoidable in surrogate mother arrangements are questions such as : "Did I get a good one?" We see similar behavior with respect to the adoption of children: comparatively speaking, there is no shortage of black, Mexican-American, mentally retarded, or older children seeking homes; the shortage is in attractive, intelligent-looking Caucasian babies.[9] Similarly, surrogate mother arrangements involve more than just the desire to have a child. The desire is for a certain type of child.

But, it may be objected, don't all parents voice these same concerns in the normal course of having children? Not exactly. No one doubts or minimizes the pain and disappointment parents feel when they learn that their child is born with some genetic or congenital birth defect. But this is different from the surrogate mother situation, where neither the surrogate mother nor the adopting parents may feel responsible, and both sides may feel that they have a legitimate excuse not to assume responsibility for the child. The surrogate mother might blame the biological father for having "defective sperm," as the adopting parents might blame the surrogate mother for a "defective ovum" or for improper care of the fetus during pregnancy. The adopting parents desire a normal child, not *this* child in any condition, and the surrogate mother doesn't want it in any event. So both sides will feel threatened by the birth of an "undesirable child." Like bruised fruit in the produce bin of a supermarket, this child is likely to become an object of avoidance.

Certainly, in the natural course of having children a mother may doubt whether she wants a child if the father has died before its birth; parents may shy away from a defective infant, or be distressed at the thought of multiple births. Nevertheless, I believe they are more likely to accept these contingencies as a matter of fate. I do not think this is the case with surrogate mother arrangements. After all, in the surrogate mother arrangement the adopting parents can blame someone outside the marital relationship. The surrogate mother has been hosting this child all along, and she is delivering it. It certainly *looks* far more like a commodity than the child that arrives in the natural course within the family unit.

A Dangerous Agenda

Another social problem which arises out of the first, is the fear that surrogate mother arrangements will fall prey to eugenic concerns.[10] Surrogate mother contracts typically have clauses requiring genetic tests of the fetus and stating that the surrogate mother must have an abortion (or keep the child herself) if the child does not pass these tests.[11]

In the last decade we have witnessed a renaissance of interest in eugenics. This, coupled with advances in biomedical technology, has created a host of abuses and new moral problems. For example, genetic counseling clinics now face a dilemma: amniocentesis, the same procedure that identifies whether a fetus suffers from certain genetic defects, also discloses the sex of a fetus. Genetic counseling clinics have reported that even when the fetus is normal, a disproportionate number of mothers abort female children.[12] Aborting normal fetuses simply because the prospective parents desire children of a certain sex is one result of viewing children as commodities. The recent scandal at the Repository for Germinal Choice, the so-called "Nobel Sperm Bank," provides another chilling example. Their first "customer" was, unbeknownst to the staff, a woman who "had lost custody of two other children because they were abused in an effort to 'make them smart.' "[13] Of course, these and similar evils may occur whether or not surrogate mother arrangements are allowed by law. But to the extent that they promote the view of children as commodities, these arrangements contribute to these problems. There is nothing wrong with striving for betterment, as long as it does not result in intolerance to that which is not perfect. But I fear that the latter attitude will become prevalent.

Sanctioning surrogate mother arrangements can also exert pressures upon the family structure. First, as was noted earlier, there is nothing technically to prevent the use of surrogate mother arrangements by single males desiring to become parents. Indeed, single females can already do this with AID or even without it. But even if legislation were to limit the use of the surrogate mother arrangements to infertile couples, other pressures would occur: namely the intrusion of a third adult into the marital community.[14] I do not think that society is ready to accept either single parenting or quasi-adulterous arrangements as normal.

Another stress on the family structure arises within the family of the surrogate mother. When the child is surrendered to the adopting parents it is removed not only from the surrogate mother, but also from her family. They too have interests to be considered. Do not the siblings of that child have an interest in the fact that their little baby brother has been "given" away?[15] One woman, the mother of a medical student who had often donated sperm for artificial insemination, expressed her feelings to me eloquently. She asked, "I wonder how many grandchildren I have that I have never seen and never been able to hold or cuddle."

Intrafamily tensions can also be expected to result in the family of the adopting parents due to the asymmetry of relationship the adopting parents will have toward the child. The adopting mother has no biological relationship to the child, whereas the adopting father is also the child's biological father. Won't this unequal biological claim on the child be used as a wedge in child-rearing arguments? Can't we imagine the father saying, "Well, he is my son, not yours"? What if the couple eventually gets divorced? Should custody in a subsequent divorce between the adopting mother and the biological father be treated simply as a normal child custody dispute? Or should the biological relationship between father and child weigh more heavily? These questions do not arise in typical adoption situations since both parents are equally unrelated biologically to the child. Indeed, in adoption there is symmetry. The surrogate mother situation is more analogous to second marriages, where the children of one party by a prior marriage are adopted by the new spouse. Since asymmetry in second marriage situations causes problems, we can anticipate similar difficulties arising from surrogate mother arrangements.

There is also the worry that the offspring of a surrogate mother arrangement will be deprived of important information about his or her heritage. This also happens with adopted children or children conceived by AID,[16] who lack information about their biological parents, which could be important to them medically. Another less popularly recognized problem is the danger of half-sibling marriages,[17] where the child of the surrogate mother unwittingly falls in love with a half sister or brother. The only way to avoid these problems is to dispense with the confidentiality of parental records; however, the natural parents may not always want their identity disclosed.

The legalization of surrogate mother arrangements may also put undue pressure upon poor women to use their bodies in this way to support themselves and their families. Analogous problems have arisen in the past with the use of paid blood donors.[18] And occasionally the press reports someone desperate enough to offer to sell an eye or some other organ.[19] I believe that certain things should be viewed as too important to be sold as commodities , and I hope that we have advanced from the time when parents raised children for profitable labor, or found themselves forced to sell their children.

While many of the social dilemmas I have outlined here have their analogies in other present-day occurrences such as divorced families or in adoption, every addition is hurtful. Legalizing surrogate mother arrangements will increase the frequency of these problems and put more stress on our society's shared moral values.[20]

A Tale for Our Time

An infertile couple might prefer to raise a child with a biological relationship to the husband, rather than to raise an adopted child who has no biological relationship to either the husband or the wife. But does the marginal increase in joy that they might therefore experience outweigh the potential pain that they, or the child conceived in such arrangements, or others might suffer? Does their preference outweigh the social costs and problems that the legalization of surrogate mothering might well engender? I honestly do not know. I don't even know on what hypothetical scale such interests could be weighed and balanced. But even if we could weigh such interests, and even if personal preference outweighed the costs, I still would not be able to say that we could justify achieving those ends by these means; that ethically it would be permissible for a person to create a child, not because she desired it, but because it could be useful to her.

Edmond Cahn has termed this ignoring of means in the attainment of ends the "Pompey syndrome":[21]

> I have taken the name from young Sextus Pompey, who appears in Shakespeare's *Antony and Cleopatra* in an incident drawn directly from Plutarch. Pompey, whose navy has won control of the seas around Italy, comes to negotiate peace with the Roman triumvirs Mark Antony, Octavius Caesar, and Lepidus, and they meet in a roistering party on Pompey's ship. As they carouse, one of Pompey's lieutenants draws him aside and whispers that he can become lord of all the world if he will only grant the lieutenant

leave to cut first the mooring cable and then the throats of the triumvirs. Pompey pauses, then replies in these words:

> Ah, this thou shouldst have done,
> And not have spoke on't!
> In me 'tis villainy:
> In thee't had been good service.
> Thou must know tis not my profit that does
>   lend mine honour;
> Mine honour, it. Repent that e'er thy tongue
> Hath so betrayed thine act; being done un-
>   known;
> I should have found it afterwards well done,
> But must condemn it now. Desist, and drink.

Here we have the most pervasive of moral syndromes, the one most characteristic of so-called respectable men in a civilized society. To possess the end and yet not be responsible for the means, to grasp the fruit while disavowing the tree, to escape being told the cost until someone else has paid it irrevocably; this is the Pompey syndrome and the chief hypocrisy of our time.

Notes

1. See Philip J. Parker, "Motivation of Surrogate Mothers: Initial Findings," *American Journal of Psychiatry* 140:1 (January 1983), 117–18; see also Doe v. Kelley, Circuit Court of Wayne County Michigan (1980) reported in 1980 Rep. on Human Reproduction and Law II-A-1.

2. See, e.g., C. M. v C. C., 152 N.J. Supp. 160, 377 A2d 821 (1977); "Why She Went to 'Nobel Sperm Bank' for Child," *Los Angeles Herald Examiner*, Aug. 6, 1982, p. A9; "Womb for Rent," *Los Angeles Herald Examiner*, Sept. 21, 1981, p. A3.

3. See also Richard McCormick, "Reproductive Technologies: Ethical Issues" in *Encyclopedia of Bioethics*, edited by Walter Reich, Vol. 4 (New York: The Free Press, 1978) pp. 1454, 1459; Robert Snowden and G. D. Mitchell, *The Artificial Family* (London: George Allen & Unwin, 1981), p. 71.

4. See e.g., Alexander Peters, "The Brave New World: Can the Law Bring Order Within Traditional Concepts of Due Process?" *Suffolk Law Review* 4 (1970), 894, 901–02; Roderie Gorney, "The New Biology and the Future of Man," *UCLA Law Review* 15 (1968), 273, 302; J. G. Castel, "Legal Implications of Biomedical Science and Technology in the Twenty-First Century," *Canadian Bar Review* 51 (1973), 119, 127.

5. See Harry Nelson, "Maintaining Dead to Serve as Blood Makers Proposed: Logical, Sociologist Says," *Los Angeles Times*, February 26, 1974 p. II-1;

Hans Jonas, "Against the Stream: Comments on the Definition and Redefinition of Death," in *Philosophical Essays: From Ancient Creed to Technological Man* (Chicago: University of Chicago Press, 1974), pp. 132–140.

6. See Leo Alexander, "Medical Science under Dictatorship," *New England Journal of Medicine* 241:2 (1949), 39; United States v. Brandt, Trial of the Major War Criminals, International Military Tribunal: Nuremberg, 14 November 1945–1 October 1946.

7. Bob Dvorchak, "Surrogate Mothers: Pregnant Idea Now a Pregnant Business," *Los Angeles Herald Examiner*, December 27, 1983, p. A1.

8. "Surrogate's Baby Born with Deformities Rejected by All," *Los Angeles Times*, January 22, 1983, p. I-17; "Man Who Hired Surrogate Did Not Father Ailing Baby," *Los Angeles Herald Examiner*, February 3, 1983, p. A-6.

9. See, e.g., Adoption in America, Hearing before the Subcommittee on Aging, Family and Human Services of the Senate Committee on Labor and Human Resources, 97th Congress, 1st Session (1981), p. 3 (comments of Senator Jeremiah Denton) and pp. 16–17 (statement of Warren Master, Acting Commissioner of Administration for Children, Youth and Families, HHS).

10. Cf. "Discussion: Moral, Social and Ethical Issues," in *Law and Ethics of A.I.D. and Embryo Transfer* (1973) (comments of Himmelweit), reprinted in Michael Shapiro and Roy Spece. *Bioethics and Law* (St. Paul: West Publishing Company, 1981), p. 548.

11. See, e.g., Lane (*Newsday*), "Womb for Rent," *Tucson Citizen* (Weekender), June 7, 1980, p. 3: Susan Lewis, "Baby Bartering? Surrogate Mothers Pose Issues for Lawyers, Courts," *The Los Angeles Daily Journal*, April 20, 1981; see also Elaine Markoutsas, "Women Who Have Babies for Other Women," *Good Housekeeping* 96 (April 1981), 104.

12. See Morton A. Stenchever, "An Abuse of Prenatal Diagnosis," *Journal of the American Medical Association* 221 (1972), 408, Charles Westoff and Ronald R. Rindfus, "Sex Preselection in the United States: Some Implications," *Science* 184 (1974), 633, 636; see also Phyllis Battelle, "Is It a Boy or a Girl"? *Los Angeles Herald Examiner*, Oct. 8, 1981, p. A17.

13. "2 Children Taken from Sperm Bank Mother," *Los Angeles Times*, July 14, 1982; p. I-3; "The Sperm-Bank Scandal," *Newsweek* 24 (July 26, 1982).

14. See Helmut Thielicke, *The Ethics of Sex*, John W. Doberstein, trans. (New York: Harper & Row, 1964).

15. According to one newspaper account, when a surrogate mother informed her nine-year-old daughter that the new baby would be given away, the daughter replied, "Oh, good. If it's a girl we can keep it and give Jeffrey [her two-year-old half brother] away," "Womb for Rent," *Los Angeles Herald Examiner*, Sept. 21, 1981, p. A3.

16. See, e.g., Lorraine Dusky, "Brave New Babies"? *Newsweek* 30 (December 6, 1982). Also testimony of Suzanne Rubin before the California Assembly Committee on Judiciary, Surrogate Parenting Contracts, Assembly Publication No. 962, pp. 72–75 (November 19, 1982).

17. This has posed an increasing problem for children conceived through AID. See, e.g., Martin Curie-Cohen, et al., "Current Practice of Artificial Insemination by Donor in the United States," *New England Journal of Medicine* 300 (1979), 585–89.

18. See, e.g., Richard M. Titmuss, *The Gift Relationship: From Human Blood to Social Policy* (New York: Random House, 1971).

19. See, e.g., "Man Desperate for Funds: Eye for Sale at $35,000," *Los Angeles Times*, February 1, 1975, p. II-1; "100 Answer Man's Ad for New Kidney," *Los Angeles Times*, September 12, 1974, p. I-4.

20. See generally Guido Calabresi, "Reflections on Medical Experimentation in Humans," *Daedalus* 98 (1969), 387–93; also see Michael Shapiro and Roy Spece, "On Being 'Unprincipled on Principle': The Limits of Decision Making 'On the Merits' " in *Bioethics and Law*, pp. 67–71.

21. Edmond Cahn, "Drug Experiments and the Public Conscience," in *Drugs in Our Society*, edited by Paul Talalay (Baltimore: The Johns Hopkins Press, 1964), pp. 255, 258–61.

Ruling on Baby M

New Jersey Superior Court, Judge Harvey R. Sorkow

Background Note. On March 30, 1986, Dr. Elizabeth Stern, a 41-year-old professor of pediatrics, and her husband William accepted from Mary Beth Whitehead a baby who had been born four days earlier. The child's biological mother was Mrs. Whitehead, but she had been engaged by the Sterns as a surrogate mother. Even so, it was not until almost exactly a year later that the Sterns were able to claim permanent legal custody of the child.

The Sterns, working through the Infertility Center of New York, had first met with Mrs. Whitehead and her husband Richard in January of 1985. Mrs. Whitehead, who already had a son and a daughter, had indicated her willingness to become a surrogate mother by signing up at the Infertility Center. "What brought her there was empathy with childless couples who were infertile," her attorney later stated. Her own sister had been unable to conceive.

According to court testimony, the Sterns considered Mrs. Whitehead a "perfect person" to bear a child for them. Mr. Stern said that it was "compelling" for him to have children, for he had no relatives "anywhere in the world." He and his wife planned to have children, but they put off attempts to conceive until his wife completed her medical residency in 1981. However, in 1979 she was diagnosed as having an eye condition that indicated that she probably had multiple sclerosis. When she learned that the symptoms of the disease might be worsened by pregnancy and that she might become temporarily or even permanently paralyzed, the Sterns "decided the risk wasn't worth it." It was this decision that led them to the Infertility Center and to Mary Beth Whitehead.

The Sterns agreed to pay Mrs. Whitehead $10,000 to be artificially inseminated with Mr. Stern's sperm and to bear a child. Mrs. Whitehead would then turn the child over to the Sterns, and Dr. Stern would be allowed to adopt the child legally. The agreement was drawn up by Noel P. Keane, a Michigan lawyer specializing in surrogacy arrangements. Mr. Stern later testified that Mrs. Whitehead had seemed perfectly pleased with the agreement and had expressed no interest in keeping the baby she was to bear. "She said she would not come to our doorstep," he said. "All she wanted from us was a photograph each year and a little letter on what transpired that year."

The baby was born on March 27, 1986. According to Dr. Stern, the first indication that Mrs. Whitehead might not keep the agreement was her statement to the Sterns in the hospital two days after the baby's birth. "She said she didn't know if 'I can go through with it,' " Dr. Stern testified. Although Mrs. Whitehead did turn over the baby to the Sterns on March 30, she called a few hours later. "She said she didn't know if she could live any more," Dr. Stern said.

She called again the next morning and asked to see the baby, and she and her sister arrived at the Sterns's house before noon.

According to Dr. Stern, Mrs. Whitehead told her that she "woke up screaming in the middle of the night" because the baby was gone, that her husband was threatening to leave her, and that she had "considered taking a bottle of Valium." Dr. Stern quoted Mrs. Whitehead as saying, " 'I just want her for a week, and I'll be out of your lives forever.' " The Sterns allowed Mrs. Whitehead to take the baby home with her.

Mrs. Whitehead then refused to return the baby voluntarily and took the infant with her to the home of her parents in Florida. The Sterns obtained a court order, and on July 31 the child was seized from Mrs. Whitehead. The Sterns were granted temporary custody. Then Mr. Stern, as the father of the child, and Mrs. Whitehead, as the mother, each sought permanent custody from the Superior Court of the State of New Jersey.

The seven-week trial attracted considerable attention, for the legal issues were virtually without precedent. Mrs. Whitehead was the first to challenge the legal legitimacy of a surrogate agreement in a United States court. She argued that the agreement was "against public policy" and violated New Jersey prohibitions against selling babies. In contrast, Mr. Stern was the first to seek a legal decision to uphold the "specific performance" of the terms of a surrogate contract. In particular, he argued that Mrs. Whitehead should be ordered to uphold her agreement and to surrender her parental rights and permit his wife to become the baby's legal mother. In addition to the contractual issue, the judge had to deal with the "best interests" of the child as required by New Jersey child-custody law. In addition to being a vague concept, the "best interest" standard had never been applied in a surrogacy case.

On March 31, 1987, Judge Harvey R. Sorkow announced his decision. He upheld the legality of the surrogate-mother agreement between the Sterns and Mrs. Whitehead and dismissed all arguments that the contract violated public policy or prohibitions against selling babies. Immediately after reading his decision, Judge Sorkow summoned Elizabeth Stern into his chambers and allowed her to sign documents permitting her to adopt the baby she and her husband called Melissa. The court decision effectively stripped Mary Beth Whitehead of all parental rights concerning this same baby, the one she called Sara. The child was known in court and to the public as Baby M.

The court decision was made too late for a discussion of it to be included in the introduction to this chapter.

The Issue

The primary issue to be determined by this litigation is what are the best interests of a child until now called Baby M. All other concerns raised by counsel constitute commentary.

. . .

Jurisdiction

There can be no solution satisfactory to all in this kind of case. Justice, our desired objective, to the child and the mother, to the child and the father, cannot be obtained for both parents. The court will seek to achieve justice for the child. This court's fact finding and application of relevant law must mitigate against the heartfelt desires of one or the other of the natural parents.

Where courts are forced to choose between a parent's rights and a child's welfare, the choice is and must be the child's welfare and best interest by virtue of the court's responsibility as *parens patriae.*

Findings

. . .

It took years of legislative debate and judicial inquiry to define and develop today's laws of abortion and artificial insemination. The issues and dimensions of surrogacy are still evolving but it is necessary that laws be adopted to give our society a sense of definition and direction if the concept is to be allowed to further develop. With an increasing number of surrogate births, legislation can avoid harm to society, the family and the child. . . . Many questions must be answered; answers must come from legislation. If there is no law then society will suffer the negative aspects of this alternative reproduction vehicle that appears to hold out so much hope to the childless who make up a substantial segment of our society.

. . .

The four experts called by the parties, both hypothetical and clinical, all conclude that Mrs. Stern has multiple sclerosis—albeit, in a mild form and the possibility of progression is limited to unknown.

. . .

With regard to Mrs. Stern's disease, all the experts called on this issue conclude that her decision not to become pregnant in light of her knowledge of her disease, her experienced symptomology, the accepted medical understanding of the medical profession at the time that risk of exacerbation was attendant to pregnancy was a medically reasonable and understandable decision.

. . .

It is argued that the child will not be protected. So long as there is no legislation and some court action in surrogacy arrangements is required, the child born of surrogacy will be protected in New Jersey. If there is compliance with the contract terms, adoption will be necessary; hence court inquiry about best interests must take place. If there is noncompliance with the contract, as in this case, best interest is still litigated with protection to the child.

. . .

The second argument against surrogacy is that the surrogate mother will be exploited. To the contrary. It is the private adoption that has that great potential, if not fact, for the exploitation of the mother. In the private adoption, the woman is already pregnant. The biological father may be unknown or at best uninterested in his obligation. The woman may want to keep the child but cannot do so for financial reasons. There is the risk of illegal consideration being paid to the mother. In surrogacy, none of these "downside" elements appear. The arrangement is made when the desire and intention to have a family exist on the couple's part. The surrogate has an opportunity to consult, take advice and consider her act and is not forced into the relationship. She is not yet pregnant.

The third argument is that to produce or deal with a child for money denigrates human dignity. To that premise, this court urgently agrees. The 13th Amendment to the United States Constitution is still valid law. The law of adoption in New Jersey does prohibit the exchange of any consideration for obtaining a child. The fact is, however, that the money to be paid to the surrogate is not being paid for the surrender of the child to the father. . . . The biological father pays the surrogate for her willingness to be impregnated and carry his child to term. At birth, the father does not purchase the child. It is his own biological genetically related child. He cannot purchase what is already his.

The fourth argument against surrogacy is that it is a concept running contrary to the laws of adoption in New Jersey. It is in this court's view that the laws of adoption in this state do not apply to surrogacy contracts.

. . .

The fifth argument against surrogacy is that it will undermine traditional notions of family. How can that be when the childless husband and wife so very much want a child?

. . .

The final and sixth argument suggests an elite upper economic group of people will use the lower economic group of women to "make their babies." This argument is insensitive and offensive to the intense drive to procreate naturally and when that is impossible, to use what lawful means is possible to gain a child.

. . .

It must be reasoned that if one has a right to procreate coitally, then one has the right to reproduce noncoitally. If it is the reproduction that is protected, then the means of reproduction are also to be protected. The value and interests underlying the creation of family are the same by whatever means obtained. This court holds that the protected means extends to the use of surrogates. . . .

While a state could regulate, indeed should and must regulate the circumstances under which parties enter into reproductive contracts, it could not ban or refuse to enforce such transactions altogether without compelling reason. It might even be argued that refusal to enforce these contracts and prohibition of money payments would constitute an unconstitutional interference with procreative liberty since it would prevent childless couples from obtaining the means with which to have families.

. . .

For the foregoing reasons, this court concludes and holds that the surrogate parenting agreement is a valid and enforceable contract pursuant to the Laws of New Jersey. The rights of the parties to contract are constitutionally protected under the 14th Amendment of the United States Constitution.

. . .

This court is satisfied by clear and convincing proof that Mr. and Mrs. Stern wanted and planned for this child. They intended to be parents of the child. They have a strong and mutually supportive relationship wherein each respects the other and there is a balancing of obligations. There is proof of a successful cooperative parenting effort. The Sterns have a private, quiet and unremarkable life which augurs well for a stable household environment. Mr. and Mrs. Stern show sensitivity to the child's physical and emotional needs. They would be supportive of education and have shown, at least in their own lives, a motivation for learning. It can be concluded that they would initiate and encourage intellectual curiosity and learning for the child. . . .

Finally, they have shown no difficulty in coping with crisis. It may be anticipated that because the child is unique and at risk, crisis for the next several years will be part of their lives. Mr. and Mrs. Stern have shown an ability to deal with such exigencies. It is for all these reasons, it is because of all the facts found by this court as the trier of fact that we find by clear and convincing evidence, indeed by a measure of evidence reaching beyond reasonable doubt that Melissa's best interest will be served by being placed in her father's sole custody.

The Right to Lesbian Parenthood

Gillian Hanscombe

Anyone daring to address the subject of human rights faces both an appalling responsibility and being accused of an unnatural arrogance of utterance. I accept these risks not because I think myself expert on the subject of human rights, but because my experience is that human rights in the domain of parenthood are so very often denied existence.

I refer to a large minority in our population, that of lesbian women and gay men. Even at the most conservative estimate—which is that at least 1 in 20 adult people are homosexual—a group comprising 5 per cent—we are dealing with a group larger than the 4 per cent ethnic minorities group which already receives, as indeed it deserves to do, special attention. Lesbian women and gay men have to date, in all matters of social policy, been traditionally regarded as a deviant group.

It is the case, nonetheless, that the pathologising of this group is increasingly questioned, not only by members of the gay community themselves, but also by the agencies of our institutional life: that is, by medical practitioners, by teachers and social workers, and by working parties of religious and/or political orientation.

I am the co-author of a book about lesbian mothers.[1] It is written for the general public, rather than for specialists, but is nevertheless the only book to date on the subject which I know of. It records the experiences of a selected group of lesbian mothers—selected to range over the varieties of social existence these parents and their children experience—from divorced women to single women who have deliberately chosen to conceive their children by artificial insemination by donor (AID).

The question asked by many heterosexual professionals who are charged with the theory or practice of social policy, is whether lesbian women, for example, should be (a) allowed, and (b) aided, to become mothers.

Objections to lesbian women being *allowed* to reproduce can only be social, since no physiological studies seeking to find physical differences between lesbian and non-lesbian women have ever succeeded in demonstrating such a difference.

Social objections fall into two categories: (a) the extent to which the psychopathology of the lesbian mother is assumed or demonstrated to deviate negatively from the norm. No studies to date have demonstrated that lesbian mothering is either significantly different from heterosexual mothering or that the lesbian mother is psychologically inadequately equipped to mother;[2] (b) the extent to which the children of lesbian mothers are assumed to fall victim to negative psychosexual developmental influences. No study to date has succeeded in demonstrating such a phenomenon.[3]

There remain social objections issuing from prejudice, which in turn issues from ignorance. Since the medical profession forms a professional part of our social policy-making institutional life, it is required that medical practitioners do not form judgments based on ignorance. A mere assumption that because, historically, lesbian women have been pathologised this somehow proves that they are 'not normal' (and that in a negative sense) is, of course, unacceptable.

A good way of thinking about this is to begin with what is known about female sexuality. In the first place, it is clear that women, unlike men, are able to separate their sexual practice from their reproductive practice. It is possible, that is, for a woman (a) to become sexually aroused and reach orgasm without any possibility that she will become pregnant and (b) for a woman to be inseminated—either naturally or artificially—and become pregnant whether or not, at the same time, she experiences any sexual pleasure. Whatever might be thought, therefore, about lesbian sexual practice, it is clear that lesbian women are able to conceive and bear children in the same way as non-lesbian women do.

Hence, attempting not to allow them to do so would be highly problematic, even apart from the

Reprinted by permission of Journal of Medical Ethics, *1983, vol. 9, 133-135.*

massive dilemma—were such a decision taken—of not being *able* to enforce the sanction. Contrary to popular prejudice, it is the case that lesbian women, like other women, are quite capable of engaging in sexual intercourse with a man and, like other women, often solely for the reason that they intend to become pregnant.

Prejudice is not only rife within what are called the 'helping professions', it is rife, too, in the courts. Lesbian mothers in dispute with husbands almost all lose custody of their children solely on the grounds of their lesbianism.[4] Because of this, as well as for many other reasons, young women in the last decade have turned increasingly to the alternative of AID. They have found, by and large, that medical practitioners are not willing to provide AID for them, again solely on the grounds of their lesbianism. They have decided, increasingly, in response to this attitude, to conduct AID by themselves, with the assistance of sympathetic men. This is neither technically difficult nor is it illegal. Many AID daughters and sons of lesbian women are now in our nurseries and schools.

There are over two million lesbian mothers in the United States. Calculations for Britain are well-nigh impossible, owing to the professional non-recognition of the existence of the group, together with the mothers' reticence in the face of prejudice. They are rightly anxious to conceal their sexuality since, like nearly all mothers, they love their children and will not willingly give them up, either to the courts or to any other social agency.

We might consider one case in particular. A lesbian woman, of middle-class background and professional standing in her own right, decided that she wanted to become a mother. It was, for her, a natural fulfillment of her womanhood, just as it is for millions of other women.

She became pregnant, deliberately, but unfortunately suffered a miscarriage, accompanied by much distress and depression. The usual practice of the hospital treating her was that, following the customary D & C, the patient should report to her own general practitioner. This she did, some six weeks later, wanting very much to know whether there were any clinical reasons why she might suffer further miscarriages. She asked the GP whether the hospital had sent her report.

'Yes, why?' came the reply.

'I want to know whether there is anything wrong with me which explains why I lost the baby,' the woman explained.

'Why do you want to know?' persisted the GP.

'Because if there isn't, I want to become pregnant again,' said the woman. 'It was so dreadful losing the baby that I wouldn't knowingly go through it again. But if I can have a normal, full-term pregnancy, I want to try.'

'But you can't have a baby,' replied the GP, appalled; 'you're not married!'

'What's that got to do with it?' asked the woman. And so ensued an embarrassing session of moralistic instruction from the GP to the silent woman. Her question remained unanswered.

She asked a friend who was a GP in a different area to write to the hospital for the information. This was done. There was no clinical reason for the miscarriage and the woman was pronounced normal and healthy.

The woman became pregnant again. But instead of feeling she could be cared for by her GP, she felt forced to opt for ante-natal care in the impersonal atmosphere of the hospital, where hundreds of women attended the clinic and where the same practitioner hardly ever appeared twice. At each visit, she was seen by different staff, which was comfortless but which at least ensured minimal questioning.

When she was nearly three months pregnant, the sister-in-charge said she must see the social worker. It was 'hospital policy'. But only, of course, for the unmarried. The woman felt angry and hurt, but didn't want to be accused of 'making trouble'. The social worker was sympathetic. 'Just for the record, do you want your baby?' she asked. 'Just for the record,' the woman replied, 'I planned my baby.'

After delivery, she and her baby were not placed in an ordinary ward, but in one where mothers with handicapped babies were placed, together with mothers who had not had normal deliveries. In addition, she was 'strongly advised' to stay for the full period, rather than to go home after 48 hours. And yet both she and her baby were fit and healthy.

This mother keeps away from the 'helping

professions'. She is not open with her present GP, her child's school or the para-medical services, either about the circumstances of her child's birth or about her own sexuality. When she is offered contraception during her cervical smear tests, she simply declines it, not daring to explain that she is one of thousands of lesbian women who don't need it.

This woman is a proud and independent mother.[5] And her story is only one among scores. There is the mother who was refused AID by her local medical services and who then answered an advertisement in a lonely hearts column in order to find a man who would make her pregnant. She charted her ovulation cycle, and when she was fertile, dated the man, who only and clearly wanted casual sex. Her 'experiment' worked and she bore a healthy child. There is the mother who came home from work one day to find a weeping partner who had to tell her that both her children—a son aged nine and a daughter aged seven—had been taken into care, because someone had told the social worker that the two women were lesbians.[6]

Hardly any histories of lesbian mothers and their children are on the record. But they are amongst us and they deserve the same care from professional carers as do other mothers and their children.

There are, too, gay men who parent and there are lesbian women and gay men who, though not biological parents themselves, are necessarily involved in childcare by virtue of their partners' parenthood. And there are men who donate semen for the insemination of women who take on themselves the responsibility of conception in order to exercise their right to reproduce and to bring up children. None of the considered and intricate planning undertaken by all these people is mentioned in the vast literature about the family, either in professional or popular publications. Hardly any of this material finds its way into discussions and seminars about family policy, about education, about poverty and so on.

In addition, cruel and heartless lobbying from powerful religious and political quarters—aimed against the human rights of adult homosexual women and men—is ongoing, despite its lack of scientific objectivity. Such pressure is also richly funded. The onus is therefore on the rational, well-informed and compassionate professionals in our caring institutions to consider how they will respond to those of our number born to homosexual parents. Removing the right to reproduce is both immoral and impractical. Neglecting the need of parents for normal support is both discriminatory and cruel. Removing their children from the natural custody of their parents—merely on grounds of the parents' sexuality—is a monstrous interference, with consequences for the children which are no better than the fate of children who are unwanted by their natural mothers. What is needed is education, not legislation.

There are no data—scientific, psychological, or social—which could support the thesis that homosexual people should not have the right to reproduce and to bring up their children. There are only differing opinions and prejudices, which are not capable of sustaining the rigorous intellectual analysis upon which any given body of knowledge must rest. Hitler didn't like homosexuals. Or the handicapped. Or Jews. His answer was to attempt to exterminate them. Our cruelties are not so extreme. What we do is simply to ignore groups of people whose existence troubles us.

I submit, humbly but confidently, that using an argument to exclude adult people from parenthood which is based solely on the definition of an individual's sexual practice, is untenable and uncivilised. Adult people have in their gift the right to dispose of their own reproductive potential as they themselves think suitable. And the rest of us share, all of us, in the responsibility to care for all those committed to parenting and for the children for whom they care.

References and Notes

1. Hanscombe G E, Forster J. *Rocking the cradle.* London: Peter Owen, 1981 and Sheba Feminist Publishers, 1982.

2. Green R. Sexual identity of 37 children raised by homosexual or transexual parents. *American journal of psychiatry* 1978; 6: 692–697.

3. See project comparing the psychosexual development of lesbians' children with that of single non-lesbians' children, undertaken by Michael Rutter, Susan Golombok and Ann Spencer, of the Institute of Psychiatry in London. Not all the data is

yet published—to my present knowledge—but see reference (1) 85–87.

4. In February of this year the Court of Appeal ruled in favour of a lesbian mother retaining custody of her two daughters. The case made newspaper headlines, not least because such rulings have been so rare.

5. Identity and details withheld.

6. Identities and details withheld.

Artificial Insemination and Donor Responsibility _____

Ronald Munson

When Onan cast his seed on the ground, according to the Biblical account, that was the end of the possibility that his sperm might generate offspring. Modern biomedical technology has substantially altered the situation. Sperm cast into a sterile plastic container may immediately be used in an attempt to fertilize an ovum of a woman who has requested the procedure. Or the sperm might be frozen and later used toward the same end.

Onan may have had responsibilities to his God, but neither he nor anyone else had any particular moral responsibilities concerning the use of his cast-off sperm. By contrast, artificial insemination (AI) presents a great variety of moral, legal, and social issues. Some of the questions concern individual rights and responsibilities: Can a child born from AI legitimately demand to know the name of her biological father? Should any woman be permitted to be inseminated "on demand"? Should self-described lesbians be acknowledged as having a right to have children by AI? Should a woman be allowed to order sperm donated by a man who approximates her ideal (ethnic group, hair and eye color, height, body type, intelligence, physical attractiveness, sexual orientation)?

Other questions concern the proper role and responsibilities of sperm banks as social institutions: How thoroughly must sperm donors be screened for genetic diseases? Should acknowledged homosexuals be permitted to be sperm donors? What physical, educational, or general social traits (if any) should individuals possess to qualify as donors? Should national records be maintained and shared to prevent the marriage or mating of individuals born from AI with the same biological father (that is, the same anonymous donor)?

My concern here clearly cannot be with all of the issues raised by AI. I wish to limit consideration to a single, although central, issue. The question can be formulated in this way: *Are there any special moral difficulties associated with the donation of sperm for use in AI?* In particular, does the sperm donor have any special responsibilities or rights? If the sperm donor is exactly similar to the blood donor or organ donor, then there will be no special moral difficulties associated with the role. The responsibilities of each sort of donor will be the same. Yet if there are morally relevant features that distinguish donating sperm from donating blood, it is possible that the sperm donor may have rights or responsibilities not shared by the blood donor.

Before addressing the question directly, it is worth considering the issues involved in two court cases concerning AI. The legal issues show that the moral issues are not purely speculative ones.

1. Two Court Cases

Since the turn of the century, a variety of legal issues have been discussed in connection with AI. Most of them have concerned inheritance and legitimacy, but two relatively recent court decisions raise issues that bear more directly on moral rights and responsibilities. One is the 1968 California Supreme Court decision in the case of *People* v. *Sorenson*.[1] The Sorensons, a married couple, agreed that Mrs. Sorenson would be artificially inseminated by a physician employing the sperm of an anonymous donor. The procedure was carried out, Mrs. Sorenson became pregnant, and a child was born. Four years afterwards, the couple separated, and

Mrs. Sorenson took custody of the child. She requested child-support payments, but Mr. Sorenson refused to pay on the grounds that he was not the father of the child.

The court rejected Mr. Sorenson's argument and held that he was liable for child support. According to the court, "the word 'father' is construed to include a husband who, unable to accomplish his objective of creating a child by using his own semen, purchases semen from a donor and uses it to inseminate his wife to achieve his purpose."[2] Furthermore, the court held that the donor could not be regarded as the father, for "he is no more responsible for the use made of his sperm than is the donor of blood or a kidney."[3] For the court, then, the "natural father" of the child was the husband who consented to his wife's being inseminated with donor sperm. The sperm donor was explicitly held to be no different from a blood donor or an organ donor.

A more unusual court case also focused on the question of identifying the "natural father" of a child conceived by AI. The case of *CM* v. *CC* in the New Jersey Juvenile and Domestic Relations Court involved a situation considered to be without legal precedent.[4] The woman in the case, CC, wished to have a child, but she neither wished to marry at the time nor to have intercourse before marriage. Her male friend, CM, whom she was dating exclusively, offered to provide the sperm to be used in AI. The physician at the sperm bank to which CC applied for assistance refused to perform the procedure, but CC acquired sufficient information to inseminate herself. This she did, with the cooperation of CM, and became pregnant by that means. Three months before the birth of the child, CC and CM severed their relationship.

After the child was born, CC refused to allow CM to visit, and CM turned to the court to claim visitation rights. The issue, as the court saw it, was whether CM should be recognized as the natural father of the child, given that his sperm had been "transferred to CC by other than natural conventional means." If so, then CM would have visitation rights, for courts have repeatedly held that the natural fathers of illegitimate children have such a right.

In making its decision, the court reasoned that if a child is conceived by intercourse between two unmarried people, the fact that they are un-married does not alter the fact that the man is the father. Similarly, if a child is conceived between two unmarried people by employing the sperm of the man, the fact that the sperm was delivered by artificial means does not alter the fact that the man is the father. CM was a willing participant in CC's becoming pregnant, and in the circumstances, the manner in which the sperm was "delivered" was irrelevant. The court accordingly granted CM visitation rights, but it also enjoined him with the parental obligation of providing "support and maintenance of the child and payment of any expenses incurred in his birth."[5]

2. Donors as Supplying a Product to Be Used by Others

In the Sorenson case, the court held that the sperm donor was no more responsible for the use made of his sperm than a blood donor is for the use made of his blood. In either case, the donor is only supplying a product that is to be used by others. Presumably, then, if there are relevant moral differences between blood transfusions and AI, the differences are ones connected with the actions. Consequently, only the agents who perform the actions or consent to them are the proper subjects of moral evaluation.

The court was concerned primarily with the question of legal paternity, and it would be wrong to read the decision as implying that blood donors have no moral responsibilities so neither do sperm donors. This view of the moral situation is obviously too simple.

A person who knowingly sells a quantity of rat poison to a reputed bluebeard is not guilty of any ensuing act of poisoning by his customer, but he is surely guilty of something. Similarly, someone who donates blood knowing that it is going to be used to lengthen the life of someone who is being tortured to death bears some degree of blame for contributing to the action. Likewise, a sperm donor who sells sperm that he suspects is going to be used to impregnate a woman against her will is surely blameworthy in some way and to some extent.

Such cases make it plain that a person who knowingly supplies the material conditions necessary for an immoral act does not escape all responsibility for the act merely because he does not perform it himself. Under appropriate conditions, supplying materials is one way of acquiring responsibility. In this respect, there is no morally relevant difference between being a blood donor and being a sperm donor. In either case, the donor has some responsibility for the use to which his contributed product is put. This also means that he has some responsibility for finding out how it will be used before he contributes (or sells) it.

Some have contended that AI is inherently immoral, for it requires masturbation, which violates the "natural end" of sex. On this view, the very act of donating sperm would be wrong. However, if AI is not in itself wrong and masturbation is not in itself wrong (views I accept but will not argue for), then whatever responsibilities a sperm donor may have, they do not stem from contributing to or performing an invariably wrong act.

3. Donors as Responsible for the Quality of the Product

So far in discussing blood and sperm donors we have focused on the material supplied for use in an action performed by another. Thus, potential wrongfulness in both instances is acquired only at secondhand, since it depends on the actions of those who make use of the materials. However, there is a way in which wrongfulness may attach directly to the action of a donor.

Suppose that a donor falsifies his genetic history or lies about being the carrier of a heritable genetic defect (such as Tay-Sachs disease). In such an instance, he is directly responsible for the birth of a child with the associated relevant genetic defect. The physician who performs the insemination has not acted wrongly. Rather, the blame attaches to the donor. The donor has knowingly provided a defective and potentially deadly product.

Here again there is no disanalogy between sperm donation and blood donation. Before the procedure for testing blood for the presence of AIDS antibodies was introduced, someone who had been diagnosed as having AIDS could have concealed that fact and quite knowingly put others at risk of dying from the disease communicated via his blood.

So far as blameworthiness is concerned, there seems to be no real difference between donating blood and donating sperm. In both instances, wrongfulness may be attributed directly to the action of a donor.

4. Sperm Donation and Sexual Intercourse

The comparison between donating blood and donating sperm has produced results that support the view that there are no special moral problems or responsibilities connected with sperm donation. But perhaps by focusing on the fact that both are donations of a product we have been led to overlook significant disanalogies between the two sorts of acts.

Certainly there are important differences between donating blood and "donating" sperm through intercourse. The most significant difference is connected with the potential outcome of the acts. While donating blood is at most a contribution toward someone's interest (health, well-being, treatment, etc.), "donating" sperm may lead to the conception and birth of another human being—a dependent child. The biological difference between blood and sperm makes the acts of giving quite different. Thus, in considering AI, it may be more reasonable to compare the results of sperm donation to the results of sexual intercourse, rather than to the results of blood donation.

The responsibility for a child normally falls to the biological parents. Exceptions to this are made in law only in special circumstances. For example, a child conceived by a woman as a result of an adulterous relationship may be considered the legal progeny of the woman's husband for certain purposes. However, except in such cases, responsibility is typically assigned to both biological parents, and whether or not they are married to one another is irrelevant. Thus, if we take seriously the fact that AI and intercourse may lead to the same outcome, should we not say that the sperm donor is responsible for the child conceived from his sperm?

This view seems both counterintuitive and simplistic. But why should this be? Are there really morally relevant differences between delivering sperm by intercourse and delivering it by AI? The question is one that merits an answer if we are to avoid an uncritical dogmatism that assumes that the answer is obvious and needs no argument to support it.

At least two differences between the two sorts of cases stand out, and prima facie they may seem to explain why we are unwilling to count the sperm donor as the, so to speak, moral father of a child, even though he may be the biological father. First, it might be argued that the sperm donor has no intention of impregnating the woman who might receive his sperm. She is, most likely, a total stranger, someone he has never met and probably never will meet. Thus, it is totally ridiculous to suggest that he could have the intention of making her pregnant or becoming a father. Most likely, the donor has only the intention of making money by being paid a fee for donating his sperm. Or, at best, the sperm donor, like the blood donor, has the intention of providing a material that may be of assistance to someone who has a specific need that he is in a position to satisfy.

The obvious flaw in this argument is that men who "deliver" sperm by having sex do not always have the intention of impregnating their partners. The news has been out for some time that men engage in intercourse for a variety of reasons, and impregnating the female is not invariably one of them. Consequently, the man who delivers sperm through intercourse may be just as lacking in intention as the sperm donor may be imagined to be. In neither case need pregnancy have anything to do with the aim of action, and intention cannot be the grounds for holding that the man who engages in intercourse is the biological father who must accept attendant responsibilities, while the man who donates his sperm is the biological father who has no such responsibilities.

Second, it might be held that the likelihood of producing a pregnancy marks the difference between intercourse-and-responsibility and sperm donation-and-no-responsibility. After all, in having sex there is always a real probability of the female partner's becoming pregnant. The probability might be lowered by birth-control procedures, including vasectomy, but some degree of probability always remains. If we assume that the male knows that there is at least some risk, no matter how small, of pregnancy resulting from intercourse, then it is reasonable to hold him responsible if it occurs. By contrast, a sperm donor has no way of knowing what is going to be done with his sperm. It might be used for research purposes, it might be discarded after its "shelf-life" has passed, it might be mixed with the husband's sperm, or it might be used as merely one of a series of inseminations in which the sperm of others is also employed.

Once again, however, such a contrast is more apparent than real. Ordinarily, the sperm donor can be assumed to know that there is at least some degree of probability that his sperm will be used in AI. In this respect, then, he is in exactly the same position as the man who engages in intercourse, and there is no morally relevant difference (based on likelihood of pregnancy) between the cases.

However, let us assume that the sperm donor is completely ignorant of the likelihood that his sperm will be used to produce a pregnancy. This ignorance does not alter the fact that there is a certain degree of probability that someone will become pregnant by means of his sperm. Notice, though, that it is also possible for a male engaging in intercourse to be ignorant of the fact that there is a probability that his partner will become pregnant. (He may simply be ignorant of the realities of sex or he may hold certain false beliefs. For example, he may think that it is impossible for a nursing mother to become pregnant, or he may believe that his vasectomy guarantees that he is incapable of insemination.)

It is difficult to imagine a situation in which we would hold that ignorance on the part of the male who engages in intercourse excuses him from the responsibilities that attach to being the biological father of a resulting child. But if ignorance in the intercourse case is not a reason for setting aside the responsibilities of the biological father, then there seems to be no reason why it should be in the sperm-donation case.

Are we thus forced to accept the counterintuitive conclusion that since the sperm donor is the biological father, then he must also be the moral father? We are not if we can show that being the biological father is not a sufficient condition for being the moral father.

Under ordinary conditions, we are inclined to identify the biological father with the moral father. The reason for this lies in the general principle that someone who causes something to happen is responsible for its happening. Indeed, the question "Who is responsible for this?" asked about the occurrence of an event is a request for the identity of a person or persons who can be considered candidates for praise or blame. We expect and require that people, as we say, accept the consequences of their actions.

If a woman becomes pregnant as a result of having sex with A, we hold A responsible (partially) for the child, just because A is the cause of the pregnancy. It is irrelevant that the woman also had sex with B and C. They might have been responsible for the pregnancy, but as a matter of fact they were not. A is not responsible because he has genetic characteristics that are different from B and C or anything of the kind. A is responsible, we hold, because he is causally responsible, because the pregnancy resulted from his actions. We then expect and require him to accept the consequences of his actions. We thus identify him as both the biological and the moral father of the child.

By contrast with the actions of A in our example, the sperm donor does nothing to impregnate the recipient of the sperm. He is *not responsible* for her becoming pregnant, even though it is his sperm that makes her pregnant. He is the biological father, just as is A, but he is not the moral father, for unlike A, he is not the causal agent. Not being the causal agent, the sperm donor is not appropriately placed to "accept the consequences of his actions," when this means accepting responsibility for the child produced by the use of his sperm. The donor's actions consist only in donating (selling) his sperm, and as we discussed earlier, some responsibilities attach to such actions, but the responsibility of being a moral father is not among them.

In saying that the donor is not the causal agent of the pregnancy, I do not mean to deny that he is part of the causal complex. If "the cause" of an event is the entire set of conditions sufficient for the occurrence of the event, then the donor provides what is usually called a contributory condition. In this respect, his role is no different from that of the person who supplied the pigments Michaelangelo used to paint the Sistine ceiling. Just as it would be absurd to identify the paint supplier as responsible for the paintings, it would be absurd to identify the sperm donor as responsible for the child. (It is tempting to say that the donor's sperm is a necessary condition for the occurrence of the pregnancy, but that is not correct. Sperm is a necessary condition, but not *his* sperm. At most, he supplies a necessary condition relative to that particular set of conditions that is jointly sufficient.)

It is in causal agency that we can locate the relevant moral difference between being a sperm donor whose sperm is used in AI and someone who impregnates a woman through intercourse. However, this seems to require us to conclude that the physician who uses the sperm to perform AI is the moral father of the child. Since the physician causes the pregnancy, it would seem to follow that he or she is responsible for it.

This particular counterintuitive outcome indicates that the AI situation is more complicated than we have allowed for so far. We have assumed that an action that causes an outcome entails a responsibility for the outcome. This is true so far as causal responsibility is concerned; however, causal responsibility is, at most, a necessary condition for moral responsibility. If a terrorist has filled a hospital ward with methane gas and by unsuspectingly turning on the light I cause the gas to explode, I am causally responsible for the explosion. That is, I performed the action that completed the causal chain. However, moral responsibility lies with the terrorist who filled the room with explosive gas.

The physician who performs AI is causally responsible for a woman's becoming pregnant. It is his act that makes her pregnant. However, she does not become pregnant because, to use an apt phrase from the last century, he "has his way with her." She becomes pregnant because the physician is not merely acting with her consent, but acting as her agent. She is as morally responsible for her own pregnancy as the terrorist is morally responsible for the explosion.

It is true that the physician must agree to act as the agent and, in doing so, accepts certain responsibilities. The physician must be assured that the woman is in a state of health compatible with being pregnant, that she genuinely wants to be pregnant, that she is not having a baby merely to sell for profit, and so on. Additional responsibilities attach to how the physician performs the task—has a serious effort been made to choose a sperm donor free of genetic disease, is the procedure performed in accordance with professional standards, and has meaningful consent been secured? However, in acting as the woman's agent, the physician is in no way responsible for the child that is conceived. The real causal agent is the woman herself.

What about the circumstance in which a male

marriage partner agrees to the AI of his wife, with her consent, by the use of donor sperm? Does the husband then have no responsibilities, since he has not acted as a causal agent? The reasoning of the court in *Sorenson* seems quite correct in such a case. The husband, as one of the parties to the initial agreement, explicitly assumes responsibility for the child. He acknowledges himself to be the moral father. If he later changes his mind, he is still responsible because of his original commitment. His wife becomes pregnant as though by his word, and he can no more cease to be the moral father than he could if he were also the biological father. If the wife acts as a result of the agreement with her husband, then to some degree he too is causally responsible for the birth of the child.

It is now easy to see why the courts in *Sorenson* and in *CM* v. *CC* adopted different views toward the sperm donors. In *Sorenson*, the husband was a causal agent in the sense described above, for his wife became pregnant as though by his word. Accordingly, the anonymous sperm donor played no role at all as a causal agent. By contrast, in *CM* v. *CC*, CM cooperated with CC in her becoming pregnant, and each played the same sort of causal role they would have played had actual intercourse taken place. CM was a sperm "donor" only in a Pickwickian sense.

A general result that follows from the position we have argued for is the recognition that being a biological father is not sufficient condition for being a moral or social father. We must now acknowledge that the special circumstances of AI make the role of biological father irrelevant to assigning responsibilities for the care of a child after it is born. The biological father in AI also has no rights as moral or social father. Since he played no role as a causal agent in the conception of the child, he can make no claim on the child, nor can the child or the child's representatives make any claim on him.

The exception to this concerns the area in which the sperm donor does have responsibilities. If he has in ignorance or through deception been responsible for the birth of a child with a genetic disorder, then he is liable to be held at least morally accountable for his action of contributing sperm. If he acted in ignorance, the only claim on him might be to provide medical information that might be of help to the child. If he acted with the intent to deceive, then we might believe that he

should be liable for more than our moral condemnation. We might argue, for example, that he should be forced to pay an indemnity.

Conclusion

The question we began with was whether a sperm donor has any special responsibilities or rights. In particular, we asked, are there any morally relevant differences between the sperm donor and the blood donor? Prima facie it seemed that there might be, for donating blood does not lead to the same sort of potential outcome that donating sperm does, for sperm may result in the birth of a dependent child.

What we have found is that there is no reason to hold that a sperm donor is the moral father of the child conceived by this sperm. Being the biological father, we argued, is not sufficient condition for being the moral father. The sperm donor is not a *causal agent* in the conception of the child and so is not responsible for the child. Further, although the physician who inseminates plays a causal role, he or she is not responsible for the child either. Causal responsibility is only a necessary condition for moral responsibility, and the physician is acting as the agent of the woman who has requested AI. A husband who agrees that his wife will have a child by AI is also acting as a causal agent, and in his agreement he has committed himself to becoming the moral father of the child. His wife has become pregnant by his word, rather than by his sperm.

There are differences between the sperm donor and the blood donor, but the differences are not morally relevant ones. Both have responsibilities, but they are responsibilities that come from providing a product. The fact that sperm can be used to produce a child and blood cannot is not morally significant.

References

1. The People v. Falmer J. Sorenson. Supreme Court of California, Cr. 11708 (Feb. 26, 1968). 437 P. 2d 495.
2. Op. cit., 500.
3. Op. cit., 498.
4. C. M. v. C. C. Juvenile and Domestic Relations Court, Cumberland County, N.J., 152 N.J. Super. 160 (July 19, 1977). 377A. 2d 821.
5. Op. cit., 825.

Instruction on Respect for Human Life in Its Origin and on the Dignity of Procreation: Replies to Certain Questions of the Day

Congregation for the Doctrine of the Faith

Background Note. The following "Instruction" was issued on February 22, 1987. It was approved and ordered published by Pope John Paul II and thus may be taken as representing the official position of the Roman Catholic Church on the issues addressed. The document was actually published on March 10, 1987, too late to be discussed in the introduction to this chapter.

The document takes the position that a number of current or potential practices connected with reproductive technology are morally illegitimate. Included are the following:

Prenatal diagnosis by amniocentesis or ultrasound for the purpose of identifying impaired fetuses so that abortion can be performed;
Therapeutic intervention that may cause a risk to a fetus disproportionate to a potential benefit;
Experimentation on a living embryo that is not directly therapeutic;
Keeping alive human embryos for experimental or commercial purposes;
Destroying human embryos produced by in vitro techniques for the purpose of either research or procreation;
Cross-species fertilization involving human and animal gametes;
The gestation of a human embryo in an animal uterus or an artificial uterus;
The use of human genetic material in procedures like cloning, parthenogenesis, and twin fission (the splitting of gametes);
Attempts to manipulate genetic material for the purpose of sex selection or to promote desirable characteristics;
Artificial insemination involving unmarried individuals or the artificial insemination of an unmarried woman or a widow, even if the sperm is that of her deceased husband;
Acquiring sperm by means of masturbation;
Surrogate motherhood.

Some techniques and practices, according to the document, are morally legitimate. Included are the following:

Medical intervention to remove the causes of infertility;
The prescription of drugs to promote fertility;
Prenatal diagnosis with the aim of promoting the welfare of the fetus;
Prenatal therapeutic intervention (including genetic manipulation) with the aim of healing the developing embryo or fetus;
Prenatal research that is limited to monitoring or observing the embryo.

The document also makes a number of specific recommendations to governments to establish laws and policies governing reproductive technologies. It asks that civil laws be passed to prohibit the donation of sperm or ova between unmarried people. Laws should "expressly forbid" the use of living embryos for experimentation and protect them from mutilation and destruction. Further, legislation should prohibit "embryo banks, postmortem insemination and 'surrogate motherhood.' "

Some Roman Catholic theologians disagreed sharply with parts of the document. "The document argues that a child can be born only from a sexual act," Richard A. McCormick pointed out. "The most that can be argued is that a child should be born within a marriage from a loving act. Sexual intercourse is not the only loving act." Some suggested that individuals would make up their own minds on the issues, quite apart from the Vatican position. The significance of the document to non-Catholics is that the positions taken and the arguments for them are likely to affect the character of the discussion about reproductive technology and have an impact on legislation that will place restraints on research and practices many currently consider legitimate.

Foreword

The Congregation for the Doctrine of the Faith has been approached by various Episcopal Conferences or individual Bishops, by theologians, doctors and scientists, concerning biomedical techniques which make it possible to intervene in the initial phase of the life of a human being and in the very processes of procreation and their conformity with the principles of Catholic morality. The present Instruction, which is the result of wide consultation and in particular of a careful evaluation of the declarations made by Episcopates, does not intend to repeat all the Church's teaching on the dignity of human life as it originates and on procreation, but to offer, in the light of the previous teaching of the Magisterium, some specific replies to the main questions being asked in this regard.

The exposition is arranged as follows: an *introduction* will recall the fundamental principles, of an anthropological and moral character, which are necessary for a proper evaluation of the problems and for working out replies to those questions; the *first part* will have as its subject respect for the human being from the first moment of his or her existence; the *second part* will deal with the moral questions raised by technical interventions on human procreation; the *third part* will offer some orientations on the relationships between moral law and civil law in terms of the respect due to human embryos and fetuses* and as regards the legitimacy of techniques of artificial procreation.

Introduction

1. Biomedical Research and the Teaching of the Church

The gift of life which God the Creator and Father has entrusted to man calls him to appreciate the inestimable value of what he has been given and to take responsibility for it: this fundamental principle must be placed at the center of one's reflection in order to clarify and solve the moral problems raised by artificial interventions on life as it originates and on the processes of procreation.

Thanks to the progress of the biological and medical sciences, man has at his disposal ever more effective therapeutic resources; but he can also acquire new powers, with unforeseeable consequences, over human life at its very beginning and in its first stages. Various procedures now make it possible to intervene not only in order to assist but also to dominate the processes of procreation. These techniques can enable man to "take in hand his own destiny," but they also expose him "to the temptation to go beyond the limits of a reasonable dominion over nature."[1] They might constitute progress in the service of man, but they also involve serious risks. Many people are therefore expressing an urgent appeal that in interventions on procreation the values and rights of the

---

*   The terms "zygote," "pre-embryo," "embryo" and "fetus" can indicate in the vocabulary of biology successive stages of the development of a human being. The present Instruction makes free use of these terms, attributing to them an identical ethical relevance, in order to designate the birth (whether visible or not) of human generation, from the first moment of its existence until birth. The reason for this usage is clarified by the text (cf*I, 1).

human person be safeguarded. Requests for clarification and guidance are coming not only from the faithful but also from those who recognize the Church as "an expert in humanity"[2] with a mission to serve the "civilization of love"[3] and of life.

The Church's Magisterium does not intervene on the basis of a particular competence in the area of the experimental sciences; but having taken account of the data of research and technology, it intends to put forward, by virtue of its evangelical mission and apostolic duty, the moral teaching corresponding to the dignity of the person and to his or her integral vocation. It intends to do so by expounding the criteria of moral judgment as regards the applications of scientific research and technology, especially in relation to human life and its beginnings. These criteria are the respect, defense and promotion of man, his "primary and fundamental right" to life,[4] his dignity as a person who is endowed with a spiritual soul and with moral responsibility[5] and who is called to beatific communion with God.

The Church's intervention in this field is inspired also by the love which she owes to man, helping him to recognize and respect his rights and duties. This love draws from the fount of Christ's love: as she contemplates the mystery of the Incarnate Word, the Church also comes to understand the "mystery of man";[6] by proclaiming the Gospel of salvation, she reveals to man his dignity and invites him to discover fully the truth of his own being. Thus the Church once more puts forward the divine law in order to accomplish the work of truth and liberation.

For it is out of goodness—in order to indicate the path of life—that God gives human beings his commandments and the grace to observe them; and it is likewise out of goodness—in order to help them persevere along the same path—that God always offers to everyone his forgiveness. Christ has compassion on our weaknesses: he is our Creator and Redeemer. May his spirit open men's hearts to the gift of God's peace and to an understanding of his precepts.

2. Science and Technology at the Service of the Human Person

God created man in his own image and likeness: "male and female he created them" (Gen

1:27), entrusting to them the task of "having dominion over the earth" (Gen 1:28). Basic scientific research and applied research constitute a significant expression of this dominion of man over creation. Science and technology are valuable resources for man when placed at his service and when they promote his integral development for the benefit of all; but they cannot of themselves show the meaning of existence and of human progress. Being ordered to man, who initiates and develops them, they draw from the person and his moral values the indication of their purpose and the awareness of their limits.

It would on the one hand be illusory to claim that scientific research and its applications are morally neutral; on the other hand one cannot derive criteria for guidance from mere technical efficiency, from research's possible usefulness to some at the expense of others, or, worse still, from prevailing ideologies. Thus science and technology require, for their own intrinsic meaning, an unconditional respect for the fundamental criteria of the moral law: that is to say, they must be at the service of the human person, of his inalienable rights and his true and integral good according to the design and will of God.[7]

The rapid development of technological discoveries gives greater urgency to this need to respect the criteria just mentioned: science without conscience can only lead to man's ruin. "Our era needs such wisdom more than bygone ages if the discoveries made by man are to be further humanized. For the future of the world stands in peril unless wiser people are forthcoming."[8]

3. Anthropology and Procedures in the Biomedical Field

Which moral criteria must be applied in order to clarify the problems posed today in the field of biomedicine? The answer to this question presupposes a proper idea of the nature of the human person in his bodily dimension.

For it is only in keeping with his true nature that the human person can achieve self-realization as a "unified totality":[9] and this nature is at the same time corporal and spiritual. By virtue of its substantial union with a spiritual soul, the human body cannot be considered as a mere complex of tissues, organs and functions, nor can it be evaluated in the same way as the body of animals; rather it is a constitutive part of the person who manifests and expresses himself through it.

The natural moral law expresses and lays down the purposes, rights and duties which are based upon the bodily and spiritual nature of the human person. Therefore this law cannot be thought of as simply a set of norms on the biological level; rather it must be defined as the rational order whereby man is called by the Creator to direct and regulate his life and actions and in particular to make use of his own body.[10]

A first consequence can be deduced from these principles: An intervention on the human body affects not only the tissues, the organs and their functions but also involves the person himself on different levels. It involves therefore, perhaps in an implicit but nonetheless real way, a moral significance and responsibility. Pope John Paul II forcefully reaffirmed this to the World Medical Association when he said: "Each human person, in his absolutely unique singularity, is constituted not only by his spirit, but by his body as well. Thus, in the body and through the body, one touches the person himself in his concrete reality. To respect the dignity of man consequently amounts to safeguarding this identity of the man 'corpore et anima unus,' as the Second Vatican Council says (*Gaudium et Spes*, 14, par. 1). It is on the basis of this anthropological vision that one is to find the fundamental criteria for decision-making in the case of procedures which are not strictly therapeutic, as, for example, those aimed at the improvement of the human biological condition."[11]

Applied biology and medicine work together for the integral good of human life when they come to the aid of a person stricken by illness and infirmity and when they respect his or her dignity as a creature of God. No biologist or doctor can reasonably claim, by virtue of his scientific competence, to be able to decide on people's origin and destiny. This norm must be applied in a particular way in the field of sexuality and procreation, in which man and woman actualize the fundamental values of love and life.

God, who is love and life, has inscribed in man and woman the vocation to share in a special way in his mystery of personal communion and in his work as Creator and Father.[12] For this reason marriage possesses specific goods and values in its union and in procreation which cannot be likened to those existing in lower forms of life. Such values and meanings are of the personal order and determine from the moral point of view the meaning and limits of artificial interventions on procreation and on the origin of human life. These interventions are not to be rejected on the grounds that they are artificial. As such, they bear witness to the possibilities of the art of medicine. But they must be given a moral evaluation in reference to the dignity of the human person, who is called to realize his vocation from God to the gift of love and the gift of life.

4. Fundamental Criteria for a Moral Judgment

The fundamental values connected with the techniques of artificial human procreation are two: the life of the human being called into existence and the special nature of the transmission of human life in marriage. The moral judgment on such methods of artificial procreation must therefore be formulated in reference to these values.

Physical life, with which the course of human life in the world begins, certainly does not itself contain the whole of a person's value, nor does it represent the supreme good of man who is called to eternal life. However it does constitute in a certain way the "fundamental" value of life, precisely because upon this physical life all the other values of the person are based and developed.[13] The inviolability of the innocent human being's right to life "from the moment of conception until death"[14] is a sign and requirement of the very inviolability of the person to whom the Creator has given the gift of life.

By comparison with the transmission of other forms of life in the universe, the transmission of human life has a special character of its own, which derives from the special nature of the human persons. "The transmission of human life is entrusted by nature to a personal and conscious act and as such is subject to the all-holy laws of God: immutable and inviolable laws which must be recognized and observed. For this reason one cannot use means and follow methods which

could be licit in the transmission of the life of plants and animals."[15]

Advances in technology have now made it possible to procreate apart from sexual relations through the meeting *in vitro* of the germ-cells previously taken from the man and the woman. But what is technically possible is not for that very reason morally admissible. Rational reflection on the fundamental values of life and of human procreation is therefore indispensable for formulating a moral evaluation of such technological interventions on a human being from the first stages of his development.

5. Teachings of the Magisterium

On its part, the Magisterium of the Church offers to human reason in this field too the light of Revelation: the doctrine concerning man taught by the Magisterium contains many elements which throw light on the problems being faced here.

From the moment of conception, the life of every human being is to be respected in an absolute way because man is the only creature on earth that God has "wished for himself"[16] and the spiritual soul of each man is "immediately created" by God;[17] his whole being bears the image of the Creator. Human life is sacred because from its beginning it involves "the creative action of God"[18] and it remains forever in a special relationship with the Creator, who is its sole end.[19] God alone is the Lord of life from its beginning until its end: no one can, in any circumstance, claim for himself the right to destroy directly an innocent human being.[20]

Human procreation requires on the part of the spouses responsible collaboration with the fruitful love of God;[21] the gift of human life must be actualized in marriage through the specific and exclusive acts of husband and wife, in accordance with the laws inscribed in their persons and in their union.[22]

Part I: Respect for Human Embryos

Careful reflection on this teaching of the Magisterium and on the evidence of reason, as mentioned above, enables us to respond to the numerous moral problems posed by technical interventions upon the human being in the first phases of his life and upon the processes of his conception.

1. What Respect Is Due to the Human Embryo, Taking into Account His Nature and Identity?

The human being must be respected—as a person—from the very first instant of his existence.

The implementation of procedures of artificial fertilization has made possible various interventions upon embryos and human fetuses. The aims pursued are of various kinds: diagnostic and therapeutic, scientific and commercial. From all of this, serious problems arise. Can one speak of a right to experimentation upon human embryos for the purpose of scientific research? What norms or laws should be worked out with regard to this matter? The response to these problems presupposes a detailed reflection on the nature and specific identity—the word "status" is used—of the human embryo itself.

At the Second Vatican Council, the Church for her part presented once again to modern man her constant and certain doctrine according to which: "Life once conceived, must be protected with the utmost care; abortion and infanticide are abominable crimes." More recently the *Charter of the Rights of the Family*, published by the Holy See,[23] confirmed that "Human life must be absolutely respected and protected from the moment of conception."[24]

This Congregation is aware of the current debates concerning the beginning of human life, concerning the individuality of the human being and concerning the identity of the human person. The Congregation recalls the teachings found in the Declaration on Procured Abortion: "From the time that the ovum is fertilized, a new life is begun which is neither that of the father nor of the mother: it is rather the life of a new human being with his own growth. It would never be made human if it were not human already. To this perpetual evidence . . . modern genetic science brings valuable confirmation. It has demonstrated that, from the first instant, the programme is fixed as to what this living being will be: a man, this individual-man with his characteristic aspects already well determined. Right from fertilization is

begun the adventure of a human life, and each of its great capacities requires time . . . to find its place and to be in a position to act."[25] This teaching remains valid and is further confirmed, if confirmation were needed, by recent findings of human biological science which recognize that in the zygote* resulting from fertilization the biological identity of a new human individual is already constituted.

Certainly no experimental datum can be in itself sufficient to bring us to the recognition of a spiritual soul; nevertheless, the conclusions of science regarding the human embryo provide a valuable indication for discerning by the use of reason a personal presence at the moment of the first appearance of a human life: how could a human individual not be a human person? The Magisterium has not expressly committed itself to an affirmation of a philosophical nature, but it constantly reaffirms the moral condemnation of any kind of procured abortion. This teaching has not been changed and is unchangeable.[26]

Thus the fruit of human generation, from the first moment of its existence, that is to say from the moment the zygote has formed, demands the unconditional respect that is morally due to the human being in his bodily and spiritual totality. The human being is to be respected and treated as a person from the moment of conception; and therefore from that same moment his rights as a person must be recognized, among which in the first place is the inviolable right of every innocent human being to life.

The doctrinal reminder provides the fundamental criterion for the solution of the various problems posed by the development of the biomedical sciences in this field: since the embryo must be treated as a person, it must also be defended in its integrity, tended and cared for, to the extent possible, in the same way as any other human being as far as medical assistance is concerned.

2. Is Prenatal Diagnosis Morally Licit?

If prenatal diagnosis respects the life and integrity of the embryo and the human fetus and is directed towards its safeguarding or healing as an individual, then the answer is affirmative.

---

*   The zygote is the cell produced when the nuclei of the two gametes have fused.

For prenatal diagnosis makes it possible to know the condition of the embryo and of the fetus when still in the mother's womb. It permits, or makes it possible to anticipate earlier and more effectively, certain therapeutic, medical or surgical procedures.

Such diagnosis is permissible, with the consent of the parents after they have been adequately informed, if the methods employed safeguard the life and integrity of the embryo and the mother, without subjecting them to disproportionate risks.[27] But this diagnosis is gravely opposed to the moral law when it is done with the thought of possibly inducing an abortion depending upon the results: a diagnosis which shows the existence of a malformation or a hereditary illness must not be the equivalent of a death-sentence. Thus a woman would be committing a gravely illicit act if she were to request such a diagnosis with the deliberate intention of having an abortion should the results confirm the existence of a malformation or abnormality. The spouse or relatives or anyone else would similarly be acting in a manner contrary to the moral law if they were to counsel or impose such a diagnostic procedure on the expectant mother with the same intention of possibly proceeding to an abortion. So too the specialist would be guilty of illicit collaboration if, in conducting the diagnosis and in communicating its results, he were deliberately to contribute to establishing or favoring a link between prenatal diagnosis and abortion.

In conclusion, any directive or program of the civil and health authorities or of scientific organizations which in any way were to favor a link between prenatal diagnosis and abortion, or which were to go as far as directly to induce expectant mothers to submit to prenatal diagnosis planned for the purpose of eliminating fetuses which are affected by malformations or which are carriers of hereditary illness, is to be condemned as a violation of the unborn child's right to life and as an abuse of the prior rights and duties of the spouses.

3. Are Therapeutic Procedures Carried Out on the Human Embryo Licit?

As with all medical interventions on patients, *one must uphold as licit procedures carried out on the human embryo which respect the life and integrity of the embryo and do not involve disproportionate risks for it but are directed towards its healing, the improvement of its condition of health, or its individual survival.*

Whatever the type of medical, surgical or other therapy, the free and informed consent of the parents is required, according to the deontological rules followed in the case of children. The application of this moral principle may call for delicate and particular precautions in the case of embryonic or fetal life.

The legitimacy and criteria of such procedures have been clearly stated by Pope John Paul II: "A strictly therapeutic intervention whose explicit objective is the healing of various maladies such as those stemming from chromosomal defects will, in principle, be considered desirable, provided it is directed to the true promotion of the personal well-being of the individual without doing harm to his integrity or worsening his conditions of life. Such an intervention would indeed fall within the logic of the Christian moral tradition."[28]

4. How Is One to Evaluate Morally Research and Experimentation* on Human Embryos and Fetuses?

Medical research must refrain from operations on live embryos, unless there is a moral certainty of not causing harm to the life or integrity of the unborn child and the mother, and on condition that the parents have given their free and informed consent to the procedure. It follows that all research, even when limited to the simple observation of the embryo, would be-

---

*   Since the terms "research" and "experimentation" are often used equivalently and ambiguously, it is deemed necessary to specify the exact meaning given them in this document.

1. By *research* is meant any inductive-deductive process which aims at promoting the systematic observation of a given phenomenon in the human field or at verifying a hypothesis arising from previous observations.

2. By *experimentation* is meant any research in which the human being (in the various stages of his existence: embryo, fetus, child or adult) represents the object through which or upon which one intends to verify the effect, at present unknown or not sufficiently known, of a given treatment (e.g. pharmacological, teratogenic, surgical, etc.).

come illicit were it to involve risk to the embryo's physical integrity or life by reason of the methods used or the effects induced.

As regards experimentation, and presupposing the general distinction between experimentation for purposes which are not directly therapeutic and experimentation which is clearly therapeutic for the subject himself, in the case in point one must also distinguish between experimentation carried out on embryos which are still alive and experimentation carried out on embryos which are dead. *If the embryos are living, whether viable or not, they must be respected just like any other human person; experimentation on embryos which is not directly therapeutic is illicit.*[29]

No objective, even though noble in itself, such as a foreseeable advantage to science, to other human beings or to society, can in any way justify experimentation on living human embryos or fetuses, whether viable or not, either inside or outside the mother's womb. The informed consent ordinarily required for clinical experimentation on adults cannot be granted by the parents, who may not freely dispose of the physical integrity or life of the unborn child. Moreover, experimentation on embryos and fetuses always involves risk, and indeed in most cases it involves the certain expectation of harm to their physical integrity or even their death.

To use human embryos or fetuses as the object or instrument of experimentation constitutes a crime against their dignity as human beings having a right to the same respect that is due to the child already born and to every human person.

The Charter of the Rights of the Family published by the Holy See affirms: "Respect for the dignity of the human being excludes all experimental manipulation or exploitation of the human embryo."[30] The practice of keeping alive human embryos in vivo or in vitro for experimental or commercial purposes is totally opposed to human dignity.

In the case of experimentation that is clearly therapeutic, namely, when it is a matter of experimental forms of therapy used for the benefit of the embryo itself in a final attempt to save its life, and in the absence of other reliable forms of therapy, recourse to drugs or procedures not yet fully tested can be licit.[31]

The corpses of human embryos and fetuses, whether they have been deliberately aborted or not, must be respected just as the remains of other human beings. In particular, they cannot be subjected to mutilation or to autopsies if their death has not yet been verified and without the consent of the parents or of the mother. Furthermore, the moral requirements must be safeguarded that there be no complicity in deliberate abortion and that the risk of scandal be avoided. Also, in the case of dead fetuses, as for the corpses of adult persons, all commercial trafficking must be considered illicit and should be prohibited.

5. How Is One to Evaluate Morally the Use for Research Purposes of Embryos Obtained by Fertilization 'In Vitro'?

Human embryos obtained in vitro are human beings and subjects with rights: their dignity and right to life must be respected from the first moment of their existence. *It is immoral to produce human embryos destined to be exploited as disposable "biological material."*

In the usual practice of in vitro fertilization, not all of the embryos are transferred to the woman's body; some are destroyed. Just as the Church condemns induced abortion, so she also forbids acts against the life of these human beings. *It is a duty to condemn the particular gravity of the voluntary destruction of human embryos obtained 'in vitro' for the sole purpose of research, either by means of artificial insemination of by means of "twin fission."* By acting in this way the researcher usurps the place of God; and, even though he may be unaware of this, he sets himself up as the master of the destiny of others inasmuch as he arbitrarily chooses whom he will allow to live and whom he will send to death and kills defenseless human beings.

Methods of observation or experimentation which damage or impose grave and disproportionate risks upon embryos obtained in vitro are morally illicit for the same reasons. Every human being is to be respected for himself, and cannot be reduced in worth to a pure and simple instrument for the advantage of others. *It is therefore not in conformity with the moral law deliberately to expose to death human embryos obtained 'in vitro'.* In consequence of the fact that they have been produced in vitro, those embryos which are not transferred into the body of the mother and are called "spare" are exposed to an absurd fate, with no possibility of their being offered safe means of survival which can be licitly pursued.

6. What Judgment Should Be Made on Other Procedures of Manipulating Embryos Connected with the "Techniques of Human Reproduction"?

Techniques of fertilization in vitro can open the way to other forms of biological and genetic manipulation of human embryos, such as attempts or plans for fertilization between human and animal gametes and the gestation of human embryos in the uterus of animals, or the hypothesis or project of constructing artificial uteruses for the human embryos. *These procedures are contrary to the human dignity proper to the embryo, and at the same time they are contrary to the right of every person to be conceived and to be born within marriage and from marriage.*[32] *Also, attempts or hypotheses for obtaining a human being without any connection with sexuality through "twin fission," cloning or parthenogenesis are to be considered contrary to the moral law, since they are in opposition to the dignity both of human procreation and of the conjugal union.*

The *freezing of embryos,* even when carried out in order to preserve the life of an embryo—cryo-preservation—*constitutes an offense against the respect due to human beings* by exposing them to grave risks of death or harm to their physical integrity and depriving them, at least temporarily, of maternal shelter and gestation, thus placing them in a situation in which further offenses and manipulation are possible.

Certain attempts to influence chromosomic or genetic inheritance are not therapeutic but are aimed at producing human beings selected according to sex or other predetermined qualities. These manipulations are contrary to the personal dignity of the human being and his or her integrity and identity. Therefore in no way can they be justified on the grounds of possible beneficial consequences for future humanity.[33] Every person must be respected for himself: in this consists the dignity and right of every human being from his or her beginning.

Part II: Interventions upon Human Procreation

By "artificial procreation" or "artificial fertilization" are understood here the different technical procedures directed towards obtaining a human conception in a manner other than the sexual union of man and woman. This Instruction deals with fertilization of an ovum in a test-tube (in vitro fertilization) and artificial insemination through transfer into the woman's genital tracts of previously collected sperm.

A preliminary point for the moral evaluation of such technical procedures is constituted by the consideration of the circumstances and consequences which those procedures involve in relation to the respect due the human embryo. Development of the practice of in vitro fertilization has required innumerable fertilizations and destructions of human embryos. Even today, the usual practice presupposes a hyper-ovulation on the part of the woman: a number of ova are withdrawn, fertilized and then cultivated in vitro for some days. Usually not all are transferred into the genital tracts of the woman; some embryos, generally called "spare," are destroyed or frozen. On occasion, some of the implanted embryos are sacrificed for various eugenic, economic or psychological reasons. Such deliberate destruction of human beings or their utilization for different purposes to the detriment of their integrity and life is contrary to the doctrine on procured abortion already recalled.

The connection between in vitro fertilization and the voluntary destruction of human embryos occurs too often. This is significant: through these procedures, with apparently contrary purposes, life and death are subjected to the decision of man, who thus sets himself up as the giver of life and death by decree. This dynamic of violence and domination may remain unnoticed by those very individuals who, in wishing to utilize this procedure, become subject to it themselves. The facts recorded and the cold logic which links them must be taken into consideration for a moral judgment on IVF and ET (in vitro fertilization and embryo transfer): the abortion-mentality which has made this procedure possible thus leads, whether one wants it or not, to man's domination over the life and death of his fellow human beings and can lead to a system of radical eugenics.

Nevertheless, such abuses do not exempt one from a further and thorough ethical study of the techniques of artificial procreation considered in themselves, abstracting as far as possible from the destruction of embryos produced in vitro.

The present Instruction will therefore take into consideration in the first place the problems posed by heterologous artificial fertilization (II, 1–3),* and subsequently those linked with homologous artificial fertilization (II, 4–6).**

Before formulating an ethical judgment on each of these procedures, the principles and values which determine the moral evaluation of each of them will be considered.

---

*   By the term heterologous artificial fertilization or procreation, the Instruction means techniques used to obtain a human conception artificially by the use of gametes coming from at least one donor other than the spouses who are joined in marriage. Such techniques can be of two types:

a. Heterologous IVF and ET: the technique used to obtain a human conception through the meeting in vitro of gametes taken from at least one donor other than the two spouses joined in marriage.

b. Heterologous artificial insemination: the technique used to obtain a human conception through the transfer into the genital tracts of the woman of the sperm previously collected from a donor other than the husband.

** By artificial homologous fertilization or procreation, the Instruction means the technique used to obtain a human conception using the gametes of the two spouses joined in marriage. Homologous artificial fertilization can be carried out by two different methods:

a. Homologous IVF and ET: the technique used to obtain a human conception through the meeting in vitro of the gametes of the spouses joined in marriage.

b. Homologous artificial insemination: the technique used to obtain a human conception through the transfer into the genital tracts of a married woman of the sperm previously collected from her husband.

A. Heterologous Artificial Fertilization

1. Why Must Human Procreation Take Place in Marriage?   *Every human being is always to be accepted as a gift and blessing of God. However, from the moral point of view a truly responsible procreation vis-a-vis the unborn child must be the fruit of marriage.*

For human procreation has specific characteristics by virtue of the personal dignity of the parents and of the children: the procreation of a new person, whereby the man and the woman collaborate with the power of the Creator, must be the fruit and the sign of the mutual self-giving of the spouses, of their love and of their fidelity.[34] *The fidelity of the spouses in the unity of marriage involves reciprocal respect of their right to become a father and a mother only through each other.*

The child has the right to be conceived, carried in the womb, brought into the world and brought up within marriage: it is through the secure and recognized relationship to his own parents that the child can discover his own identity and achieve his own proper human development.

The parents find in their child a confirmation and completion of their reciprocal self-giving: the child is the living image of their love, the permanent sign of their conjugal union, the living and indissoluble concrete expression of their paternity and maternity.[35]

By reason of the vocation and social responsibilities of the person, the good of the children and of the parents contributes to the good of civil society; the vitality and stability of society require that children come into the world within a family and that the family be firmly based on marriage.

The tradition of the Church and anthropological reflection recognize in marriage and in its indissoluble unity the only setting worthy of truly responsible procreation.

2. Does Heterologous Artificial Fertilization Conform to the Dignity of the Couple and to the Truth of Marriage?   Through IVF and ET and heterologous artificial insemination, human conception is achieved through the fusion of gametes of at least one donor other than the spouses who are united in marriage. *Heterologous artificial fertilization is contrary to the unity of marriage, to the dignity of the spouses, to the vocation proper to parents,* *and to the child's right to be conceived and brought into the world in marriage and from marriage.*[36]

Respect for the unity of marriage and for conjugal fidelity demands that the child be conceived in marriage; the bond existing between husband and wife accords the spouses, in an objective and inalienable manner, the exclusive right to become father and mother solely through each other.[37] Recourse to the gametes of a third person, in order to have sperm or ovum available, constitutes a violation of the reciprocal commitment of the spouses and a grave lack in regard to that essential property of marriage which is its unity.

Heterologous artificial fertilization violates the rights of the child; it deprives him of his filial relationship with his parental origins and can hinder the maturing of his personal identity. Furthermore, it offends the common vocation of the spouses who are called to fatherhood and motherhood: it objectively deprives conjugal fruitfulness of its unity and integrity; it brings about and manifests a rupture between genetic parenthood, gestational parenthood and responsibility for upbringing. Such damage to the personal relationships within the family has repercussions on civil society: what threatens the unity and stability of the family is a source of dissension, disorder and injustice in the whole of social life.

These reasons lead to a negative moral judgment concerning heterologous artificial fertilization: consequently fertilization of a married woman with the sperm of a donor different from her husband and fertilization with the husband's sperm of an ovum not coming from his wife are morally illicit. Furthermore, the artificial fertilization of a woman who is unmarried or a widow, whoever the donor may be, cannot be morally justified.

The desire to have a child and the love between spouses who long to obviate a sterility which cannot be overcome in any other way constitute understandable motivations; but subjectively good intentions do not render heterologous artificial fertilization conformable to the objective and inalienable properties of marriage or respectful of the rights of the child and of the spouses.

3. Is "Surrogate"* Motherhood Morally Licit? *No, for the same reasons which lead one to reject heterologous artificial fertilization: for it is contrary*

to the unity of marriage and to the dignity of the procreation of the human person.

Surrogate motherhood represents an objective failure to meet the obligations of maternal love, of conjugal fidelity and of responsible motherhood; it offends the dignity and the right of the child to be conceived, carried in the womb, brought into the world and brought up by his own parents; it sets up, to the detriment of families, a division between the physical, psychological and moral elements which constitute those families.

B. Homologous Artificial Fertilization

Since heterologous artificial fertilization has been declared unacceptable, the question arises of how to evaluate morally the process of homologous artificial fertilization: IVF and ET and artificial insemination between husband and wife. First a question of principle must be clarified.

4. What Connection Is Required from the Moral Point of View between Procreation and the Conjugal Act?

a. The Church's teaching on marriage and human procreation affirms the "inseparable connection, willed by God and unable to be broken by man on his own initiative, between the two meanings of the conjugal act: the unitive meaning and the procreative meaning. Indeed, by its intimate structure, the conjugal act, while most closely uniting husband and wife, capacitates them for

---

*   By "surrogate mother" the Instruction means:

a. the woman who carries in pregnancy an embryo implanted in her uterus and who is genetically a stranger to the embryo because it has been obtained through the union of the gametes of "donors." She carries the pregnancy with a pledge to surrender the baby once it is born to the party who commissioned or made the agreement for the pregnancy.

b. the woman who carries in pregnancy an embryo to whose procreation she has contributed the donation of her own ovum, fertilized through insemination with the sperm of a man other than her husband. She carries the pregnancy with a pledge to surrender the child once it is born to the party who commissioned or made the agreement for the pregnancy.

the generation of new lives, according to laws inscribed in the very being of man and of woman."[38] This principle, which is based upon the nature of marriage and the intimate connection of the goods of marriage, has well-known consequences on the level of responsible fatherhood and motherhood. "By safeguarding both these essential aspects, the unitive and the procreative, the conjugal act preserves in its fullness the sense of true mutual love and its ordination towards man's exalted vocation to parenthood."[39]

The same doctrine concerning the link between the meanings of the conjugal act and between the goods of marriage throws light on the moral problem of homologous artificial fertilization, since "it is never permitted to separate these different aspects to such a degree as positively to exclude either the procreative intention or the conjugal relation."[40]

Contraception deliberately deprives the conjugal act of its openness to procreation and in this way brings about a voluntary dissociation of the ends of marriage. Homologous artificial fertilization, in seeking a procreation which is not the fruit of a specific act of conjugal union, objectively effects an analogous separation between the goods and the meanings of marriage.

Thus, fertilization is licitly sought when it is the result of a "conjugal act which is per se suitable for the generation of children to which marriage is ordered by its nature and by which the spouses become one flesh."[41] But from the moral point of view procreation is deprived of its proper perfection when it is not desired as the fruit of the conjugal act, that is to say of the specific act of the spouses' union.

b. The moral value of the intimate link between the goods of marriage and between the meanings of the conjugal act is based upon the unity of the human being, a unity involving body and spiritual soul.[42] Spouses mutually express their personal love in the "language of the body," which clearly involves both "spousal meanings" and parental ones.[43] The conjugal act by which the couple mutually express their self-gift at the same time expresses openness to the gift of life. It is an act that is inseparably corporal and spiritual. It is in their bodies and through their bodies that the spouses consummate their marriage and are able to become father and mother. In order to respect the language of their bodies and their natural generosity, the conjugal union must take place with respect for its openness to procreation; and the procreation of a person must be the fruit and the result of married love. The origin of the human being thus follows from a procreation that is "linked to the union, not only biological but also spiritual, of the parents, made one by the bond of marriage."[44] Fertilization achieved outside the bodies of the couple remains by this very fact deprived of the meanings and the values which are expressed in the language of the body and in the union of human persons.

c. Only respect for the link between the meanings of the conjugal act and respect for the unity of the human being make possible procreation in conformity with the dignity of the person. In his unique and irrepeatable origin, the child must be respected and recognized as equal in personal dignity to those who give him life. The human person must be accepted in his parents' act of union and love; the generation of a child must therefore be the fruit of that mutual giving[45] which is realized in the conjugal act wherein the spouses cooperate as servants and not as masters in the work of the Creator who is Love.[46]

In reality, the origin of a human person is the result of an act of giving. The one conceived must be the fruit of his parents' love. He cannot be desired or conceived as the product of an intervention of medical or biological techniques; that would be equivalent to reducing him to an object of scientific technology. No one may subject the coming of a child into the world to conditions of technical efficiency which are to be evaluated according to standards of control and dominion.

The moral relevance of the link between the meanings of the conjugal act and between the goods of marriage, as well as the unity of the human being and the dignity of his origin, demand that the procreation of a human person be brought about as the fruit of the conjugal act specific to the love between spouses. The link between procreation and the conjugal act is thus shown to be of great importance on the anthropological and moral planes, and it throws light on the positions of the Magisterium with regard to homologous artificial fertilization.

5. Is Homologous 'In Vitro' Fertilization Morally Licit? The answer to this question is strictly dependent on the principles just mentioned. Certainly one cannot ignore the legitimate aspirations of sterile couples. For some, recourse to homologous IVF and ET appears to be the only way of fulfilling their sincere desire for a child. The question is asked whether the totality of conjugal life in such situations is not sufficient to insure the dignity proper to human procreation. It is acknowledged that IVF and ET certainly cannot supply for the absence of sexual relations[47] and cannot be preferred to the specific acts of conjugal union, given the risks involved for the child and the difficulties of the procedure. But it is asked whether, when there is no other way of overcoming the sterility which is a source of suffering, homologous in vitro fertilization may not constitute an aid, if not a form of therapy, whereby its moral licitness could be admitted.

The desire for a child—or at the very least an openness to the transmission of life—is a necessary prerequisite from the moral point of view for responsible human procreation. But this good intention is not sufficient for making a positive moral evaluation of in vitro fertilization between spouses. The process of IVF and ET must be judged in itself and cannot borrow its definitive moral quality from the totality of conjugal life of which it becomes part nor from the conjugal acts which may precede or follow it.[48]

It has already been recalled that, in the circumstances in which it is regularly practiced, IVF and ET involves the destruction of human beings, which is something contrary to the doctrine on the illicitness of abortion previously mentioned.[49] But even in a situation in which every precaution were taken to avoid the death of human embryos, homologous IVF and ET dissociates from the conjugal act the actions which are directed to human fertilization. For this reason the very nature of homologous IVF and ET also must be taken into account, even abstracting from the link with procured abortion.

Homologous IVF and ET is brought about outside the bodies of the couple through actions of third parties whose competence and technical activity determine the success of the procedure. Such fertilization entrusts the life and identity of the embryo into the power of doctors and biologists and establishes the domination of technology over the origin and destiny of the human person. Such a relationship of domination is in itself contrary to the dignity and equality that must be common to parents and children.

Conception in vitro is the result of the technical action which presides over fertilization. *Such fertilization is neither in fact achieved nor positively willed as the expression and fruit of specific acts of the conjugal union. In homologous IVF and ET, therefore, even if it is considered in the context of 'de facto' existing sexual relations, the generation of the human person is objectively deprived of its proper perfection: namely, that of being the result and fruit of a conjugal act in which the spouses can become "cooperators with God for giving life to a new person."*[50]

These reasons enable us to understand why the act of conjugal love is considered in the teaching of the Church as the only setting worthy of human procreation. For the same reasons the so-called "simple case," i.e. a homologous IVF and ET procedure that is free of any compromise with the abortive practice of destroying embryos and with masturbation, remains a technique which is morally illicit because it deprives human procreation of the dignity which is proper and connatural to it.

Certainly, homologous IVF and ET fertilization is not marked by all that ethical negativity found in extra-conjugal procreation; the family and marriage continue to constitute the setting for the birth and upbringing of the children. Nevertheless, in conformity with the traditional doctrine relating to the goods of marriage and the dignity of the person, *the Church remain opposed from the moral point of view to homologous 'in vitro' fertilization. Such fertilization is in itself illicit and in opposition to the dignity of procreation and of the conjugal union, even when everything is done to avoid the death of the human embryo.*

Although the manner in which human conception is achieved with IVF and ET cannot be approved, every child which comes into the world must in any case be accepted as a living gift of the divine Goodness and must be brought up with love.

6. How Is Homologous Artificial Insemination to Be Evaluated from the Moral Point of View? *Homologous artificial insemination within marriage cannot be admitted except for those cases in* *which the technical means is not a substitute for the conjugal act but serves to facilitate and to help so that the act attains its natural purpose.*

The teaching of the Magisterium on this point has already been stated.[51] This teaching is not just an expression of particular historical circumstances but is based on the Church's doctrine concerning the connection between the conjugal union and procreation and on a consideration of the personal nature of the conjugal act and of a human procreation. "In its natural structure, the conjugal act is a personal action, a simultaneous and immediate cooperation on the part of the husband and wife, which by the very nature of the agents and the proper nature of the act is the expression of the mutual gift which, according to the words of Scripture, brings about union 'in one flesh.' "[52] Thus moral conscience "does not necessarily proscribe the use of certain artificial means destined solely either to the facilitating of the natural act or to insuring that the natural act normally performed achieves its proper end."[53] If the technical means facilitates the conjugal act or helps it to reach its natural objectives, it can be morally acceptable. If, on the other hand, the procedure were to replace the conjugal act, it is morally illicit.

Artificial insemination as a substitute for the conjugal act is prohibited by reason of the voluntarily achieved dissociation of the two meanings of the conjugal act. Masturbation, through which the sperm is normally obtained, is another sign of this dissociation: even when it is done for the purpose of procreation, the act remains deprived of its unitive meaning: "It lacks the sexual relationship called for by the moral order, namely the relationship which realizes 'the full sense of mutual self-giving and human procreation in the context of true love.' "[54]

7. What Moral Criterion Can Be Proposed with Regard to Medical Intervention in Human Procreation? The medical act must be evaluated not only with reference to its technical dimension but also and above all in relation to its goal which is the good of persons and their bodily and psychological health. The moral criteria for medical intervention in procreation are deduced from the dignity of human person ~f their sexuality and of their origin.

Medicine which seeks to be ordered to the integral good of the person must respect the specifically human values of sexuality.[55] *The doctor is at the service of persons and of human procreation. He does not have the authority to dispose of them or to decide their fate. A medical intervention respects the dignity of persons when it seeks to assist the conjugal act either in order to facilitate its performance or in order to enable it to achieve its objective once it has been normally performed.*[56]

On the other hand, it sometimes happens that a medical procedure technologically replaces the conjugal act in order to obtain a procreation which is neither its result nor its fruit. In this case the medical act is not, as it should be, at the service of conjugal union but rather appropriates to itself the procreative function and thus contradicts the dignity and the inalienable rights of the spouses and of the child to be born.

The humanization of medicine, which is insisted upon today by everyone, requires respect for the integral dignity of the human person first of all in the act and at the moment in which the spouses transmit life to a new person. It is only logical therefore to address an urgent appeal to Catholic doctors and scientists that they bear exemplary witness to the respect due to the human embryo and to the dignity of procreation. The medical and nursing staff of Catholic hospitals and clinics are in a special way urged to do justice to the moral obligations which they have assumed, frequently also, as part of their contract. Those who are in charge of Catholic hospitals and clinics and who are often Religious will take special care to safeguard and promote a diligent observance of the moral norms recalled in the present Instruction.

8. The Suffering Caused by Infertility in Marriage *The suffering of spouses who cannot have children or who are afraid of bringing a handicapped child into the world is a suffering that everyone must understand and properly evaluate.*

On the part of the spouses, the desire for a child is natural: it expresses the vocation to fatherhood and motherhood inscribed in conjugal love. This desire can be even stronger if the couple is affected by sterility which appears incurable. Nevertheless, marriage does not confer upon the spouses the right to have a child, but only the right to perform those natural acts which are per se ordered to procreation.[57]

A true and proper right to a child would be contrary to the child's dignity and nature. The child is not an object to which one has a right, nor can he be considered as an object of ownership: rather, a child is a gift, "the supreme gift"[58] and the most gratuitous gift of marriage, and is a living testimony of the mutual giving of his parents. For this reason, the child has the right, as already mentioned, to be the fruit of the specific act of the conjugal love of his parents; and he also has the right to be respected as a person from the moment of his conception.

Nevertheless, whatever its cause or prognosis, sterility is certainly a difficult trial. The community of believers is called to shed light upon and support the suffering of those who are unable to fulfill their legitimate aspiration to motherhood and fatherhood. Spouses who find themselves in this sad situation are called to find in it an opportunity for sharing in a particular way in the Lord's Cross, the source of spiritual fruitfulness. Sterile couples must not forget that "even when procreation is not possible, conjugal life does not for this reason lose its value. Physical sterility in fact can be for spouses the occasion for other important services to the life of the human person, for example, adoption, various forms of educational work, and assistance to other families and to poor or handicapped children."[59]

Many researchers are engaged in the fight against sterility. While fully safeguarding the dignity of human procreation, some have achieved results which previously seemed unattainable. Scientists therefore are to be encouraged to continue their research with the aim of preventing the causes of sterility and of being able to remedy them so that sterile couples will be able to procreate in full respect for their own personal dignity and that of the child to be born.

Part III: Moral and Civil Law
The Values and Moral Obligations That Civil Legislation Must Respect and Sanction in This Matter

The inviolable right to life of every innocent human individual and the rights of the family and of the institution of marriage constitute funda-

mental moral values, because they concern the natural condition and integral vocation of the human person; at the same time they are constitutive elements of civil society and its order.

For this reason the new technological possibilities which have opened up in the field of biomedicine require the intervention of the political authorities and of the legislator, since an uncontrolled application of such techniques could lead to unforeseeable and damaging consequences for civil society. Recourse to the conscience of each individual and to the self-regulation of researchers cannot be sufficient for insuring respect for personal rights and public order. If the legislator responsible for the common good were not watchful, he could be deprived of his prerogatives by researchers claiming to govern humanity in the name of the biological discoveries and the alleged "improvement" processes which they would draw from those discoveries. "Eugenism" and forms of discrimination between human beings could come to be legitimized: this would constitute an act of violence of and serious offense to the equality, dignity and fundamental rights of the human person.

The intervention of the public authority must be inspired by the rational principles which regulate the relationships between civil law and moral law. The task of the civil law is to insure the common good of people through the recognition of and the defense of fundamental rights and through the promotion of peace and of public morality.[60] In no sphere of life can the civil law take the place of conscience or dictate norms concerning things which are outside its competence. It must sometimes tolerate, for the sake of public order, things which it cannot forbid without a greater evil resulting. However, the inalienable rights of the person must be recognized and respected by civil society and the political authority. These human rights depend neither on single individuals nor on parents; nor do they represent a concession made by society and the state: they pertain to human nature and are inherent in the person by virtue of the creative act from which the person took his or her origin.

Among such fundamental rights one should mention in this regard: a) every human being's right to life and physical integrity from the moment of conception until death; b) the rights of the family and of marriage as an institution and, in this area, the child's right to be conceived, brought into the world and brought up by his parents. To each of these two themes it is necessary here to give some further consideration.

In various states certain laws have authorized the direct suppression of innocents: the moment a positive law deprives a category of human beings of the protection which civil legislation must accord them, the state is denying the equality of all before the law. When the state does not place its power at the service of the rights of each citizen, and in particular of the more vulnerable, the very foundations of a state based on law are undermined. The political authority consequently cannot give approval to the calling of human beings into existence through procedures which would expose them to those very grave risks noted previously. The possible recognition by positive law and the political authorities of techniques of artificial transmission of life and the experimentation connected with it would widen the breach already opened by the legalization of abortion.

As a consequence of the respect and protection which must be insured for the unborn child from the moment of his conception, the law must provide appropriate penal sanctions for every deliberate violation of the child's rights. The law cannot tolerate—indeed it must expressly forbid—that human beings, even at the embryonic stage, should be treated as objects of experimentation, be mutilated or destroyed with the excuse that they are superfluous or incapable of developing normally.

The political authority is bound to guarantee to the institution of the family, upon which society is based, the juridical protection to which it has a right. From the very fact that it is at the service of people, the political authority must also be at the service of the family. Civil law cannot grant approval to techniques of artificial procreation which, for the benefit of third parties (doctors, biologists, economic or governmental powers), take away what is a right inherent in the relationship between spouses; and therefore civil law cannot legalize the donation of gametes between persons who are not legitimately united in marriage.

Legislation must also prohibit, by virtue of the support which is due to the family, embryo banks, post mortem insemination and "surrogate motherhood."

It is part of the duty of the public authority to insure that the civil law is regulated according to the fundamental norms of the moral law in matters concerning human rights, human life and the institution of the family. Politicians must commit themselves, through their interventions upon public opinion, to securing in society the widest possible consensus on such essential points and to consolidating this consensus wherever it risks being weakened or is in danger of collapse.

In many countries, the legalization of abortion and juridical tolerance of unmarried couples makes it more difficult to secure respect for the fundamental rights recalled by this Instruction. It is to be hoped that states will not become responsible for aggravating these socially damaging situations of injustice. It is rather to be hoped that nations and states will realize all the cultural, ideological and political implications connected with the techniques of artificial procreation and will find the wisdom and courage necessary for issuing laws which are more just and more respectful of human life and the institution of the family.

The civil legislation of many states confers an undue legitimation upon certain practices in the eyes of many today; it is seen to be incapable of guaranteeing that morality which is in conformity with the natural exigencies of the human person and with the "unwritten laws" etched by the Creator upon the human heart. All men of good will must commit themselves, particularly within their professional field and in the exercise of their civil rights, to insuring the reform of morally unacceptable civil laws and the correction of illicit practices. In addition, "conscientious objection" vis-à-vis such laws must be supported and recognized. A movement of passive resistance to the legitimation of practices contrary to human life and dignity is beginning to make an ever sharper impression upon the moral conscience of many, especially among specialists in the biomedical sciences.

Conclusion

The spread of technologies of intervention in the processes of human procreation raises very serious moral problems in relation to the respect due to the human being from the moment of conception, to the dignity of the person, of his or her sexuality, and of the transmission of life.

With this Instruction the Congregation for the Doctrine of the Faith, in fulfilling its responsibility to promote and defend the Church's teaching in so serious a matter, addresses a new and heartfelt invitation to all those who, by reason of their role and their commitment, can exercise a positive influence and insure that, in the family and in society, due respect is accorded to life and love. It addresses this invitation to those responsible for the formation of consciences and of public opinion, to scientists and medical professionals, to jurists and politicians. It hopes that all will understand the incompatibility between recognition of the dignity of the human person and contempt for life and love, between faith in the living God and the claim to decide arbitrarily the origin and fate of a human being.

In particular, the Congregation for the Doctrine of the Faith addresses an invitation with confidence and encouragement to theologians, and above all to moralists, that they study more deeply and make ever more accessible to the faithful the contents of the teaching of the Church's Magisterium in the light of a valid anthropology in the matter of sexuality and marriage and in the context of the necessary interdisciplinary approach. Thus they will make it possible to understand ever more clearly the reasons for and the validity of this teaching. By defending man against the excesses of his own power, the Church of God reminds him of the reasons for his true nobility; only in this way can the possibility of living and loving with that dignity and liberty which derive from respect for the truth be insured for the men and women of tomorrow. The precise indications which are offered in the present Instruction therefore are not meant to halt the effort of reflection but rather to give it a renewed impulse in unrenounceable fidelity to the teaching of the Church.

In the light of the truth about the gift of human life and in the light of the moral principles which flow from the truth, everyone is invited to act in the area of responsibility proper to each and, like the good Samaritan, to recognize as a neighbor even the littlest among the children of men (Cf. Lk 10: 29–37). Here Christ's words find a new and particular echo: "What you do to one of the least of my brethren, you do unto me" (Mt 25: 40).

During an audience granted to the undersigned Prefect after the plenary session of the Congregation for the Doctrine of the Faith, the Supreme Pontiff, John Paul II, approved this Instruction and ordered it to be published.

Given at Rome, from the Congregation for the Doctrine of the Faith, February 22, 1987, The Feast of the Chair of St. Peter, the Apostle.

JOSEPH Card. RATZINGER
Prefect

ALBERTO BOVONE
Titular Archbishop
Of Caesarea in Numidia
Secretary

Notes

1. Pope John Paul II, Discourse to those taking part in the 81st Congress of the Italian Society of Internal Medicine and the 82d Congress of the Italian Society of General Surgery, 27 October 1980: AAS 72 (1980) 1126.

2. Pope Paul VI, discourse to the General Assembly of the United Nations Organization, 4 Oct., 1965: AAS 57 (1965) 878; Encyclical Populorum Progresso, 13: AAS 59 (1967) 263.

3. Pope Paul VI, Homily during the Mass closing the Holy Year, 25 December 1975: AAS 68 (1976) 145; Pope John Paul II, Encyclical Dives in Misericordia, 30: AAS 72 (1980) 1224.

4. Pope John Paul II, Discourse to those taking part in the 35th General Assembly of the World Medical Association, 29 Oct., 1983: AAS 76 (1984) 390.

5. Cf. Declaration Dignitatis Humanae, 2.

6. Pastoral Constitution Gaudium et Spes, 22; Pope John Paul II, Encyclical Redemptor Hominis, 8: AAS 71 (1979) 270–272.

7. Cf. Pastoral Constitution Gaudium et Spes, 35.

8. Pastoral Constitution Gaudium et Spes, 15; cf. also Pope Paul VI, Encyclical Populorum Progresso, 20: AAS 59 (1967) 267; Pope John Paul II, Encyclical Redemptor Hominis, 15: AAS 71 (1979) 286–289; Apostolic Exhortation Familiaris Consortio, 8: AAS 74 (1982) 89.

9. Pope John Paul II, Apostolic Exhortation Familiaris Consortio, 11: AAS 74 (1982) 92.

10. Cf. Pope Paul VI, Encyclical Humanae Vitae, 10: AAS 60 (1968) 487–488.

11. Pope John Paul II, Discourse to the members of the 35th General Assembly of the World Medical Association, 29 Oct., 1983: AAS 76 (1984) 393.

12. Cf. Pope John Paul II, Apostolic Exhortation Familiaris Consortio, 11: AAS 74 (1982) 91–92; cf, also Pastoral Constitution Gaudium et Spes, 50.

13. Sacred Congregation for the Doctrine of the Faith, Declaration on Procured Abortion, 9, AAS 66 (1974) 736–737.

14. Pope John Paul II, Discourse to those taking part in the 35th General Assembly of the World Medical Association, 29 October 1983: AAS 76 (1984) 390.

15. Pope John XXIII, Encyclical Mater et Magistra, III: AAS 53 (1961) 447.

16. Pastoral Constitution Gaudium et Spes, 24.

17. Cf. Pope Pius XII, Encyclical Humani Generis: AAS 42 (1950) 575; Pope Paul VI, Professio Fidei: AAS 60 (1968) 436.

18. Pope John XXIII, Encyclical Mater et Magistra, III: AAS 53 (1961) 447; cf. Pope John Paul II, Discourse to priests participating in a seminar on "Responsible Procreation," 17 Sept., 1983, Insegnamenti di Giovanni Paolo II, VI, 2 (1983) 562: "At the origin of each human person there is a creative act of God: no man comes into existence by chance; he is always the result of the creative love of God."

19. Cf. Pastoral Constitution Gaudium et Spes, 24.

20. Cf. Pope Pius XII, Discourse to the Saint Luke Medical-Biological Union, 12 Nov., 1944: Discorsi e Radiomessaggi VI (1944–1945) 191–192.

21. Cf. Pastoral Constitution Gaudium et Spes, 50.

22. Cf. Pastoral Constitution Gaudium et Spes, 51: "When it is a question of harmonizing married love with the responsible transmission of life, the moral character of one's behavior does not depend only on the good intention and the evaluation of the motives: the objective criteria must be used, criteria drawn from the nature of the human person and human acts, criteria which respect the total meaning of mutual self-giving and human procreation in the context of true love."

23. Pastoral Constitution Gaudium et Spes, 51.

24. Holy See, Charter of the Rights of the Family, 4; L'Osservatore Romano, 25 November 1983.

25. Sacred Congregation for the Doctrine of the Faith, Declaration on Procured Abortion, 12–13: AAS 66 (1974) 738.

26. Cf. Pope Paul VI, Discourse to participants in the 23d National Congress of Italian Catholic Jurists, 9 Dec., 1972: AAS 64 (1972) 777.

27. The obligation to avoid disproportionate risks involves an authentic respect for human beings and the uprightness of therapeutic intentions. It implies that the doctor "above all . . . must carefully evaluate the possible negative consequences which the necessary use of a particular exploratory technique may have upon the unborn child and avoid recourse to diagnostic procedures which do not offer sufficient guarantees of their honest purpose and substantial harmlessness. And if, as often happens in human choices, a degree of risk must be undertaken, he will take care to assure that it is justified by a truly urgent need for the diagnosis and by the importance of the results that can be achieved by it for the benefit of the unborn child himself." (Pope John Paul II, Discourse to Participants in the Pro-Life Movement Congress, 3 December 1982: Insegnamenti di Giovanni Paolo II, V, 3 [1982] 1512). This clarification concerning "proportionate risk" is also to be kept in mind in the following sections of the present Instruction, whenever this term appears.

28. Pope John Paul II, Discourse to the Participants in the 35th General Assembly of the World Medical Association, 29 Oct., 1983: AAS 76 (1984) 392.

29. Cf. Pope John Paul II, Address to a Meeting of the Pontifical Academy of Sciences, 23 Oct., 1982: AAS 75 (1983) 37: "I condemn, in the most explicit and formal way, experimental manipulation of the human embryo, since the human being, from conception to death, cannot be exploited for any purpose whatsoever."

30. Holy See, Charter of the Rights of the Family, 4b: L'Osservatore Romano, 25 Nov., 1983.

31. Cf. Pope John Paul II, Address to the Participants in the Convention of the Pro-Life Movement, 3 December 1982: Insegnamenti di Giovanni Paolo II, V, 3 (1982) 1511: "Any form of experimentation on the fetus that may damage its integrity or worsen its condition is unacceptable, except in the case of a final effort to save it from death." Sacred Congregation for the Doctrine of the Faith, Declaration on Euthanasia, 4: AAS 72 (1980) 550: "In the absence of other sufficient remedies, it is permitted, with the patient's consent, to have recourse to the means provided by the most advanced medical techniques, even if these means are still at the experimental stage and are not without a certain risk."

32. No one, before coming into existence, can claim a subjective right to begin to exist; nevertheless, it is legitimate to affirm the right of the child to have a fully human origin through conception in conformity with the personal nature of the human

being. Life is a gift that must be bestowed in a manner worthy both of the subject receiving it and of the subjects transmitting it. This statement is to be borne in mind also for what will be explained concerning artificial human procreation.

33. Cf. Pope John Paul II, Discourse to those taking part in the 35th General Assembly of the World Medical Association, 29 Oct., 1983: AAS 76 (1984) 391.

34. Cf. Pastoral Constitution on the Church in the Modern World, Gaudium et Spes, 50.

35. Cf. Pope John Paul II, Apostolic Exhortation Familiaris Consortio, 14: AAS 74 (1982) 96.

36. Cf. Pope Pius XII, Discourse to those taking part in the 4th International Congress of Catholic Doctors, 29 Sept., 1949: AAS 41 (1949) 559. According to the plan of the Creator, "A man leaves his father and his mother and cleaves to his wife, and they become one flesh" (Gen 2:24). The unity of marriage, bound to the order of creation, is a truth accessible to natural reason. The Church's Tradition and Magisterium frequently make reference to the Book of Genesis, both directly and through the passages of the New Testament that refer to it: Mt 19:4–6; Mk 10:5–8; Eph 5:31. Cf. Athenagoras, Legato pro christianis, 33: PG 6, 965–967; Sr. Chrysostom, In Matthaeum homiliae, LXII, 19, 1: PG 58 597; St. Leo the Great, Epist. ad Rusticum, 4: PL 54, 1204; Innocent III, Epist. Gaudemus in Domino: DS 778; Council of Lyons II, IV Session: DS 860; Council of Trent, XXIV Session: DS 1798, 1802; Pope Leo XIII, Encyclical Arcanum Divinae Sapientiae: AAS 12 (1879/80) 388–391; Pope Pius XI, Encyclical Casti Connubii: AAS 22 (1930) 546–547; Second Vatican Council, Gaudium et Spes, 48; Pope John Paul II, Apostolic Exhortation Familiaris Consortio, 19: AAS 74 (1982) 101–102; Code of Canon Law, Can. 1056.

37. Cf. Pope Pius XII, Discourse to those taking part in the 4th International Congress of Catholic Doctors, 29 Sept., 1949; AAS 4 (1949) 560; Discourse to those taking part in the Congress of the Italian Catholic Union of Midwives, 29 Oct., 1951: AAS 43 (1951) 850; Code of Canon law, Can. 1134.

38. Pope Paul VI, Encyclical Letter Humanae Vitae, 12: AAS 60 (1968) 448–489.

39. Loc. cit., ibid., 489.

40. Pope Pius XII, Discourse to those taking part in the Second Naples World Congress on Fertility and Human Sterility, 19 May, 1956: AAS 48 (1956) 470.

41. Code of Canon Law, Can. 1061. According to this Canon, the conjugal act is that by which the marriage is consummated if the couple "have performed (it) between themselves in a human manner."

42. Cf. Pastoral Constitution Gaudium et Spes, 14.

43. Cf. Pope John Paul II, General Audience on 16 Jan., 1980: Insegnamenti di Giovanni Paolo II, III, 1 (1980) 148–152.

44. Pope John Paul II, Discourse to those taking part in the 35th General Assembly of the World Medical Association, 29 Oct., 1983: AAS 76 (1984) 393.

45. Cf. Pastoral Constitution Gaudium et Spes, 51.

46. Cf. Pastoral Constitution Gaudium et Spes, 50.

47. Cf. Pope Pius XII, Discourse to those taking part in the 4th International Congress of Catholic Doctors, 29 Sept., 1949: AAS 41 (1949) 560: "It would be erroneous . . . to think that the possibility of resorting to this means (artificial fertilization) might render valid a marriage between persons unable to contract it because of the *impedimentum impotentiae.*"

48. A similar question was dealt with by Pope Paul VI, Encyclical Humanae Vitae, 14: AAS 60 (1968) 490–491.

49. Cf. supra: I, 1 ff.

50. Pope Paul II, Apostolic Exhortation Familiaris Consortio, 14: AAS 74 (1982) 96.

51. Cf. response of the Holy Office, 17 March, 1897: DS 3323; Pope Pius XII, Discourse to those taking part in the 4th International Congress of Catholic Doctors, 29 Sept., 1949: AAS 41 (1949) 560; Discourse to the Italian Catholic Union of Midwives, 29 Oct., 1951: AAS 43 (1951) 840; Discourse to those taking part in the Second Naples World Congress on Fertility and Human Sterility, 19 May, 1956: AAS 48 (1956) 471–473; Discourse to those taking part in the 7th International Congress of the International Society of Hematology, 12 Sept., 1958: AAS 50 (1958) 733; Pope John XXIII, Encyclical Mater et Magistra, III: AAS 53 (1961) 447.

52. Pope Pius XII, Discourse to the Italian Catholic Union of Midwives, 29 Oct., 1951: AAS 43 (1951) 850.

53. Pope Pius XII, Discourse to those taking part in the 4th International Congress of Catholic Doctors, 29 Sept., 1949: AAS 41 (1949) 560.

54. Sacred Congregation for the Doctrine of the Faith, Declaration on Certain Questions Concerning Sexual Ethics, 9: AAS 68 (1976) 86, which quotes

the Pastoral Constitution Gaudium et Spes, 51. Cf. Decree of the Holy Office, 2 Aug., 1929: AAS 21 (1929) 490; Pope Pius XII, Discourse to those taking part in the 26th Congress of the Italian Society of Urology, 8 Oct., 1953: AAS 45 (1953) 678.

55. Cf. Pope John XXIII, Encyclical Mater et Magistra, III: AAS 53 (1961) 447.

56. Cf. Pope Pius XII, Discourse to those taking part in the 4th International Congress of Catholic

Doctors, 29 Sept., 1949: AAS 41 (1949), 560.

57. Cf. Pope Pius XII, Discourse to those taking part in the Second Naples World Congress on Fertility and Human Sterility, 19 May, 1956: AAS 48 (1956) 471–473.

58. Pastoral Constitution Gaudium et Spes, 50.

59. Pope John Paul II, Apostolic Exhortation Familiaris Consortio, 14: AAS 74 (1982) 97.

60. Cf. Declaration Dignitatis Humanae, 7.

Sterilization of the Mentally Retarded: A Decision for the Courts

George J. Annas

In the most notorious case involving sterilization of a mentally retarded person, the United States Supreme Court upheld a Virginia statute that was the basis for sterilizing Carrie Buck, a "feeble-minded eighteen-year-old" who was "the daughter of a feeble-minded mother and the mother of an illegitimate feeble-minded child." Oliver Wendell Holmes, speaking for the Court, argued:

> It is better for all the world, if instead of waiting to execute degenerate offspring for crime, or let them starve for their imbecility, society can prevent those who are manifestly unfit from continuing their kind. . . . Three generations of imbeciles are enough (*Buck* v. *Bell*, 274 U.S. 200[1927]).

After an orgy of eugenic sterilizations, the pendulum has swung back to the point where this opinion represents neither good law nor good genetics. On the way, in 1942, the same Supreme Court concluded in a different context that the right to procreate was a basic constitutional right. Sterilization "forever deprived" an individual of this right, which is "fundamental to the very existence and survival of the race" (*Skinner* v. *Oklahoma*, 316 U.S. 535 [1942]).

At least three approaches are now possible. One—the majority approach—is for courts in states that have no specific statutes authorizing sterilization simply to declare that it cannot be done on individuals who cannot personally consent to it. Another is for courts individually to evaluate cases in which sterilization of a mentally retarded individual is contemplated, and to authorize it only if it is in the person's "best interests." And the third is for courts to adopt a "*Quinlan*-type approach" by defining the test to be applied in making a decision to sterilize and permitting the family of the incompetent and their physician (with or without the help of a review committee) to make the decision without resort to the courts. (See George J. Annas, "In re Quinlan: Legal Comfort for Doctors," *Hastings Center Report*, June 1976, pp. 29–31.)

If any court could be expected to take a *Quinlan* approach it would be the New Jersey Supreme Court, the same court that wrote the *Quinlan* decision. Thus it will undoubtedly surprise some *Quinlan* enthusiasts that this court opted for the second choice, requiring a court to decide if an incompetent may be sterilized.

Reprinted with permission of the author and the publisher from Hastings Center Report, 11 *(August 1981) 18–19 © Institute of Society, Ethics and the Life Sciences, 360 Broadway, Hastings-on-Hudson, N.Y. 10706.*

The Case of Lee Ann Grady

The case that brought the issue to the New Jersey Supreme Court involved Lee Ann Grady, a nineteen-year-old with Down's syndrome. She is the oldest of three children, lives at home with them and her parents, and has never been institutionalized. Her IQ is in the "upper 20s to upper 30s range." She can converse, count to some extent, and recognize letters of the alphabet. She can dress and bathe herself. Her life expectancy and physical maturation are normal; however, her mental deficiency has prevented the normal emotional and social development of sexuality. If she becomes pregnant, she will not understand her condition, and she will not be capable of caring for a baby alone.

Because of her sexual development, her parents have provided her with birth control pills for the past four years, although there is no evidence that she has ever engaged in sexual activity or has any interest in it. At the age of twenty she will leave her special class in the public school system. Her parents would like to have her placed in a sheltered work group, and eventually in a group home for retarded adults so that she can begin a more independent life and have a place to live after they die. They believe that dependable and continuous contraception is a prerequisite to this change; and they and their doctor sought to have her sterilized, using a tubal ligation, at the Morristown Memorial Hospital. The hospital refused without court approval, and a lawsuit followed. (*In the Matter of Lee Ann Grady*, 426 A. 2d 467 [N.J., 1981]).

The Appeal

The lower court granted the parents' application; and the public advocate and attorney general, both invited to appear by the trial judge, appealed. The appeals court begins its analysis by recognizing that "sterilization [destroys] an important part of a person's social and biological identity"; and rejects any notion that it might assign fewer rights to the mentally retarded than to other citizens. The court declines to classify the proposed sterilization as either voluntary (since she could not understand the problem or the proposed solution) or compulsory (since no one is actually objecting to the procedure on her behalf). Instead it defines a new category: a procedure "lacking personal consent because of a legal disability."

Following closely the logic of the *Quinlan* case, the court concludes that the right to prevent contraception through sterilization is one of the privacy rights protected by the U.S. Constitution, and declines to discard it for the mentally retarded "solely on the basis that [their] condition prevents conscious exercise of the choice." As in *Quinlan*, this court sees its task as fashioning a way to preserve the right of choice for incompetent persons. Unlike *Quinlan*, however, the court refuses to permit the person's parents and a court-appointed guardian to make the decision. Instead it insists that only the court can make this decision for an incompetent. The reasons for this departure from *Quinlan* are instructive.

The court gives two reasons for distinguishing this case from *Quinlan*. First, it sees the alternatives in *Quinlan* as "much more clear cut": indefinite life in a coma versus natural death. It believes such a choice is "not conducive to detached evaluation and resolution by the person exercising it in behalf of the patient," but that the decision relies more "on instinct than reasoned calculation." Second, there was no history of abuse in *Quinlan*-type decisions. In contrast, many choices are open to Lee Ann Grady; and there is a history of horrible abuses in this area.

The court notes that similar decisions in adoption and child custody cases are routinely made by the courts, and holds that, under its inherent *parens patriae* power, the courts have the authority to protect incompetents who cannot protect themselves because of an innate legal disability. This power has been applied in medical cases, including authorizations to treat children over the parents' objection, kidney and bone marrow transplant cases, and in the *Quinlan* case itself.

The court understands that its decision is *not* Lee Ann's, but

> . . . it is a genuine choice . . . designed to further the same interests she might pursue had she the ability to decide herself. We believe that having the choice made in her behalf produces a more just and compassionate result than leaving Lee Ann with no way of exercising a constitutional

right. *Our Court should accept the responsibility of providing her with a choice* to compensate for her inability to exercise personally an important constitutional right. (Emphasis supplied.)

Standards for Decision

Having decided that a court is a proper decision maker, the appeals court considered the standards and procedures to be employed. The court stops short of requiring a showing of "strict necessity," but does enunciate very strict criteria that must be met before sterilization can be authorized. The Court must appoint a guardian *ad litem* to represent the interests of the ward, and "should receive" independent medical and psychological evaluations by qualified professionals. The trial judge must personally meet with the individual before concluding that the person lacks capacity to make a decision about sterilization and that the incapacity is unlikely to change. This incapacity must be proven by clear and convincing evidence. Finally, the court must be persuaded, also by clear and convincing evidence, that the sterilization is in the person's *best interests*. In making this determination, the court must consider the

- Possibility of pregnancy;
- Possibility of physical and mental harm from pregnancy and from sterilization;
- Likelihood of sexual activity;
- Inability of the person to understand contraception;
- Feasibility of a less drastic means of contraception;
- Possibility of postponing sterilization;
- Ability of the person to care for a child, or the possibility of marriage at a future date with ability of the couple to care for the child;
- Evidence of relevant medical advances;
- Demonstration that the proponents of sterilization are seeking it in good faith for the primary concern of the person and not their own or the public's convenience.

This list is not meant to be inclusive, and "the ultimate criterion is the best interests of the incom-

petent person." Because the trial court did not apply the stringent "clear and convincing" standard of proof (it used the more traditional "preponderance of evidence" standard) to the best interests conclusion, the case was remanded for further proceedings.

Protecting Individual Rights

The court finds a new substantive right—the right to sterilization—and seeks to protect incompetents from its arbitrary use by demanding strict due process protection. This is far superior to a blanket prohibition of sterilization, and much more protective of individual rights than permitting families to make this decision on their own. The basis on which *Quinlan* is distinguished is instructive. It supports the notion that a terminally ill patient in a chronic vegetative state has suffered a form of "death" and therefore has no good options. Since the only two choices for such a patient are both so bleak, the court thinks that "instinct" rather than logic must be called upon to make this choice. If the court's words are taken seriously, New Jersey courts might be inclined to require a court decision in cases like *Saikewicz*, where the choices are much more complex, since an individual presumably has a greater interest in preserving life than in preserving an ability to procreate.

The second distinction from *Quinlan*, the history of abuse, seems to indicate that should abuses in other areas of medical care for incompetents come to light, courts will step in to protect this class of persons. If *Quinlan* was read by some as a judicial retreat from protecting incompetent individuals, the New Jersey courts have clearly signaled that this "retreat" was made under very specific circumstances from which we cannot generalize.

If a structural problem exists with the decision, it is in the role of the guardian *ad litem*. The court defines the guardian's role as "representing the interests of his ward." This seems inappropriate for a proceeding in which the judge, not the guardian, will make the judgment as to whether the sterilization is in the person's best interests. Since the petitioners will always be arguing in favor of the sterilization, it would make more sense if the guardian *ad litem* were required to present all of the arguments against sterilization to the best of his ability. As Professor Charles Baron of Boston College Law School has argued, "Without advocates on both sides of the issue to develop the record, the court is too likely to face mental set and path-of-least-resistance pitfalls. . . . [A] general pattern will seem to emerge from the evidence; an accustomed label is waiting for the case, and without awaiting further proofs, this label is promptly assigned to it." (Charles Baron, "Voluntary Sterilization of the Mentally Retarded" in Aubrey Milunsky, George J. Annas, editors, *Genetics and the Law*, New York: Plenum, 1976, pp. 273–74.)

The New Jersey model is as good as anything that exists, but it stands almost alone in the country. Since most courts will not act without them, statutes should be enacted in each state to prohibit sterilization of the mentally retarded and other incompetent individuals except when a court finds, after an adversary hearing, that the sterilization is in the best interests of the individual. Such a procedure permits sterilization in cases where a compelling case can be made, and protects potential victims from sterilization abuse for the benefit of others.

Decision Scenario 1 ....

"I'm sorry we can't help you," Patricia Spring said. "But what you want is simply against our policy."

Charles Blendon and Carla Neuman didn't try to hide their disappointment. The San Diego Reproductive Clinic had been their last hope. They very badly wanted to have a child, but Carla's fallopian tubes had been surgically removed as part of a successful effort to treat precancerous growths.

"In fact," Patricia Spring said, "you don't meet at least two of our criteria."

"We can afford to pay," Charles Blendon said.

"That's not it. First of all, Carla is thirty-eight, and we set thirty-five as the upper limit. And second, you two are not married, and we require that the donor and the patient be husband and wife."

"Who makes those rules?" Carla Neuman asked. "It seems to me that if we want to have a child, then that's our business and nobody else's."

"The Clinic makes the rules," Patricia Spring said. "You see, there is some greater risk of birth defects in women who are over the age of thirty-five. There are sound medical reasons for our criteria."

"But what if we're willing to take the risk?" Charles Blendon asked.

"You can't take a risk that is likely to affect an unborn child."

"But I'm willing to have tests," Carla Neuman said. "And neither of us is against abortion. If there is something wrong with the fetus, then I'll have an abortion."

"And just what sort of medical basis is there for the marriage requirement?" Charles Blendon asked. "It seems to me that the Clinic is just imposing its own moral standards on Carla and me."

"Look," Patricia Spring said, "I know you're both upset and disappointed. I sympathize with you. But the Clinic operates in a community, and our criteria reflect both good medical judgment and the standards of the community."

"Does the Clinic receive any public money," Carla Neuman asked.

"We have some research grants."

"Then it seems to me that we have grounds for a suit," Carla said. "The Clinic is discriminating against us because we aren't married, and it's denying us the right to take a risk we're willing to take."

"I can only tell you what our criteria are," Patricia Spring said. "I can't arrange for you to be accepted as a patient here, and there's nothing you or I can do about it."

"That remains to be seen," Charles Blendon said.

Is the Clinic justified in setting an age limit on the women it will accept as patients? If so, why?

How might a rule utilitarian justify the Clinic's requirement that a couple be married in order for the woman to be accepted as a patient?

Does the fact that the Clinic receive public funds provide any reason to believe that its services should be open to everyone?

On what grounds might Kass and Krimmel object to the very existence of such a clinic?

Decision Scenario 2 ·······································

In January of 1985, the British High Court took custody of a five-day-old girl, the first child known to be born in Britain to a woman paid to be a surrogate mother.

An American couple, known only as "Mr. and Mrs. A," were reported to have paid about $7,500 to a twenty-eight-year-old woman who allowed herself to be artificially inseminated with sperm from Mr. A. The woman, Kim Cotton, was prevented from turning the child over to Mr. and Mrs. A by a court order issued because of the uncertainty over the legal status of a surrogate mother.

The court permitted "interested parties, including the natural father" to apply for custody of the child. Mr. A applied, and judge Sir John Latey ruled that the couple could take the baby girl out of the country, because they could offer her the chance of "a very good upbringing."

Are there any moral reasons that might have made the court hesitate before turning over the child to her biological father? For example, could it be persuasively argued that Kim Cotton was, in effect, selling her baby to Mr. and Mrs. A?

Kim Cotton agreed to be a surrogate mother for the sake of the money. Is surrogate pregnancy a practice that tends to exploit the poor? Or is it a legitimate way to earn money by providing a needed service?

Is serving as a surrogate mother essentially the same as prostitution? If it is not, then what are the relevant differences?

On what grounds do Kass and Krimmel oppose the practice of surrogate pregnancy? How persuasive are the arguments?

Decision Scenario 3 ·······································

Dr. Charles Davis quickly scanned the data sheet on his desk, then looked at the woman seated across from him. Her name was Nancy Callahan. She was twenty-five years old and worked as a print conservator at an art museum.

"I see that you aren't married," Dr. Davis said.

"That's right," Nancy Callahan said. "That's basically the reason I'm here." When Dr. Davis looked puzzled, she added, "I still want to have a child."

Dr. Davis nodded and thought for a moment. Nancy Callahan was the first unmarried person to come to the Bayside Fertility Clinic to request AID. As the legal owner and operator of the Clinic, as well as the Chief of Medical Services, Dr. Davis was the one ultimately responsible for the Clinic's policies.

"I hope you understand that I have to ask you some personal questions," Dr. Davis said.

"Of course."

"You're not engaged or planning to get married?"

"No. At least not at the moment. I don't want to rule out the possibility that I will want to get married someday."

"Don't you know anybody you would want to have a child with in the ordinary sexual way?"

"I might be able to find someone," Nancy Callahan said. "But you see, I don't want to get involved with anybody right now. I'm ready to be a mother, but I'm not ready to get into the kind of situation that having a child in what you call 'the ordinary sexual way' would require."

"I see."

"I hope you do. This is something I really want to do. I think I'll be a good mother. I want a child very much, and I can afford to support one."

"It's just somewhat unusual," Dr. Davis said."

"But it's not illegal, is it?"

"No," Dr. Davis said. "It's not illegal."

"So what's the problem? I'm healthy. I'm financially sound and mentally stable, and I'm both able and eager to accept the responsibility of being a mother."

"It's just that at the moment the policy of our Clinic requires that patients be married and that both husbands and wives agree to the insemination procedure."

"But there's nothing magical about a policy," Nancy Callahan said. "It can be changed for good reasons, can't it?"

"Perhaps so," said Dr. Davis.

Suppose that Ms. Callahan is a lesbian. Should this be a relevant consideration in deciding whether she should receive AID? Why, according to Hanscombe, should it not be?

What utilitarian argument can be advanced in favor of the Clinic's policy?

Does the natural law view support such a policy?

How might it be argued that respect for Ms. Callahan's autonomy makes it wrong to deny her the service she requests, while providing it to a married woman?

Decision Scenario 4 ....

"My husband and I have talked over the matter in great detail," Marge Gower said. "We don't care about the sex of the child, but we know exactly the kinds of features we want to try for."

"Mrs. Gower," Dr. Louise Singh said. "You've got to understand that we're not running a mail-order catalog business for babies."

"I'm not trying to order a *baby.* I just want to tell you what I'm looking for in a sperm donor. I want somebody who is at least six feet tall, muscular—not fat—has light-colored hair and is very good looking. Also, I want some proof that he has a good sense of humor and is intelligent. He has to have at least a college degree. I'll leave all the rest to you. I mean, things about health."

"Thank you," said Dr. Singh. "But I really don't think I can go along with that."

"I don't see why not. If I were going to have a child in the usual way and I were deliberately going to get pregnant, I would certainly choose somebody like I described."

"But you aren't doing it in the usual way. You're going to be using donor semen."

"But who is going to choose the donor? You are, aren't you?"

"I plan to. I'll select somebody from our list of applicants who resembles you and your husband in a general way."

"I don't see why you should have that kind of power," Mrs. Gower said. "It's going to be my baby. I think I have the right to say what the father should be like."

"That's against Reproductive Medicine's policy."

"Well, that's too bad. Just tell me who to talk to to get the policy changed. I'm going to have a baby like my husband and I want. As long as I have to have artificial insemination, I want to get the most good out of it."

On what grounds might a utilitarian support the claim that Dr. Singh ought to be wholly responsible for choosing the sperm donor?

On what grounds might a utilitarian support the claim that Mrs. Gower and her husband ought to be able to select the features that a sperm donor should have?

Would it be better for the potential recipient of artificial insemination if the sperm donor were known personally to her and her husband? What are some of the problems caused by anonymity?

Might the choice of a sperm donor by the physician be regarded as an unacceptable form of paternalism? (See the discussion of paternalism in Chapter 4.)

Consider the issue involved here from the standpoint of the potential sperm donor. Should a sperm donor have some control over the use of his sperm in artificial insemination? Mrs. Gower argues that since the child will be hers, she should be the one who specifies what traits the donor should have. Since, biologically speaking, the child will equally be the offspring of the sperm donor, should he be able to specify the traits the sperm recipient should have?

Decision Scenario 5 ....

"I'm going to sell my sperm for the simple reason that I need the money," John Lolton said. "It's no big deal."

"I think it is," Mary Cooper said. "You seem to think it's like selling your blood, but it isn't. If somebody is transfused with your blood, that's an end to things. But if a woman is inseminated with your sperm, a child may result."

"I don't have any responsibilities for what people do with my sperm," Lolton replied. "It's just a product."

"Not so," Cooper said. "It's a product all right, but if it's used in artificial insemination, that means that you're the father of a child. And if

you're the father of a child, that means you have to be willing to accept responsibility for that child."

"That is absolute nonsense," Lolton said.

If sperm is just a product, is Lolton correct in saying that he has no responsibilities for its use?

State as explicitly as possible Cooper's argument that a sperm donor is responsible for any child resulting from AI using his donated sperm.

According to Munson, why is being the biological father of a child born as a result of AI not a sufficient condition for being the moral father of the child?

Decision Scenario 6 ....

"Now Ms. Ralston, I don't know if you fully realize the consequences of tubal ligation," Dr. Swabey said.

"I'm perfectly aware of them," Teri Ralston said. "It means that ova will no longer come down the fallopian tubes and be available for fertilization. It means that I will never get pregnant, and I believe the operation is best thought of as irreversible."

Dr. Swabey was somewhat taken aback. The young woman seated in his office seemed intelligent and well informed. However, he was almost certain that what she wanted would be a big mistake.

"That's all quite right," he said. "But now here you are, twenty-eight years old, coming to me and asking to be sterilized. You may think that's what you want, that may *be* what you want. But that's what you want right now. You may change your mind next week or next year. You may meet a man you want to have children with, and you won't be able to have any. You'll be sorry you ever chose this path."

Teri Ralston shook her head. "I'm not likely to change my mind. I know I never want to have children. It just doesn't fit into my life style."

"That's what you say now, but I'm talking about the future."

"That's what I say now, and that's what I'll

say later," Teri Ralston insisted. "You see, Dr. Swabey, I know what I want to do with my life. I don't want to have children—ever—and I don't want to run the risk of getting pregnant. I don't believe in abortions unless they are absolutely necessary, and I want to do what I can to see that one isn't ever necessary in my case."

"I suppose I understand your views," Dr. Swabey said. "But I never sterilize a woman as young as you are, unless there are medical indications of the need to do so."

"What do you mean?"

"Well, say, if you were the carrier of a genetic disease, then I would agree to sterilize you."

"But you won't do it just on the basis of my own ideas about my life."

"No, I won't."

Is there any reason to believe that Teri Ralston's decision to be sterilized is anything but voluntary?

Is there any reason to believe that Dr. Swabey is violating Ms. Ralston's individual autonomy in refusing to perform a sterilization procedure?

On what grounds might a rule utilitarian argue in favor of the position taken by Dr. Swabey?

On what grounds might a defender of the natural law theory object to Teri Ralston's decision?

Decision Scenario 7 ··

Louise Tredle was twenty years old and retarded. Her IQ measured less than thirty on the WAIS, and she had difficulty understanding even very simple concepts.

Louise Tredle was also a mother. Her child was four years old. Both he and Louise lived with Louise's widowed mother. The child's father was unknown.

Mrs. Tredle never felt it was safe to leave Louise and the child by themselves. Louise could be trusted to perform routine chores, but she simply was not able to protect either herself or the child from the hazards of ordinary life. Because of this, Mrs. Tredle couldn't take a job outside the home. She was forced to operate the household on the money she got from social security and from payments made by state and federal welfare agencies.

When Mrs. Tredle found out that Louise had started stopping in at a neighborhood bar on her way back from the grocery store, Mrs. Tredle became fearful. Louise was sexually naive, and her intelligence level made her easy to take advantage of. Mrs. Tredle was very much afraid that Louise would become pregnant again. For Mrs. Tredle, abortion was out of the question, and she didn't know if she would be able to take care of another child.

Mrs. Tredle decided that she would have to try to get Louise sterilized. Only then would there be full protection for Louise and the rest of the family. Dr. Feldman, the physician who had arranged for Louise to be declared legally incompetent, also arranged for Mrs. Tredle to talk to someone in a community legal services organization. After Mrs. Tredle explained the situation, Mr. Olson, one of the agency's lawyers, took the necessary steps to set up a court hearing.

Mrs. Tredle testified at the court hearing. She explained her fears and tried to make the judge see that she was just not able to take responsibility for Louise and her child and, perhaps, another child. She explained the difficulty of watching Louise all the time and trying to make sure she didn't become sexually involved with anyone.

Mr. Olson arranged for a psychiatrist to examine Louise, and the psychiatrist testified that Louise was indeed of subnormal intelligence and unable to function in an ordinary responsible way. Louise herself was questioned by the court. She responded to questions about how she liked being a mother by saying that she liked it very much and that she loved her child. When she was asked if she knew what sterilization was, she said that she knew it meant she wouldn't be able to have children. She also said that she didn't want that to happen to her.

To Mrs. Tredle's surprise, the judge ruled against her request. In the court's opinion, Louise's wish not to lose the capacity to have children outweighed all other considerations. The court refused to approve sterilization.

What sort of evidence should be considered to show that sterilization is in the best interest of the individual? (See the discussion by Annas.)

Would a Quinlan-type approach to the decision be more likely to emphasize considerations other than the best interest of the person?

According to Rawls, what features must a paternalistic action have to justify it as legitimate? Does the fact that Mrs. Tredle will gain benefits from having Louise sterilized necessarily mean that such an action cannot be justified?

Would a utilitarian consider Louise's mental limitations and Mrs. Tredle's situation and wishes relevant to deciding whether a decision to sterilize Louise would be justified?

Does the fact that Louise knows that sterilization means she won't be capable of having more children show that she is sufficiently informed to make her wish not to lose that capacity equivalent to a refusal to give consent?

PART IV

RESOURCES

CHAPTER 8

ALLOCATING SCARCE MEDICAL RESOURCES

CASE PRESENTATION
Selection Committee for Dialysis

In 1966 Brattle, Texas, proper had a population of about ten thousand people. In Brattle County there were twenty thousand more people who lived on isolated farms deep within the pine forests, or in crossroads towns with a filling station, a feed store, one or two white, frame churches, and maybe twenty or twenty-five houses.

Brattle was the marketing town and county seat, the place all the farmers, their wives, and children went to on Saturday afternoon. It was also the medical center because it had the only hospitals in the county. One of them, Conklin Clinic, was hardly more than a group of doctors' offices. But Crane Memorial Hospital was quite a different sort of place. Occupying a relatively new three-story brick building in downtown Brattle, the hospital offered new equipment, a well-trained staff, and high quality medical care.

This was mostly due to the efforts of Dr. J. B. Crane, Jr. The hospital was dedicated to the memory of his father, a man who practiced medicine in Brattle County for almost fifty years. Before Crane became a memorial hospital, it was Crane Clinic. But J. B. Crane, Jr., after returning from the Johns Hopkins Medical School, was determined to expand the clinic and transform it into a modern hospital. The need was there, and private inves-

tors were easy to find. Only a year after his father's death, Dr. Crane was able to offer Brattle County a genuine hospital.

It was only natural that when the County Commissioner decided that Brattle County should have a dialysis machine, he would turn to Dr. Crane's hospital. The machine was bought with county funds, but Crane Memorial Hospital would operate it under a contract agreement. The hospital was guaranteed against loss by the county, but the hospital was also not permitted to make a profit on dialysis. Furthermore, although access to the machine was not restricted to county residents, residents were to be given priority.

Dr. Crane was not pleased with this stipulation. "I don't like to have medical decisions influenced by political considerations," he told the Commissioner. "If a guy comes in and needs dialysis, I don't want to tell him that he can't have it because somebody else who doesn't need it as much is on the machine and that person is a county resident."

"I don't know what to tell you," the Commissioner said. "It was county tax money that paid for the machine, and the County Council decided that the people who supplied the money ought to get top priority."

"What about the kind of case that I mentioned?" Dr. Crane asked. "What about somebody who could wait for dialysis who is a resident as opposed to somebody who needs it immediately who's not a resident?"

"We'll just leave that sort of case to your discretion," the Commissioner said. "People around here have confidence in you and your doctors. If you say they can wait, then they can wait. I know you won't let them down. Of course if somebody died while some outsider was on the machine . . . Well, that would be embarrassing for all of us, I guess."

Dr. Crane was pleased to have the dialysis machine in his hospital. Not only was it the only one in Brattle County, but none of the neighboring counties had even one. Only the big hospitals in places like Dallas, Houston, and San Antonio had the machines. It put Crane Memorial up in the top rank.

Dr. Crane was totally unprepared for the problem when it came. He hadn't known there were so many people with chronic renal disease in Brattle County. But when news spread that there was a kidney machine available at Crane Memorial Hospital, twenty-three people applied for the dialysis program. Some were Dr. Crane's own patients or patients of his associates on the hospital staff. But a number of them were ones referred to the hospital by other physicians in Brattle and surrounding towns. Two of them were from neighboring Lopez County.

Working at a maximum, the machine could accommodate fourteen patients. But the staff decided that maximum operation would be likely to lead to dangerous equipment malfunctions and breakdowns. They settled on ten as the number of patients that should be admitted to the program.

Dr. Crane and his staff interviewed each of the program's applicants, reviewed their medical history, and got a thorough medical workup on each. They persuaded two of the patients to continue to commute to Houston, where they were already in dialysis. In four cases, renal disease had already progressed to the point that the staff decided that the patients could not benefit sufficiently from the program to make them good medical risks. In one other case, a patient suffering intestinal cancer and in generally poor health was rejected as a candidate. Two people were not in genuine need of dialysis but could be best treated by a program of medication.

That left fourteen candidates for the ten positions. Thirteen were from Brattle County and one from Lopez County.

"This is not a medical problem," Dr. Crane told the Commissioner. "And I'm not going to take the responsibility of deciding which people to condemn to death and which to give an extra chance at life."

"What do you want me to do?" the Commissioner asked. "I wouldn't object if you made the decision. I mean, you wouldn't have to tell everybody about it. You could just decide."

"That's something I won't do," Dr. Crane said. "All of this has to be open and aboveboard. It's got to be fair. If I decide, then everybody will think I am favoring my own patients or just taking the people who can pay the most money."

"I see what you mean. If I appoint a selection committee, will you serve on it?"

"I will. So long as my vote is the same as everybody else's."

"That's what I'll do then," the Commissioner said.

The Brattle County Renal Dialysis Selection Committee was appointed and operating within the week. In addition to Dr. Crane, it was made up of three people chosen by the Commissioner. Amy Langford, a Brattle housewife in her middle fifties whose husband owned the largest automobile and truck agency in Brattle County, was one member. Reverend David Johnson was another member. He was the only black on the committee and the pastor of the largest predominantly black church in Brattle. The last member was Jacob Sims, owner of a hardware store in the nearby town of Silsbee. He was the only member of the committee not from the town of Brattle.

"Now I'm inclined to favor this fellow," said Mr. Sims at the Selection Committee's first meeting. "He's twenty-four years old, he's married and has a child two years old."

"You're talking about James Nelson?" Mrs. Langford asked. "I had some trouble with him. I've heard that he used to drink a lot before he got sick, and from the looks of his record he's had a hard time keeping a job."

"That's hard to say," said Reverend Johnson. "He works as a pulp-wood hauler, and people who do that change jobs a lot. You just have to go where the work is."

"That's right," said Mr. Sims. "One thing, though. I can't find any indication of his church membership. He says he's a Methodist, but I don't see where he's told us what his church is."

"I don't either," said Mrs. Langford. "And he's not a member of the Masons or the Lions Club or any other sort of civic group. I wouldn't say he's made much of a contribution to this community."

"That's right," said Reverend Johnson. "But let's don't forget that he's got a wife and baby depending on him. That child is going to need a father."

"I think he is a good psychological candidate," said Dr. Crane. "That is, I think if he starts the program he'll stick to it. I've talked with his wife, and I know she'll encourage him."

"We should notice that he's a high school dropout," Mrs. Langford said. "I don't think we can ever expect him to make much of a contribution to this town or to the county."

Do you want to vote on this case?" asked Mr. Sims, the chairman of the committee.

"Let's talk about all of them, then go back and vote," Reverend Johnson suggested.

Everyone around the table nodded in agreement. The files were arranged by date of application, and Mr. Sims picked up the next one from the stack in front of him.

"Alva Algers," he said. "He's a fifty-three-year-old lawyer with three grown children. His wife is still alive, and he's still married to her. He's Secretary of the Layman's Board of the Brattle Episcopal Church, a member of the Rotary Club and the Elks. He used to be a scoutmaster."

"From the practical point of view," said Dr. Crane, "he would be a good candidate. He's intelligent and educated and understands what's involved in dialysis."

"I think he's definitely the sort of person we want to help," said Mrs. Langford. "He's the kind of person that makes this a better town. I'm definitely in favor of him."

"I am too," said Reverend Johnson. "Even if he does go to the wrong church."

"I'm not so sure," said Mr. Sims. "I don't think fifty-three is old—I'd better not, because I'm fifty-two myself. Still, his children are grown, he's

led a good life. I'm not sure I wouldn't give the edge to some younger fellow."

"How can you say that," Mrs. Langford said. "He's got a lot of good years left. He's a person of good character who might still do a lot for other people. He's not like that Nelson, who's not going to do any good for anybody except himself."

"I guess I'm not convinced that lawyers and members of the Rotary Club do a lot more good for the community than drivers of pulp-wood trucks," Mr. Sims said.

"Perhaps we ought to go on to the next candidate," Reverend Johnson said.

"We have Mrs. Holly Holton, a forty-three-year-old housewife from Mineral Springs," Mr. Sim said.

"That's in Lopez County, isn't it?" Mrs. Langford asked. "I think we can just reject her right off. She didn't pay the taxes that bought the machine, and our county doesn't have any responsibility for her."

"That's right," said Reverend Johnson.

Mr. Sims agreed and Dr. Crane raised no objection.

"Now," said Mr. Sims, "here's Alton Conway. I believe he's our only black candidate."

"I know him well," said Reverend Johnson. "He owns a dry cleaning business, and people in the black community think very highly of him."

"I'm in favor of him," Mrs. Langford said. "He's a married man and seems quite settled and respectable."

"I wouldn't want us to take him just because he's black," Reverend Johnson said. "But I think he's got a lot in his favor."

"Well," said Mr. Sims, "unless Dr. Crane wants to add anything, let's go on to Nora Bainridge. She's a thirty-year-old divorced woman whose eight-year-old boy lives with his father over in Louisiana. She's a waitress at the Pep Cafe."

"She is a very vital woman," said Dr. Crane. "She's had a lot of trouble in her life, but I think she's a real fighter."

"I don't believe she's much of a churchgoer," said Reverend Johnson. "At least she doesn't give us a pastor's name."

"That's right, said Mrs. Langford. "And I just wonder what kind of morals a woman like her has. I mean, being divorced and working as a waitress and all."

"I don't believe we're trying to award saint-hood here," said Mr. Sims.

"But surely moral character is relevant," said Mrs. Langford.

"I don't know anything against her moral character," said Mr. Sims. "Do you?"

"I'm only guessing," said Mrs. Langford. "But I wouldn't say that a woman of her background and apparent character is somebody we ought to give top priority to."

"I don't want to be the one to cast the first stone," said Reverend Johnson. "But I wouldn't put her at the top of our list either."

"I think we had better be careful not to discriminate against people who are poor and uneducated," said Dr. Crane.

"I agree," said Mrs. Langford. "But surely we have to take account of a person's worth."

"Can you tell us how we can measure a person's worth?" asked Mr. Sims.

"I believe I can," Mrs. Langford said. "Does the person have a steady job? Is he or she somebody we would be proud to know? Is he a church-goer? Does he or she do things for other people? We can see what kind of education the person has had, and consider whether he is somebody we would like to have around."

"I guess that's some of it all right," said Mr. Sims. "But I don't like to rely on things like education, money, and public service. A lot of people just haven't had a decent chance in this world. Maybe they were born poor or have had a lot of bad luck. I'm beginning to think that we ought to make our choices just by drawing lots."

"I can't approve of that," said Reverend Johnson. "That seems like a form of gambling to me. We ought to choose the good over the wicked, reward those who have led a virtuous life."

"I agree," Mrs. Langford said. "Choosing by drawing straws or something like that would mean we are just too cowardly to make decisions. We would be shirking our responsibility. Clearly, some people are more deserving than others, and we ought to have the courage to say so."

"All right," said Mr. Sims. "I guess we'd better get on with it then. Simon Gootz is a forty-eight-year-old baker. He's got a wife and four children. Owns his own bakery—probably all of us have been there. He's Jewish."

"I'm not sure he's the sort of person who can

stick to the required diet and go through the dialysis program," Dr. Crane said.

"I'll bet his wife and children would be a good incentive," said Mrs. Langford.

"There's not a Jewish church in town," said Reverend Johnson. "So of course we can't expect him to be a regular churchgoer."

"He's an immigrant," said Mr. Sims. "I don't believe he has any education to speak of, but he did start that bakery and build it up from nothing. I think that says a lot about his character."

"I think we can agree he's a good candidate," said Mrs. Langford.

"Let's just take one more before we break for dinner," Mr. Sims said. "Rebecca Scarborough. She's a sixty-three-year-old widow. Her children are all grown and living somewhere else."

"She's my patient," Dr. Crane said. "She's a tough and resourceful old woman. I believe she can follow orders and stand up to the rigors of the program, and her health in general is good."

Reverend Johnson said, "I just wonder if we shouldn't put a lady like her pretty far down on our list. She's lived a long life already, and she hasn't got anybody depending on her."

"I'm against that," Mrs. Langford said. "Everybody knows Mrs. Scarborough. Her family has been in this town for ages. She's one of our most substantial citizens. People would be scandalized if we didn't select her."

"Of course I'm not from Brattle," said Mr. Sims. "And maybe that's an advantage here, because I don't see that she's got much in her favor except being from an old family."

"I think that's worth something," said Mrs. Langford.

"I'm not sure it's enough, though," said Reverend Johnson.

After dinner at the Crane Memorial Hospital cafeteria, the Selection Committee met again to discuss the seven remaining candidates. It was past ten o'clock before their final decisions were made. James Nelson, the pulp-wood truck driver, Holly Holton, the housewife from Mineral Springs, and Nora Bainridge, the waitress, were all rejected as candidates. Mrs. Scarborough was rejected also. The lawyer, Alva Algers, the dry cleaner, Alton Conway, and the baker, Simon Gootz, were selected to participate in the dialysis program. Others selected were a retired secondary school teacher, an assembly-line worker at the Rigid Box Company, a Brattle County Sheriff's Department patrolman, and a twenty-seven-year-old woman file clerk in the office of the Texas Western Insurance Company.

Dr. Crane was glad that the choices were made so that the program could begin operation. But he was not pleased with the selection method and resolved to talk to his own staff and with the County Commissioner about devising some other kind of selection procedure.

Without giving any reasons, Mr. Sims sent a letter to the County Commissioner resigning from the Renal Dialysis Selection Committee.

Mrs. Langford and Reverend Johnson also sent letters to the Commissioner. They thanked him for appointing them to the Committee and indicated their willingness to continue to serve.

SOCIAL CONTEXT: ORGAN TRANSPLANTS

In 1984 an intense media campaign in the St. Louis area succeeded in raising over 265 thousand dollars to pay for the liver transplant needed by a small girl in neighboring Cahokia, Illinois.

The campaign is only one of many that have been mounted throughout the country in recent years. It is relatively easy for the public to identify with the plight of a single individual who is in need of a transplant organ and to respond with an outpouring of sympathy and cash contributions. What the public generally does not recognize is that allocation decisions are made daily that take away the last vestige of hope from some people in need of life-saving organ transplants. It is easy to think that a cash donation to save the life of a particular individual solves the problems posed by organ transplants, but the actual issues are much broader in scope and much more intractable.

Replacing damaged, diseased, or defective organs by surgically transplanting donor organs has become increasingly common during the last decade. Although the trans-

planting of kidneys began as early as the 1950s, the list of organs now transplanted with a relatively significant degree of success has been expanded to include corneas, bone marrow, bone and skin grafts, livers, pancreases, and hearts. New techniques of management and the development of drugs to suppress part of the immune response promise to make possible even more transplants in the future. (See the Introduction for more details.)

Most transplant surgery is extremely expensive. A liver transplant, for example, may cost in the range of 100 to 250 thousand dollars. Currently, Medicare pays for kidney transplants but will not pay for procedures (such as liver transplants) that are still regarded as too experimental. (In 1982 Medicare spent some 1.8 billion dollars on the End-Stage Renal Disease Program. Some analysts believe that the costs of the program could be lowered by increasing the number of kidney transplants and so decreasing the use of dialysis. The quality of life of renal transplant recipients is generally thought to be better, also.) More than half of U.S. insurance companies are willing to cover the costs of liver, heart, kidney, and bone marrow transplants, and some state Medicaid programs cover the costs of most transplants. However, individuals without insurance or without the proper kind of insurance and who do not qualify for Medicaid are generally unable to afford the cost of a needed organ transplant. A kidney transplant is the exception, for the Medicare program will pay the costs, regardless of the age of the recipient.

The second major problem, after cost, is the availability of donor organs. The increase in the number of transplant operations performed has resulted in a condition of chronic scarcity for most organs. Kidneys, hearts, and livers are always in short supply, for there is no way in which they can be preserved in usable condition for more than a few hours at most.

A total of about ten thousand people in the United States are waiting for organ transplants. In 1984, some seven thousand patients received kidney transplants, but eight thousand others were left waiting for kidneys to become available. Hundreds more are currently in need of livers, pancreases, and hearts, and many of these people are likely to die before appropriate organs become available. Those in need of a kidney or pancreas can rely on dialysis and insulin injections to treat their diseases, but those in need of a liver or heart have almost no alternative treatment. For them the lack of a suitable transplant organ spells almost certain death.

Given the currently limited supply of transplant organs, we face two key questions today: How can the supply of organs be increased? How are those who will actually receive organs be selected from the pool of candidates?

The obvious answer to the first question is that the supply of organs can be increased by increasing donations. The overwhelming majority of organs that could be used for transplant are not salvaged from the recently dead. According to one estimate, only about 15 percent of available organs are retrieved. Most people are simply buried with all their organs. This is true even in states that print an organ donation card on the back of driver's licenses. Most often, physicians and hospital administrators are reluctant to intrude on a family's grief by asking that a deceased patient's organs be donated for use as transplants. (Even if a patient has signed an organ donation card, the permission of the immediate family is required, in most cases, before the organs can be removed.)

In an attempt to overcome this reluctance, state laws in Oregon and New York now require that hospitals ask families for organ donations whenever a patient is declared dead. The families are not required to agree to the request, and if it is known that the patient was opposed to organ transplants, then the request does not have to be made. However, some experts believe that merely asking for donations is likely to increase considerably the number of donations. At present, only about four thousand people a year donate their organs, and if organs could be retrieved after brain death, this alone would increase the number of donors to twenty thousand. A national policy of requesting organ donations, perhaps one administered through the Department of Health and Human Services, would be likely to do a great deal to reduce the chronic shortage of transplant organs.

Another possibility for increasing the organ supply is to permit organs to be offered for sale on the open market. Before death, an individual might arrange payment for the posthumous use of one or more of his organs. Or after the individual's death, his survivors might sell his organs to those in need of them. In a variation of this proposal, donors or their families might receive certain forms of tax credits, or a donor might be legally guaranteed that if a family member or friend required a transplant organ, then that person would be given priority in the distribution. Under either plan, there would be a strong incentive to make organs available for transplant.

The public reaction to any plan for marketing organs has been strongly negative. People generally regard the prospect of individuals in need of transplants bidding against one another in an "organ auction" as ghoulish and morally repugnant, and this attitude extends to all forms of the market approach. Legislation is currently before the U.S. Congress to make the sale of organs for transplant illegal.

A third possibility would be to allow living individuals to sell their nonvital organs to those in need of transplants. Taking hearts and livers from living people is illegal, for it would involve suicide by the individual and homicide by the surgeon who removed them. However, kidneys occur in pairs, and we already permit individuals to donate one of their kidneys to a family member—indeed, we celebrate those who do. It is only a short step from the heroic act of giving away a kidney to the commercial act of selling one.

Such a procedure would be in keeping with the generally acknowledged principle that people ought to be free to do what they wish with their own bodies. However, the decisive disadvantage to allowing such transactions as a matter of social policy is that it would be the poor who would be most likely to suffer from it. It is all too easy to imagine a mother wishing to improve the lives and opportunities of her children deciding to sell a kidney to help make that possible. That the economically advantaged should thrive by literally exploiting the bodies of the poor is morally repulsive. It is no answer to object that someone should be permitted to do as he wishes with his body to provide for the welfare of his family. If selling a kidney and putting his own life and health at risk is the only option open to someone with that aim, then this in itself constitutes a prima facie case for major social reform.

A final possibility that has been widely discussed as a means of increasing the number of organs available for transplant is the adoption of a policy of "presumed consent." That is, a state or federal law would allow hospitals to take it for granted that a recently deceased person has tacitly consented to having any needed organs removed, unless the person had indicated otherwise or unless the family objects. The burden of securing consent would be removed from physicians and hospitals, but the burden of denying consent would be imposed on individuals or their families. To withdraw consent would require a positive action.

A policy of presumed consent has been adopted by several European countries. Critics of the policy point out that this has not, in general, done much to reduce the shortage of transplant organs in those countries. Although legally empowered to remove without out a family's permission, physicians continue to be reluctant to do so. It is doubtful that a policy of presumed consent would be any more successful in this country. Also, if families are to be given the opportunity to deny consent, they must be notified of the death of the patient, and in many cases this would involve not only complicated practical arrangements, but also a considerable loss of time. Thus, it is somewhat doubtful that presumed consent would do a great deal to increase the number of usable transplant organs.

In the view of many observers, the present system of organ procurement by voluntary donation is the best system. It appeals to the best in people, rather than to greed and self-interest, it avoids exploiting the poor, and it is efficient. Many believe that without any fundamental alterations in the system it is possible to increase the number of available organs. As one observer commented, there is no shortage of donors, just a shortage of askers. If so, then a policy of requiring that the next of kin be asked to donate organs holds the promise of relieving the chronic shortage. As mentioned earlier, this is a policy already adopted by at least two states, but to be wholly effective, the policy should be nationwide.

Whatever the future may promise, the fact remains that at the present there is a limited supply of transplant organs, and the demand exceeds the supply. Thus, the key question today is "How are organs to be distributed when they become available?" There are currently no national policies or procedures for answering this question. Typically, such decisions are made in accordance with policies adopted by particular regional or hospital-based transplant programs.

In a characteristic instance, a member of a hospital staff notifies someone in a transplant program of a potential donor, often a patient recently declared brain-dead. Someone from the program then approaches the family to secure consent. If consent is granted, the organs are removed and arrangements made to transplant them as soon as possible. Patients who are judged to be most in need medically and who have a good (not necessarily perfect) tissue match with the donor organ are chosen as the recipients.

Medical need is not the only factor considered in all instances, however. Decisions are also based on the patient's general medical condition, how much he might be expected to benefit from the transplant, his age, his ability to pay for the operation, whether he has a family that will assist him during recovery, and whether he belongs to the constituency that the hospital is committed to serving. In addition, other factors, such as the individual's "social worth" (education, occupation, accomplishments), may be taken into account.

Some of these factors, particularly the patient's social worth and ability to pay, have been strongly criticized as morally irrelevant to deciding who is to receive a transplant organ. In an attempt to formulate acceptable guidelines for making such decisions, some states have established commissions to study the issues and make recommendations. A good example is the Massachusetts Task Force on Organ Transplantation. The group met for a year to consider the problems posed by distribution and fairness and in 1984 issued a unanimous report that included the following recommendations:

Transplant surgery should be provided "to those who can benefit most from it in terms of probability of living for a sig-

nificant period of time with a reasonable prospect for rehabilitation."

Decisions should not be based on "social worth" criteria.

Age may be considered as a factor in the selection process, but only to the extent that age is relevant to life expectancy and prospects for rehabilitation. Age must not be the only factor considered.

If not enough organs are available for all those who might benefit from them, then final selections should be made by some random process (e.g., a lottery or first-come, first-served basis).

Transplants should be provided to residents of New England on the basis of need, regardless of their ability to pay, so long as this does not adversely affect health-care services with a higher priority. Those who are not residents of New England should be accepted as transplant candidates only after they have demonstrated their ability to pay for the procedure.

It is likely that the guidelines currently being developed by a Presidential commission will resemble those of the Massachusetts Task Force. The obvious difference will be the lack of a state or regional constituency requirement. What remains to be seen is whether the commission will recommend that federal funds be used to pay for organ transplants for all who are in need of them but cannot afford them.

The particular issues that surround the allocation of organs are part of the general problem of fairly and equitably distributing scarce resources that is dealt with in the readings in this chapter.

CASE PRESENTATION
Policy Decision and the Neonatal Unit

Jake Hanna (as we will call him) stood by the admitting desk in the emergency room of Commerce County Hospital and couldn't believe what was happening. It was like being trapped in a nightmare.

Less than ten miles away, his wife Christine lay in a recovery room at Valley View Hospital. She had just given birth to their first child and was still groggy from the anesthesia.

Martha, as they had already decided to name their daughter before her birth, had been premature. She was almost six weeks early, and both Jake and Chris had been surprised when Chris began to experience labor pains. At first they didn't know what the pains were; then they decided that to be safe, they had better get Chris to the hospital Chris's obstetrician had told them to go to. They were lucky to have gotten to Valley View in time, because the birth was a difficult one, and Chris had needed help and reassurance.

In another respect, they hadn't been so lucky. Valley View was a small private hospital with restricted facilities. It had an emergency room, but no intensive care or neonatal units.

And Martha needed help. She was small and underdeveloped. Her heart sounds were weak and slightly irregular, she was having difficulty breathing, and her blood chemistry was unbalanced and showed inadequate kidney function. If she was to have a good chance at living, she needed special treatment and continuous monitoring.

"You need to get her into a special facility," Dr. Birk told Jake. "We're doing all we can for her here, but that's not very much. We aren't even set up to do dialysis. We simply don't have the equipment or the personnel to provide her with the kind of care she needs."

"Where could she go?" Jake asked.

"Commerce County Hospital—it's the only place in the area with a neonatal setup."

"Can you make the arrangements?"

"I'm sorry, I can't. They won't take referrals anymore. Somebody on their staff has to do the admitting. I think they're trying to cut back on their program."

"Can I get her in?"

"I'm not sure," Dr. Birk said. "but she needs to be there. They may take her as a walk-in. So you're going to have to go in person and take the baby with you. Do you have a friend or family member here?"

"Chris's mother is with her. But isn't it dangerous to move the baby?"

"Not really. She's in a stable condition, and if you take her you'll save a lot of time. She needs help as fast as she can get it."

With Martha wrapped in a grey hospital blanket and held by Chris's mother, Jake drove the ten miles to Commerce County Hospital and double-parked at the emergency entrance. He literally ran through the wide doors.

He explained to the clerk at the admitting desk that Dr. Birk had said that the baby needed to be in a neonatal unit at once. The clerk said that he had no authority to make that kind of admission and told Jake to sit down while he paged Dr. Donna Chavez, the director of the unit.

The wait seemed interminable to Jake, but in less than ten minutes Dr. Chavez appeared in the emergency room. Jake walked over to her, and while they stood by the admitting desk with a dozen people waiting for their names to be called, he explained the problem once again.

When Jake had finished, Dr. Chavez shook her head. "We can't admit the child," she said. "I'm sorry, but we just can't do it."

"Why not?" Jake asked. "Don't you have room or something?"

"That's not the problem. We actually have enough space."

"Then what is it?"

"This is going to be hard for you to understand," Dr. Chavez said. "But the hospital has adopted a new policy. At no time can we have more than twenty patients in the neonatal unit, and that's the number we have now. The problem is with costs."

"But I'm willing to pay, and I have insurance."

"It's not particular costs, Mr. Hanna. It's the cost of the whole unit, and Commerce has just decided to cut back on its size. That's why they've imposed a twenty-infant limit."

"But what about my child?" Jake asked. "She needs help, and she needs it right now."

"I'm very, very sorry," Dr. Chavez said. "If the decision were mine alone, I would admit her at once. But as things are, I simply have to follow the hospital's policy guidelines."

"So you refuse to take her?"

"I must. I don't have any real choice in the matter."

"What am I supposed to do? Just let her die?"

"I suggest you take the child back to Valley View. They will do everything they can, and with luck things will work out for her. I certainly hope so."

Jake thought he had never had a nightmare as bad as this. He had never before felt so helpless, so powerless. There was no way he could force them to admit Martha, and there was nothing he could do for her himself. It surprised him that he didn't feel particularly angry at Dr. Chavez or at the hospital. He was simply too numb to feel much of anything.

Jake said nothing more to Dr. Chavez. He went out to the car and drove back to Valley View. Mrs. Williams cried all the way back, and Jake wished that he could.

Inside the emergency room at Valley View, a nurse took the baby from Mrs. Williams. They took Martha to a small treatment room and gave her oxygen to help her breathing.

Jake and Mrs. Williams sat in the waiting area. They agreed that there was no need to tell Chris anything yet. She was asleep and no purpose would be served by waking her.

Three hours later, a doctor Jake had never seen before came to tell him that Martha was dead.

INTRODUCTION

The story of Robin Cook's novel *Coma* takes place in a large Boston hospital at the present time. What sets the novel apart from dozens of others with similar settings and characters is the fact that the plot hinges on the operations of a large-scale black market in transplant organs. For enormous fees, the criminals running the operation will supply corneas, kidneys, or hearts to those who can pay the price.

Cook claims that the inspiration for his novel came from an advertisement in a California newspaper. The anonymous ad offered to sell for five thousand dollars any organ that a reader wanted to buy. Thus, Cook's novel seems to be rooted firmly in the world we know today and not just a leap into the speculative realms of science fiction.

Organ transplants have attracted a considerable amount of attention in the last few years. Not only are transplants dramatic, often offering last-minute salvation from an almost certain death, but the very possibility of organ transplants is bright with promise. We can easily imagine a future in which any injured or diseased organ can be replaced almost as easily as the parts on a car. The present state of biomedical technology makes this more than a distant dream, although not a current reality.

The basic problem with organ transplants is the phenomenon of tissue rejection by the immune system. Alien proteins trigger the body's defense mechanisms. In the past, the proteins in the transplanted tissues were matched as carefully as possible with those of the recipient, then powerful immunosuppressive drugs were used in an effort to allow the host body to accommodate itself to the foreign tissue. These drugs left the body open to infections that it could normally cope with without much difficulty.

Increased use of the drug cyclosporine has done a great deal to increase the success of organ transplants. Cyclosporine selectively inhibits only part of the immune system and leaves enough of the system sufficiently functional to fight off most of the infections that were once fatal to large numbers of transplant recipients. Also, although tissue matching is still important, particularly for kidneys, the matches do not have to be as close as before. Now almost four out of five transplanted kidneys function after one year; in the 1970s only about 50 percent did. Since 1970, the one-year survival rate for children with liver transplants has increased from 38 to 70 percent, and there is good reason to believe that if children survive as long as one year, they have a genuine chance to live a normal life. More than 70 percent of heart-transplant recipients now live for at least one year, a major increase from the 20 percent of the 1970s.

Because of the relatively high rate of success in organ transplants, the need for organs (kidneys in particular) is always greater than the supply. (The black market operation in Cook's novel may not be wholly unrealistic.) In such a situation, where scarcity and need conflict, it is frequently necessary to decide who among the candidates for a transplant will receive an available organ. Relatively objective considerations such as the "goodness" of tissue matching, the size of the organ, and the general medical condition of the candidates may rule out some individuals. But it does happen that choices have to be made.

Who should make such choices? Should they be made by a physician, following his or her own intuitions? Should they be made by a committee or board? If so, who should be on the committee? Should a patient have a representative to speak for his or her interest—someone to "make a case" for receiving the transplant organ?

Should the decision be made in accordance with a set of explicit criteria? If so, then what criteria are appropriate? Are matters such as age, race, sex, and place of residence irrelevant? Should the character and accomplishments of the candidates be given any weight? Should people be judged by their estimated "worth to the community"? Should

the fact that someone is a parent be given any weight?

These are just some of the questions that are relevant to the general issue of deciding how to allocate medical goods in situations in which the available supply is surpassed by a present need. Transplant organs are just an example of one type of goods. In the future, with the improvement of transplant technology, the allocation of organs will no doubt become an even more frequent problem than it is at present. It is, of course, already a morally serious problem.

It was not organ transplants that first called public attention to the issue of resource allocation. This occurred most dramatically in the early 1960s when the Artificial Kidney Center in Seattle, Washington, initiated an effective large-scale treatment program for people with renal diseases. Normal kidneys filter waste products from the blood that have accumulated as a result of ordinary cellular metabolism—salt, urea, creatinine, potassium, uric acid, and other substances. These waste products are sent from the kidneys to the bladder, where they are then secreted as urine. Kidney failure, which can result from one of a number of diseases, allows waste products to build up in the blood. This can cause high blood pressure and even heart failure, tissue edema (swelling), and muscular seizure. If unremedied, the condition results in death.

When renal failure occurs, hemodialysis is a way of cleansing the blood of waste products by passing it through a cellophanelike tube immersed in a chemical bath. The impurities in the blood pass through the membrane and into the chemical bath by osmosis, and the purified blood is then returned to the patient's body.

At the beginning of the Seattle program, there were many more candidates for dialysis than there were units ("kidney machines") to accommodate them. As a response to this situation, the Kidney Center set up a committee to select those patients who would receive treatment. (See the Case Presentation for an account of how such a committee might work.) In effect, the committee was offering to some a better chance for life than they would have without access to dialysis equipment.

As other centers and hospitals established renal units, they faced the same painful decisions that Seattle did. Almost always there were many more patients needing hemodialysis than there was equipment available to treat them. It was partly in response to this situation that Section 299-1 of Public Law 92-603 was passed by Congress in 1972. Those that require hemodialysis or kidney transplants are now eligible for Medicare payments that cover as much as 80 percent of the costs involved.

More than seventy thousand patients are now receiving dialysis supported by Medicare. Present costs are over 1.8 billion dollars a year, and the patient load is expected to increase at a rate of some 20 percent a year. Although those in the End-Stage Renal Disease Program constitute only one quarter of 1 percent of those receiving benefits under Medicare B (which covers outpatient treatment), their benefits make up some 10 percent of the budget.

Quite apart from the cost, which is much higher than originally expected, dialysis continues to present moral difficulties. Resources are still finite so that at a given time more patients may both need and want dialysis than can be accommodated. Hence the need to make choices among patients is still present. It brings with it all the problems that we mentioned above.

In addition, because more dialysis equipment is available and is financially available to virtually everyone, physicians face a serious difficulty. Even if a physician believes that a patient is not likely to gain benefits from dialysis to an extent to justify the expense, should he recommend the patient for dialysis anyway? Not to do so may mean almost certain death for the patient in the near future, yet the social cost (measured in terms of the cost of equipment and its operation, hospital facilities, and the time of physicians, nurses, and technicians) may be immense. It can be as much as seventy-five to one hundred thousand dollars a year for a single person.

It is important to notice that dialysis does not solve all the problems for patients with terminal kidney diseases. Although time spent on the machine varies, some patients spend five hours, three days a week, attached to the machine. Medical and psychological problems are typical even when the process works at its most efficient. Prolonged dialysis can produce neurological disorders, severe headaches, gastrointestinal bleeding, and bone diseases. Psychological and physical stress is always present, and particularly before dialysis treatments, severe depression is common. A 1971 study showed that 5 percent of dialysis patients take their own lives, and a number of others simply drop out of treatment programs and allow themselves to die. For these reasons, strong motivation, psychological stability, age, and a generally sound physical condition are factors considered important in deciding whether to admit a person to dialysis.

The characteristics required to make someone a "successful" dialysis patient are to some extent "middle-class virtues." A patient must not only be motivated to save his life, but he must also understand the need for the dialysis, be capable of adhering to a strict diet, show up for scheduled dialysis sessions, and so on. As a consequence, where decisions about whether to admit a patient to dialysis are based on estimates of the likelihood of the patient's doing what is required, members of the white middle class have a definite edge over others. Selection criteria that are apparently objective may actually involve hidden class or racial bias.

Various ways of dealing with both the costs and the personal problems presented by dialysis are currently under discussion. In the view of some, increasing the number of kidney transplants would do the most to improve the lives of patients and to reduce the cost of the kidney program. (This would have the result of increasing even more the demand for transplant organs. See the Social Context section for a discussion of proposals for doing this.) Others have pressed for training more patients to perform home dialysis, which is substantially cheaper than dialysis performed in clinics or hospitals. However, those who are elderly, live alone, or lack adequate facilities are not likely to be able to use and maintain the complicated equipment involved. Other things being equal, should such people be given priority for transplants?

The problems of transplants and dialysis are ones that involve decisions that affect individuals in a direct and immediate way—either a person is accepted into a dialysis program or he is not. As we will see in the next chapter, there are a number of broader social issues connected with providing and distributing medical resources. But our concern here is with the sort of decision making that involves the welfare of particular people in specific situations. The situations are ones in which there is not enough of what is needed to go around. The basic question, of course, is who shall get it and who shall go without?

Any commodity or service that can be in short supply relative to the need for it raises the issue of fair and justifiable distribution. Decisions that control the supply itself, that determine, for example, what proportion of the federal budget will be spent on medical care, are generally referred to as *macroallocation* decisions. These are the large-scale decisions that do not involve individuals in a direct way. Similarly, deciding what proportion of the money allocated to health care should be spent on dialysis is another example of a macroallocation decision.

By contrast, *microallocation* decisions are ones that directly impinge on individuals. Thus, when one donor heart is available, and six people in need of a transplant make a claim on it, the decision as to who gets the heart is a microallocation decision. In Chapter 9, in discussing the claim to health care, we will focus more on macroallocation, but in this chapter we will be concerned mostly with microallocation. (The distinction between macroallocation and microallocation is often less clear than the explanation here suggests. After all, there are many levels of decision making in the distribution of resources, and the terms macro and micro are relative ones.)

Although the examples we have considered have been restricted to transplant organs and dialysis machines, the question of fair distribution can be raised just as appropriately about cardiac resuscitation teams, microsurgical teams, space in burn units or intensive-care wards, hospital beds, drugs and vaccines, medical-evacuation helicopters, operating rooms, physicians' time, and all other medical goods and services that are in limited supply with respect to the demand for them. Earlier, in connection with transplants, we considered some of the more specific questions that have to be asked about distribution. The questions generally fall into two categories: Who shall decide? What criteria or standards should be employed in making the allocation decision? These are the questions that must be answered whenever there is scarcity relative to needs and wants.

ETHICAL THEORIES AND THE ALLOCATION OF MEDICAL RESOURCES

An analogy that is frequently used in the discussion of the distribution of limited medical resources compares such a situation to the plight of a group of people adrift in a lifeboat. If some of the group are sacrificed, then the others will have a much better chance of surviving. But who should be sacrificed?

One answer to this question is that no one should be. Simply by virtue of being human, each person in the lifeboat has an equal worth. An action that involved sacrificing anyone for the good of the others in the boat would not be morally defensible. This suggests that the only right course of action would be simply to do nothing.

This point of view is one that may be regarded as compatible with Kant's ethical principles. Because each individual may be considered to have inherent value, considerations such as talent, intelligence, age, social worth, and so on are morally irrelevant. Accordingly, there seem to be no grounds for distinguishing those who are to be sacrificed from those who may be saved. In the medical context, this would mean that when there are not enough goods and services to go around, then no one should receive them.

This is not a result that is dictated by Kant's principles, however. One might also argue that the fact that every person is equal to every other in dignity and worth does not require the sacrifice of all. A random procedure—such as drawing straws—might be used to determine who is to have an increased chance of survival. In such a case, each person is being treated as having equal value, and the person who loses might be regarded as exercising his autonomy by sacrificing himself or herself. The maxim underlying the sacrifice would, apparently, be one that would meet the test of the categorical imperative. Any rational person might be expected to sacrifice himself in such a situation and under the conditions in which the decision was made. In the case of medical resouces, a random procedure would seem to be a morally legitimate procedure.

The natural law view and Ross's would seem to support a similar line of argument. Although we all have a duty, on these views, to preserve our lives, this does not mean that we do not sometimes have to risk them. Just such a risk might be involved in agreeing to abide by the outcome of a random procedure to decide who will be sacrificed and who saved.

Utilitarianism does not dictate a specific answer to the question of who, if anyone, should be saved. It does differ radically in one respect, however, from those moral views that ascribe an intrinsic value to each human life. The principle of utility suggests that we ought to take into account the consequences of sacrificing some people rather than others. Who, for example, is more likely to make a contribution to the general welfare of the society, an accountant or a nurse? This approach opens the way to considering the "social worth" of people and makes morally relevant such characteristics as education, occupation, age, record of accomplishment, and so on.

To take this approach would require working out a set of criteria that would assign value to various properties of people. Those to be sacrificed would be those whose point total put them at the low end of the ranking. Here, then, a typical "calculus of utilities" would be relied on to solve the decision problem. Decisions about the allocation of medical resources would follow exactly the same pattern.

This approach is not one required by the principle of utility, however. Someone might argue that a policy formulated along those lines would have so many harmful social consequences that some other solution would be preferable. Thus, a utilitarian might argue that a better policy would be one based on some random process. In connection with medical goods and services, a "first-come, first-served" approach might be superior. (This, at least, is a possible option for rule utilitarianism. It could be argued that an act utilitarian would be forced to adopt the first approach.)

Rawls's principles of justice seem clearly

to rule out distributing medical resources on the grounds of "social worth." Where special benefits are to be obtained, those benefits must be of value to all and open to all. It is compatible with Rawls's view, of course, that there should be no special medical resources. But if there are and they must be distributed under conditions of scarcity, then some genuinely fair procedure, such as random selection, must be the procedure used.

No ethical theory that we have considered gives a straightforward answer to the question of who shall make the selection. Where a procedure is random or "first-come, first-served," the decision-making process requires only establishing the right kind of social arrangements to implement the policy. Only when social worth must be judged and considered as a relevant factor in decision making does the procedure assume importance. (This is assuming that medical decisions about appropriateness have already been made, decisions that establish a class of candidates for the limited resources.)

A utilitarian answer as to who shall make the allocation decision might be that the decision should be made by those who are in a good position to judge the likelihood of an individual's contributing to the welfare of the society as a whole. Since physicians are not uniquely qualified to make such judgments, leaving decisions to an individual physician or a committee of physicians would not be the best approach. A better one would probably be to rely on a committee composed of a variety of people representative of the society.

There are many more questions of a moral kind connected with the allocation of scarce resources than we have mentioned here. We have not, for example, considered whether an individual should be allowed to make a case for receiving resources. Nor have we examined any of the problems with employing specific criteria for selection for treatment (such as requiring that a person be a resident of a certain community or state). We have, however, touched upon enough of the basic issues that it should be easy to see how other appropriate questions might be asked.

THE SELECTIONS

Nicholas Rescher in his essay makes a useful distinction between two kinds of criteria: criteria of inclusion (for the selection of candidates) and criteria of comparison (for selection of recipients). Rescher argues that three areas need to be considered in establishing a class of candidates: (1) constituency (Is the person a member of the community the institution is designed to serve?); (2) progress of science (Can new knowledge be gained from the case?); and (3) success (Is the treatment of the person likely to be effective?).

Five factors, Rescher claims, ought to be considered in deciding upon recipients of the goods or services: (1) the likelihood of successful treatment compared with others in the group; (2) the life-expectancy of the person; (3) the person's family role; (4) the potential of the person in making future contributions; and (5) the person's record of services or contributions.

Rescher argues that it is necessary to have a rational selection system, but he admits that the exact manner in which a system takes into account relevant factors cannot be fixed and exact. In his view, which is basically a utilitarian one, an acceptable selection system might be one that makes use of point ratings of the factors mentioned above. This would establish a smaller group, but as a final step, he suggests, the best procedure might well be to make use of a chance factor (such as a lottery) to choose recipients.

Childress's essay is explicitly critical of the utilitarian approach that would make "social worth" the source of selection criteria. Such criteria, Childress argues, lead us to value only the person who is a conformist. What is more, they have the effect of reducing people to their social roles. Childress favors some sort of random selection procedure ("first-come, first-served," or a lottery). Only an approach of this kind, he argues, preserves an individual's "personal and transcendent dignity, which on the utilitarian approach would be submerged in his social role and function." Also, Childress suggests, the random approach contributes to the preservation of such values as the maintenance of trust between patient and physician.

It can be argued that Childress is wrong to identify the utilitarian approach with the use of criteria based on social roles. As we mentioned earlier, it seems possible for rule utilitarianism to endorse the random approach advocated by Childress, although for very different reasons. Yet Childress's criticisms do hit at the utilitarian solutions recommended by Rescher.

George Annas takes a position on transplant selection that introduces a modification of the first-come, first-served principle endorsed by Childress. He reviews four approaches to rationing scarce medical resources—market, selection committee, lottery, and customary—and finds each has disadvantages so serious as to make them all unacceptable. An acceptable approach, he suggests, is one that combines efficiency, fairness, and a respect for the value of life. Because candidates should both want a transplant and be able to derive significant benefits from one, the first phase of selection should involve a screening process that is based exclusively on medical criteria that are objective and as free as possible of judgments about social worth.

Since selection might still have to be made from this pool of candidates, it might be done by social-worth criteria or by lottery. However, social-worth criteria seem arbitrary, and a lottery would be unfair to those who are in more immediate need of a transplant, ones who might die quickly without it. After reviewing the relevant considerations, a committee operating at this stage might allow those in immediate need of a transplant to be moved to the head of a waiting list. To those not in immediate need, organs would be distributed in a first-come, first-served fashion. Although absolute equality is not embodied in this process, the procedure is sufficiently flexible to recognize that some may have needs that are greater (more immediate) than others.

The Allocation of Exotic Medical Lifesaving Therapy

Nicholas Rescher

I. The Problem

Technological progress has in recent years transformed the limits of the possible in medical therapy. However, the elevated state of sophistication of modern medical technology has brought the economists' classic problem of scarcity in its wake as an unfortunate side product. The enormously sophisticated and complex equipment and the highly trained teams of experts requisite for its utilization are scarce resources in relation to potential demand. The administrators of the great medical institutions that preside over these scarce resources thus come to be faced increasingly with the awesome choice: *Whose life to save?*

A (somewhat hypothetical) paradigm example of this problem may be sketched within the following set of definitive assumptions: We suppose that persons in some particular medically morbid condition are "mortally afflicted": It is virtually certain

Reprinted from Ethics 79 *(April 1969), by permission of The University of Chicago Press and the author.*
© *The University of Chicago Press.*

that they will die within a short time period (say ninety days). We assume that some very complex course of treatment (e.g., a heart transplant) represents a substantial probability of life prolongation for persons in this mortally afflicted condition. We assume that the facilities available in terms of human resources, mechanical instrumentalities, and requisite materials (e.g., hearts in the case of a heart transplant) make it possible to give a certain treatment—this "exotic (medical) lifesaving therapy," or ELT for short—to a certain, relatively small number of people. And finally we assume that a substantially greater pool of people in the mortally afflicted condition is at hand. The problem then may be formulated as follows: How is one to select within the pool of afflicted patients the ones to be given the ELT treatment in question; how to select those "whose lives are to be saved"? Faced with many candidates for an ELT process that can be made available to only a few, doctors and medical administrators confront the decision of who is to be given a chance at survival and who is, in effect, to be condemned to die.

As has already been implied, the "heroic" variety of spare-part surgery can pretty well be assimilated to this paradigm. One can foresee the time when heart transplantation, for example, will have become pretty much a routine medical procedure, albeit on a very limited basis, since a cardiac surgeon with the technical competence to transplant hearts can operate at best a rather small number of times each week and the elaborate facilities for such operations will most probably exist on a modest scale. Moreover, in "spare-part" surgery there is always the problem of availability of the "spare parts" themselves. A report in one British newspaper gives the following picture: "Of the 150,000 who die of heart disease each year [in the U.K.], Mr. Donald Longmore, research surgeon at the National Heart Hospital [in London] estimated that 22,000 might be eligible for heart surgery. Another 30,000 would need heart and lung transplants. But there are probably only between 7,000 and 14,000 potential donors a year."[1] Envisaging this situation in which at the very most something like one in four heart-malfunction victims can be saved, we clearly confront a problem in ELT allocation.

A perhaps even more drastic case in point is afforded by long-term haemodialysis, an ongoing process by which a complex device—an "artificial kidney machine"—is used periodically in cases of chronic renal failure to substitute for a nonfunctional kidney in "cleaning" potential poisons from the blood. Only a few major institutions have chronic haemodialysis units, whose complex operation is an extremely expensive proposition. For the present and foreseeable future the situation is that "the number of places available for chronic haemodialysis is hopelessly inadequate."[2]

The traditional medical ethos has insulated the physician against facing the very existence of this problem. When swearing the Hippocratic Oath, he commits himself to work for the benefit of the sick in "whatsoever house I enter."[3] In taking this stance, the physician substantially renounces the explicit choice of saving certain lives rather than others. Of course, doctors have always in fact had to face such choices on the battlefield or in times of disaster, but there the issue had to be resolved hurriedly, under pressure, and in circumstances in which the very nature of the case effectively precluded calm deliberation by the decision maker as well as criticism by others. In sharp contrast, however, cases of the type we have postulated in the present discussion arise predictably, and represent choices to be made deliberately and "in cold blood."

It is, to begin with, appropriate to remark that this problem is not fundamentally a medical problem. For when there are sufficiently many afflicted candidates for ELT then—so we may assume— there will also be more than enough for whom the purely medical grounds for ELT allocation are decisively strong in any individual case, and just about equally strong throughout the group. But in this circumstance a selection of some afflicted patients over and against others cannot *ex hypothesi* be made on the basis of purely medical considerations.

The selection problem, as we have said, is in substantial measure not a medical one. It is a problem *for* medical men, which must somehow be solved by them, but that does not make it a medical issue—any more than the problem of hospital building is a medical issue. As a problem it belongs to the category of philosophical problems— specifically a problem of moral philosophy or ethics. Structurally, it bears a substantial kinship with those issues in this field that revolve about the notorious whom-to-save-on-the-lifeboat and whom-to-throw-to-the-wolves-pursuing-the-sled questions. But whereas questions of this just-indicated sort are artificial, hypothetical, and far-fetched, the ELT issue poses a *genuine* policy question for the responsible administrators in medical institutions, indeed a question that threatens to become commonplace in the foreseeable future.

Now what the medical administrator needs to have, and what the philosopher is presumably *ex officio* in a position to help in providing, is a body of *rational guidelines* for making choices in these literally life-or-death situations. This is an issue in which many interested parties have a substantial stake, including the responsible decision maker who wants to satisfy his conscience that he is acting in a reasonable way. Moreover, the family and associates of the man who is turned away—to say nothing of the man himself—have the right to an acceptable explanation. And indeed even the general public wants to know that what is being done is fitting and proper. All of these interested parties are entitled to insist that a reasonable code of operating principles provides a defensible rationale for making the life-and-death choices involved in ELT.

II. The Two Types of Criteria

Two distinguishable types of criteria are bound up in the issue of making ELT choices. We shall call these *Criteria of Inclusion* and *Criteria of Comparison,* respectively. The distinction at issue here requires some explanation. We can think of the selection as being made by a two-stage process: (1) the selection from among all possible candidates (by a suitable screening process) of a group to be taken under serious consideration as candidates for therapy, and then (2) the actual singling out, within this group, of the particular individuals to whom therapy is to be given. Thus the first process narrows down the range of comparative choices by eliminating *en bloc* whole categories of potential candidates. The second process calls for a more refined, case-by-case comparison of those candidates that remain. By means of the first set of criteria one forms a selection group; by means of the second set, an actual selection is made within this group.

Thus what we shall call a "selection system" for the choice of patients to receive therapy of the ELT type will consist of criteria of these two kinds. Such a system will be acceptable only when the reasonableness of its component criteria can be established.

III. Essential Features of an Acceptable ELT Selection System

To qualify as reasonable, an ELT selection must meet two important "regulative" requirements: it must be *simple* enough to be readily intelligible, and it must be *plausible,* that is, patently reasonable in a way that can be apprehended easily and without involving ramified subtleties. Those medical administrators responsible for ELT choices must follow a modus operandi that virtually all the people involved can readily understand to be acceptable (at a reasonable level of generality, at any rate). Appearances are critically important here. It is not enough that the choice be made in a *justifiable* way; it must be possible for people—*plain* people—to "see" (i.e., understand without elaborate teaching or indoctrination) that *it is justified,* insofar as any mode of procedure can be justified in cases of this sort.

One "constitutive" requirement is obviously an essential feature of a reasonable selection system: all of its component criteria—those of inclusion and those of comparison alike—must be reasonable in the sense of being *rationally defensible*. The ramifications of this requirement call for detailed consideration. But one of its aspects should be noted without further ado: it must be *fair*—it must treat relevantly like cases alike, leaving no room for "influence" or favoritism, etc.

IV. The Basic Screening Stage: Criteria of Inclusion (and Exclusion)

Three sorts of considerations are prominent among the plausible criteria of inclusion/exclusion at the basic screening stage: the constituency factor, the progress-of-science factor, and the prospect-of-success factor.

A. The Constituency Factor

It is a "fact of life" that ELT can be available only in the institutional setting of a hospital or medical institute or the like. Such institutions generally have normal clientele boundaries. A veterans' hospital will not concern itself primarily with treating nonveterans, a children's hospital cannot be expected to accommodate the "senior citizen," an army hospital can regard college professors as outside its sphere. Sometimes the boundaries are geographic—a state hospital may admit only residents of a certain state. (There are, of course, indefensible constituency principles—say race or religion, party membership, or ability to pay; and there are cases of borderline legitimacy, e.g., sex.[4]) A medical institution is justified in considering for ELT only persons within its own constituency, provided this constituency is constituted upon a defensible basis. Thus the haemodialysis selection committee in Seattle "agreed to consider only those applications who were residents of the state of Washington. . . . They justified this stand on the grounds that since the basic research . . . had been done at . . . a state-supported institution—the people whose taxes had paid for the research should be its first beneficiaries."[5]

While thus insisting that constituency considerations represent a valid and legitimate factor in ELT selection, I do feel there is much to be said for minimizing their role in life-or-death cases. Indeed a refusal to recognize them at all is a significant part of medical tradition, going back to the very oath of Hippocrates. They represent a departure from the ideal arising with the institutionalization of medicine, moving it away from its original status as an art practiced by an individual practitioner.

B. The Progress-of-Science Factor

The needs of medical research can provide a second valid principle of inclusion. The research interests of the medical staff in relation to the specific nature of the cases at issue is a significant consideration. It may be important for the progress of medical science—and thus of potential benefit to many persons in the future—to determine how effective the ELT at issue is with diabetics or persons over sixty or with a negative RH factor.

Considerations of this sort represent another type of legitimate factor in ELT selection.

A very definitely *borderline* case under this head would revolve around the question of a patient's willingness to pay, not in monetary terms, but in offering himself as an experimental subject, say by contracting to return at designated times for a series of tests substantially unrelated to his own health, but yielding data of importance to medical knowledge in general.

C. The Prospect-of-Success Factor

It may be that while the ELT at issue is not without *some* effectiveness in general, it has been established to be highly effective only with patients in certain specific categories (e.g., females under forty of a specific blood type). This difference in effectiveness—in the absolute or in the probability of success—is (we assume) so marked as to constitute virtually a difference in kind rather than in degree. In this case, it would be perfectly legitimate to adopt the general rule of making the ELT at issue available only or primarily to persons in this substantial-promise-of-success category. (It is on grounds of this sort that young children and persons over fifty are generally ruled out as candidates for haemodialysis.)

We have maintained that the three factors of constituency, progress of science, and prospect of success represent legitimate criteria of inclusion for ELT selection. But it remains to examine the considerations which legitimate them. The legitimating factors are in the final analysis practical or pragmatic in nature. From the practical angle it is advantageous—indeed to some extent necessary—that the arrangements governing medical institutions should embody certain constituency principles. It makes good pragmatic and utilitarian sense that progress-of-science considerations should be operative here. And, finally, the practical aspect is reinforced by a whole host of other considerations—including moral ones—in supporting the prospect-of-success criterion. The workings of each of these factors are of course conditioned by the ever-present element of limited availability. They are operative only in this context, that is, prospect of success is a legitimate consideration at all only because we are dealing with a situation of scarcity.

V. The Final Selection Stage: Criteria of Selection

Five sorts of elements must, as we see it, figure primarily among the plausible criteria of selection that are to be brought to bear in further screening the group constituted after application of the criteria of inclusion: the relative-likelihood-of-success factor, the life-expectancy factor, the family role factor, the potential-contributions factor, and the services-rendered factor. The first two represent the *biomedical* aspect, the second three the *social* aspect.

A. The Relative-Likelihood-of-Success Factor

It is clear that the relative likelihood of success is a legitimate and appropriate factor in making a selection within the group of qualified patients that are to receive ELT. This is obviously one of the considerations that must count very significantly in a reasonable selection procedure.

The present criterion is of course closely related to item C of the preceding section. There we were concerned with prospect-of-success considerations categorically and *en bloc*. Here at present they come into play in a particularized case-by-case comparison among individuals. If the therapy at issue is not a once-and-for-all proposition and requires ongoing treatment, cognate considerations must be brought in. Thus, for example, in the case of a chronic ELT procedure such as haemodialysis it would clearly make sense to give priority to patients with a potentially reversible condition (who would thus need treatment for only a fraction of their remaining lives).

B. The Life-Expectancy Factor

Even if the ELT is "successful" in the patient's case he may, considering his age and/or other aspects of his general medical condition, look forward to only a very short probable future life. This is obviously another factor that must be taken into account.

C. The Family Role Factor

A person's life is a thing of importance not only to himself but to others—friends, associates, neighbors, colleagues, etc. But his (or her) relationship to his immediate family is a thing of unique intimacy and significance. The nature of his relationship to his wife, children, and parents, and the issue of their financial and psychological dependence upon him, are obviously matters that deserve to be given weight in the ELT selection process. Other things being anything like equal, the mother of minor children must take priority over the middle-aged bachelor.

D. The Potential Future-Contributions Factor (Prospective Service)

In "choosing to save" one life rather than another, "the society," through the mediation of the particular medical institution in question—which should certainly look upon itself as a trustee for the social interest—is clearly warranted in considering the likely pattern of future *services to be rendered* by the patient (adequate recovery assumed), considering his age, talent, training, and past record of performance. In its allocations of ELT, society "invests" a scarce resource in one person as against another and is thus entitled to look to the probable prospective "return" on its investment.

It may well be that a thoroughly egalitarian society is reluctant to put someone's social contribution into the scale in situations of the sort at issue. One popular article states that "the most difficult standard would be the candidate's value to society," and goes on to quote someone who said: "You can't just pick a brilliant painter over a laborer. The average citizen would be quickly eliminated."[6] But what if it were not a brilliant painter but a brilliant surgeon or medical researcher that was at issue? One wonders if the author of the *obiter dictum* that one "can't just pick" would still feel equally sure of his ground. In any case, the fact that the standard is difficult to apply is certainly no reason for not attempting to apply it. The problem of ELT selection is inevitably burdened with difficult standards.

Some might feel that in assessing a patient's value to society one should ask not only who if permitted to continue living can make the greatest contribution to society in some creative or constructive way, but also who by dying would leave behind the greatest burden on society in assuming the discharge of their residual responsibilities.[7] Certainly the philosophical utilitarian would give equal weight to both these considerations. Just here is where I would part ways with orthodox utilitarianism. For—though this is not the place to do so—I should be prepared to argue that a civilized society has an obligation to promote the furtherance of positive achievements in cultural and related areas even if this means the assumption of certain added burdens.[8]

E. The Past Services-Rendered Factor (Retrospective Service)

A person's services to another person or group have always been taken to constitute a valid basis for a claim upon this person or group—of course a moral and not necessarily a legal claim. Society's obligation for the recognition and reward of services rendered—an obligation whose discharge is also very possibly conducive to self-interest in the long run—is thus another factor to be taken into account. This should be viewed as a morally necessary correlative of the previously considered factor of *prospective* service. It would be morally indefensible of society in effect to say: "Never mind about services you rendered yesterday—it is only the services to be rendered tomorrow that will count with us today." We live in very future-oriented times, constantly preoccupied in a distinctly utilitarian way with future satisfactions. And this disinclines us to give much recognition to past services. But parity considerations of the sort just adduced indicate that such recognition should be given *on grounds of equity.* No doubt a justification for giving weight to services rendered can also be attempted along utilitarian lines. ("The reward of past services rendered spurs people on to greater future efforts and is thus socially advantageous in the long-run future.") In saying that past services should be counted "on grounds of equity"—rather than "on grounds of utility"—I take the view that even if this utilitarian defense could somehow be shown to be fallacious, I should still be prepared to maintain the propriety of taking services rendered into account. The position does not rest on a utilitarian basis and so would not collapse with the removal of such a basis.[9]

As we have said, these five factors fall into three groups: the biomedical factors *A* and *B*, the familial factor *C*, and the social factors *D* and *E*. With items *A* and *B* the need for a detailed analysis of the medical considerations comes to the fore.

The age of the patient, his medical history, his physical and psychological condition, his specific disease, etc., will all need to be taken into exact account. These biomedical factors represent technical issues: they call for the physicians' expert judgment and the medical statisticians' hard data. And they are ethically uncontroversial factors—their legitimacy and appropriateness are evident from the very nature of the case.

Greater problems arise with the familial and social factors. They involve intangibles that are difficult to judge. How is one to develop subcriteria for weighing the relative social contributions of (say) an architect or a librarian or a mother of young children? And they involve highly problematic issues. (For example, should good moral character be rated a plus and bad a minus in judging services rendered?) And there is something strikingly unpleasant in grappling with issues of this sort for people brought up in times greatly inclined towards maxims of the type "Judge not!" and "Live and let live!" All the same, in the situation that concerns us here such distasteful problems must be faced, since a failure to choose to save some is tantamount to sentencing all. Unpleasant choices are intrinsic to the problem of ELT selection; they are of the very essence of the matter.[10]

But is reference to all these factors indeed inevitable? The justification for taking account of the medical factors is pretty obvious. But why should the social aspect of services rendered and to be rendered be taken into account at all? The answer is that they must be taken into account not from the *medical* but from the *ethical* point of view. Despite disagreement on many fundamental issues, moral philosophers of the present day are pretty well in consensus that the justification of human actions is to be sought largely and primarily—if not exclusively—in the principles of utility and of justice.[11] But utility requires reference of services to be rendered and justice calls for a recognition of services that have been rendered. Moral considerations would thus demand recognition of these two factors. (This, of course, still leaves open the question of whether the point of view provides a valid basis of action: Why base one's actions upon moral principles?—or, to put it bluntly—Why be moral? The present paper is, however, hardly the place to grapple with so fundamental an issue, which has been canvassed in the literature of philosophical ethics since Plato.)

VI. More than Medical Issues Are Involved

An active controversy has of late sprung up in medical circles over the question of whether non-physician laymen should be given a role in ELT selection (in the specific context of chronic haemodialysis). One physician writes: "I think that the assessment of the candidates should be made by a senior doctor on the [dialysis] unit, but I am sure that it would be helpful to him—both in sharing responsibility and in avoiding personal pressure—if a small unnamed group of people [presumably including laymen] officially made the final decision. I visualize the doctor bringing the data to the group, explaining the points in relation to each case, and obtaining their approval of his order of priority."[12]

Essentially this procedure of a selection committee of laymen has for some years been in use in one of the most publicized chronic dialysis units, that of the Swedish Hospital of Seattle, Washington.[13] Many physicians are apparently reluctant to see the choice of allocation of medical therapy pass out of strictly medical hands. Thus in a recent symposium on the "Selection of Patients for Haemodialysis,"[14] Dr. Ralph Shakman writes: "Who is to implement the selection? In my opinion it must ultimately be the responsibility of the consultants in charge of the renal units . . . I can see no reason for delegating this responsibility to lay persons. Surely the latter would be better employed if they could be persuaded to devote their time and energy to raise more and more money for us to spend on our patients."[15] Other contributors to this symposium strike much the same note. Dr. F. M. Parsons writes: "In an attempt to overcome . . . difficulties in selection some have advocated introducing certain specified lay people into the discussions. Is it wise? I doubt whether a committee of this type can adjudicate as satisfactorily as two medical colleagues, particularly as successful therapy involves close cooperation between doctor and patient."[16] And Dr. M. A. Wilson writes in the same symposium: "The

suggestion has been made that lay panels should select individuals for dialysis from among a group who are medically suitable. Though this would relieve the doctor-in-charge of a heavy load of responsibility, it would place the burden on those who have no personal knowledge and have to base their judgments on medical or social reports. I do not believe this would result in better decisions for the group or improve the doctor-patient relationship in individual cases."[17]

But no amount of flag waving about the doctor's facing up to his responsibility—or prostrations before the idol of the doctor-patient relationship and reluctance to admit laymen into the sacred precincts of the conference chambers of medical consultations—can obscure the essential fact that ELT selection is not a wholly medical problem. When there are more than enough places in an ELT program to accommodate all who need it, then it will clearly be a medical question to decide who does have the need and which among these would successfully respond. But when an admitted gross insufficiency of places exists, when there are ten or fifty or one hundred highly eligible candidates for each place in the program, then it is unrealistic to take the view that purely medical criteria can furnish a sufficient basis for selection. The question of ELT selection becomes serious as a phenomenon of scale—because, as more candidates present themselves, strictly medical factors are increasingly less adequate as a selection criterion precisely because by numerical category-crowding there will be more and more cases whose "status is much the same" so far as purely medical considerations go.

The ELT selection problem clearly poses issues that transcend the medical sphere because—in the nature of the case—many residual issues remain to be dealt with once all of the medical questions have been faced. Because of this there is good reason why laymen as well as physicians should be involved in the selection process. Once the medical considerations have been brought to bear, fundamental social issues remain to be resolved. The instrumentalities of ELT have been created through the social investment of scarce resources, and the interests of the society deserve to play a role in their utilization. As representatives of their social interests, lay opinions should function to complement and supplement medical views once the proper arena of medical considerations is left behind.[18] Those physicians who have urged the presence of lay members on selection panels can, from this point of view, be recognized as having seen the issue in proper perspective.

One physician has argued against lay representation on selection panels for haemodialysis as follows: "If the doctor advises dialysis and the lay panel refuses, the patient will regard this as a death sentence passed by an anonymous court from which he has no right of appeal."[19] But this drawback is not specific to the use of a lay panel. Rather, it is a feature inherent in every *selection procedure*, regardless of whether the selection is done by the head doctor of the unit, by a panel of physicians, etc. No matter who does the selecting among patients recommended for dialysis, the feelings of the patient who has been rejected (and knows it) can be expected to be much the same, provided that he recognizes the actual nature of the choice (and is not deceived by the possibly convenient but ultimately poisonous fiction that because the selection was made by physicians it was made entirely on medical grounds).

In summary, then, the question of ELT selection would appear to be one that is in its very nature heavily laden with issues of medical research, practice, and administration. But it will not be a question that can be resolved on solely medical grounds. Strictly social issues of justice and utility will invariably arise in this area—questions going outside the medical area in whose resolution medical laymen can and should play a substantial role.

VII. The Inherent Imperfection (Non-Optimality) of Any Selection System

Our discussion to this point of the design of a selection system for ELT has left a gap that is a very fundamental and serious omission. We have argued that five factors must be taken into substantial and explicit account:

A. *Relative likelihood of success*   Is the chance of the treatment's being "successful" to be rated as high, good, average, etc.?[20]

B. *Expectancy of future life*   Assuming the "suc-cess" of the treatment, how much longer does the patient stand a good chance (75 per cent or better) of living—considering his age and general condition?

C. *Family role*   To what extent does the patient have responsibilities to others in his immediate family?

D. *Social contributions rendered*   Are the patient's past services to his society outstanding, substantial, average, etc.?

E. *Social contributions to be rendered*   Considering his age, talents, training, and past record of performance, is there a substantial probability that the patient will—*adequate recovery being assured*—render in the future services to his society that can be characterized as outstanding, substantial, average, etc.?

This list is clearly insufficient for the construction of a reasonable selection system, since that would require not only *that these factors be taken into account* (somehow or other), but—going beyond this—would specify *a specific set of procedures for taking account of them*. The specific procedures that would constitute such a system would have to take account of the interrelationship of these factors (e.g., *B* and *E*), and to set out exact guidelines as to the relevant weight that is to be given to each of them. This is something our discussion has not as yet considered.

In fact, I should want to maintain that there is no such thing here as a single rationally superior selection system. The position of affairs seems to me to be something like this: (1) It is necessary (for reasons already canvassed) to *have* a system, and to have a system that is rationally defensible, and (2) to be rationally defensible, this system must take the factors *A–E* into substantial and explicit account. But (3) the exact manner in which a rationally defensible system takes account of these factors cannot be fixed in any one specific way on the basis of general considerations. Any of the variety of ways that give *A–E* "their due" will be acceptable and viable. One cannot hope to find within this range of workable systems some one that is *optimal* in relation to the alternatives. There is no one system that does "the (uniquely) best"—only a variety of systems that do "as well as one can expect to do" in cases of this sort.

The situation is structurally very much akin to that of rules of partition of an estate among the relations of a decedent. It is important *that there be* such rules. And it is reasonable that spouse, children, parents, siblings, etc., be taken account of in these rules. But the question of the exact method of division—say that when the decedent has neither living spouse nor living children then his estate is to be divided, dividing 60 per cent between parents, 40 per cent between siblings versus dividing 90 per cent between parents, 10 per cent between siblings—cannot be settled on the basis of any general abstract considerations of reasonableness. Within broad limits, a *variety* of resolutions are all perfectly acceptable—so that no one procedure can justifiably be regarded as "the (uniquely) best" because it is superior to all others.[21]

VIII. A Possible Basis for a Reasonable Selection System

Having said that there is no such thing as *the optimal* selection system for ELT, I want now to sketch out the broad features of what I would regard as *one acceptable* system.

The basis for the system would be a point rating. The scoring here at issue would give roughly equal weight to the medical considerations (*A* and *B*) in comparison with the extramedical considerations (*C* = family role, *D* = services rendered, and *E* = services to be rendered), also giving roughly equal weight to the three items involved here (*C*, *D*, and *E*). The result of such a scoring procedure would provide the essential *starting point* of our ELT selection mechanism. I deliberately say "starting point" because it seems to me that one should not follow the results of this scoring in an *automatic* way. I would propose that the actual selection should only be guided but not actually be dictated by this scoring procedure, along lines now to be explained.

IX. The Desirability of Introducing an Element of Chance

The detailed procedure I would propose—not of course as optimal (for reasons we have seen), but as eminently acceptable—would combine the scoring procedure just discussed with an element of chance. The resulting selection system would function as follows:

1. First the criteria of inclusion of Section IV above would be applied to constitute a *first phase selection group*—which (we shall suppose) is substantially larger than the number *n* of persons who can actually be accommodated with ELT.

2. Next the criteria of selection of Section V are brought to bear via a scoring procedure of the type described in Section VIII. On this basis a *second phase selection group* is constituted which is only *somewhat* larger—say by a third or a half—than the critical number *n* at issue.

3. If this second phase selection group is relatively homogeneous as regards rating by the scoring procedure—that is, if there are no really major disparities within this group (as would be likely if the initial group was significantly larger than *n*)—then the final selection is made by *random* selection of *n* persons from within this group.

This introduction of the element of chance—in what could be dramatized as a "lottery of life and death"—must be justified. The fact is that such a procedure would bring with it three substantial advantages.

First, as we have argued above (in Section VII), any acceptable selection system is inherently non-optimal. The introduction of the element of chance prevents the results that life-and-death choices are made by the automatic application of an admittedly imperfect selection method.

Second, a recourse to chance would doubtless make matters easier for the rejected patient and those who have a specific interest in him. It would surely be quite hard for them to accept his exclusion by relatively mechanical application of objective criteria in whose implementation subjective judgment is involved. But the circumstances of life have conditioned us to accept the workings of chance and to tolerate the element of luck (good or bad): human life is an inherently contingent process. Nobody, after all, has an absolute right to ELT—but most of us would feel that we have "every bit as much right" to it as anyone else in significantly similar circumstances. The introduction of the element of chance assures a like handling of like cases over the widest possible area that seems reasonable in the circumstances.

Third (and perhaps least), such a recourse to random selection does much to relieve the administrators of the selection system of the awesome burden of ultimate and absolute responsibility.

These three considerations would seem to build up a substantial case for introducing the element of chance into the mechanism of the system for ELT selection in a way limited and circumscribed by other weightier considerations, along some such lines as those set forth above.[22]

It should be recognized that this injection of *man-made* chance supplements the element of *natural* chance that is present inevitably and in any case (apart from the role of chance in singling out certain persons as victims for the affliction at issue). As F. M. Parsons has observed: "any vacancies [in an ELT program—specifically haemodialysis] will be filled immediately by the first suitable patients, even though their claims for therapy may subsequently prove less than those of other patients refused later."[23] Life is a chancy business and even the most rational of human arrangements can cover this over to a very limited extent at best.

Notes

1. Christine Doyle, "Spare-Part Heart Surgeons Worried by Their Success," *Observer*, May 12, 1968.

2. J. D. N. Nabarro, "Selection of Patients for Haemodialysis," *British Medical Journal* (March 11, 1967), p. 623. Although several thousand patients die in the U.K. each year from renal failure—there are about thirty new cases per million of population—only 10 per cent of these can for the foreseeable future be accommodated with chronic haemodialysis. Kidney transplantation—itself a very tricky procedure—cannot make a more than minor contribution here. As this article goes to press, I learn that patients can be maintained in home dialysis at an operating cost about half that of maintaining them in a hospital dialysis unit (roughly an $8,000 minimum). In the United States, around 7,000 patients with terminal uremia who could benefit from haemodialysis evolve yearly. As of mid-1968, some 1,000 of these can be accommodated in existing hospital units. By June 1967, a world-wide total of some 120 patients were in treatment by home dialysis. (Data from a forthcoming paper, "Home Dialysis," by C. M.

Conty and H. V. Murdaugh. See also R. A. Baillod *et al.*, "Overnight Haemodialysis in the Home," *Proceedings of the European Dialysis and Transplant Association*, VI [1965], 99 ff.)

3. For the Hippocratic Oath see *Hippocrates: Works* (Loeb ed.; London, 1959), I, p. 298.

4. Another example of borderline legitimacy is posed by an endowment "with strings attached," e.g., "In accepting this legacy the hospital agrees to admit and provide all needed treatment for any direct descendant of myself, its founder."

5. Shana Alexander, "They Decide Who Lives, Who Dies," *Life*, LIII (November 9, 1962), 102–25 (see p. 107).

6. Lawrence Lader, "Who Has the Right To Live?" *Good Housekeeping* (January 1968), p. 144.

7. This approach could thus be continued to embrace the previous factor, that of family role, the preceding item (C).

8. Moreover a doctrinaire utilitarian would presumably be willing to withdraw a continuing mode of ELT such as haemodialysis from a patient to make room for a more promising candidate who came to view at a later stage and who could not otherwise be accommodated. I should be unwilling to adopt this course, partly on grounds of utility (with a view to the demoralization of insecurity), partly on the non-utilitarian ground that a "moral commitment" has been made and must be honored.

9. Of course the difficult question remains of the relative weight that should be given to prospective and retrospective service in cases where these factors conflict. There is good reason to treat them on a par.

10. This in the symposium on "Selection of Patients for Haemodialysis," *British Medical Journal* (March 11, 1967), pp. 622–24. F. M. Parsons writes: "But other forms of selecting patients [distinct from first come, first served] are suspect in my view if they imply evaluation of man by man. What criteria could be used? Who could justify a claim that the life of a mayor would be more valuable than that of the humblest citizen of his borough? Whatever we may think as individuals none of us is indispensable." But having just set out this hard-line view he immediately backs away from it: "On the other hand, to assume that there was little to choose between Alexander Fleming and Adolf Hitler . . . would be nonsense, and we should be naive if we were to pretend that we could not be influenced by their achievements and characters if we had to choose between the two of them. Whether we like it or not we cannot escape the fact that this kind of selection for long-term haemodialysis will be

required until very large sums of money become available for equipment and services [so that *everyone* who needs treatment can be accommodated]."

11. The relative fundamentality of these principles is, however, a substantially disputed issue.

12. J. D. N. Nabarro, *op. cit.*, p. 622.

13. See Shana Alexander, *op. cit.*

14. *British Medical Journal* (March 11, 1967), pp. 622–24.

15. *Ibid.*, p. 624. Another contributor writes in the same symposium, "The selection of the few [to receive haemodialysis] is proving very difficult—a true 'Doctor's Dilemma'—for almost everybody would agree that this must be a medical decision, preferably reached by consultation among colleagues" (Dr. F. M. Parsons, *ibid.*, p. 623).

16. "The Selection of Patients for Haemodialysis," *op. cit.* (n. 10 above), p. 623.

17. Dr. Wilson's article concludes with the perplexing suggestion—wildly beside the point given the structure of the situation at issue—that "the final decision will be made by the patient." But this contention is only marginally more ludicrous than Parsons's contention that in selecting patients for haemodialysis "gainful employment in a well chosen occupation is necessary to achieve the best results" since "only the minority wish to live on charity" (*ibid.*).

18. To say this is of course not to deny that such questions of applied medical ethics will invariably involve a host of medical considerations—it is only to insist that extra-medical considerations will also invariably be at issue.

19. M. A. Wilson, "Selection of Patients for Haemodialysis," *op. cit.*, p. 624.

20. In the case of an ongoing treatment involving complex procedure and dietary and other mode-of-life restrictions—and chronic haemodialysis definitely falls into this category—the patient's psychological makeup, his willpower to "stick with it" in the face of substantial discouragements—will obviously also be a substantial factor here. The man who gives up, takes not his life alone, but (figuratively speaking) also that of the person he replaced in the treatment schedule.

21. To say that acceptable solutions can range over broad limits is *not* to say that there are no limits at all. It is an obviously intriguing and fundamental problem to raise the question of the factors that set these limits. This complex issue cannot be dealt with adequately here. Suffice it to say that

considerations regarding precedent and people's expectations, factor of social utility, and matters of fairness and sense of justice all come into play.

22. One writer has mooted the suggestion that: "Perhaps the right thing to do, difficult as it may be to accept, is to select [for haemodialysis] from among the medical and psychologically qualified patients on a strictly random basis" (S. Gorovitz, "Ethics and the Allocation of Medical Resources," *Medical Research Engineering*, V [1966], p. 7). Outright random selection would, however, seem indefensible because of its refusal to give weight to considerations which, under the circumstances, *deserve* to be given weight. The proposed procedure of superimposing a certain degree of randomness upon the rational-choice criteria would seem to combine the advantages of the two without importing the worst defects of either.

23. "Selection of Patients for Haemodialysis," *op. cit.*, p. 623. The question of whether a patient for chronic treatment should ever be terminated from the program (say if he contracts cancer) poses a variety of difficult ethical problems with which we need not at present concern ourselves. But it does seem plausible to take the (somewhat anti-utilitarian) view that a patient should not be terminated simply because a "better qualified" patient comes along later on. It would seem that a quasi-contractual relationship has been created through established expectations and reciprocal understandings, and that the situation is in this regard akin to that of the man who, having undertaken to sell his house to one buyer, cannot afterward unilaterally undo this arrangement to sell it to a higher bidder who "needs it worse" (thus maximizing the over-all utility).

24. I acknowledge with thanks the help of Miss Hazel Johnson, Reference Librarian at the University of Pittsburgh Library, in connection with the bibliography.

Bibliography[24]

S. Alexander. "They Decide Who Lives, Who Dies," *Life*, LIII (November 9, 1962), 102–25.

C. Doyle. "Spare-Part Heart Surgeons Worried by Their Success," *Observer* (London), May 12, 1968.

J. Fletcher. *Morals and Medicine.* London, 1955.

S. Gorovitz. "Ethics and the Allocation of Medical Resources," *Medical Research Engineering*, V (1966), 5–7.

L. Lader. "Who Has the Right To Live?" *Good Housekeeping* (January, 1968), pp. 85 and 144–50.

J. D. N. Nabarro, F. M. Parsons, R. Shakman, and M. A. Wilson. "Selection of Patients for Haemodialysis," *British Medical Journal* (March 11, 1967), pp. 622–24.

H. M. Schmeck, Jr. "Panel Holds Life-or-Death Vote in Allotting of Artificial Kidney," *New York Times*, May 6, 1962, pp. 1, 83.

G. E. W. Wolstenholme and M. O'Connor (eds.). *Ethics in Medical Progress.* London, 1966.

Who Shall Live When Not All Can Live?

James F. Childress

Who shall live when not all can live? Although this question has been urgently forced upon us by the dramatic use of artificial internal organs and organ transplantations, it is hardly new. George Bernard Shaw dealt with it in "The Doctor's Dilemma":

> *Sir Patrick.* Well, Mr. Savior of Lives: which is it to be? that honest decent man Blenkinsop, or that rotten blackguard of an artist, eh?
> *Ridgeon.* It's not an easy case to judge, is it? Blenkinsop's an honest decent man; but is he any use? Dubedat's a rotten blackguard; but he's a genuine source of pretty and pleasant and good things.
> *Sir Patrick.* What will he be a source of for that poor innocent wife of his, when she finds him out?
> *Ridgeon.* That's true. Her life will be a hell.
> *Sir Patrick.* And tell me this. Suppose you had this choice put before you: either to go through life and find all the pictures bad but all the men and women good, or go through life and find all the pictures good and all the men and women rotten. Which would you choose?[1]

A significant example of the distribution of scarce medical resources is seen in the use of penicillin shortly after its discovery. Military officers had to determine which soldiers would be treated—those with venereal disease or those wounded in combat.[2] In many respects such decisions have become routine in medical circles. Day after day physicians and others make judgments and decisions "about allocations of medical care to various segments of our population, to various types of hospitalized patients, and to specific individuals,"[3] for example, whether mental illness or cancer will receive the higher proportion of available funds. Nevertheless, the dramatic forms of "Scarce Life-Saving Medical Resources" (hereafter

abbreviated as SLMR) such as hemodialysis and kidney and heart transplants have compelled us to examine the moral questions that have been concealed in many routine decisions. I do not attempt in this paper to show how a resolution of SLMR cases can help us in the more routine ones which do not involve a conflict of life with life. Rather I develop an argument for a particular method of determining who shall live when not all can live. No conclusions are implied about criteria and procedures for determining who shall receive medical resources that are not directly related to the preservation of life (e.g. corneal transplants) or about standards for allocating money and time for studying and treating certain diseases.

Just as current SLMR decisions are not totally discontinuous with other medical decisions, so we must ask whether some other cases might, at least by analogy, help us develop the needed criteria and procedures. Some have looked at the principles at work in our responses to abortion, euthanasia, and artificial insemination.[4] Usually they have concluded that these cases do not cast light on the selection of patients for artificial and transplanted organs. The reason is evident: in abortion, euthanasia, and artificial insemination, there is no conflict of life with life for limited but indispensable resources (with the possible exception of therapeutic abortion). In current SLMR decisions, such a conflict is inescapable, and it makes them so morally perplexing and fascinating. If analogous cases are to be found, I think that we shall locate them in moral conflict situations.

Analogous Conflict Situations

An especially interesting and pertinent one is *U.S. v. Holmes.*[5] In 1841 an American ship, the

Reprinted with the permission of the publisher from Soundings, An Interdisciplinary Journal 53, *no. 4 (Winter 1970). Editor's Note: The footnotes in this reading have been renumbered.*

William Brown, which was near Newfoundland on a trip from Liverpool to Philadelphia, struck an iceberg. The crew and half the passengers were able to escape in the two available vessels. One of these, a longboat, carrying too many passengers and leaking seriously, began to founder in the turbulent sea after about twenty-four hours. In a desperate attempt to keep it from sinking, the crew threw overboard fourteen men. Two sisters of one of the men either jumped overboard to join their brother in death or instructed the crew to throw them over. The criteria for determining who should live were "not to part man and wife, and not to throw over any women." Several hours later the others were rescued. Returning to Philadelphia, most of the crew disappeared, but one, Holmes, who had acted upon orders from the mate, was indicted, tried, and convicted on the charge of "unlawful homicide."

We are interested in this case from a moral rather than a legal standpoint, and there are several possible responses to and judgments about it. Without attempting to be exhaustive I shall sketch a few of these. The judge contended that lots should have been cast, for in such conflict situations, there is no other procedure "so consonant both to humanity and to justice." Counsel for Holmes, on the other hand, maintained that the "sailors adopted the only principle of selection which was possible in an emergency like theirs, —a principle more humane than lots."

Another version of selection might extend and systematize the maxims of the sailors in the direction of "utility"; those are saved who will contribute to the greatest good for the greatest number. Yet another possible option is defended by Edmond Cahn in *The Moral Decision.* He argues that in this case we encounter the "morals of the last day." By this phrase he indicates that an apocalyptic crisis renders totally irrelevant the normal differences between individuals. He continues:

> In a strait of this extremity, all men are reduced—or raised, as one may choose to denominate it—to members of the genus, mere congeners and nothing else. Truly and literally, all were "in the same boat," and thus none could be saved separately from the others. I am driven to conclude that otherwise—that is, if none sacrifice themselves of free will to spare the others—they must all wait and die together. For where all have become congeners, pure and simple, no one can save himself by killing another.[6]

Cahn's answer to the question "who shall live when not all can live" is "none" unless the voluntary sacrifice by some persons permits it.

Few would deny the importance of Cahn's approach although many, including this writer, would suggest that it is relevant mainly as an affirmation of an elevated and, indeed, heroic or saintly morality which one hopes would find expression in the voluntary actions of many persons trapped in "borderline" situations involving a conflict of life with life. It is a maximal demand which some moral principles impose on the individual in the recognition that self-preservation is not a good which is to be defended at all costs. The absence of this saintly or heroic morality should not mean, however, that everyone perishes. Without making survival an absolute value and without justifying all means to achieve it, we can maintain that simply letting everyone die is irresponsible. This charge can be supported from several different standpoints, including society at large as well as the individuals involved. Among a group of self-interested individuals, none of whom volunteers to relinquish his life, there may be better and worse ways of determining who shall survive. One task of social ethics, whether religious or philosophical, is to propose relatively just institutional arrangements within which self-interested and biased men can live. The question then becomes: which set of arrangements—which criteria and procedures of selection—is most satisfactory in view of the human condition (man's limited altruism and inclination to seek his own good) and the conflicting values that are to be realized?

There are several significant differences between the *Holmes* and SLMR cases, a major one being that the former involves *direct* killing of another person, while the latter involves only *permitting* a person to die when it is not possible to save all. Furthermore, in extreme situations such as Holmes, the restraints of civilization have been stripped away and something approximating a state of nature prevails, in which life is "solitary, poor, nasty, brutish and short." The state of nature does not mean that moral standards are irrelevant and that might should prevail, but it does suggest that much of the matrix which normally supports morality has been removed. Also, the necessary but unfortunate decisions about who shall live and die are made by men who are existentially and personally involved in the outcome. Their survival too is at stake. Even though the institutional role of sailors seems to require greater sacrificial actions, there is obviously no assurance that they will adequately assess the number of sailors required to man the vessel or that they will impartially and objectively weigh the common good at stake. As the judge insisted in his defense of casting lots in the *Holmes* case: "In no other than this [casting lots] or some like way are those having equal rights put upon an equal footing, and in no other way is it possible to guard against partiality and oppression, violence, and conflict." This difference should not be exaggerated since self-interest, professional pride, and the like obviously affect the outcome of many medical decisions. Nor do the remaining differences cancel *Holmes'* instructiveness.

Criteria of Selection for SLMR

Which set of arrangements should be adopted for SLMR? Two questions are involved: Which standards and criteria should be used? and, Who should make the decision? The first question is basic, since the debate about implementation, e.g. whether by a lay committee or physician, makes little progress until the criteria are determined.

We need two sets of criteria which will be applied at two different stages in the selection of recipients of SLMR. First, medical criteria should be used to exclude those who are not "medically acceptable." Second, from this group of "medically acceptable" applicants, the final selection can be made. Occasionally in current American medical practice, the first stage is omitted, but such an omission is unwarranted. Ethical and social responsibility would seem to require distributing these SLMR only to those who have some reasonable prospect of responding to the treatment. Furthermore, in transplants such medical tests as tissue and blood typing are necessary, although they are hardly fully developed.

"Medical acceptability" is not as easily determined as many non-physicians assume since there is considerable debate in medical circles about the relevant factors (e.g., age and complicating diseases). Although ethicists can contribute little or nothing to this debate, two proposals may be in order. First, "medical acceptability" should be used only to determine the group from which the final selection will be made, and the attempt to establish fine degrees of prospective response to treatment should be avoided. Medical criteria, then, would exclude some applicants but would not serve as a basis of comparison between those who pass the first stage. For example, if two applicants for dialysis were medically acceptable, the physicians would *not* choose the one with the *better* medical prospects. Final selection would be made on other grounds. Second, psychological and environmental factors should be kept to an absolute minimum and should be considered only when they are without doubt critically related to medical acceptability (e.g., the inability to cope with the requirements of dialysis which might lead to suicide).

The most significant moral questions emerge when we turn to the final selection. Once the pool of medically acceptable applicants has been defined and still the number is larger than the resources, what other criteria should be used? How should the final selection be made? First, I shall examine some of the difficulties that stem from efforts to make the final selection in terms of social value; these difficulties raise serious doubts about the feasibility and justifiability of the utilitarian approach. Then I shall consider the possible justification for random selection or chance.

Occasionally criteria of social worth focus on past contributions but most often they are primarily future-oriented. The patient's potential and probable contribution to the society is stressed, although this obviously cannot be abstracted from his present web of relationships (e.g., dependents) and occupational activities (e.g., nuclear physicist). Indeed, the magnitude of his contribution to society (as an abstraction) is measured in terms of these social roles, relations, and functions. Enough has already been said to suggest the tremendous range of factors that affect social value or worth.[7] Here we encounter the first major difficulty of this approach: How do we determine the relevant criteria of social value?

How does one quantify and compare the needs of the spirit (e.g., education, art, religion), political life, economic activity, technological development? Joseph Fletcher suggests that "some day we may learn how to 'quantify' or 'mathematicate' to 'computerize' the value problem in selection, in the same careful and thorough way that diagnosis has been."[8] I am not convinced that we can ever quantify values, or that we should attempt to do so. But even if the various social and human needs, in principle, could be quantified, how do we determine how much weight we will give to each one? Which will have priority in case of conflict? Or even more basically, in the light of which values and principles do we recognize social "needs"?

One possible way of determining the values which should be emphasized in selection has been proposed by Leo Shatin.[9] He insists that our medical decisions about allocating resources are already based on an unconscious scale of values (usually dominated by material worth). Since there is really no way of escaping this, we should be self-conscious and critical about it. How should we proceed? He recommends that we discover the values that most people in our society hold and then use them as criteria for distributing SLMR. These values can be discovered by attitude or opinion surveys. Presumably if fifty-one percent in this testing period put a greater premium on military needs than technological development, military men would have a greater claim on our SLMR than experimental researchers. But valuations of what is significant change, and the student revolutionary who was denied SLMR in 1970 might be celebrated in 1990 as the greatest American hero since George Washington.

Shatin presumably is seeking criteria that could be applied nationally, but at the present, regional and local as well as individual prejudices tincture the criteria of social value that are used in selection. Nowhere is this more evident than in the deliberations and decisions of the anonymous selection committee of the Seattle Artificial Kidney Center where such factors as church membership and Scout leadership have been deemed significant for determining who shall live.[10] As two critics conclude after examining these criteria and procedures, they rule out "creative nonconformists, who rub the bourgeoisie the wrong way but who historically have contributed so much to the making of America. The Pacific Northwest is no place for a Henry David Thoreau with bad kidneys."[11]

Closely connected to this first problem of determining social values is a second one. Not only is it difficult if not impossible to reach agreement on social values, but it is also rarely easy to predict what our needs will be in a few years and what the consequences of present actions will be. Furthermore it is difficult to predict which persons will fulfill their potential function in society. Admissions committees in colleges and universities experience the frustrations of predicting realization of potential. For these reasons, as someone has indicated, God might be a utilitarian, but we cannot be. We simply lack the capacity to predict very accurately the consequences which we then must evaluate. Our incapacity is never more evident than when we think in societal terms.

Other difficulties make us even less confident that such an approach to SLMR is advisable. Many critics raise the spectre of abuse, but this should not be overemphasized. The fundamental difficulty appears on another level: the utilitarian approach would in effect reduce the person to his social role, relations, and functions. Ultimately it dulls and perhaps even eliminates the sense of the person's transcendence, his dignity as a person which cannot be reduced to his past or future contribution to society. It is not at all clear that we are willing to live with these implications of utilitarian selection. Wilhelm Kolff, who invented the artificial kidney, has asked: "Do we really subscribe to the principle that social standing should determine selection? Do we allow patients to be treated with dialysis only when they are married, go to church, have children, have a job, a good income and give to the Community Chest?"[12]

The German theologian Helmut Thielicke contends that any search for "objective criteria" for selection is already a capitulation to the utilitarian point of view which violates man's dignity.[13] The solution is not to let all die, but to recognize that SLMR cases are "borderline situations" which inevitably involve guilt. The agent, however, can have courage and freedom (which, for Thielicke, come from justification by faith) and can

> go head anyway and seek for criteria for deciding the question of life or death in the matter of the artificial kidney. Since these criteria are . . . questionable, necessarily alien to the meaning of human existence, the decision to which they lead can be little more than that arrived at by casting lots.[14]

The resulting criteria, he suggests, will probably be very similar to those already employed in American medical practice.

He is most concerned to preserve a certain *attitude* or *disposition* in SLMR—the sense of guilt which arises when man's dignity is violated. With this sense of guilt, the agent remains "sound and healthy where it really counts."[15] Thielicke uses man's dignity only as a judgmental, critical, and negative standard. It only tells us how all selection criteria and procedures (and even the refusal to act) implicate us in the ambiguity of the human condition and its metaphysical guilt. This approach is consistent with his view of the task of theological ethics: "to teach us how to understand and endure—not "solve"—the borderline situation."[16] But ethics, I would contend, can help us discern the factors and norms in whose light relative, discriminate judgments can be made. Even if all actions in SLMR should involve guilt, some may preserve human dignity to a greater extent than others. Thielicke recognizes that a decision based on any criteria is "little more than that arrived at by casting lots." But perhaps selection by chance would come the closest to embodying the moral and nonmoral values that we are trying to maintain (including a sense of man's dignity).

The Values of Random Selection

My proposal is that we use some form of randomness or chance (either natural, such as "first come, first served," or artificial, such as a lottery) to determine who shall be saved. Many reject randomness as a surrender to non-rationality when responsible and rational judgments can and must be made. Edmond Cahn criticizes "Holmes' judge" who recommended the casting of lots because, as Cahn puts it, "the crisis involves stakes too high for gambling and responsibilities too deep for destiny."[17] Similarly, other critics see randomness as a surrender to "non-human" forces which necessarily vitiates human values (e.g., it is important to have persons rather than impersonal forces determining who shall live). Sometimes they are identified with the outcome of the process (e.g., the features such as creativity and fullness of being which make human life what it is are to be considered and respected in the decision). Regarding the former, it must be admitted that the use of chance seems cold and impersonal. But presumably the

defenders of utilitarian criteria in SLMR want to make their application as objective and impersonal as possible so that subjective bias does not determine who shall live.

Such criticism, however, ignores the moral and nonmoral values which might be supported by selection by randomness or chance. A more important criticism is that the procedure that I develop draws the relevant moral context too narrowly. That context, so the argument might run, includes the society and its future and not merely the individual with his illness and claim upon SLMR. But my contention is that the values and principles at work in the narrower context may well take precedence over those operative in the broader context both because of their weight and significance and because of the weaknesses of selection in terms of social worth. As Paul Freund rightly insists, "The more nearly total is the estimate to be made of an individual, and the more nearly the consequence determines life and death, the more unfit the judgment becomes for human reckoning. . . . Randomness as a moral principle deserves serious study."[18] Serious study would, I think point toward its implementation in certain conflict situations, primarily because it preserves a significant degree of *personal dignity by providing equality* of opportunity. Thus it cannot be dismissed as a "non-rational" and "non-human" procedure without an inquiry into the reasons, including human values, which might justify it. Paul Ramsey stresses this point about the *Holmes* case:

> Instead of fixing our attention upon "gambling" as the solution—with all the frivolous and often corrupt associations the word raises in our minds—we should think rather of equality of opportunity as the ethical substance of the relations of those individuals to one another that might have been guarded and expressed by casting lots.[19]

The individual's personal and transcendent dignity, which on the utilitarian approach would be submerged in his social role and function, can be protected and witnessed to by a recognition of his equal right to be saved. Such a right is best preserved by procedures which establish equality of opportunity. Thus selection by chance more closely approximates the requirements established by human dignity than does utilitarian calculation. It is not infallibly just, but it is preferable to the alternatives of letting all die or saving only those who have the greatest social responsibilities and potential contribution.

This argument can be extended by examining values other than individual dignity and equality of opportunity. Another basic value in the medical sphere is the relationship of trust between physician and patient. Which selection criteria are most in accord with this relationship of trust? Which will maintain, extend, and deepen it? My contention is that selection by randomness or chance is preferable from this standpoint too.

Trust, which is inextricably bound to respect for human dignity, is an attitude of expectation about another. It is not simply the expectation that another will act toward him in certain ways—which will respect him as a person. As Charles Fried writes:

> Although trust has to do with reliance on a disposition of another person, it is reliance on a disposition of a special sort: the disposition to act morally, to deal fairly with others, to live up to One's undertakings, and so on. Thus to trust another is first of all to expect him to accept the principle of morality in his dealings with you, to respect your status as a person, your personality.[20]

This trust cannot be preserved in life-and-death situations when a person expects decisions about him to be made in terms of his social worth, for such decisions violate his status as a person. An applicant rejected on grounds of inadequacy in social value or virtue would have reason for feeling that his "trust" had been betrayed. Indeed, the sense that one is being viewed not as an end in himself but as a means in medical progress or the achievement of a greater social good is incompatible with attitudes and relationships of trust. We recognize this in the billboard which was erected after the first heart transplants: "Drive Carefully. Christiaan Barnard Is Watching You." The relationship of trust between the physician and patient is not only an instrumental value in the sense of being an important factor in the patient's treatment. It is also to be endorsed because of its intrinsic worth as a relationship.

Thus the related values of individual dignity and trust are best maintained in selection by chance. But other factors also buttress the argument for this approach. Which criteria and procedures would men agree upon? We have to suppose a hypothetical situation in which several men are going to determine for themselves and their families the criteria and procedures by which they would want to be admitted to and excluded from SLMR if the need arose.[21] We need to assume two restrictions and then ask which set of criteria and procedures would be chosen as the most rational and, indeed, the fairest. The restrictions are these: (1) That men are *self-interested.* They are interested in their own welfare (and that of members of their families), and this, of course, includes survival. Basically, they are not motivated by altruism. (2) Furthermore, they are ignorant of their own talents, abilities, potential, and probable contribution to the social good. They do not know how they would fare in a competitive situation, e.g., the competition for SLMR in terms of social contribution. Under these conditions which institution would be chosen—letting all die, utilitarian selection, or the use of chance? Which would seem the most rational? the fairest? By which set of criteria would they want to be included in or excluded from the list of those who will be saved? The rational choice in this setting (assuming self-interest and ignorance of one's competitive success) would be random selection or chance since this alone provides equality of opportunity. A possible response is that one would prefer to take a "risk" and therefore choose the utilitarian approach. But I think not, especially since I added that the participants in this hypothetical situation are choosing for their children as well as for themselves; random selection or chance could be more easily justified to the children. It would make more sense for men who are self-interested but uncertain about their relative contribution to society to elect a set of criteria which would build in equality of opportunity. They would consider selection by chance as relatively just and fair.

An important psychological point supplements earlier arguments for using chance or random selection. The psychological stress and strain among those who are rejected would be greater if the rejection is based on insufficient social worth than if it is based on chance. Obviously stress and strain cannot be eliminated in these borderline situations, but they would almost certainly be increased by the opprobrium of being judged relatively "unfit" by society's agents using society's values. Nicholas Rescher makes this point very effectively:

> . . . a recourse to chance would doubtless make matters easier for the rejected patient and those who have a specific interest in him. It would surely be quite hard for them to accept his exclusion by relatively mechanical application of objective criteria in whose implementation subjective judgment is involved. But the circumstances of life have conditioned us to accept the workings of chance and to tolerate the element of luck (good or bad): human life is an inherently contingent process. Nobody, after all, has an absolute right to ELT [Exotic Lifesaving Therapy]—but most of us would feel that we have "every bit as much right" to it as anyone else in significantly similar circumstances.[22]

Although it is seldom recognized as such, selection by chance is already in operation in practically every dialysis unit. I am not aware of any unit which removed some of its patients from kidney machines in order to make room for later applicants who are better qualified in terms of social worth. Furthermore, very few people would recommend it. Indeed, few would even consider removing a person from a kidney machine on the grounds that a person better qualified *medically* had just applied. In a discussion of the treatment of chronic renal failure by dialysis at the University of Virginia Hospital Renal Unit from November 15, 1965 to November 15, 1966, Dr. Harry Abram writes: "Thirteen patients sought treatment but were not considered because the program had reached its limit of nine patients."[23] Thus, in practice and theory, natural chance is accepted at least within certain limits.

My proposal is that we extend this principle (first come, first served) to determine who among the medically acceptable patients shall live or that we utilize artificial chance such as a lottery or randomness. "First come, first served" would be more feasible than a lottery since the applicants make their claims over a period of time rather than as a group at one time. This procedure would be in accord with at least one principle in our present practices and with our sense of individual dignity, trust, and fairness. Its significance in relation to these values can be underlined by asking how the decision can be justified to the rejected applicant. Of course, one easy way of avoiding this task is to maintain the traditional cloak of secrecy, which works to a great extent because patients are often not aware that they are being considered for SLMR in addition to the usual treatment. But whether public justification is instituted or not is not the significant question; it is rather what reasons for rejection would be most acceptable to the unsuccessful applicant. My contention is that rejection can be accepted more readily if equality of opportunity, fairness, and trust are preserved, and that they are best preserved by selection by randomness or chance.

This proposal has yet another advantage since it would eliminate the need for a committee to examine applicants in terms of their social value. This onerous responsibility can be avoided.

Finally, there is a possible indirect consequence of widespread use of random selection which is interesting to ponder, although I do *not* adduce it as a good reason for adopting random selection. It can be argued, as Professor Mason Willrich of the University of Virginia Law School has suggested, that SLMR cases would practically disappear if these scarce resources were distributed randomly rather than on social worth grounds. Scarcity would no longer be a problem because the holders of economic and political power would make certain that they would not be excluded by a random selection procedure; hence they would help to redirect public priorities or establish private funding so that life-saving medical treatment would be widely and perhaps universally available.

In the framework that I have delineated, are the decrees of chance to be taken without exception? If we recognize exceptions, would we not open Pandora's box again just after we had succeeded in getting it closed? The direction of my argument has been against any exceptions, and I would defend this as the proper way to go. But let me indicate one possible way of admitting exceptions while at the same time circumscribing them so narrowly that they would be very rare indeed.

An obvious advantage of the utilitarian approach is that occasionally circumstances arise which make it necessary to say that one man is practically indispensable for a society in view of a particular set of problems it faces (e.g., the President when the nation is waging a war for survival). Certainly the argument to this point has stressed that the burden of proof would fall on those who think that the social danger in this instance is so great that they simply cannot abide by the outcome of a lottery or a first come, first served policy. Also, the reason must be negative rather than positive; that is, we depart from chance in this instance not because we want to take advantage of this person's potential contribution to the improvement of our society, but because his immediate loss would possibly (even probably) be disastrous (again, the President in a grave national emergency). Finally, social value (in the negative sense) should be used as a standard of exception in dialysis, for example, only if it would provide a reason strong enough to warrant removing another person from a kidney machine if all machines were taken. Assuming this strong reluctance to remove anyone once the commitment has been made to him, we would be willing to put this patient ahead of another applicant for a vacant machine only if we would be willing (in circumstances in which all machines are being used) to vacate a machine by removing someone from it. These restrictions would make an exception almost impossible.

While I do not recommend this procedure of recognizing exceptions, I think that one can defend it while accepting my general thesis about selection by randomness or chance. If it is used, a lay committee (perhaps advisory, perhaps even stronger) would be called upon to deal with the alleged exceptions since the doctors or others would in effect be appealing the outcome of chance (either natural or artificial). This lay committee would determine whether this patient was so indispensable at this time and place that he had to be saved even by sacrificing the values preserved by random selection. It would make it quite clear that exception is warranted, if at all, only as the "lesser of two evils." Such a defense would be recognized only rarely, if ever, primarily because chance and randomness preserve so many important moral and nonmoral values in SLMR cases.

Notes

1. George Bernard Shaw, *The Doctor's Dilemma* (New York, 1941), pp. 132–133.

2. Henry K. Beecher, "Scarce Resources and Medical Advancement," *Daedalus* (Spring 1969), pp. 279–280.

3. Leo Shatin, "Medical Care and the Social Worth of a Man," *American Journal of Orthopsychiatry*, 36 (1967), 97.

4. Harry S. Abram and Walter Wadlington, "Selection of Patients for Artificial and Transplant Organs," *Annals of Internal Medicine*, 69 (September 1968), 615–620.5.

5. *United States v. Holmes* Fed Cas. 360 (C.C.E.D. Pa 1842). All references are to the text of the trial as reprinted in Philip E. Davis, ed. *Moral Duty and Legal Responsibility: A Philosophical-Legal Casebook* (New York, 1966), pp. 102–118.

6. *The Moral Decision* (Bloomington, Ind., 1955) p. 71.

7. I am excluding from consideration the question of the ability to pay because most of the people involved have to secure funds from other sources, public or private, anyway.

8. Joseph Fletcher, "Donor Nephrectomies and Moral Responsibility," *Journal of the American Medical Women's Association*, 23 (Dec. 1968), p. 1090.

9. Leo Shatin, *op. cit.*, pp. 96–101.

10. For a discussion of the Seattle selection committee, see Shana Alexander, "They Decide Who Lives, Who Dies," *Life*, 53 (Nov. 9, 1962), 102. For an examination of general selection practices in dialysis see "Scarce Medical Resources," *Columbia Law Review* 69:620 (1969) and Harry S. Abram and Walter Wadlington, op. cit.

11. David Sanders and Jesse Dukeminier, Jr., "Medical Advance and Legal Lag: Hemodialysis and Kidney Transplantation," *UCLA Law Review* 15:367 (1968) 378.

12. "Letters and Comments," *Annals of Internal Medicine*, 61 (Aug. 1964), 360. Dr. G. E. Schreiner contends that "if you really believe in the right of society to make decisions on medical availability on these criteria you should be logical and say that when a man stops going to church or is divorced or loses his job, he ought to be removed from the programme and somebody else who fulfills these criteria substituted. Obviously no one faces up to this logical consequence." (G. E. W. Wolstenholme and Maeve O'Connor, ed. *Ethics in Medical Progress: With Special Reference to Transplantation*, A Ciba Foundation Symposium [Boston, 1966], p. 127.)

13. Helmut Thielicke, "The Doctor as Judge of Who Shall Live and Who Shall Die," *Who Shall Live?* ed. by Kenneth Vaux (Philadelphia, 1970), p. 172.

14. Ibid., pp. 173–174.

15. Ibid., p. 173.

16. Thielicke, *Theological Ethics, Vol. I, Foundations* (Philadelphia, 1966), p. 602.

17. Cahn, op. cit., p. 71.

18. Paul Freund, "Introduction," *Daedalus* (Spring 1969), xiii.

19. Paul Ramsey, *Nine Modern Moralists* (Englewood Cliffs, N.J., 1961), p. 245.

20. Charles Fried, "Privacy," In *Law, Reason, and Justice,* ed. by Graham Hughes (New York, 1969), p. 52.

21. My argument is greatly dependent on John Rawls's version of justice as fairness, which is a reinterpretation of social contract theory. Rawls, however, would probably not apply his ideas to "borderline situations." See "Distributive Justice: Some Addenda," Natural Law Forum, 13 (1968), 53. For Rawls's general theory, see "Justice as Fairness," Philosophy, Politics and Society (Second Series), ed. by Peter Laslett and W. G. Runciman (Oxford, 1962), pp. 132–157 and his other essays on aspects of this topic.

22. Nicholas Rescher, "The Allocation of Exotic Medical Lifesaving Therapy," *Ethics* 79 (1969): 173–180.

23. Harry S. Abram, M.D., "The Psychiatrist, the Treatment of Chronic Renal Failure, and the Prolongation of Life: II" *American Journal of Psychiatry* 126:157–167 (1969), 158.

The Prostitute, the Playboy, and the Poet: Rationing Schemes for Organ Transplantation

George J. Annas

In the public debate about the availability of heart and liver transplants, the issue of rationing on a massive scale has been credibly raised for the first time in United States medical care. In an era of scarce resources, the eventual arrival of such a discussion was, of course, inevitable.[1] Unless we decide to ban heart and liver transplantation, or make them available to everyone, some rationing scheme must be used to choose among potential transplant candidates. The debate has existed throughout the history of medical ethics. Traditionally it has been stated as a choice between saving one of two patients, both of whom require the immediate assistance of the only available physician to survive.

National attention was focused on decisions regarding the rationing of kidney dialysis machines when they were first used on a limited basis in the late 1960s. As one commentator described the debate within the medical profession:

"Shall machines or organs go to the sickest, or to the ones with most promise of recovery; on a first-come, first-served basis; to the most 'valuable' patient (based on wealth, education, position, what?); to the one with the most dependents; to women and children first; to those who can pay; to whom? Or should lots be cast, impersonally and uncritically?"[2]

In Seattle, Washington, an anonymous screening committee was set up to pick who among competing candidates would receive the life-saving technology. One lay member of the screening committee is quoted as saying:

"The choices were hard . . . I remember voting against a young woman who was a known prostitute. I found I couldn't vote for her, rather than another candidate, a young wife and mother. I also voted against a young man who, until he learned he had renal failure, had been a ne'er do-well, a real playboy. He promised he would reform his character, go back to school, and so on, if only he were selected for treatment. But I felt I'd lived long enough to know that a person like that won't really do what he was promising at the time."[3]

When the biases and selection criteria of the committee were made public, there was a general

Reprinted by permission of the author and The American Journal of Public Health, *Vol. 75, no. 2, 1985, pp. 187–189.*

negative reaction against this type of arbitrary device. Two experts reacted to the "numbing accounts of how close to the surface lie the prejudices and mindless cliches that pollute the committee's deliberations," by concluding that the committee was "measuring persons in accordance with its own middle-class values." The committee process, they noted, ruled out "creative nonconformists" and made the Pacific Northwest "no place for a Henry David Thoreau with bad kidneys."[4]

To avoid having to make such explicit, arbitrary, "social worth" determinations, the Congress, in 1972, enacted legislation that provided federal funds for virtually all kidney dialysis and kidney transplantation procedures in the United States.[5] This decision, however, simply served to postpone the time when identical decisions will have to be made about candidates for heart and liver transplantation in a society that does not provide sufficient financial and medical resources to provide all "suitable" candidates with the operation.

There are four major approaches to rationing scarce medical resources: the market approach; the selection committee approach; the lottery approach; and the "customary" approach.[1]

The Market Approach

The market approach would provide an organ to everyone who could pay for it with their own funds or private insurance. It puts a very high value on individual rights, and a very low value on equality and fairness. It has properly been criticized on a number of bases, including that the transplant technologies have been developed and are supported with public funds, that medical resources used for transplantation will not be available for higher priority care, and that financial success alone is an insufficient justification for demanding a medical procedure. Most telling is its complete lack of concern for fairness and equity.[6]

A "bake sale" or charity approach that requires the less financially fortunate to make public appeals for funding is demeaning to the individuals involved, and to society as a whole. Rationing by financial ability says we do not believe in equality, but believe that a price can and should be placed on human life and that it should be paid by the individual whose life is at stake. Neither belief is tolerable in a society in which income is inequitably distributed.

The Committee Selection Process

The Seattle Selection Committee is a model of the committee process. Ethics Committees set up in some hospitals to decide whether or not certain handicapped newborn infants should be given medical care may represent another.[7] These committees have developed because it was seen as unworkable or unwise to explicitly set forth the criteria on which selection decisions would be made. But only two results are possible, as Professor Guido Calabresi has pointed out: either a pattern of decision-making will develop or it will not. If a pattern does develop (e.g., in Seattle, the imposition of middle-class values), then it can be articulated and those decision "rules" codified and used directly, without resort to the committee. If a pattern does not develop, the committee is vulnerable to the charge that it is acting arbitrarily, or dishonestly, and therefore cannot be permitted to continue to make such important decisions.[1]

In the end, public designation of a committee to make selection decisions on vague criteria will fail because it too closely involves the state and all members of society in explicitly preferring specific individuals over others, and in devaluing the interests those others have in living. It thus directly undermines, as surely as the market system does, society's view of equality and the value of human life.

The Lottery Approach

The lottery approach is the ultimate equalizer which puts equality ahead of every other value. This makes it extremely attractive, since all comers have an equal chance at selection regardless of race, color, creed, or financial status. On the other hand, it offends our notions of efficiency and fairness since it makes *no* distinctions among such things as the strength of the desires of the candidates, their potential survival, and their quality of life. In this sense it is a mindless method of trying to solve society's dilemma which is caused by its unwillingness or inability to spend enough resources to make a lottery unnecessary. By making this macro spending decision evident to all, it also undermines society's view of the pricelessness of human life. A first-come, first-served system is a type of natural lottery since referral to a transplant program is generally random in time. Nonetheless, higher income groups have quicker access to referral networks and thus have an inherent advantage over the poor in a strict first-come, first-served system.[8,9]

The Customary Approach

Society has traditionally attempted to avoid explicitly recognizing that we are making a choice not to save individual lives because it is too expensive to do so. As long as such decisions are not explicitly acknowledged, they can be tolerated by society. For example, until recently there was said to be a general understanding among general practitioners in Britain that individuals over age 55 suffering from end-stage kidney disease not be referred for dialysis or transplant. In 1984, however, this unwritten practice became highly publicized, with figures that showed a rate of new cases of end-stage kidney disease treated in Britain at 40 per million (versus the US figure of 80 per million) resulting in 1500–3000 "unnecessary deaths" annually.[10] This has, predictably, led to movements to enlarge the National Health Service budget to expand dialysis services to meet this need, a more socially acceptable solution than permitting the now publicly recognized situation to continue.

In the US, the customary approach permits individual physicians to select their patients on the basis of medical criteria or clinical suitability. This, however, contains much hidden social worth criteria. For example, one criterion, common in the transplant literature, requires an individual to have sufficient family support for successful aftercare. This discriminates against individuals without families and those who have become alienated from their families. The criterion may be relevant, but it is hardly medical.

Similar observations can be made about medical criteria that include IQ, mental illness, criminal records, employment, indigency, alcoholism, drug addiction, or geographical location. Age is perhaps more difficult, since it may be impressionistically related to outcome. But it is not medically logical to assume that an individual who is 49 years old is necessarily a better medical candidate for a transplant than one who is 50 years old. Unless specific examination of the characteristics of older persons that make them less desirable candidates is undertaken, such a cut off is arbitrary, and thus devalues the lives of older citizens. The same can be said of blanket exclusions of alcoholics and drug addicts.

In short, the customary approach has one great advantage for society and one great disadvantage: it gives us the illusion that we do not have to make choices; but the cost is mass deception, and when this deception is uncovered, we must deal with it either by universal entitlement or by choosing another method of patient selection.

A Combination of Approaches

A socially acceptable approach must be fair, efficient, and reflective of important social values. The most important values at stake in organ transplantation are fairness itself, equity in the sense of equality, and the value of life. To promote efficiency, it is important that no one receive a transplant unless they want one and are likely to obtain significant benefit from it in the sense of years of life at a reasonable level of functioning.

Accordingly, it is appropriate for there to be an initial screening process that is based *exclusively* on medical criteria designed to measure the probability of a successful tranplant, i.e., one in which the patient survives for at least a number of years and is rehabilitated. There is room in medical criteria for social worth judgments, but there is probably no way to avoid this completely. For example, it has been noted that "in many respects social and medical criteria are inextricably intertwined" and that therefore medical criteria might "exclude the poor and disadvantaged because health and socioeconomic status are highly interdependent."[11] Roger Evans gives an example. In the End Stage Renal Disease Program, "those of lower socioeconomic status are likely to have multiple comorbid health conditions such as diabetes, hepatitis, and hypertension" making them both less desirable candidates and more expensive to treat.[11]

To prevent the gulf between the haves and have nots from widening, we must make every reasonable attempt to develop medical criteria that are objective and independent of social worth categories. One minimal way to approach this is to require that medical screening be reviewed and approved by an ethics committee with significant public representation, filed with a public agency, and made readily available to the public for comment. In the event that more than one hospital in a state or region is offering a particular transplant service, it would be most fair and efficient for the individual hospitals to perform the initial medical screening themselves (based on the uniform, objective criteria), but to have all subsequent non-medical selection done by a method approved by a single selection committee composed of representatives of all hospitals engaged in a particular transplant procedure, as well as significant representation of the public at large.

As this implies, after the medical screening is performed, there may be more acceptable candidates in the "pool" than there are organs or surgical teams to go around. Selection among waiting candidates will then be necessary. This situation occurs now in kidney transplantation, but since the organ matching is much more sophisticated than in hearts and livers (permitting much more precise matching of organ and recipient), and since dialysis permits individuals to wait almost indefinitely for an organ without risking death, the situations are not close enough to permit use of the same matching criteria. On the other hand, to the extent that organs are specifically tissue- and size-matched and fairly distributed to the best matched candidate, the organ distribution system itself will resemble a natural lottery.

When a pool of acceptable candidates is developed, a decision about who gets the next available, suitable organ must be made. We must choose between using a conscious, value-laden, social worth selection criterion (including a committee to make the actual choice), or some type of random device. In view of the unacceptability and arbitrariness of social worth criteria being applied, implicitly or explicitly, by committee, this method is neither viable nor proper. On the other hand, strict adherence to a lottery might create a situation where an individual who has only a one-in-four chance of living five years with a transplant (but who could survive another six months without one) would get an organ before an individual

who could survive as long or longer, but who will die within days or hours if he or she is not immediately transplanted. Accordingly, the most reasonable approach seems to be to allocate organs on a first-come, first-served basis to members of the pool but permit individuals to "jump" the queue if the second level selection committee believes they are in immediate danger of death (but still have a reasonable prospect for long-term survival with a transplant) and the person who would otherwise get the organ can survive long enough to be reasonably assured that he or she will be able to get another organ.

The first-come, first-served method of basic selection (after a medical screen) seems the preferred method because it most closely approximates the randomness of a straight lottery without the obviousness of making equity the only promoted value. Some unfairness is introduced by the fact that the more wealthy and medically astute will likely get into the pool first, and thus be ahead in line, but this advantage should decrease sharply as public awareness of the system grows. The possibility of unfairness is also inherent in permitting individuals to jump the queue, but some flexibility needs to be retained in the system to permit it to respond to reasonable contingencies.

We will have to face the fact that should the resources devoted to organ transplantation be limited (as they are now and are likely to be in the future), at some point it is likely that significant numbers of individuals will die in the pool waiting for a transplant. Three things can be done to avoid this: 1) medical criteria can be made stricter, perhaps by adding a more rigorous notion of "quality" of life to longevity and prospects for rehabilitation; 2) resources devoted to transplantation and organ procurement can be increased; or 3) individuals can be persuaded not to attempt to join the pool.

Of these three options, only the third has the promise of both conserving resources and promoting autonomy. While most persons medically eligible for a transplant would probably want one, some would not—at least if they understood all that was involved, including the need for a lifetime commitment to daily immunosuppression medications, and periodic medical monitoring for rejection symptoms. Accordingly, it makes public policy sense to publicize the risks and side effects of transplantation, and to require careful explanations of the procedure be given to prospective patients *before* they undergo medical screening. It is likely that by the time patients come to the transplant center they have made up their minds and would do almost anything to get the transplant. Nonetheless, if there are patients who, when confronted with all the facts, would voluntarily elect not to proceed, we enhance both their own freedom and the efficiency and cost-effectiveness of the transplantation system by screening them out as early as possible.

Conclusion

Choices among patients that seem to condemn some to death and give others an opportunity to survive will always be tragic. Society has developed a number of mechanisms to make such decisions more acceptable by camouflaging them. In an era of scarce resources and conscious cost containment, such mechanisms will become public, and they will be usable only if they are fair and efficient. If they are not so perceived, we will shift from one mechanism to another in an effort to continue the illusion that tragic choices really don't have to be made, and that we can simultaneously move toward equity of access, quality of services, and cost containment without any challenges to our values. Along with the prostitute, the playboy, and the poet, we all need to be involved in the development of an access model to extreme and expensive medical technologies with which we can live.

Notes

1. Calabresi G, Bobbitt P: *Tragic Choices.* New York: Norton, 1978.
2. Fletcher J: Our shameful waste of human tissue. *In:* Cutler DR (ed): The Religious Situation. Boston: Beacon Press, 1969; 223–252.
3. Quoted in Fox R, Swazey J: *The Courage to Fail.* Chicago: Univ of Chicago Press, 1974; 232.
4. Sanders & Dukeminier: Medical advance and legal lag: hemodialysis and kidney transplantation. UCLA L Rev 1968; 15:357.
5. Rettig RA: The policy debate on patient care financing for victims of end stage renal disease. Law & Contemporary Problems 1976; 40:196.
6. President's Commission for the Study of Ethical Problems in Medicine: *Securing Access to Health Care.* US Govt Printing Office, 1983; 25.
7. Annas GJ: Ethics committees on neonatal care: substantive protection or procedural diversion? Am J Public Health 1984; 74:843–845.
8. Bayer R: Justice and health care in an era of cost containment: allocating scarce medical resources. Soc Responsibility 1984; 9:37–52.
9. Annas GJ: Allocation of artificial hearts in the year 2002: *Minerva v National Health Agency.* Am J Law Med 1977; 3:59–76.
10. Commentary: UK's poor record in treatment of renal failure. Lancet July 7, 1984; 53.
11. Evans R: Health care technology and the inevitability of resource allocation and rationing decisions, Part II. JAMA 1983; 249:2208, 2217.

Decision Scenario 1 ··

"What do you mean you don't know who he is?" asked Dr. Bridewell, the head of the Oakbrook Hospital Renal Unit.

"He was unconscious when the police brought him to the ER. We started the IV, stopped his bleeding, and patched him up. But he still hasn't recovered consciousness. The police think it was a hit-and-run driver." Dr. Kathy McDowell spoke in a precise, matter-of-fact voice. Dr. Bridewell always frightened her, but she was determined not to show it.

"He didn't have any identification?"

"That's right. They think that either the driver robbed him or somebody else who came along did. Anyway, he was wearing jeans and a sweatshirt, nothing that gives any clue as to his background. There is one thing we do know definitely."

"What's that?" asked Dr. Bridewell.

"Both of his kidneys were hopelessly damaged, but his general physical condition is good. We think he's a good candidate for a transplant."

"Then you know we've got a guy whose brain waves we're waiting to flatten out?"

"Dr. Liebsbaum told me."

"He ought to keep his mouth shut," Dr. Bridewell said. "Oh, don't take that seriously. I'm just upset because this faces us with a big problem. We're only going to have one kidney to transplant. The other one's shot."

"That's all we want," said McDowell.

Bridewell ignored her. "You did a tissue check?" he asked.

"It's close enough."

"Too bad. What I mean is that I've got another candidate. Now we have to decide which of the two gets the kidney."

"Who's the other candidate?"

"A Mrs. Benson. She's a woman in her early sixties who's active in local affairs. She was on the school board. Her husband's a rich lawyer, and both of them move in high social circles. She does a lot of work now with a foundation that's supposed to help minority children in school. She also happens to be a pretty good candidate physically for a transplant."

"So you'll choose her over my patient?" McDowell felt herself getting angry.

"I didn't say that. How old is this guy?"

"I would estimate that he's in his early or middle thirties. He seems to be in good physical condition."

"But we don't know anything about him," said Dr. Bridewell. "He might just be a drifter passing through town. He's probably not a member of the community that this hospital is supposed to serve, the one that pays bills and makes donations."

"Not that we know of," Dr. McDowell admitted. "But he might be. He might be a person of great value. Maybe he's even a physician."

"But we don't know for sure, do we?" said Dr. Bridewell.

Suppose you are Dr. Bridewell and have to decide between the unknown man and Mrs. Benson. On what grounds might you make your decision?

In the absence of any information about "social worth" and "family role," is it possible to apply Rescher's criteria in this case?

Does Childress's position suggest that the best way to solve the problem is just by tossing a coin?

Suppose the unknown patient regains consciousness and reveals that he is a state senator, the father of a two-year-old child, and a writer of detective novels. Might this information alter the way in which the decision would be made according to Childress? Might it alter the outcome of a decision based on the use of Rescher's criteria?

Decision Scenario 2 ••

"It will be at least two weeks before that melts," Miller said. He stood at the top of the trail looking down into the snow-blocked canyon.

"There's no way to go around?" Jennifer Martin asked. Backpacking up the steep mountain trail had been a grand adventure until the spring snowslide had isolated their little group. Now things were awful. Carl had lost his footing and tumbled down a steep slope, breaking a rib and ripping open his left side. Then Alice had gotten sick and was running a high fever. Doug Miller thought it might be pneumonia. Both Carl and Alice lay in their sleeping bags on the floor of the drafty line shack at the top of the trail.

"That's the only way in or out," Miller said. "And the snow is too loose and filled with pockets to support anybody. At least we have enough food."

"But we really need to do something for Carl and Alice," said Jennifer. "I didn't want to say this where they could hear me, but without treatment both of them have a good chance of dying."

"I thought you brought enough supplies for treatment. We all thought it was wonderful to have our own doctor along."

"Both need antibiotic therapy," Jennifer said. "Infection is the great risk in each case. And I just don't have enough antibiotics to treat both of them. One maybe."

"We can't do that," Miller said. "Can't you just split what there is between them?"

"Yes, but that would probably do little good. With antibiotics you've got to kill all the bugs to keep the infection under control. Partial treatment is like trying to put out a house fire with a cup of water."

"So partial treatment of both might not help either?"

"It would help some but probably not enough," Jennifer said.

"Then it seems to me that we shouldn't treat either of them. That's the only fair thing to do."

"Then both will probably die."

"Are you willing to make the decision?" Miller asked. "Are you willing to say, 'I'm going to treat you, but I'm not going to treat the other person'?"

"I don't want to do that. And I don't want to give partial treatment either. I want to be able to save at least one of them."

"How are you going to choose?" asked Miller. "I think Carl is a nicer person than Alice, but Alice is a chemist, and society would probably regard her as more valuable. After all, Carl is just an unsuccessful poet and a bookstore clerk."

"Maybe we should explain the situation to them," Jennifer said. "Maybe one of them will volunteer to let the other use all of the antibiotics."

"I think that's cruel," Miller said. "I'll go back to my original suggestion that we don't give either of them any drugs."

What do you consider to be the right thing to do in this situation? Justify your decision.

What might a utilitarian argue?

Should Alice and Carl be consulted? If so, does the categorical imperative require that each agree to give up his or her claim to the antibiotics for the sake of the other?

Does the duty to preserve one's life (in Kant's theory or natural law) require that Carl and Alice demand the antibiotics for themselves?

What light (if any) does a case such as this throw on the question of establishing a policy for allocating scarce resources?

Decision Scenario 3 ··

Valdez Regional Hospital is the primary medical facility for the residents of Valdez County, Arizona. Its intensive care unit is the only one available in the entire county, and the closest comparable unit is eighty-five miles away in Somora County.

The Valdez ICU is a twelve-bed facility and, from the statistical point of view, it is generally adequate to serve the needs of its patient population. That is, the cost of adding extra equipment and staff to increase the size of the facility is much greater than its actual use would justify.

Valdez's ICU policy, which is similar to policies of hospitals everywhere, requires that the staff make the effort to keep at least one of the twelve beds free for use in a genuine emergency.

On a bright, clear afternoon one day after Christmas, sixty-eight-year-old Harry Aveni was brought to the emergency room of Valdez after he had collapsed on the patio of his house. Mr. Aveni had been brought to the emergency room twice before. Both were episodes of congestive heart failure, and this third occasion was no different. Mr. Aveni had broken his diet during the holidays and consumed an unaccustomed amount of salt.

Mr. Aveni responded well to emergency treatment. The fluid surrounding his heart was withdrawn, a glycoside medication was administered, and his condition seemed to stabilize. Then that evening, there was a sudden onset of fibrillation—his heart started beating erratically. Again, Mr. Aveni responded well to treatment, and after emergency defibrillation, his condition again stabilized.

"He needs to be put into the ICU," Dr. Ellen Gracian said. "We can't care for him sufficiently on the wards, because he's got to have constant monitoring."

"I don't think Dr. Franklin is going to want to admit him," the nurse said. "There's only one bed left."

Dr. Gracian immediately left the floor and went to the ICU director's office. She explained what she wanted and waited while he seemed to be thinking it over.

"I don't think I can admit him," Dr. Franklin said. "Here we have an elderly gentleman who has now gone through three episodes of congestive failure and also seems to have something wrong to cause the fibrillation. He didn't stick to his diet, and in general his days are likely to be in the rather small numbers."

"But if he doesn't have intensive care, the numbers may be even smaller," Dr. Gracian said.

"That's no doubt true. But as things are, we've got eleven people who need to stay right where they are for God knows how long, and we've got just one bed at our disposal."

"But that's all I need, just one bed."

"I understand that," said Dr. Franklin. "But let's suppose we install your patient in the ICU and fifteen minutes after we put him there an eighteen-year-old accident victim is brought in. She's going to have to have emergency treatment, then close and constant monitoring, or she's likely to die."

"But you don't know that somebody like that is going to come in," Dr. Gracian said. "And Mr. Aveni is here right now and is in need right now."

"I'm sorry," said Dr. Franklin. "But the chances are very good that somebody is going to need that bed, somebody we can do more for than we can do for your patient. Somebody who's got a better chance to live a longer and more normal life."

"I see," Dr. Gracian said. "But I thought we were in the business of saving lives."

"We are. But we can't save them all, and that's where the problems come in."

What argument can be made from the point of view of an act utilitarian to support Dr. Franklin's decision?

Would a selection procedure of the sort favored by Childress secure a bed in the ICU for Mr. Aveni?

Is the fact that Mr. Aveni broke his diet and so is, in some sense, responsible for being in immediate need relevant to deciding whether he should be admitted to the ICU?

Would any of the criteria presented by Rescher lead to the selection of Mr. Aveni over an eighteen-year-old accident victim?

Would Annas's recognition of immediate need as a justification for selection in transplants also justify granting intensive care to Mr. Aveni?

Decision Scenario 4 ••

The microsurgical team at Benton Public Hospital consisted of twenty-three people. Five were surgeons, three were anesthesiologists, three were internists, two were radiologists, and the remaining members were various sorts of nurses and technicians.

Early Tuesday afternoon on a date late in March, the members of the team that had to be sterile were scrubbing while the others were preparing to start operating on Mr. Hammond Cox. Mr. Cox was a fifty-nine-year-old unmarried black man who worked as a janitor in a large apartment building. While performing his duties, Mr. Cox had caught his hand in the mechanism of a commercial trash compactor. The bones of his wrist had been crushed and the blood vessels severed.

The head of the team, Dr. Herbert Lagorio, believed that it was possible to restore at least partial functioning to Mr. Cox's hand. Otherwise, the hand would have to be amputated.

Mr. Cox had been drunk when the accident happened. When the police ambulance brought him to the emergency room, he was still so drunk

that a decision was made to delay surgery for almost an hour to give him a chance to burn up some of the alcohol he had consumed. As it was, administering anesthesia to Mr. Cox would incur a greater than average risk. Furthermore, blood tests had shown that Mr. Cox already suffered from some degree of liver damage. In both short- and long-range terms, Mr. Cox was not a terribly good surgical risk.

Dr. Lagorio was already scrubbed when Dr. Carol Levine, a resident in emergency medicine, had him paged.

"This had better be important," he told her. "I've got a guy prepped and waiting."

"I know you do," Dr. Levine said. "But there's something you ought to know about before you start."

"Tell me quickly."

"They just brought in a thirty-five-year-old white female with a totally severed right hand. She's a biology professor at Columbia and was working late in her lab when some maniac looking for drugs came in and attacked her with a cleaver."

"What shape is the hand in?"

"Excellent. The campus cops were there within minutes, and there was ice in the lab. One of the cops had the good sense to put the hand in a plastic bag and bring it with her."

"Is she in good general health?"

"It seems excellent," Dr. Levine said.

"This is a real problem."

"You can't do two cases at once?"

"No way. We need everybody we've got to do one."

"How about sending her someplace else?"

"No place else is set up to do what has to be done," Dr. Lagorio said.

"So what are you going to do?"

"That's what I've got to decide," Dr. Lagorio said.

Does a "first-come, first-served" criterion like that defended by Childress require that Mr. Cox receive the surgery?

Does a "social-value" criterion require that the biology professor receive the surgery?

Can the chance of a successful outcome in each case be used as a criterion without violating the notion that all people are of equal inherent worth?

In your view, who should have the potential benefits of the surgery? Give reasons to support your view.

Decision Scenario 5 ....

"Your baby's pituitary gland is not fully developed," Dr. Robert Amatin said.

Clarissa Austin nodded to show that she understood that at least something was wrong with her child. She had already made up her mind to do whatever she had to do to see to it that her baby was all right.

"That means he's not getting enough of a hormone—a chemical—produced there," Dr. Amatin went on. "He won't undergo the normal course of development without that chemical."

"Can you give it to him?"

Dr. Amatin avoided answering the question directly. "A transplant is the best hope," he said. "If we can surgically remove the malformed pituitary and attach a new one, then the baby has a very good chance of being normal."

"I'll be happy to give my permission, if that's what you're waiting for," Clarissa said.

"It's not that simple," Dr. Amatin said. He looked uncomfortable. "It really comes down to a matter of money."

"I don't have much money," Clarissa said. "You know my bills are being paid by Medicaid."

"I know that, and the government won't pay for transplant organs."

"How much does it cost?"

"I've got a family right now that says it wants five thousand dollars for the pituitary of their baby. She just died this morning."

"I can't get money like that," Clarissa said.

"I can ask them to come up and talk to you.

Maybe they would take less, or maybe you could work out some kind of deferred payment with them."

"What if I can't?"

Dr. Amatin shook his head. "I can't arrange for a transplant without an organ, and I suspect they will just try to find somebody else to sell it to."

"That don't seem fair," Clarissa said. "Just because I haven't got the money, my little baby is going to have to be some kind of cripple and maybe die."

Does the possibility of such situations demonstrate that the present policy of relying on donated organs is a superior one?

If organs are sold on the open market, are such situations inevitable?

What other organ procurement policy, besides voluntary donation and organ sales, might be worth considering as a means to increase the number of transplant organs available?

Is Ms. Austin correct in saying that it would be unfair for her child not to have the organ because she cannot afford to pay the asking price? After all, surely it is not unfair for her child not to have, say, a silver drinking cup because she cannot afford to pay the asking price.

On what grounds does Annas object to the market approach?

CHAPTER 9

THE CLAIM TO HEALTH CARE

SOCIAL CONTEXT: THE CRISIS IN AMERICAN HEALTH CARE

A crisis exists in a social institution when there are factors present that tend to destroy the institution or render it ineffective in achieving its goals. Two major factors have led some observers to say that the American health-care system is in a state of crisis: the increasing cost to the society of health care, and the failure to deliver health care to those who need it at prices they can afford. Let us examine each of these factors briefly and then turn to some solutions that have been offered.

COST OF HEALTH CARE

After defense, health care is the most expensive item in the federal budget, and the average American must work over one month a year to pay for medical insurance, physician's fees, and the cost of hospitalization.

In recent years, policy analysts have issued strong warnings about the need to take measures to curb the rising cost of health care. In 1960 health expenditures in the United States amounted to some 27 billion dollars, while by 1983 (the last year for which complete figures are available), expenditures had climbed to 356 billion dollars. Per capita, this represents an increase from 145 dollars to 1,500 dollars. As a percent of the gross national product, the cost of health care has more than doubled, from 5.3 percent to 10.8 percent.

Future increases are expected to resemble past ones. Costs in 1990 are projected to be 690 billion dollars, and those in the year 2000 are estimated to be 1.9 trillion dollars. This amounts to a 50 billion dollar average increase per year and a doubling of costs every six years.

The spiraling costs of health care are seen by most analysts as threatening the economic welfare of the country. The $1,500 per person that the U.S. spends on health costs is not matched by other industrialized nations. Japan spends $500, Great Britain $400, France $800, and West Germany $900. Because the United States spends such a large percentage of its GNP on health care, the costs of U.S. goods will be comparatively higher than those of other exporting nations. Consequently, the United States will not be as effective a competitor in world trade and will be faced with an ever more serious balance of payments problem and with the loss of even more domestic industries.

Other serious problems are connected with increasing health-care costs. The Medicare system, which was established in 1965 to provide medical care for the elderly and the handicapped, cost almost 59 billion dollars in 1983. Some studies have predicted that unless some effective way is found to limit health costs, the system will be bankrupt in a very few years. Yet the most recent attempt to limit costs by employing a prospective payment plan (see the discussion of DRGs below) has consequences that threaten to alter both the availability and quality of care. Furthermore, increasing health-care costs in all areas, not just Medicare, may initiate a round of inflation and recession and severely weaken the entire economy.

Various explanations have been given for the spiraling costs of health care. Stanley Hwang suggests that one factor is the lack of financial accountability from those responsible for operating the health-care system. Most Americans are covered by employee group insurance that pays physicians and hospitals on a fee-for-service basis. The system serves to hide the cost of medical care from the consumer. Because the consumer gets a relatively unlimited amount of medical services for a fixed premium, and because the premium itself is hidden in the form of direct and indirect payroll deductions, the consumer has no incentive to avoid unnecessary or quite expensive medical services. Physicians and hospitals have no incentive to trim costs because the consumer is not concerned, and insurers respond to rising costs by passing them on in the form of increased premiums. In such a situation, no one is forced to be concerned about costs.

Quite apart from various flaws in the way in which the health-care system operates, other factors having to do with a changing population and the state of medicine itself are no doubt responsible to some extent for increasing costs. Here are three of them:

> As children born during the baby boom of the 1940s have reached adulthood, there has been an increase in the median age of the population. An aging population requires more medical care and more expensive medical care than a population with a lower median age.
>
> Improvements in medical technology now make it possible to provide a greater number of services to hospitalized patients. This also means that more people are likely to be hospitalized in order to receive the services.
>
> Improvements in medical treatments now make it possible to provide treatment for illnesses that once would not have been treated. The very availability of such treatments means increasing the hospital population, and the very success of such treatments means that more people will be alive who can benefit from additional care.

While the major item responsible for increasing the expense of health care in general is hospital costs, all of these factors significantly contribute to the overall costs.

Such considerations as the ones we have mentioned here have persuaded nearly everyone concerned with the formulation and implementation of health-care policies that the current state of affairs needs to be changed. There is a general belief that if it is not, the health-care system will become so economically unrealistic that it will collapse.

HEALTH-CARE DELIVERY

Despite the great economic investment in health care, some 25 million people, about 10 percent of the population, received no care at all during 1982. About 6 percent of American families, almost four million, reported that they were in need of care but could not get it.

Although efforts over the past two decades have improved access to health care for low-income and minority groups, it is obvious that a significant portion of the population is still not receiving needed care. The situation seems to be growing worse. For one thing, the tightening of federal and state regulations determining eligibility for Medicaid and Medicare has led to a sharp decline in the percentage of poor people receiving benefits. Furthermore, the number of people without medical insurance has now reached 35 million, up from 29 million in 1979. As a result, one in every six Americans lacks the coverage necessary to pay the expenses that accompany serious illness or injury. This consequence is partly due to the loss of jobs in industries that provided insurance coverage for their workers.

The loss of the ability to pay for medical care by low-income people has put great stress on university and public hospitals that have traditionally provided care for the indigent. Such hospitals have historically recouped the cost of caring for the poor by cost-shifting—that is by charging higher rates to those who can afford to pay or who have an insurer that will pay. However, because of increasing costs, the federal government, Health Maintenance Organizations, business groups with insurance programs, and private insurance companies have started resisting paying inflated rates for some patients. The private organizations are concerned with limiting their expenditures and increasing their profits. They reject the idea that they should, directly or indirectly, subsidize medical care for the poor.

According to one estimate, fewer than 9 percent of the nation's hospitals account for 40 percent of the care given to the poor. The percentage figure may shrink and public hospitals become even more overburdened. If university hospitals are denied a means of passing on the costs of caring for patients unable to pay, they may be forced to reduce the number of such patients cared for to be able to continue to support their teaching and research missions. Also, investor-owned hospital cooperations, which operate hospitals with the aim of making profits, are increasingly reluctant to accept patients who are uninsured or who are unable to pay for the full cost of their care. Such hospitals typically send such patients to public hospitals. Even when patients enter the hospital as emergency cases, they are moved to public facilities as soon as possible. (Critics have charged that some patients are moved too soon, putting their lives and safety at risk.)

The current pattern of change suggests that before long the care of the poor will be primarily the responsibility of public hospitals. Some policy analysts fear that this will lead to a two-tier medical system in which the poor will receive second-class care, while those able to pay will receive the best care available. However, if the poor are to receive any care at all, public hospitals will have to receive additional financing from some source. Several states have introduced measures to tax the revenues of hospitals and use the money to compensate hospitals that care for a disproportionate number of indigent patients. This solution is not regarded as satisfactory by some analysts, for it leads hospitals that are taxed to increase their fees to pass on their costs to paying patients. The only reasonable solution, according to some, is for the state and federal governments to face up to the task of caring for the poor and establish programs and appropriate tax money for that purpose.

Some advocates for the poor see two recent proposals as particularly threatening. Under current federal regulations, hospitals receiving building funds under the Hill-Burton Act must provide "uncompensated services" equal to 3 percent of their annual operating costs or 10 percent of the money they have received, whichever is less. The hospitals must also post signs and issue public notices indicating that free care is available to those without financial means. Currently, some 4,653 health-care facilities are obligated to provide free care. However, under a new regulation proposed by the Reagan administration, 2,444 (53 percent) of these facilities could be certified as a "public facility" and exempted from the rule specifying the amount of free care they must offer.

Critics have claimed that the new regulation would lead to a reduction in the amount of medical care provided to the poor. They charge that many hospitals already fail to abide by the requirement to provide free care and do not advertise its availability. The government, the critics say, has done little to insure compliance, and under the new regulation, hospitals are likely to care for even fewer poor patients.

The second proposal is to modify the Medicaid program, the public assistance program explicitly designed to provide the poor with medical care. The major portion of the 37 billion dollars spent on medical assistance programs in 1973 was spent for Medicaid. Recent emphasis on cost containment has led to the proposal that the cost of Medicaid be controlled by requiring that the family members of recipients bear part of the cost when they are financially able to do so. In March of 1983, the Department of Health and Human Services announced that states could require "adult family members to support adult relatives without violating the Medicaid statute." Some states have enacted such laws, and it is possible that the requirement might be made a federal one. In the view of critics, the requirement is an attempt to make the poor take care of the poor, and it may have the result of reducing to poverty the families of those already impoverished. The requirement raises both constitutional and moral issues. Is it legitimate, for example, to impose a financial burden on the adult and independent children of a parent on Medicaid?

The failure of the current medical system to supply an adequate level of health care (a "decent minimum," as it is often phrased) to everyone in the society who is in need of it is the result of a tangled web of social and economic factors. Some of the factors that make health care so expensive are also ones that restrict access to it. The following are among those that are frequently mentioned:

Reductions in funding for community clinics, prenatal care centers, and pediatric clinics that were established in the 1960s have forced many to close or to cut back severely on services. This has deprived many people in the lower socioeconomic groups of a major source of care. It has also led many to turn to hospitals for care, and hospital care is much more expensive. Also, medical problems that might have been avoided if treated early at clinics become more serious and require longer hospital stays. It has been repeatedly shown that the money spent on prenatal care is more than repaid by reducing the risk that infants will require special care.

Overspecialization by physicians leaves general social needs unsatisfied. It has been claimed that virtually every medical specialty has an oversupply. Specialists are more expensive to educate, and in practice they charge higher fees for what is often the same care provided by nonspecialists. The financial and social incentives that encourage specialization are costly, and they also leave too few physicians in general-care practice.

Although there is no shortage of physicians, a serious social problem is caused by their distribution. Most have chosen to live and practice in major metropolitan areas. As a consequence, many rural areas and small towns have been left totally without professional medical care. Furthermore, even physicians in cities have chosen to locate in certain areas only. This means that predominately poor neighborhoods, which are also most likely to be black or hispanic, may be without the services of a physician. Such neighborhoods may also be without a nearby hospital or clinic.

In 1983, physicians' fees amounted to over 147 billion dollars, more than 41 percent of the total health-care expenditures. In the view of some, physicians are paid too much for their services, and the cost of their services is a barrier to those of low or moderate income who are in need of care.

Factors such as these are often mentioned to support the claim that the American health-care system is not adequately serving the needs of the people. The charge is made that we live in a system in which there are still two kinds of medicine—one for the rich and one for the poor. And it too often happens that the medicine for the poor is none at all.

POSSIBLE SOLUTIONS AND ACTUAL PROBLEMS

A recent analysis of public opinion polls revealed that Americans hold inconsistent attitudes about health-care costs. In particular:

> Increasing costs are regarded by both the public and elected officials as the major problem in health care. Yet the problem does not appear in rankings of the top ten problems facing the country.
>
> People report that they are deeply disturbed by the rising cost of health care, yet they are not disturbed by the proportion of the economy devoted to it. Most believe we spend too little on health care, rather than too much.
>
> Most people say they believe that present health-care arrangements are not satisfactory, yet they do not wish to change the way in which they receive care.
>
> Most people are unwilling to give up their own physicians, but they favor requiring low-income people to use HMOs (see below) or clinics.

The authors of the analysis point out that public opinion is only one of the many factors that influence health-care policy. However, as they also note, there are practical and political limits on the changes that will be accepted by the society. Mostly, people are unwilling to see any changes that would produce a major alteration in the way in which they currently arrange for their own medical care. However, people are willing to approve of a variety of cost-containment programs that would make a cumulative difference in slowing or halting the increase in costs.

In fact, recent changes in the ways in which health care is paid for have not been ones requiring a major restructuring of social arrangements, and they have mostly been accepted without complaint by the public. However, the most significant change involves the way in which Medicare payments are made, and it is possible that it has not been in effect long enough for the public to realize its consequences. As we shall see, it has some major difficulties associated with it.

Medicare and Diagnosis Related Groups (DRGs)

In 1983 about 60 billion dollars were spent under the Medicare program to provide medical services for the elderly. In 1970 its cost was 7.5 billion. To attempt to gain control over escalating costs, in March of 1983 Congress approved a plan for paying hospitals a predetermined price for each Medicare patient. At the heart of this "prospective payment plan" are the Diagnosis Related Groups (DRGs), for they determine the price Medicare will pay.

The DRGs consist of 468 categories, and associated with each category is an index number that represents the relative amount of medical resources required to treat a patient with that diagnosis. The patient's diagnosis at the time of discharge from the hospital (the patient's DRG) determines the payment the hospital will receive. The actual payment is determined by multiplying the index number by the average dollar cost per patient at hospitals within the geographical region.

If the actual cost of treating a patient exceeds the DRG-determined price by more than 150 percent, Medicare will consider the patient a statistical "outlier" and pay 60 percent of the costs above the 150 percent. In such a case, the hospital must take a loss amounting to the difference between 100 and 150 percent plus 40 percent of the amount above 150 percent.

Under the traditional "retrospective payment" plan, hospitals were simply reimbursed for the actual cost of treating a Medicare patient. Neither the patient nor the hospital had an incentive to control costs, and the DRG plan is intended to introduce a motive for cost containment. If hospital costs are higher than the DRG amount, the hospital will lose money. However, if the costs are lower, the hospital will receive the allowable amount.

In the long run, however, hospitals cannot gain from reducing their costs. If they lower their overall costs to make up the difference in those cases in which the actual costs of treating Medicare patients are not fully paid for by the DRG amounts, they will lower the average cost per patient in their region. An annual review of regional rates will reflect this, and the next year's DRG payments will be even smaller. Hospitals are thus forced to cut costs, but they are not actually rewarded for it.

Some who object to the prospective payment plan argue that the elderly, who are the great majority of Medicare recipients, may not be provided with the highest quality care. To be sure that they do not lose money, hospitals will be tempted to spend no more in caring for a Medicare patient than they can expect to be reimbursed for. Thus, laboratory tests and treatments that might be helpful might not be offered. Given an option, hospitals may choose the least expensive methods, supplies, and devices. (Hip-replacement joints might come in deluxe and Medicare models.) Thus, people who can afford to pay for the best of care will get it, while those wholly dependent on Medicare may not.

Danielle Dolenc and Charles Dougherty, along with other critics, have called attention to additional potentially negative aspects of DRGs:

Patients may be discharged from hospitals before they are fit, because they have reached the point at which hospitals will lose money if their stay is prolonged.

Hospitals may be discouraged from treating patients who may not respond to treatment in a way average for their DRG. Similarly, hospitals may avoid admitting patients in DRGs they judge to be artificially low.

University hospitals and hospitals that specialize in certain diseases or draw from special populations usually treat a higher proportion of seriously ill patients with longer lengths of stay. Consequently, the DRG payments, based on averages, do not provide them with complete compensation.

Rural and inner-city hospitals, which typically accept all patients in all categories, may not be able to get the proper "case mix" to insure their financial stability. Hospitals may tend to identify the DRGs that produce the greatest profit and admit a disproportionate number of patients in those categories.

Ancillary services, such as physical therapy, that do not yield an adequate financial return may be phased out.

Patients may have some cause to worry that their diagnoses and treatments are determined, at least to some extent, by the DRG and the need to control costs, rather than by unhampered medical judgment.

The development of medical technology may be slowed down. DRGs reward only short-run cost effectiveness, and new technology is typically more expensive in the beginning. Also, with university hospitals losing money on their sicker and longer-term patients, money that currently goes to research and teaching will not be available. Academic medicine seems almost certain to suffer.

DRGs are likely to be an effective means of controlling costs, but as these considerations indicate, they are associated with some serious potential drawbacks. To some extent, the liabilities are features of the current program, rather than of the basic DRG concept. Some analysts believe that it may be possible to alter the current program in ways that will correct many of its major shortcomings. The basic question is, if the drawbacks are corrected, will DRGs continue to be effective in controlling costs?

It seems quite likely that private insurers and group health organizations will follow the lead of Medicare and adopt prospective payment plans. The potential that such plans offer for controlling costs is too great to be overlooked. Thus it is reasonable to expect that in the future virtually all health care in the United States will be under the control of DRGs. This prospect makes it crucially important to find ways to eliminate or reduce the actual shortcomings and potential hazards that DRGs possess. Otherwise, there is a serious risk that the entire medical system will decline in both the quantity and quality of service it can provide.

Physicians' Fee Schedule

Under development by the Department of Health and Human Services is a proposal to establish a fee schedule for physicians providing services to Medicare patients. In 1984 almost 20 percent of the 75 billion dollars spent on physicians' services was paid for by Medicare. Bringing fees under control by means of a program comparable to DRG

schedules for hospitals is seen as the next obvious step in Medicare cost containment.

At present there is little competition among physicians in setting fees. Current Medicare policy is to pay "current and prevailing" charges, and this has the consequence of perpetuating fee disparities that exist among specialties and geographical regions. Thus the current system is regarded as inherently inflationary, for when fees are raised by increasing the customary rates, Medicare payments are raised to match them. As with DRGs, variations in fees would have to be tied to such factors as cost differences associated with living in rural or urban areas.

In 1984 physicians' fees were frozen by Medicare so that by late 1985 physicians were getting only 25 to 30 percent of the amounts actually billed. For this reason, physicians themselves might not be opposed to altering the ways in which they are reimbursed by Medicare. Also, physicians in some specialties might benefit by fee schedules. Studies show that surgeons, in particular, are overpaid in comparison with those in other medical specialties. Fee schedules could raise the rates for those in internal medicine and family practice.

Mandated fee schedules threaten access to medical care and the quality of the care delivered for the same reasons that DRG-based hospital payments threaten them. Here again the question is whether it is possible to control costs without unacceptably compromising the strengths of the present system.

Health-Care Organizations

In the last decade, the United States has moved toward establishing Health Maintenance Organizations (HMOs). An HMO is a medical plan in which an individual pays a fixed annual fee to an organized group of physicians. The group then undertakes to supply the individual with most kinds of needed medical services, at no additional charge.

HMOs hold out the possibility of lowered medical costs. They avoid unnecessary tests and procedures because the profit of the group is determined by the money remaining after the expenses of patients have been paid. Better patient care may result because the HMO organization encourages patients to consult a physician at the beginning of an illness rather than waiting until it grows serious.

In a variation on the HMO concept, some businesses and unions have established contracts with physicians to provide medical services for their employees or members. These Preferred Provider Organizations (PPOs) have the advantage of allowing individuals to choose their physicians from a list of those who have entered into the arrangement. In this way a major complaint against HMOs, that the individual is required to receive care from a group and has no physician of his own, is avoided.

HMOs and PPOs have made a contribution to reducing health-care costs. To some extent, however, this has been achieved by providing less than a full range of services. As businesses and other contracting organizations begin to demand more services for their members, the cost of providing them will rise.

Critics have also pointed out that health-care organizations also have inherent weaknesses. There is the possibility that they will encourage physicians to provide inferior care in order to maximize their own profits. Furthermore, patients may be dissatisfied with the care they receive, for physicians are empowered to turn down their requests for medical services if the physician believes they are unnecessary.

It is still too early to tell how successful health-care organizations will be in providing high-quality care at a reasonable price. However, experiences in California suggest that such organizations can work very well. The Kaiser plan, which was started in 1945, owns twenty-three hospitals and one hundred fifty-eight clinics and has 20 percent of the residents of the San Francisco area as members. Over six million people in California are members of either the Kaiser plan or the Ross-Loos plan. In the view of some analysts, health-care organizations offer the best approach to providing national health insurance that attempts to meet the medical needs of all citizens.

Alternative Solutions

Some have argued that more radical solutions to the health-care problems of the United States are required than would be provided by health-care organizations, employee-option insurance, or particular cost-containment policies. Some claim that the entire medical-delivery system of the country needs to be totally altered. Only then, they say, can costs be controlled, medical needs met, and justice done. The following are among the many recommendations that have been made:

Issue health stamps to those whose income shows them to be in need. Health-stamp recipients could then shop around for medical services. This would introduce an element of competition among health-care providers and lead to a reduction in costs.

Place all pharmaceutical and medical-equipment manufacturers under public ownership. By eliminating excessive profits, the costs of drugs and equipment would come closer to reflecting their true development and production costs.

"Draft" physicians and assign them to work in rural areas or in inner-city neighborhoods where physicians are nonexistent or in short supply.

Limit by law the number of people allowed to enter a medical specialty. Or, alternatively, make it illegal to use public funds to finance specialty training.

Educate great numbers of additional physicians, nurses, and other health-care professionals and require that they put in a term of service in assigned areas.

Eliminate all fee-for-service transactions between physicians and patients and remove the profit motive from health care.

Place all hospitals and clinics under community control.

Require that everyone pay premiums for a national health insurance program, but allow claims beyond a certain limit only by those who cannot afford to pay.

Not all of these proposals are equally sound, of course. Some are politically and socially unrealistic at the present time. They are suggestive, however, and they do provide alternative views about how a system that is almost universally regarded as dangerously unworkable might be modified. That such proposals should be made is itself evidence that the health-care system is indeed in crisis.

CASE PRESENTATION
The Dumping of Mrs. Smith

Mrs. Helen Smith (as we will call her) was a fifty-year-old overweight black woman with diabetes and hypertension. Until recently, she had been hospitalized for treatment at Central Medical City, a private facility.

Now Mrs. Smith was in the emergency room of Chicago's Cook County Hospital. Clutching a grocery bag filled with bottles of outdated medicines and a sheaf of unfilled prescriptions, she waited patiently until a physician could see her.

In addition to her grocery bag, Mrs. Smith carried with her a note from her previous physician that she turned over to the clerk at the admissions desk. The note said only: "Please assume medical care of Mrs. Smith. She is no longer eligible for medical assistance and cannot afford to see me." No records had been sent with her, no information about her medical problems, no results of tests that might have been done, no list of medications prescribed. Thus, the emergency-room physician would be denied access to data crucial to providing Mrs. Smith with the best mode of medical treatment.

Mrs. Smith had been dumped. That is, she

had been turned out of a private hospital for lacking the means to pay for her medical care, although still in need of it. Mrs. Smith was ambulatory and so could be discharged with the advice that she go to Cook County Hospital or to some other public facility that would have to accept her. Had she not been ambulatory, she would still have been dumped, but the process would have been more complicated. The private hospital would have had to call and arrange for her transfer. She would then have been delivered to the public hospital in an ambulance.

Over five hundred patients a month are now transferred to Cook County Hospital from private hospitals in the Chicago area. In 1983, only about sixty or seventy a month were transferred. What is true of Cook County Hospital is true of public hospitals nationwide. A recent study shows that private hospitals provide two to three times less care that is uncompensated ("charity cases") than do public institutions, and the number of patients transferred has dramatically increased.

Because physicians and administrators in private hospitals are under pressure to reduce their costs and increase profits, they are also under pressure to reduce the number of nonpaying or low-paying patients that they treat. It is this situation that encourages the dumping of patients into public hospitals.

Some critics of dumping have presented evidence to show that patients are often transferred before they have been medically stabilized. Thus, treatment needed by such patients is often delayed, and the patients are put in risk of their very lives. Furthermore, critics charge, physicians at private hospitals sometimes misrepresent the medical status of patients by withholding relevant data about them. In some cases, if the patient's true condition were known, the public hospital would refuse to accept the transfer.

Mrs. Smith needed immediate medical treatment and received it. Because her medical history was lacking, she did not receive the best kind of treatment for her condition. Yet she was among the luckier of those who are dumped.

INTRODUCTION

It has been estimated that it was not until the middle 1930s that the intervention of a physician in the treatment of an illness was likely to affect the outcome in a substantial way. The change was brought about by the discovery and development of antibiotic agents such as penicillin and sulfa drugs. They made it possible, for the first time, both to control infection and to provide specific remedies for a variety of diseases. Additional advances in treatment modalities, procedures, and technology have helped establish contemporary medicine as an effective enterprise.

Before these dramatic changes occurred, there was little reason for anyone to be particularly concerned with the question of the distribution of medical care within society. The situation in the United States has altered significantly, and a number of writers have recently argued that everyone ought to be guaranteed at least some form of medical care. In part this is a reflection of the increased effectiveness of contemporary medicine, but it is

also no doubt due to a growing awareness of the serious difficulties faced by disadvantaged groups within society.

In the last chapter we discussed one aspect of the problem of the distribution of medical resources—that of allocating limited resources among competing individuals in a particular situation. Here we need to call attention to some of the broader social issues. These are ones that transcend moral decisions about particular people and raise questions about the basic aims and obligations of society.

A great number of observers believe that the United States is currently faced with a health-care crisis. Some of the reasons supporting this belief, as well as some proposed solutions, are outlined in the Social Context part of this chapter, and we need not repeat them here. But one element of the crisis is often said to be the lack of any program to provide health care for everyone in the society. That there should be people forced to do without needed health care for primarily financial reasons has seemed to some a morally intolerable state of affairs.

This point of view has frequently been based on the claim that everyone has a *right* to health care. Thus, it has been argued, society has a duty to provide that care, and if it does not, then it is sanctioning a situation that is inherently wrong. To remedy the situation requires redesigning the health-care system and present practices to see to it that all who need and want health care have access to it.

The language of "rights" is very slippery. To understand and evaluate arguments that involve claiming (or denying) rights to health care it is important to understand the nature of the claim. The word "rights" is used in several distinct ways, and a failure to be clear about the use in any given case leads only to unproductive confusion.

The following distinctions may help capture some of the more important sorts of things that people have in mind when they talk about rights.

CLAIM-RIGHTS, LEGAL RIGHTS, AND STATUTORY RIGHTS

Suppose I own a copy of the book *Anne of Green Gables*. If so, then I may be said to have a *right* to do with the book whatever I choose. Other people may be said to have a *duty* to recognize my right in appropriate ways. Thus, if I want to read the book, burn it, or sell it, others have a duty not to interfere with me. If I lend the book to someone, then he has a duty to return it.

It is generally agreed in the philosophy of law that a claim-right to something serves as a ground for other people's duties. A *claim-right*, then, always entails a duty or duties on the part of someone else. Right and duty thus go together like parent and child—one is not possible without the other.

Generally speaking, *legal rights* are claim-rights. Someone has a legal right when someone else has a definable duty, and legal remedies are available when the duty is not performed. Either the person can be forced to perform the duty, or damages of some sort can be collected for failure to perform. If I pay someone to put a new roof on my house by a certain date, she has contracted a duty to perform the work we have agreed to. If the task is not performed, then I can turn to the legal system for enforcement or damages.

Statutory rights are claim-rights that are explicitly recognized in legal statutes or laws. They impose duties on certain classes of people under specified conditions. A hospital contractor, for example, has a duty to meet certain building codes. If he fails to meet them, he is liable to legal penalties. But not all legal rights are necessarily statutory rights. Such considerations as "customary and established practices" may sometimes implicitly involve a legally enforceable claim-right.

MORAL RIGHTS

Generally speaking, a *moral right* is one that is stated in or derived from the principles of a moral theory. More specifically, to say that someone has a moral right to certain goods or manner of treatment is to say that others have a moral duty to see to it that she receives what she has a right to. A moral right is a certain kind of claim-right. Here, though, the source of justification for the right and for the corresponding duty lies in moral principles and not in the laws or practices of a society.

According to Ross, for example, people have a right to expect benevolent treatment from others—we have a duty to treat other people benevolently. This is a right that is not recognized by our legal system. We may, if we wish, treat others in a harsh and unsympathetic manner and in doing so violate no law.

Of course many rights and duties that are based upon the principles of moral theories are also embodied in our laws. Thus, to take Ross again as an example, we have a prima facie duty not to injure or kill anyone. This duty, along with its correlative right to be free from injury or death at the hands of another, is reflected in the body of statutory law and common law that deals with bodily harm done to others and with killing.

The relationship between ethical theories and the laws of a society is complicated and controversial. The fundamental question is always the extent to which laws should reflect or be based upon an ethical theory. In a society such as ours, it does not seem proper that an ethical theory accepted by only a part of the people should determine the laws that govern us all. It is for this reason that some object to laws regulating sexual activity, pornography, and abortion. These are considered best regarded as a part of personal morality.

At the same time, however, it seems that we must rely upon ethical theories as a basis for evaluating laws. Unless we are prepared to say that what is legal is, in itself, what is right, we must recognize the possibility of laws that are bad or unjust. But what makes a law bad? A possible answer is that a law is bad when it violates a right derived from the principles of an ethical theory. Similarly, both laws and social practices may be criticized for failing to recognize a moral right. A moral theory, then, can serve as the basis for a demand for the reform of laws and practices.

Clearly there is no sharp line separating the moral and the legal. Indeed, virtually all of the moral theories we discussed in the introductory chapter have been used by philosophers and other thinkers as the basis for principles applying to society as a whole. Within such frameworks as utilitarianism, natural law theory, and Rawls's theory of a just society, legal and social institutions are assigned roles and functions in accordance with more general moral principles.

POLITICAL RIGHTS

Not everyone attempts to justify claims to rights by referring such claims directly to a moral theory. Efforts are frequently made to provide justification by relying upon principles or commitments that are generally acknowledged as basic to our society. (Of course, to answer how these are justified may force us to invoke moral principles.) Our society, for example, is committed to individual autonomy and equality, among other values. It is by reference to commitments of this sort that we evaluate proposals and criticize practices.

From this point of view, to recognize health care as a right is to acknowledge it as a *political* right. This means showing that it is required by our political commitments or principles. Of course, this may also mean resolving any conflicts that may arise from other rights that also seem to be demanded by our principles. But this is a familiar state of affairs. We are all aware that the Constitutional guarantee of freedom of speech, for example, is not absolute and unconditional. It can conflict with other rights or basic commitments, and we look to the courts to provide us with guidelines to resolve the conflicts.

With the distinctions that we have discussed in mind, let us return now to the question of a general right to health care. What can those who make such a claim be asserting?

Obviously everyone in our society is free to seek health care and, when the proper arrangements are made, to receive it. That is, health care is a service available in society, and people may avail themselves of it. At the same time, however, no physician or hospital has a duty to provide health care that is sought. The freedom to seek does not imply that others have a duty to provide what we seek.

There is not in our society a legally recognized claim-right to health care. Even if I am sick, no one has a legal duty to see to it that I receive treatment for my illness. (A few states, such as New York, do impose legal duies on physicians and hospitals to treat people faced with life-threatening emergencies. Even this is not generally the case, however.) I may request care, or I may attempt to persuade a physician that it is his or her moral duty to provide me with care. But I have no legal right to health care, and if someone refuses to provide it, I cannot seek a legal remedy.

Of course I may contract with a physician, clinic, or hospital for care, either in general or for a certain ailment. If I do this, then the other party acquires a legally enforceable duty to provide me the kind of care that we agreed upon. In this respect, contracting for health care is not relevantly different from contracting for a new roof on my house.

Those who assert that health care is a right cannot be regarded as merely making the obviously false claim that there is a legal right to care. Their claim, rather, must be interpreted as one of a moral or political sort. They might be taken as asserting something like "Everyone in the society *ought* to be entitled to health care, regardless of his or her financial condition."

Anyone making such a claim must be prepared to justify it by offering reasons and evidence in support of it. The ultimate source of the justification is most likely to be the principles of a moral theory. For example, Kant's principle that every person is of inherent and equal worth might be used to support the claim that every person has an equal right to medical care, simply by virtue of being a person.

Justification might also be offered in terms of principles that express the aims and commitments of the society. A society that endorses justice and equality, it might be argued, must be prepared to offer health care to all if it offers it to anyone.

However justification is offered, it is clear that to claim that health care is a right is to go beyond merely expressing an attitude. It is to say more than something like "Everyone would like to have health care" or "Everyone needs health care." It is true that the language of "rights" is frequently used in a rhetorical way to encourage us to recognize the wants and needs of people—or even other creatures, such as animals and trees. This is a perfectly legitimate way of talking. But, at bottom, to urge that something be considered a right is to make a claim requiring justification in terms of some set of legal, social, or moral principles.

Why not recognize health care for all as a right? Certainly virtually everyone would admit that in the abstract it would be a good thing. If this is so, then why should anyone wish to oppose it? Briefly stated, arguments against a right to health care are most frequently of two kinds.

First, those who subscribe to a position sometimes called "medical individualism" argue that to recognize a right to health care would have the consequence of violating the rights of physicians and other medical practitioners. Physicians, they claim, would be required to employ their intelligence, knowledge, and skills in a way dictated by society. Thus, physicians would be deprived of their autonomy and, in a very real sense, made slaves of the state.

Second, some writers have pointed out that while it is possible to admit health care to the status of a right, we must also recognize that health care is just one social good among others. Education, transportation, housing, legal assistance, and so on are other goods that are also sought and needed by members of our society. It is impossible to admit all of these (and perhaps others) to the status of rights, for the society simply cannot afford to pay for them.

The first line of argument (medical individualism) is examined in some detail in the selections of this chapter. We need not attempt to evaluate it here. It should be kept in mind, however, that medical individualism fails to recognize that the health-care situation is perhaps best regarded as one in which there is a *conflict* of rights (between patients and providers) and not just one in which the rights of physicians are being restricted.

The second line of argument does not necessarily lead to the conclusion that we should not recognize a right to health care. It does serve to warn us that we must be very careful to specify just what sort of right—if any—we want to support. Do we want to claim, for example, that everyone has a right to a certain *minimum* of health care? Or do we want to claim that everyone has a right to *equal* health care (whatever anyone can get, everyone can demand)?

Furthermore, this line of argument warns us that we have to make decisions about what we, as a society, are willing to pay for. Would we, for example, be willing to give up all public support for education in order to use the money for health care? Probably not. But we might be willing to reduce the level of support for education in order to increase that for health care. Whatever we decide, we have to face up to the problem of distributing our limited resources. This is an issue that is obviously closely connected with what sort of right to health care (or really, the right to what sort of health care) we are prepared to endorse.

THE SELECTIONS

Charles Fried's essay maintains that we cannot afford to accept the view that everyone has a right to equal health care. If everyone were given equal access to the *best* health care, Fried argues, this would absorb an intolerable portion of our gross national income. Fried is willing to grant a right to a "decent minimum" of health care to all. But, as he points out, this means that we have to face the problem of determining this minimum.

Furthermore, Fried recommends that we consider how to change the present "medical guild" so that highly paid and trained physicians might be replaced by people with less training who can provide a number of services more cheaply. Fried also suggests that we allow patients more choice in the "medical marketplace" by giving each person a certain amount of money to buy the medical services that he or she chooses. This might encourage the development of a variety of medical delivery systems suited to consumers' needs. Also those who want fancier or more individualized medical care could get it by paying additional money out of their own pocket.

The right to health care supported by Fried is a limited one. But Robert M. Sade in his essay rejects the claim to any right to health care. Sade argues that "from man's primary right—the right to his own life—derive all others." Among those that follow

from this, Sade claims, is everyone's right to pursue his own values, and "the choice of the conditions under which a physician's services are rendered belongs to the physician as a consequence of his right to support his own life."

Sade attempts to show that if there were a right on the part of the patient to a physician's care, then this would lead to an immoral result. He argues that to guarantee a right, a government must use force; thus, a physician's professional judgment ("mind") is controlled through the threat of force. No one can survive as an individual without freedom of mind.   "Thus," Sade concludes, "since the concept of medical care as the right of a patient entails the use or threat of violence against physicians, the concept is anti-mind—therefore, anti-life, therefore, immoral."

In "Social Justice and Equal Access to Health Care," Gene Outka defends a position that is at odds with those of Fried and Sade. Outka argues that concepts of justice that grant access to health care on the basis of personal merit, societal contribution, or market considerations all rely on factors that are not sufficiently relevant to the special nature of health care. Justice demands that we treat people differently only when there are relevant differences between them, and factors such as personal accomplishments, social merit, and income level are not relevant to health care.

Need, Outka claims, is the sole standard for determining who shall receive care. People who need health care are people who are ill, and being ill is the only relevant factor in determining access to care. However, because medical resources are finite, access may have to be restricted. Thus, the formal principle of justice as treating similar cases in a similar way becomes relevant. (See the discussion of this principle in the general Introduction.)

Outka suggests that restrictions might be

imposed by refusing to treat some categories of illness, by employing a procedure to select patients randomly, or by excluding some components of a comprehensive medical care system. In any case, whatever services are available to some who need them would be available to all who need them. Thus, even with restrictions, the social goal of equal access would retain its authority.

None of the selections in this chapter attempts to provide detailed answers to the multitude of questions that swarm around the issues of a public health-care policy. Yet each of them calls attention to some of the fundamental issues of rights, values, and social goals that must be resolved before any practical policy can be accepted as legitimate. If we are to recognize a right to health care, then we must be clear about exactly what is involved in recognizing such a right. Are we prepared to offer only a "decent minimum"? Does justice require that we make available to all whatever is available to any? Are we prepared to restrict the wants of some people in order to satisfy the basic needs of all people?

The issues discussed in this chapter are of more than academic interest, and they concern more than just a handful of patients and physicians. How they are resolved will affect us all, both directly and indirectly, through the character of our society.

Equality and Rights in Medical Care

Charles Fried

In this article I present arguments intended to support the following conclusions:

1. To say there is a right to health care does not imply a right to equal access, a right that whatever is available to any shall be available to all.

2. The slogan of equal access to the best health care available is just that, a dangerous slogan which could be translated into reality only if we submitted either to intolerable government controls of medical practice or to a thoroughly unreasonable burden of expense.

3. There is sense to the notion of a right to a decent standard of care for all, dynamically defined, but still not dogmatically equated with the best available.

4. We are far from affording such a standard to many of our citizens and that is profoundly wrong.

5. One of the major sources of the exaggerated demands for equality are the pretensions, inflated claims, inefficiencies, and guild-like, monopolistic practices of the health professions.

I. Background

The notion of some kind of a right to health care is not likely to be found in any but the most recent writings, not to mention legislation. After all, even the much more well-established institution of free, universal public education has not achieved the status of a federal constitutional right, is not a constitutional right by the law of many states, and stands as a right more as an inference from the practices and legislation of states, counties, and municipalities. The federal constitutional litigation regarding rights in that area has been restricted to the provision *equally* of whatever public education is in fact provided. So it should not be surprising that the notion of a right to health care is something of a novelty. Moreover, it is only fairly recently that health care could deliver a product which was as unambiguously beneficial as elementary schooling. Nevertheless, if one looks to the laws, practices, and understandings of states, counties, and municipalities, one sees growing up through the last century, and certainly in the twentieth century, an understanding which might be thought of as the inchoate recognition of a right to health care. Indeed, there are those who might say that such an inchoate recognition might be discerned as far back as Elizabethan England.

As one considers this progress, one should not misrepresent history, for in that history lies an important lesson. For the progress may represent not simply a progress in our ideas of social justice, but a progress in what medicine could do. The fact is that the increasingly general provision of medical care may be correlated as well with what medical care could accomplish as with any changing social doctrines. What could medicine accomplish a hundred or even fifty years ago? It is well known that the improvements in health that were wrought in those days were largely the result of improved sanitation, working conditions, diet, and the like. Beyond that, specifically medical ministrations could do very little. They could provide ease, amenities, relief, but rarely a cure. So society may be forgiven if it did not provide elaborate medical care to the poor until recently, since provision of medical care in essence would have meant simply the provision of amenities and placebos. And since society appeared little concerned to assure the amenities to its poor generally, it is no great surprise that it had scant inclination to provide these amenities to the sick poor.

The detailed history of the extension of medical care to the poor, and indeed to those who were not poor but lived in out-of-the-way places, has yet to be written. The emergence of a notion of a right to health care and the embodiment of such a notion in legislation and court decisions must also await difficult historical research. Nevertheless, it is worth noting that, at least in American public discourse, the idea of a right to medical care developed into something which had the appearance of inevitability only recently, in what might be called the intermediate, perhaps golden, age of modern medicine. This was a period when advances in treating acute illness, advances such as the antibiotics, could really make a large difference in prolonging life or restoring health; but the most elaborate technologies which may make only marginal improvements in situations previously thought to be hopeless had not yet been generally developed. In this recent "Golden Age" we could unambiguously afford a notion of a general right to medical care because there were a number of clear successes available to medicine, and these successes were not unduly costly. Having conquered the infectious diseases, medical science has undertaken the degenerative diseases, the malignant neoplasms, and the diseases of unknown etiology; and one must say that the ratio between expense and benefit has become exponentially more unfavorable. So it is really only now that the notion of a right to health care poses acute analytical and social problems. It is for that reason that neither history nor legal analysis will much illuminate our future course. What we do now will be a matter of our choosing, and for this reason careful analysis of the notion of a right to health care is crucial.

II. Equality and Rights: Analytical Distinctions

First, something should be said by way of at least informal definition of this term "right." A right is more than just an interest that an individual might have, a state of affairs or a state of being which an individual might prefer. A claim of right invokes entitlements; and when we speak of entitlements, we mean not those things which it would be nice for people to have, or which they would prefer to have, but which they must have, and which if they do not have they may demand, whether we like it or not. Although I would not want to say that a right is something we must recognize "no matter what," nevertheless a right is something we must accord unless _____ and what we put in to fill in the unless clause should be tightly confined and specific.

This notion of rights has interesting and not altogether obvious relations to the concept of equality, and confusions about those relations are very likely to lead to confused arguments about the very area before us—rights to health care and equality in respect to health care.

First, it should be noted that equality itself may be considered a right. Thus, a person can argue that he is not necessarily entitled to any particular thing—whether it be income, or housing, or education, or health care—but that he is entitled to equality in respect to that thing, so that whatever anyone gets he should get, too. And this is a nice example of my previous proposition about the notion of rights generally. For to recognize a right to equality may very well be—I suppose it often is—contrary to many other policies that we may have, and particularly contrary to attempts to attain some kind of efficiency. Yet, by the very notion of rights, if there is a right to equality, then granting equality cannot depend on whether or not it is efficient to do so.

Second, there is the relation between rights and equality which runs the other way, too: to say that a class of persons, or all persons, have a certain right implies that they all have that right equally. If it is said that all persons within the jurisdiction of the United States have a constitutionally protected right to freedom of speech, whatever that may mean, one thing seems clear: that this right should not depend on what it is one wants to say, who one is, and the like. Indeed, if the government against whom this right is protected were to make such distinctions, for instance, subjecting to constraints the speech of "irresponsible persons," that would be the exact concept of denial of freedom of speech to those persons.

These relations between the notion of right and of equality suggest the great importance of being very clear and precise about how a particular right is conceived: confusions in this regard are rampant in respect to health, and are the source of much pointless controversy. But because the point is quite general, let me first take an example from another area. If we were sloppy in our thinking about what the right of freedom of speech is—and many people are as sloppy about that as they are about their definition of the rights in the area which is our immediate concern—if we were sloppy about that definition, we might, for instance, consider that there has been a denial of right because some people have access to radio or television in getting their ideas across, while others have only the street-corner soapbox to broadcast their views. Indeed, there are those who might find it unjust that even on the soapbox the timid or inarticulate are much less effective than the bold or eloquent. All of these disparities, of course, may or may not be regrettable but they have nothing to do with freedom of speech as a right, given the premise that there is a right to free speech and that this right must be an equal right. It seems clear to me that it is very different from the right to be heard, believed, admired, and applauded. The right to speak freely is just that: a right to be free of constraints and impositions on whatever speaking one might wish to do, should you be able to find someone to listen.

Now this analogy is offered as more than a distant irrelevance. Is it not very similar to many things that are said in the area of health? For analogous to the claim that the right to freedom of speech really implies a right to be heard by the multitude, is the notion that whatever rights might exist in respect to health care are rights to health, rather than to health *care*. And of course the claim is equally absurd in both instances. We may sensibly guarantee that all will be equally free of constraints on the speaking they wish to do, but we should not guarantee that all will be equally effective in getting their views across. Similarly, we may or may not choose to guarantee all equality of access to health care, but we cannot possibly guarantee to all equality of health.

Consider how these clarifications operate upon the historical development I alluded to at the beginning of this analysis. The right whose recognition might be said to have been implicit in social practices throughout the past hundred years was a right not to health care as such, nor yet a right to health, but rather a right to a certain standard of health care, which was defined in terms of what medicine could reasonably do for people. It is this notion which has become so difficult in our present situation, where the apparatus of medicine has become so much more elaborate, pretentious, and costly than it was in earlier times.

Bringing together the historical and the analytical sides, we might conclude that our present dilemma comes from the fact that there are very many expensive things that medicine can do which might possibly help. And if we commit ourselves to the notion that there is a right to whatever health care might be available, we do indeed get ourselves into a difficult situation where overall national expenditure on health must reach absurd proportions—absurd in the sense that far more is devoted to health at the expense of other important social goals than the population in general wants. Indeed, more is devoted to health than the population wants relative not only to important social goals—for example, education or housing—but relative to all the other things which people would like to have money left over to pay for. And if we recognize that it would be absurd to commit our society to devote more than a certain proportion of our national income to health, while at the same time recognizing a "right to health care," we might then be caught on the other horn of the dilemma. For we might then be required to say that because a right to health care implies a right to equality of health care, then we must limit, we must lower the quality of the health care that might be purchased by some lest our commitment to equality require us to provide such care to all and thus carry us over a reasonable budget limit.

Consider the case of the artificial heart. It seems to me not too fanciful an assumption that such a device is technically feasible within a reasonable time, and likely to be hugely expensive both in terms of its actual implantation and in terms of the subsequent care required by those benefiting from the device. Now if the right to health care is taken to mean the right to whatever health care is available to anybody, and if this entails that it is a right to an equal enjoyment of whatever care anyone else enjoys, then what are we to do with respect to the artificial heart? Might we decide not to develop such a device? Though the development and experimental use of it involves an entirely tolerable burden, the general provision of the artificial heart would be an intolerable burden, and since if we provide it to any we must provide it to all, therefore perhaps we should provide it to none.

This solution seems to me to be both uncomfortable and unstable. For surely there is something odd, if not perverse, about foregoing research on such devices, not because the research might fail, but because it might succeed. Might not this research then go on under some kinds of private auspices if such a governmental decision were made? Would we then go further and forbid even private research, rather than simply refusing to fund it? I can well imagine the next step, where artificial heart research and implantation would become like abortion or sex change operations in the old days: something one went to Sweden or Denmark for. Nor is a lottery device for distributing a limited number of artificial hearts likely to be more stable or satisfactory. For there, too, would we forbid people to go outside the lottery? Would it be a crime to cross national boundaries with the intent of obtaining an artificial heart? The example makes a general point about instituting an all-inclusive "right to health care," with the necessary concomitant of an equal right to whatever health care is available. For if we really instituted such a

right and limited the provision of health care to a reasonable level, we would have to institute as well a degree of stringent state control, which it is both unlikely we can achieve and undesirable for us even to try to achieve. There is something that goes very deeply against the grain about any scheme which prohibits scientists from making discoveries which no one claims are harmful as such, but which will cause trouble because we can't give them to everybody. There is something which goes against the grain in a system which might forbid individual doctors to render a service, not because it is harmful, but because its benefits are not available to all.

Or take a much less dramatic case—dental care. It is said that ordinary basic prophylactic care is so lacking for tens of millions of our citizens that quite unnecessarily they do not have their own teeth while still in their prime. I take it that to provide the kind of elaborate dental care deployed on affluent suburban families to rural populations, and to all even poorer urban dwellers, would be a prodigiously expensive undertaking, one that would cost each of us quite heavily. But if we followed the slogan, "The best available made available to all," that is what is meant. My guess is the American people would not want to bear this burden and that as a form of transfer payment the poor would prefer just to have the money to spend on other things. But this shows the dangerousness of slogans, for perhaps the greatest part of the dental damage could be remedied at far less cost by fluoridation and by relatively routine care provided by a type of modestly trained person who is only now beginning to exist. Care of this sort can be afforded and should be provided. But this would mean abandoning the concept of equality and accepting the fact that the poor would be getting less elaborate care than those who are not poor.

Now it might be said that I am exaggerating. The case put forward is the British National Health Service, which is alleged to provide a model of high level care at reasonable costs with equality for all. But I would caution planners and enthusiasts from drawing too much from this example. The situation in Great Britain is very different in many ways. The country is smaller and more homogeneous. Moreover, even in Great Britain there are disparities between the care available between urban and rural areas; there are long waits for so-called "elective procedures"; and there is a small but significant and distinguished private sector outside of National Health which is the focus of great controversy and rancor. Finally, Great Britain is a country where a substantial portion of the citizenry is committed to the socialist ideal of equalizing incomes and nationalizing the provisions of all vital services. Surely this is a very different situation from that in the United States. Indeed, it may be that the cry for equality of access to health care bears to a general yearning for social equality much the same relation that the opposition to fetal research bears to the opposition to abortion. In each case it is a very large ideological tail wagging a relatively small and confused dog.

My point is analytical. My point is that apart from a rather general commitment to equality and, indeed, to state control of the allocation and distribution of resources, to insist on the right to health care, where that right means a right to equal access, is an anomaly. For as long as our society considers that inequalities of wealth and income are morally acceptable—acceptable in the sense that the system that produces these inequalities is in itself not morally suspect—it is anomalous to carve out a sector like health care and say that *there* equality must reign.

III. Towards a Better Definition of the Rights Involved

After all, is health care so special? Is it different from education, housing, food, legal assistance? In respect to all of these things, we recognize in our society a right, whose enjoyment may not be made wholly dependent upon the ability to pay. But just as surely in respect to all these things, we do not believe that this right entails equality of enjoyment, so that whatever diet one person or class of persons enjoys must be enjoyed by all. The argument, put forward for instance by some members of the Labor Party in Great Britain, that the independent schools in that country should be abolished because they offer a level of education better than that available in state schools, is an argument which would be found strange and repellent in the United States. Rather, in all of these areas—education, housing, food,

legal assistance—there obtains a notion of a decent, fair standard, such that when this standard is satisfied all that exists in the way of *rights* has been accorded. And it is necessarily so; were we to insist on equality all the way up, that is, past this minimum, we would have committed ourselves to a political philosophy which I take it is not the dominant one in our society.

Is health care different? Everything that can be said about health care is true of food and is at least by analogy true of education, housing, and legal assistance. The real task before us is not, therefore, I think, to explain why there must be complete equality in medicine, but the more subtle and perilous task of determining the decent minimum in respect to health which accords with sound ethical judgments, while maintaining the virtues of freedom, variety, and flexibility which are thought to flow from a mixed system such as ours. The decent minimum should reflect some conception of what constitutes tolerable life prospects in general. It should speak quite strongly to things like maternal health and child health, which set the terms under which individuals will compete and develop. On the other hand, techniques which will offer some remote relief from conditions that rarely strike in the prime of life, and which strike late in life because something must, might be thought of as too esoteric to be part of the concept of minimum decent care.

On the other hand, the notion of a decent minimum should include humane and, I would say, worthy surroundings of care for those whom we know we are not going to be able to treat. Here, it seems to me, the emphasis on technology and the attention of highly trained specialists is seriously mistaken. Not only is it unrealistic to imagine that such fancy services can be provided for everyone "as a right," but there is serious doubt whether these kinds of services are what most people really want or can benefit from.

In the end, I will concede very readily that the notion of minimum health care, which it does make sense for our society to recognize as a right, is itself an unstable and changing notion. As my initial historical remarks must have suggested, the concept of a decent minimum is always relative to what is available over all, and what the best which is available might be. I suppose (to revert to my parable of the artificial heart) that if we allowed an artificial heart to be developed under private auspices and to be available only to those who could pay for it, or who could obtain it from specialized eleemosynary institutions, then the time might well come when it would have been so perfected that it would be a reasonable component of what one would consider minimum decent care. And the process of arriving at this new situation would be a process imbued with struggle and political controversy. But since I do not believe in utopias or final solutions, a resolution of the problem of the right to health care having these kinds of tensions within it neither worries me nor leads me to suspect that I am on the wrong track. To my mind, the right track consists in identifying what it is that health care can and cannot provide, in identifying also the cost of health care, and then in deciding how much of this health care, what level of health care, we are ready to underwrite as a floor for our citizenry.

IV. Practical Proposals

Although the process of defining the decent minimum is inherently a political process, there is a great deal which analysis and research can do to make the process rational and satisfactory. Much of this is a negative service, clearing away misconceptions and fallacies. For instance, as I have already argued, to state that our objective is to provide the best medical care for all, regardless of the ability to pay, must be shown up for the misleading slogan that it is. But there are more subtle misconceptions as well. The most pervasive of these deal with the situation of the medical profession.

Many observers look at the medical profession, its history of resistance to social change, and the fact that doctors as a profession enjoy the highest incomes of any group in the nation—somewhere around $50,000 a year on the average—and they draw their own conclusions. They draw the conclusion that therefore what is needed is necessarily more regulation. They look at the oversupply of surgeons in this country. They note the obvious fact of over-recourse to surgery which seems to result, and they conclude that what is needed is more government regulation. For instance, the problems of supply would be met by a kind of doctors' draft, requiring service in underserviced rural areas. Now I would, for a moment, suggest that we consider some alternative explanations and alternative reforms. Perhaps, after all, the irrationalities in the supply of medical personnel, together with the high incomes earned, are the result not of market forces run wild, but the result of a guild system as tight and self-protective as any we know. It is, perhaps, an irony that the medical profession, having persuaded the public of the necessity of strictly limiting entry into the profession, having persuaded the public of the indispensability of highly trained specialists, is now faced with the threat of a kind of doctors' draft to make these rare specialists available to all. Perhaps clearer thinking might indicate that many of the things which highly paid and highly trained doctors do might be done by an army of less pretentious persons.

It is well known, of course, that doctors' fees as such represent the smaller portion of the total health care budget, so it might be thought that I am taking aim at an obvious, vulnerable, and somewhat irrelevant target. Yet this is not so. Though the fees of doctors represent the smaller portion of the medical budget, doctors themselves control almost all of the decisions—from the decision about hospitalization, to the decision whether to prescribe drugs by brand or generic name—which do influence the total cost of medical care. And it is in this respect that doctors have resisted most attempts to make their behavior rational and cost-effective. In general, it is said that this is because no doctor would sacrifice the individual interests of his patient, and this may be a sincere claim. But a certain skepticism is in order. What choice do the patients have to choose more economical systems of delivery? What doctor, for that matter, even gives his patient the choice between a brand and a generic prescription drug?

But it is in the choice of delivery systems themselves that the consumer is most restricted. Most consumers do not have the choice between a variety of delivery systems from prepaid group plans to the present individual fee-for-service system, with each plan costing what it really costs. If the consumer did have this choice, we might soon find out whether the alleged advantages of the fee-for-service system were something the consumer was willing to pay for. But of course we will never find this out if we are committed to underwrite, out of general revenues, the cost of this most expensive possible delivery system. "The best available to all." That is what we tend to do today for those groups whose medical care we do underwrite. The result is that we are trying to drive down the cost of this most expensive delivery system not by changing its organization but by bureaucratic control. What if, instead, each person were assured a certain amount of money to purchase medical services as he chose? If the restrictive practices of the profession itself could be avoided, would this not help a vast variety of delivery systems to grow up, all competing for the consumer's federally assured dollar? And then those who would want what might be considered as fancier or more individualized services could get them, provided only that they were willing to pay more for them.

Finally, there is a feature of our modern situation which is responsible for the present crisis in health care, and for the impossible dilemma posed by the promise of a right to health care. This is a feature of the society and the culture as a whole. I refer to our culture's inability to face and cope with the persistent facts of illness, old age, and death. Because we are little able to come to terms with the hazards which illness proposes, because the old are a burden and an embarrassment, because we pretend that death does not exist, we employ elaborate ruses to put these things out of the ambit of our ordinary lives. The reason why we hospitalize so much more than is rationally required surely goes beyond the vagaries of the health insurance system. Is it not also the result of the fact that the ill are an embarrassment to us, and that we seek to put them away, so we do not have to care for them, while assuaging our consciences that those "best qualified" to care for them are doing so? And in order that the ruse will work, we greatly overstate what it is that these "qualified"

people can do for the ill. Needless to say, they are our willing accomplices in this piece of deception. So it is with the mentally retarded, the aged, and the dying. All of these persons are defined as having an abnormal condition not only justifying but requiring their isolation from us and their care in the hands of "specialists." Perhaps it is time that we recognize that this is part of the neurosis of our age. And of course, those whom we hire to perform our proper human role toward the sick, the old, and the dying can get away with charging a very high price for relieving us of our ordinary human obligations. But is this medical care?

Finally, to avoid misunderstanding, a general theoretic point must be made. My argument must sound harsh and callous—unfeelingly, if not unerringly economic. I have elsewhere argued that it is of the essence of the physician's role and of the patient's expectations that the doctor faced with the patient's need will do everything in his power to alleviate that need.[1] I believe that. I believe that for the individual physician to do less than his best because of some economic calculation of equity or efficiency is a breach of trust. The doctor in his dealings with his patient must not act like a bureaucrat, policy maker, or legislator. But policy makers, voters, and legislators must think in different terms. It is monstrous if an individual doctor thinks like a budget officer when he cares for his patient in need; but it is chaotic and incoherent if budget officers and voters making general policy think like doctors at the bedside.

Note

1. In my book, *Medical Experimentations: Personal Integrity and Social Policy* (Amsterdam and New York: Associated Scientific Publishers/Elsevier, 1974).

Medical Care as a Right: A Refutation

Robert M. Sade

The current debate on health care in the United States is of the first order of importance to the health professions, and of no less importance to

the political future of the nation, for precedents are now being set that will be applied to the rest of American society in the future. In the enormous

Reprinted by permission from the New England Journal of Medicine 285 *(December 2, 1971): pages 1288–1292. Editor's Note: The footnotes in this reading have been renumbered.*

volume of verbiage that has poured forth, certain fundamental issues have been so often misrepresented that they have now become commonly accepted fallacies. This paper will be concerned with the most important of these misconceptions, that health care is a right, as well as a brief consideration of some of its corollary fallacies.

Rights—Morality and Politics

The concept of rights has its roots in the moral nature of man and its practical expression in the political system that he creates. Both morality and politics must be discussed before the relation between political rights and health care can be appreciated.

A "right" defines a freedom of action. For instance, a right to a material object is the uncoerced choice of the use to which that object will be put; a right to a specific action, such as free speech, is the freedom to engage in that activity without forceful repression. The moral foundation of the rights of man begins with the fact that he is a living creature: he has the right to his own life. All other rights are corollaries of this primary one; without the right to life, there can be no others, and the concept of rights itself becomes meaningless.

The freedom to live, however, does not automatically ensure life. For man, a specific course of action is required to sustain his life, a course of action that must be guided by reason and reality and has as its goal the creation or acquisition of material values, such as food and clothing, and intellectual values, such as self-esteem and integrity. His moral system is the means by which he is able to select the values that will support his life and achieve his happiness.

Man must maintain a rather delicate homeostasis in a highly demanding and threatening environment, but has at his disposal a unique and efficient mechanism for dealing with it: his mind. His mind is able to perceive, to identify percepts, to integrate them into concepts, and to use those concepts in choosing actions suitable to the maintenance of his life. The rational function of mind is volitional, however; a man must *choose* to think, to be aware, to evaluate, to make conscious decisions. The extent to which he is able to achieve his goals will be directly proportional to his commitment to reason in seeking them.

The right to life implies three corollaries: the right to select the values that one deems necessary to sustain one's own life; the right to exercise one's own judgment of the best course of action to achieve the chosen values; and the right to dispose of those values, once gained, in any way one chooses, without coercion by other men. The denial of any one of these corollaries severely compromises or destroys the right to life itself. A man who is not allowed to choose his own goals, is prevented from setting his own course in achieving those goals and is not free to dispose of the values he has earned is no less than a slave to those who usurp those rights. The right to private property, therefore, is essential and indispensable to maintaining free men in a free society.

Thus, it is the nature of man as a living, thinking being that determines his rights—his "natural rights." The concept of natural rights was slow in dawning on human civilization. The first political expression of that concept had its beginnings in 17th and 18th century England through such exponents as John Locke and Edmund Burke, but came to its brilliant debut as a form of government after the American Revolution. Under the leadership of such men as Thomas Paine and Thomas Jefferson, the concept of man as a being sovereign unto himself, rather than a subdivision of the sovereignty of a king, emperor or state, was incorporated into the formal structure of government for the first time. Protection of the lives and property of individual citizens was the salient characteristic of the Constitution of 1787. Ayn Rand has pointed out that the principle of protection of the individual against the coercive force of government made the United States the first moral society in history.[1]

In a free society, man exercises his right to sustain his own life by producing economic values in the form of goods and services that he is, or should be, free to exchange with other men who are similarly free to trade with him or not. The economic values produced, however, are not given as gifts by nature, but exist only by virtue of the thought and effort of individual men. Goods and services are thus owned as a consequence of the right to sustain life by one's own physical and mental effort.

If the chain of natural rights is interrupted, and the right to a loaf of bread, for example, is proclaimed as primary (avoiding the necessity of earning it), every man owns a loaf of bread, regardless of who produced it. Since ownership is the power of disposal,[2] every man may take his loaf from the baker and dispose of it as he wishes with or without the baker's permission. Another element has thus been introduced into the relation between men: the use of force. It is crucial to observe who has initiated the use of force: it is the man who demands unearned bread as a right, not the man who produced it. At the level of an unstructured society it is clear who is moral and who immoral. The man who acted rationally by producing food to support his own life is moral. The man who expropriated the bread by force is immoral.

To protect this basic right to provide for the support of one's own life, men band together for their mutual protection and form governments. This is the only proper function of government: to provide for the defense of individuals against those who would take their lives or property by force. The state is the repository for retaliatory force in a just society wherein the only actions prohibited to individuals are those of physical harm or the threat of physical harm to other men. The closest that man has ever come to achieving this ideal of government was in this country after its War of Independence.

When a government ignores the progression of natural rights arising from the right to life, and agrees with a man, a group of men, or even a majority of its citizens, that every man has a right to a loaf of bread, it must protect that right by the passage of laws ensuring that everyone gets his loaf—in the process depriving the baker of the freedom to dispose of his own product. If the baker disobeys the law, asserting the priority of his right to support himself by his own rational disposition of the fruits of his mental and physical labor, he will be taken to court by force or threat of force where he will have more property forcibly taken from him (by fine) or have his liberty taken away (by incarceration). Now the initiator of violence is the government itself. The degree to which a government exercises its monopoly on the retaliatory use of force by asserting a claim to the lives and property of its citizens is the degree to which it has eroded its own legitimacy. It is a frequently overlooked fact that behind every law is a policeman's gun or a soldier's bayonet. When the gun and bayonet are used to initiate violence, to take property or to restrict liberty by force, there

are no longer any rights, for the lives of the citizens belong to the state. In a just society with a moral government, it is clear that the only "right" to the bread belongs to the baker, and that a claim by any other man to that right is unjustified and can be enforced only by violence or the threat of violence.

Rights—Politics and Medicine

The concept of medical care as the patient's right is immoral because it denies the most fundamental of all rights, that of a man to his own life and the freedom of action to support it. Medical care is neither a right nor a privilege: it is a service that is provided by doctors and others to people who wish to purchase it. It is the provision of this service that a doctor depends upon for his livelihood, and is his means of supporting his own life. If the right to health care belongs to the patient, he starts out owning the services of a doctor without the necessity of either earning them or receiving them as a gift from the only man who has the right to give them: the doctor himself. In the narrative above substitute "doctor" for "baker" and "medical service" for "bread." American medicine is now at the point in the story where the state has proclaimed the nonexistent "right" to medical care as a fact of public policy, and has begun to pass the laws to enforce it. The doctor finds himself less and less his own master and more and more controlled by forces outside of his own judgment.

For instance, under the proposed Kennedy-Griffiths bill,[3] there will be a "Health Security Board," which will be responsible for administering the new controls to be imposed on doctors, hospitals and other "providers" of health care (Sec. 121). Specialized services, such as major surgery, will be done by "qualified specialists" [Sec. 22(b)(2)], such qualifications being determined by the Board (Sec. 42). Furthermore, the patient can no longer exercise his own initiative in finding a specialist to do his operation, since he must be referred to the specialist by a nonspecialist—i.e., a general practitioner or a family doctor [Sec. 22(b)]. Licensure by his own state will not be enough to be a qualified practitioner; physicians will also be subject to a second set of standards, those established by the Board [Sec. 42(a)]. Doctors will no longer be considered competent to determine their own needs for continuing education, but must meet requirements established by the Board [Sec. 42(c)]. The professional staff of a hospital will no longer be able to determine which of its members are qualified to perform which kinds of major surgery; specialty-board certification or eligibility will be required, with certain exceptions that include meeting standards established by the Board [Sec. 42(d)].

Control of doctors through control of the hospitals in which they practice will also be exercised by the Board by way of a list of requirements, the last of which is a "sleeper" that will by its vagueness allow the Board almost any regulation of the hospital: the hospital must meet "such other requirements as the Board finds necessary in the interest of quality of care and the safety of patients in the institution" [Sec. 43(i)]. Hospitals will also not be allowed to undertake construction without higher approval by a state agency or by the Board (Sec. 52).

In the name of better organization and coordination of services, hospitals, nursing homes and other providers will be further controlled through the Board's power to issue directives forcing the provider to furnish services selected by the Board [Sec. 131(a)(1),(2)] at a place selected by the Board [Sec. 131(a)(3)]. The Board can also direct these providers to form associations with one another of various sorts, including "making available to one provider the professional and technical skills of another" [Sec. 131(a)(B)], and such other linkages as the Board thinks best [Sec. 131(a)(4)(C)].

These are only a few of the bill's controls of the health-care industry. It is difficult to believe that such patent subjugation of an entire profession could ever be considered a fit topic for discussion in any but the darkest corner of a country founded on the principles of life and liberty. Yet the Kennedy-Griffiths bill is being seriously debated today in the Congress of the United States.

The irony of this bill is that, on the basis of the philosophic premises of its authors, it does provide a rationally organized system for attempting to fulfill its goals, such as "making health services available to all residents of the United States." If the government is to spend tens of billions of dollars on health services, it must assure in some way that the money is not being wasted. Every bill cur-

rently before the national legislature does, should, and must provide some such controls. The Kennedy-Griffiths bill is the closest we have yet come to the logical conclusion and inevitable consequence of two fundamental fallacies: that health care is a right, and that doctors and other health workers will function as efficiently serving as chattels of the state as they will living as sovereign human beings. It is not, and they will not.

Any act of force is anti-mind. It is a confession of the failure of persuasion, the failure of reason. When politicians say that the health system must be forced into a mold of their own design, they are admitting their inability to persuade doctors and patients to use the plan voluntarily; they are proclaiming the supremacy of the state's logic over the judgments of the individual minds of all concerned with health care. Statists throughout history have never learned that compulsion and reason are contradictory, that a forced mind cannot think effectively and, by extension, that a regimented profession will eventually choke and stagnate from its own lack of freedom. A persuasive example of this is the moribund condition of medicine as a profession in Sweden, a country that has enjoyed socialized medicine since 1955. Werkö, a Swedish physician, has stated: "The details and the complicated working schedule have not yet been determined in all hospitals and districts, but the general feeling of belonging to a free profession, free to decide—at least in principle—how to organize its work has been lost. Many hospital-based physicians regard their work now with an apathy previously unknown."[4] One wonders how American legislators will like having their myocardial infarctions treated by apathetic internists, their mitral valves replaced by apathetic surgeons, their wives' tumors removed by apathetic gynecologists. They will find it very difficult to legislate self-esteem, integrity and competence into the doctors whose minds and judgments they have throttled.

If anyone doubts that health legislation involves the use of force, a dramatic demonstration of the practical political meaning of the "right to health care" was acted out in Quebec in the closing months of 1970.[5] In that unprecedented threat of violence by a modern Western government against a group of its citizens, the doctors of Quebec were literally imprisoned in the province by Bill 41, possibly the most repressive piece of legislation ever enacted against the medical profession, and far more worthy of the Soviet Union or Red China than a western democracy. Doctors objecting to a new Medicare law were forced to continue working under penalty of jail sentence and fines of up to $500 a day away from their practices. Those who spoke out publicly against the bill were subject to jail sentences of up to a year and fines of up to $50,000 a day. The facts that the doctors did return to work and that no one was therefore jailed or fined do not mitigate the nature or implications of the passage of Bill 41. Although the dispute between the Quebec physicians and their government was not one of principle but of the details of compensation, the reaction of the state to resistance against coercive professional regulation was a classic example of the naked force that lies behind every act of social legislation.

Any doctor who is forced by law to join a group or a hospital he does not choose, or is prevented by law from prescribing a drug he thinks is best for his patient, or is compelled by law to make any decision he would not otherwise have made, is being forced to act against his own mind, which means forced to act against his own life. He is also being forced to violate his most fundamental professional commitment, that of using his own best judgment at all times for the greatest benefit of his patient. It is remarkable that this principle has never been identified by a public voice in the medical profession, and that the vast majority of doctors in this country are being led down the path to civil servitude, never knowing that their feelings of uneasy foreboding have a profoundly moral origin, and never recognizing that the main issues at stake are not those being formulated in Washington, but are their own honor, integrity and freedom, and their own survival as sovereign human beings.

Some Corollaries

The basic fallacy that health care is a right has led to several corollary fallacies, among them the following:

That health is primarily a community or social rather than an individual concern.[6] A simple calcula-

tion from American mortality statistics[7] quickly corrects that false concept: 67 per cent of deaths in 1967 were due to diseases known to be caused or exacerbated by alcohol, tobacco smoking or overeating, or were due to accidents. Each of those factors is either largely or wholly correctable by individual action. Although no statistics are available, it is likely that morbidity, with the exception of common respiratory infections, has a relation like that of mortality to personal habits and excesses.

That state medicine has worked better in other countries than free enterprise has worked here. There is no evidence to support that contention, other than anecdotal testimonials and the spurious citation of infant mortality and longevity statistics. There is, on the other hand, a good deal of evidence to the contrary.[8,9]

That the provision of medical care somehow lies outside the laws of supply and demand, and that government-controlled health care will be free care. In fact, no service or commodity lies outside the economic laws. Regarding health care, market demand, individual want, and medical need are entirely different things, and have a very complex relation with the cost and the total supply of available care, as recently discussed and clarified by Jeffers et al.[10] They point out that " 'health is purchaseable,' meaning that somebody has to pay for it, individually or collectively, at the expense of foregoing the current or future consumption of other things." The question is whether the decision of how to allocate the consumer's dollar should belong to the consumer or to the state. It has already been shown that the choice of how a doctor's services should be rendered belongs only to the doctor: in the same way the choice of whether to buy a doctor's service rather than some other commodity or service belongs to the consumer as a logical consequence of the right to his own life.

That opposition to national health legislation is tantamount to opposition to progress in health care. Progress is made by the free interaction of free minds developing new ideas in an atmosphere conducive to experimentation and trial. If group practice really is better than solo, we will find out because the success of groups will result in more groups (which has, in fact, been happening); if prepaid comprehensive care really is the best form of practice, it will succeed and the health industry will swell with new Kaiser–Permanente plans. But let one of these or any other form of practice become the law, and the system is in a straightjacket that will stifle progress. Progress requires freedom of action, and that is precisely what national health legislation aims at restricting.

That doctors should help design the legislation for a national health system, since they must live with and within whatever legislation is enacted. To accept this concept is to concede to the opposition its philosophic premises, and thus to lose the battle. The means by which nonproducers and hangers-on throughout history have been able to expropriate material and intellectual values from the producers has been identified only relatively recently: the sanction of the victim.[11] Historically, few people have lost their freedom and their rights without some degree of complicity in the plunder. If the American medical profession accepts the concept of health care as the right of the patient, it will have earned the Kennedy–Griffiths bill by default. The alternative for any health professional is to withhold his sanction and make clear who is being victimized. Any physician can say to those who would shackle his judgment and control his profession: I do not recognize your right to my life and my mind, which belong to me and me alone; I will not participate in any legislated solution to any health problem.

In the face of the raw power that lies behind government programs, nonparticipation is the only way in which personal values can be maintained. And it is only with the attainment of the highest of those values—integrity, honesty and self-esteem—that the physician can achieve his most important professional value, the absolute priority of the welfare of his patients.

The preceding discussion should not be interpreted as proposing that there are no problems in the delivery of medical care. Problems such as high cost, few doctors, low quantity of available care in economically depressed areas may be real, but it is naïve to believe that governmental solutions through coercive legislation can be anything but shortsighted and formulated on the basis of political expediency. The only long-range plan that can hope to provide for the day after tomorrow is a "nonsystem"—that is, a system that proscribes the imposition by force (legislation) of any one group's conception of the best forms of medical care. We must identify our problems and seek to solve them by experimentation and trial in an atmosphere of freedom from compulsion. Our sanction of anything less will mean the loss of our personal values, the death of our profession, and a heavy blow to political liberty.

Notes

1. Rand, A. Man's rights, Capitalism: The unknown ideal. New York, New American Library, Inc., 1967, pp 320–329.

2. Von Mises, L. Socialism: An economic and sociological analysis. New Haven, Yale University Press, 1951, pp 37–55.

3. Kennedy, E. M. Introduction of the Health Security Act. Congressional Record 116:S 14338–S 14361, 1970.

4. Werkö, L. Swedish medical care in transition. N Engl J Med 284:360–366, 1971.

5. Quebec Medicare and Medical Services Withdrawal. Toronto, Canadian Medical Association, October 19, 1970.

6. Millis, J. S. Wisdom? Health? Can society guarantee them? N Engl J Med 283:260–261, 1970.

7. Department of Health, Education, and Welfare, Public Health Service: Vital Statistics of the United States 1967. Vol II, Mortality. Part A. Washington, DC, Government Printing Office, 1969, pp 1–7.

8. Financing Medical Care: An appraisal of foreign programs. Edited by H. Shoeck. Caldwell, Idaho, Caxton Printers, Inc, 1962.

9. Lynch, M. J.; Raphael, S. S. Medicine and the State. Springfield, Illinois, Charles C. Thomas, 1963.

10. Jeffers, J. R.; Bognanno, M. F.; Bartlett, J. C. On the demand versus need for medical services and the concept of "shortage." Am J Publ Health 61:46–63, 1971.

11. Rand, A. Atlas Shrugged. New York, Random House, 1957, p 1066.

Social Justice and Equal Access to Health Care

Gene Outka

I want to consider the following question. Is it possible to understand and to justify morally a societal goal that increasing numbers of people, including Americans, accept as normative? The goal is: the assurance of comprehensive health services for every person irrespective of income or geographic location. Indeed, the goal now has almost the status of a platitude. Currently in the United States politicians in various camps give it at least verbal endorsement.[1] I do not propose to examine the possible sociological determinants in this emergent consensus. I hope to show that whatever these determinants are, one may offer a plausible case in defense of the goal on reasonable grounds. To demonstrate why appeals to the goal get so successfully under our skins, I shall have recourse to a set of conceptions of social justice. Some of the standard conceptions, found in a number of writings on justice, will do.[2] By reflecting on them it seems to me a prima facie case can be established, namely, that every person in the entire resident population should have equal access to health care delivery.

The case is prima facie only. I wish to set aside as far as possible a related question which comes readily enough to mind. In the world of "suboptimal alternatives," with the constraints, for example, that impinge on the government as it makes decisions about resource allocation, what is one to say? What criteria should be employed? Paul Ramsey in *The Patient as Person* thinks that the large question of how to choose between medical and other societal priorities is "almost, if not altogether, incorrigible to moral reasoning."[3] Whether it is or not is a matter that must be ignored for the present. One may simply observe in passing that choices are unavoidable nonetheless, as Ramsey acknowledges, even where the government allows them to be made by default, so that in some instances they are determined largely by which private pressure groups prove to be dominant. In any event, there is virtue in taking up one complicated question at a time, and we need to get the thrust of the case for equal access before us. It is

enough to observe now that Americans attach an obviously high priority to organized health care. National health expenditures for the fiscal year 1972 were $83.4 billion.[4] Even if such an enormous sum is not entirely adequate, we may still ask: How are we to justify spending whatever we do in accordance as far as possible with the goal of equal access? The answer I propose involves distinguishing various conceptions of social justice and trying to show which of these apply or fail to apply to health care considerations. . . .

Which then among the standard conceptions of social justice appear to be particularly relevant or irrelevant? Let us consider the following five:

1   To each according to his merit or desert.

2   To each according to his societal contribution.

3   To each according to his contribution in satisfying whatever is freely desired by others in the open marketplace of supply and demand.

4   To each according to his needs.

5   Similar treatment for similar cases.

In general I shall argue that the first three of these are less relevant because of certain distinctive features that health crises possess. I shall focus on crises here not because I think preventive care is unimportant (the opposite is true), but because the crisis situation shows most clearly the special significance we attach to medical treatment as an institutionalized activity or social practice, and the basic purpose we suppose it to have.

To Each According to His Merit or Desert

Meritarian conceptions, above all perhaps, are grading ones: advantages are allocated in accordance with amounts of energy expended or kinds of results achieved. What is judged is particular conduct that distinguishes persons from one another and not only the fact that all the parties are human beings. Sometimes a competitive aspect looms large.

From the *Journal of Religious Ethics,* Vol. 2, no. 1 (Spring 1974), pp. 11–32. Reprinted by permission.

In certain contexts it is illuminating to distinguish between efforts and achievements. In the case of efforts one characteristically focuses on the individual: rewards are based on the pains one takes. Some have supposed, for example, that entry into the kingdom of heaven is linked more directly to energy displayed and fidelity shown than to successful results attained.

To assess achievements is to weigh actual performance and productive contributions. The academic prize is awarded to the student with the highest grade-point average, regardless of the amount of midnight oil he or she burned in preparing for the examinations. Sometimes we may exclaim, "It's just not fair," when person X writes a brilliant paper with little effort while we are forced to devote more time with less impressive results. But then our complaint may be directed against differences in innate ability and talent which no expenditure of effort altogether removes.

After the difference between effort and achievement, and related distinctions, have been acknowledged, what should be stressed is the general importance of meritarian or desert criteria in the thinking of most people about justice. These criteria may serve to illuminate a number of disputes about the justice of various practices and institutional arrangements in our society. It may help to explain, for instance, the resentment among the working class against the welfare system. However wrongheaded or self-deceptive the resentment often is, particularly when directed toward those who want to work but for various reasons beyond their control cannot, at its better moments it involves in effect an appeal to desert considerations. "Something for nothing" is repudiated as unjust; benefits should be proportional (or at least related) to costs; those who can make an effort should do so, whatever the degree of their training or significance of their contribution to society; and so on. So, too, persons deserve to have what they have labored for; unless they infringe on the works of others their efforts and achievements are justly theirs. . . .

. . . I would simply hold now (1) that the idea of justice is not exhaustively characterized by the notion of desert, even if one agrees that the latter plays an important role; and (2) that the notion of desert is especially ill suited to play an important role in the determination of policies that should govern a system of health care.

Why is it so ill suited? Here we encounter some of the distinctive features that health crises possess. Health crises seem nonmeritarian because they occur so often for reasons beyond our control or power to predict. They frequently fall without discrimination on the (according-to-merit) just and unjust i.e., the virtuous and the wicked, the industrious and the slothful alike.

While we may believe that virtues and vices cannot depend upon natural contingencies, we are bound to admit, it seems, that many health crises do. It makes sense therefore to say that we are equal in being randomly susceptible to these crises. Even those who ascribe a prominent role to desert acknowledge that justice has also properly to do with pleas of "But I could not help it."[5] One seeks to distinguish such cases from those acknowledged to be praiseworthy or blameworthy. Then it seems unfair as well as unkind to discriminate among those who suffer health crises on the basis of their personal deserts. For it would be odd to maintain that a newborn child deserves his hemophilia or the tumor afflicting her spine.

These considerations help to explain why the following rough distinction is often made. Bernard Williams, for example, in his discussion of "equality in unequal circumstances," identifies two different sorts of inequality, inequality of merit and inequality of need, and two corresponding goods, those earned by effort and those demanded by need.[6] Medical treatment in the event of illness is located under the umbrella of need. He concludes: "Leaving aside preventive medicine, the proper ground of distribution of medical care is ill health: this is a necessary truth."[7] An irrational state of affairs is held to obtain if those whose needs are the same are treated unequally, when needs are the ground of the treatment. One might put the point this way. When people are equal in the relevant respects—in this case when their needs are the same and occur in a context of random, undeserved susceptibility—that by itself is a good reason for treating them equally.[8]

In many societies, however, a second necessary condition for the receipt of medical treatment exists de facto: the possession of money. This is not the place to consider the general question of when inequalities in wealth may be regarded as just. It is enough to note that one can plausibly appeal to all of the conceptions of justice we are embarked in sorting out. A person may be thought to be entitled to a higher income when he works more, contributes more, risks more, and not simply when he needs more. We may think it fair that the industrious should have more money than the slothful and the surgeon more than the tobacconist. The difficulty comes in the misfit between the reasons for differential incomes and the reasons for receiving medical treatment. The former may include a pluralistic set of claims in which different notions of justice must be meshed. The latter are more monistically focused on needs, and the other notions not accorded a similar relevance. Yet money may nonetheless remain as a causally necessary condition for receiving medical treatment. It may be the power to secure what one needs. The senses in which health crises are distinctive may then be insufficiently determinative for the policies which govern the actual availability of treatment. The nearly automatic links between income, prestige, and the receipt of comparatively higher quality medical treatment should then be subjected to critical scrutiny. For unequal treatment of the rich ill and the poor ill is unjust if, again, needs rather than differential income constitute the ground of such treatment.

Suppose one agrees that it is important to recognize the misfit between the reasons for differential incomes and the reasons for receiving medical treatment, and that therefore income as such should not govern the actual availability of treatment. One may still ask whether the case so far relies excessively on "pure" instances where desert considerations are admittedly out of place. That there are such pure instances, tumors afflicting the spine, hemophilia, and so on, is not denied. Yet it is an exaggeration if we go on and regard all health crises as utterly unconnected with desert. Note for example that Williams leaves aside preventive medicine. And if in a cool hour we examine the statistics, we find that a vast number of deaths occur each year due to causes not always beyond our control, e.g., automobile accidents, drugs, alcohol, tobacco, obesity, and so on. In some final reckoning it seems that many persons (though crucially, not all) have an effect on, and arguably a responsibility for, their own medical needs. Consider the following bidders for

emergency care: (1) a person with a heart attack who is seriously overweight; (2) a football hero who has suffered a concussion; (3) a man with lung cancer who has smoked cigarettes for forty years; (4) a sixty-year-old man who has always taken excellent care of himself and is suddenly stricken with leukemia; (5) a three-year-old girl who has swallowed poison left out carelessly by her parents; (6) a fourteen-year-old boy who has been beaten without provocation by a gang and suffers brain damage and recurrent attacks of uncontrollable terror; (7) a college student who has slashed his wrists (and not for the first time) from a psychological need for attention; (8) a woman raised in the ghetto who is found unconscious due to an overdose of heroin.

These cases help to show why the whole subject of medical treatment is so crucial and so perplexing. They attest to some melancholy elements in human experience. People suffer in varying ratios the effects of their natural and undeserved vulnerabilities, the irresponsibility and brutality of others, and their own desires and weaknesses. In some final reckoning, then, desert considerations seem not irrelevant to many health crises. The practical applicability of this admission, however, in the instance of health care delivery, appears limited. We may agree that it underscores the importance of preventive health care by stressing the influence we sometimes have over our medical needs. But if we try to foster such care by increasing the penalties for neglect, we normally confine ourselves to calculations about incentives. At the risk of being denounced in some quarters as censorious and puritannical, perhaps we should for example levy far higher taxes on alcohol and tobacco and pump the dollars directly into health care programs rather than (say) into highway building. Yet these steps would by no means lead necessarily to a demand that we correlate in some strict way a demonstrated effort to be temperate with the receipt of privileged medical treatment as a reward. Would it be feasible to allocate the additional tax monies to the man with leukemia before the overweight man suffering a heart attack on the ground of a difference in desert? At the point of emergency care at least, it seems impracticable for the doctor to discriminate between these cases, to make meritarian judgments at the point of catastrophe. And the number of persons who are in need of medical treatment for reasons utterly beyond their control remains a datum with tenacious relevance. There are those who suffer the ravages of a tornado, are handicapped by a genetic defect, beaten without provocation, etc. A commitment to the basic purpose of medical care and to the institutions for achieving it involves the recognition of this persistent state of affairs.

To Each According to His Societal Contribution

This conception gives moral primacy to notions such as the public interest, the common good, the welfare of the community, or the greatest good of the greatest number. Here one judges the social consequences of particular conduct. The formula can be construed in at least two ways.[9] It may refer to the interest of the social group considered collectively, where the group has some independent life all its own. The group's welfare is the decisive criterion for determining what constitutes any member's proper share. Or the common good may refer only to an aggregation of distinct individuals and considered distributively.

Either version accords such a primacy to what is socially advantageous as to be unacceptable not only to defenders of need, but also, it would seem, of desert. For the criteria of effort and achievement are often conceived along rather individualistic lines. The pains an agent takes or the results he brings about deserve recompense, whether or not the public interest is directly served. No automatic harmony then is necessarily assumed between his just share as individually earned and his proper share from the vantage point of the common good. Moreover, the test of social advantage *simpliciter* obviously threatens the agapeic concern with some minimal consideration due each person which is never to be disregarded for the sake of long-range social benefits. No one should be considered as *merely* a means or instrument.

The relevance of the canon of social productiveness to health crises may accordingly also be challenged. Indeed, such crises may cut against it in that they occur more frequently to those whose comparative contribution to the general welfare is less, e.g., the aged, the disabled, children.

Consider for example Paul Ramsey's persuasive critique of social and economic criteria for the allocation of a single scarce medical resource. He begins by recounting the imponderables that faced the widely discussed "public committee" at the Swedish Hospital in Seattle when it deliberated in the early 1960s. The sparse resource in this case was the kidney machine. The committee was charged with the responsibility of selecting among patients suffering chronic renal failure those who were to receive dialysis. Its criteria were broadly social and economic. Considerations weighed included age, sex, marital status, number of dependents, income, net worth, educational background, occupation, past performance, and future potential. The application of such criteria proved to be exceedingly problematic. Should someone with six children always have priority over an artist or composer? Were those who arranged matters so that their families would not burden society to be penalized in effect for being provident? And so on. Two critics of the committee found "a disturbing picture of the bourgeoisie sparing the bourgeoisie," and observed that "the Pacific Northwest is no place for a Henry David Thoreau with bad kidneys."[10]

The mistake, Ramsey believes, is to introduce criteria of social worthiness in the first place. In those situations of choice where not all can be saved and yet all need not die, "the equal right of every human being to live, and not relative personal or social worth, should be the ruling principle."[11] The principle leads to a criterion of "random choice among equals" expressed by a lottery scheme or a practice of "first come, first served." Several reasons stand behind Ramsey's defense of the criterion of random choice. First, a religious belief in the equality of persons before God leads intelligibly to a refusal to choose between those who are dying in any way other than random patient selection. Otherwise their equal value as human beings is threatened. Second, a moral primacy is ascribed to survival over other (perhaps superior) interests persons may have, in that it is the condition of everything else. "Life is a value incommensurate with all others, and so not negotiable by bartering one man's worth against another's."[12] Third, the entire enterprise of estimating a person's social worth is viewed with final skepticism. "We have no way of knowing how really and truly to estimate a man's societal worth or his worth to others or to himself in unfocused social situations in the ordinary lives of men in their communities."[13] This statement, incidentally, appears to allow something other than randomness in *focused* social situations; when, say, a president or prime minister and the owner of the local bar rush for the last place in the bomb shelter, and the knowledge of the former can save many lives. In any event, I have been concerned with a restricted point to which Ramsey's discussion brings illustrative support. The canon of social productiveness is notoriously difficult to apply as a workable criterion for distributing medical services to those who need them.

One can go further. A system of health care delivery that treats people on the basis of the medical care required may often go against (at least narrowly conceived) calculations of societal advantage. For example, the health care needs of people tend to rise during that period of their lives, signaled by retirement, when their incomes and social productivity are declining. More generally:

> Some 40 to 50 per cent of the American people—the aged, children, the dependent poor, and those with some significant chronic disability are in categories requiring relatively large amounts of medical care but with inadequate resources to purchase such care.[14]

If one agrees, for whatever reasons, with the agapeic judgment that each person should be regarded as irreducibly valuable, then one cannot succumb to a social productiveness criterion of human worth. Interests are to be equally considered even when people have ceased to be, or are not yet, or perhaps never will be, public assets.

To Each According to His Contribution in Satisfying Whatever Is Freely Desired by Others in the Open Marketplace of Supply and Demand

Here we have a test which, though similar to the preceding one, concentrates on what is desired de facto by certain segments of the community rather than the community as a whole, and on the relative scarcity of the service rendered. It is tantamount to the canon of supply and demand as espoused by various laissez-faire theoreticians.[15] Rewards should be given to those who by virtue of special skill, prescience, risk-taking, and the like discern what is desired and are able to take the requisite steps to bring satisfaction. A surgeon, it may be argued, contributes more than a nurse because of the greater training and skill required, burdens borne, and effective care provided, and should be compensated accordingly. So too, perhaps, a star quarterback on a pro football team should be remunerated even more highly because of the rare athletic prowess needed, hazards involved, and widespread demand to watch him play.

This formula does not then call for the weighing of the value of various contributions, and tends to conflate needs and wants under a notion of desires. It also assumes that a prominent part is assigned to consumer free choice. The consumer should be at liberty to express his preferences, and to select from a variety of competing goods and services. Those who resist many changes currently proposed in the organization and financing of health care delivery in the U.S.A.—such as national health insurance—often do so by appealing to some variant of this formula.

Yet it seems health crises are often of overriding importance when they occur. They appear therefore not satisfactorily accommodated to the context of a free marketplace where consumers may freely choose among alternative goods and services.

To clarify what is at stake in the above contention, let us examine an opposing case. Robert M. Sade, M.D., published an article in *The New England Journal of Medicine* entitled "Medical Care as a Right: A Refutation." He attacks programs of national health insurance in the name of a person's right to select one's own values, determine how they may be realized, and dispose of them if one chooses without coercion from other men. The values in question are construed as economic ones in the context of supply and demand. So we read:

> In a free society, man exercises his right to sustain his own life by producing economic values in the form of goods and services that he is, or should be, free to exchange with other men who are similarly free to trade with him or not. The economic values pro-

duced, however, are not given as gifts by nature, but exist only by virtue of the thought and effort of individual men. Goods and services are thus owned as a consequence of the right to sustain life by one's own physical and mental effort.[16]

Sade compares the situation of the physician to that of the baker. The one who produces a loaf of bread should as owner have the power to dispose of his own product. It is immoral simply to expropriate the bread without the baker's permission. Similarly, "medical care is neither a right nor a privilege: it is a service that is provided by doctors and others to people who wish to purchase it."[17] Any coercive regulation of professional practices by the society at large is held to be analogous to taking the bread from the baker without his consent. Such regulation violates the freedom of the physician over his own services and will lead inevitably to provider apathy.

The analogy surely misleads. To assume that doctors autonomously produce goods and services in a fashion closely akin to a baker is grossly oversimplified. The baker may himself rely on the agricultural produce of others, yet there is a crucial difference in the degree of dependence. Modern physicians depend on the achievements of medical technology and the entire scientific base underlying it, all of which is made possible by a host of persons whose salaries are often notably less. Moreover, the amount of taxpayer support for medical research and education is too enormous to make any such unqualified case for provider autonomy plausible.

However conceptually clouded Sade's article may be, its stress on a free exchange of goods and services reflects one historically influential rationale for much American medical practice. And he applies it not only to physicians but also to patients or "consumers."

> The question is whether the decision of how to allocate the consumer's dollar should belong to the consumer or to the state. It has already been shown that the choice of how a doctor's services should be rendered belongs only to the doctor: in the same way the choice of whether to buy a doctor's service rather than some other commodity or service belongs to the consumer as a logical consequence of the right to his own life.[18]

This account is misguided, I think, because it ignores the overriding importance that is so often attached to health crises. When lumps appear on someone's neck, it usually makes little sense to talk of choosing whether to buy a doctor's service rather than a color television set. References to just tradeoffs suddenly seem out of place. No compensation suffices, since the penalties may differ so much.

There is even a further restriction on consumer choice. One's knowledge in these circumstances is comparatively so limited. The physician makes most of the decisions: about diagnosis, treatment, hospitalization, number of return visits, and so on. In brief:

> The consumer knows very little about the medical services he is buying—probably less than about any other service he purchases. . . . While [he] can still play a role in policing the market, that role is much more limited in the field of health care than in almost any other area of private economic activity.[19]

For much of the way, then, an appeal to supply and demand and consumer choice is not quite fitting. It neglects the issue of the value of various contributions. And it fails to allow for the recognition that medical treatments may be overridingly desired. In contexts of catastrophe, at any rate, when life itself is threatened, most persons (other than those who are apathetic or seek to escape from the terrifying prospects) cannot take medical care to be merely one option among others.

To Each According to His Needs

The concept of needs is sometimes taken to apply to an entire range of interests that concern a person's "psychophysical existence."[20] On this wide usage, to attribute a need to someone is to say that the person lacks what is thought to conduce to his or her "welfare"—understood in both a physiological sense (e.g., for food, drink, shelter, and health) and a psychological one (e.g., for continuous human affection and support).

Yet even in the case of such a wide usage, what the person lacks is typically assumed to be basic. Attention is restricted to recurrent considerations rather than to every possible individual whim or frivolous pursuit. So one is not surprised to meet with the contention that a preferable rendering of this formula would be: "to each according to his essential needs."[21] This contention seems to me well taken. It implies, for one thing, that basic needs are distinguishable from felt needs or wants. For the latter may encompass expressions of personal preference unrelated to considerations of survival or subsistence, and sometimes artificially generated by circumstances of rising affluence in the society at large.

Essential needs are also typically assumed to be given rather than acquired. They are not constituted by any action for which the person is responsible by virtue of his or her distinctively greater effort. It is almost as if the designation "innocent" may be linked illuminatingly to need, as retribution, punishment, and so on, are to desert, and in complex ways, to freedom. Thus essential needs are likewise distinguishable from deserts. Where needs are unequal, one thinks of them as fortuitously distributed; as part, perhaps, of a kind of "natural lottery."[22] So very often the advantages of health and the burdens of illness, for example, strike one as arbitrary effects of the lottery. It seems wrong to say that a newborn child deserves as a reward all of his faculties when he has done nothing in particular that distinguishes him from another newborn who comes into the world deprived of one or more of them. Similarly, though crudely, many religious believers do not look on natural events as personal deserts. They are not inclined to pronounce sentences such as, "That evil person with incurable cancer got what he deserved." They are disposed instead to search for some distinction between what they may call the conditions of finitude on the one hand and sin and moral evil on the other. If the distinction is "ultimately" invalid, in this life it seems inscrutably so. Here and now it may be usefully drawn. Inequalities in the need for medical treatment are taken, it appears, to reflect the conditions of finitude more than anything else.

One can even go on to argue that among our basic or essential needs, the case of medical treatment is conspicuous in the following sense. While food and shelter are not matters about which we are at liberty to please ourselves, they are at least predictable. We can plan, for instance, to store up food and fuel for the winter. It may be held that responsibility increases along with the power to predict. If so, then many health crises seem peculi-arly random and uncontrollable. Cancer, given the present state of knowledge at any rate, is a contingent disaster, whereas hunger is a steady threat. Who will need serious medical care, and when, is then perhaps a classic example of uncertainty. . . .

. . . [J]ustice has properly to do with pleas of "But I could not help it." It seeks to distinguish such cases from those acknowledged to be praiseworthy or blameworthy. The formula "to each according to his needs" is one cogent way of identifying the moral relevance of these pleas. To ignore them may be thought to be unfair as well as unkind when they arise from the deprivation of some essential need. The move to confine the notion of justice wholly to desert considerations is thereby resisted as well. Hence we may say that sometimes "questions of social justice arise just because people are unequal in ways they can do very little to change and . . . only by attending to these inequalities can one be said to be giving their interests equal consideration.[23]

Similar Treatment for Similar Cases

This conception is perhaps the most familiar of all. Certainly it is the most formal and inclusive one. It is frequently taken as an elementary appeal to consistency and linked to the universalizability test. One should not make an arbitrary exception on one's own behalf, but rather should apply impartially whatever standards one accepts. The conception can be fruitfully applied to health care questions and I shall assume its relevance. Yet as literally interpreted, it is necessary but not sufficient. For rightly or not, it is often held to be as compatible with no positive treatment whatever as with active promotion of other peoples' interests, as long as all are equally and impartially included. Its exponents sometimes assume such active promotion without demonstrating clearly how this is built into the conception itself. Moreover, it may obscure a distinction that we have seen agapists and other make: between equal consideration and identical treatment. Needs may differ and so treatments must, if benefits are to be equalized.

I have placed this conception at the end of the list partly because it moves us, despite its formality, toward practice. Let me suggest briefly how it does so. Suppose first of all one agrees with the case so far offered. Suppose, that is, it has been shown convincingly that a need conception of justice applies with greater relevance than the earlier three when one reflects about the basic purpose of medical care. To treat one class of people differently from another because of income or geographic location should therefore be ruled out, because such reasons are irrelevant. (The irrelevance is conceptual, rather than always, unfortunately, causal.) In short, all persons should have equal access, "as needed, without financial, geographic, or other barriers, to the whole spectrum of health services."[24]

Suppose however, second, that the goal of equal access collides on some occasions with the realities of finite medical resources and needs that prove to be insatiable. That such collisions occur in fact it would be idle to deny. And it is here that the practical bearing of the formula of similar treatment for similar cases should be noticed. Let us recall Williams's conclusion: "the proper ground of distribution of medical care is ill health: this is a necessary truth." While I agree with the essentials of his argument—for all the reasons above—I would prefer, for practical purposes, a slightly more modest formulation. Illness is the proper ground for the *receipt* of medical care. However, the *distribution* of medical care in less-than-optimal circumstances requires us to face the collisions. I would argue that in such circumstances the formula of similar treatment for similar cases may be construed so as to guide actual choices in the way most compatible with the goal of equal access. The formula's allowance of no positive treatment whatever may justify exclusion of entire classes of cases from a priority list. Yet it forbids doing so for irrelevant or arbitrary reasons. So (1) if we accept the case for equal access, but (2) if we simply cannot, physically cannot, treat all who are in need, it seems more just to discriminate by virtue of categories of illness than, for example, between the rich ill and poor ill. All persons with a certain rare, noncommunicable disease would not receive priority, let us say, where the costs were inordinate, the prospects for rehabilitation remote, and for the sake of equalized benefits to many more. Or with Ramsey we may urge a policy of random patient selection when one must decide between claimants for a medical treatment unavailable to all. Or

we may acknowledge that any notion of "comprehensive benefits" to which persons should have equal access is subject to practical restrictions that will vary from society to society depending on resources at a given time. Even in a country as affluent as the United States there will surely always be items excluded, e.g., perhaps over-the-counter drugs, some teenage orthodontia, cosmetic surgery, and the like.[25] Here, too, the formula of similar treatment for similar cases may serve to modify the application of a need conception of justice in order to address the insatiability problem and limit frivolous use. In all of the foregoing instances of restriction, however, the relevant feature remains the illness, discomfort, etc. itself. The goal of equal access then retains its prima facie authoritativeness. It is imperfectly realized rather than disregarded.

• • •

Notes

1. Edward M. Kennedy, *In Critical Condition: The Crisis in America's Health Care* (New York: Simon and Schuster, 1972), pp. 234–52; Richard M. Nixon, "President's Message on Health Care System," Document No. 92–261 (March 2, 1972), House of Representatives, Washington, D.C., 1.

2. Hugo A. Bedau, "Radical Egalitarianism," pp. 168–80, in *Justice and Equality*, ed. by Hugo A. Bedau (Englewood Cliffs, N.J.: Prentice-Hall, 1971); John Hospers, *Human Conduct* (New York: Harcourt, Brace, 1961), 416–68; J. R. Lucas, "Justice," *Philosophy* 47, No. 181 (July 1972), 229–48; Ch. Perelman, *The Idea of Justice and the Problem of Argument*, trans. by John Petrie (London: Routledge and Kegan Paul, 1963); Nicholas Rescher, *Distributive Justice* (Indianapolis: Bobbs-Merrill, 1966), Gregory Vlastos, "Justice and Equality," pp. 31–72 in *Social Justice*, ed. by Richard B. Brandt (Englewood Cliffs, N.J.: Prentice-Hall, 1962).

3. Paul Ramsey, *The Patient as Person: Explorations in Medical Ethics* (New Haven: Yale University Press, 1970), p. 240.

4. Nancy Hicks, "Nation's Doctors Move to Police Medical Care," *New York Times* (Sunday, October 28, 1973), 52.

5. Lucas, 321.

6. Bernard A. O. Williams, "The Idea of Equality," pp. 116–37 in *Justice and Equality*, ed. by Hugo A. Bedau (Englewood Cliffs, N.J.: Prentice-Hall, 1971), pp. 126–37.

7. Ibid., 127.

8. See also Thomas Nagel, "Equal Treatment and Compensatory Discrimination," *Philosophy and Public Affairs* 2, No. 4, 348–63 (Summer 1973), 354.

9. Rescher, pp. 79–80.

10. Quoted in Ramsey, p. 248.

11. Ramsey, p. 256.

12. Ibid.

13. Ibid.

14. Anne R. Somers, *Health Care in Transition: Directions for the Future* (Chicago: Hospital Research and Educational Trust, 1971), p. 20.

15. Cf. Rescher, pp. 80–81.

16. Robert M. Sade, "Medical Care as a Right: a Refutation," *The New England Journal of Medicine* 285, 1288–92 (December 1971), 1289.

17. Ibid.

18. Ibid., p. 1291.

19. Charles L. Schultze, Edward R. Fried, Alice M. Rivlin, and Nancy H. Teeters, *Setting National Priorities: The 1973 Budget* (Washington, D.C.: The Brookings Institution, 1972), pp. 214–15.

20. Gene Outka, *Agape: An Ethical Analysis* (New Haven: Yale University Press, 1972), pp. 264–65.

21. Perelman, p. 22.

22. See John Rawls, *A Theory of Justice* (Cambridge: Harvard University Press, 1971), e.g. 104.

23. Benn, Stanley, I., "Egalitarianism and the Equal Consideration of Interests," pp. 152–67 in *Justice and Equality*, ed. by Hugo A. Bedau (Englewood Cliffs, N.J.: Prentice-Hall, 1971), p. 164.

24. Anne R. Somers and Herman M. Somers, "The Organization and Financing of Health Care: Issues and Directions for the Future," *American Journal of Orthopsychiatry* 42, 119–36 (January 1972), 122.

25. Anne R. Somers and Herman M. Somers, "Major Issues in National Health Insurance," *Milbank Memorial Fund Quarterly* 50, No. 2, Part 1, 177–210 (April 1972), 182.

Decision Scenario 1 ....

The Cashier's Office of Archway Memorial Hospital is, even for the wealthy and best educated, a place of frustration. Bills are presented in the form of long computer printouts, covered with unfamiliar names referring to supplies, medical treatment, and diagnostic tests. Associated with each item is a price that seems absurdly high.

For someone without any form of medical insurance, being faced with such a bill can be more than confusing. It can be frightening. And that is just the situation that Marvin Baldesi found himself in.

"Your age makes you ineligible for Medicare," said Ms. Kearney, the Archway billing officer. "And you say you aren't covered by Blue Cross or a private insurance plan."

"That's right," said Mr. Baldesi. "I own my own business. My wife and me, we run a small upholstery shop. We decided we couldn't afford to keep up our insurance."

"Normally we wouldn't have admitted you," said Ms. Kearney. "It's only because you came in as an acute emergency that you were allowed to run up such a bill."

Mr. Baldesi looked down to keep from meeting Ms. Kearney's eyes. He felt embarrassed. He had always paid his bills, and now this woman didn't bother to disguise the fact that she saw him as a deadbeat.

"I don't guess you have any money in savings?" Ms. Kearney asked.

"About fifty dollars. Just enough to keep the account open."

"Then it looks to me like you've only got two choices," Ms. Kearney said. "You've got to borrow the money or you've got to declare yourself bankrupt. If you do that, then you'll be eligible for Medicaid payments, and the hospital may be able to collect from the government. I'm not sure of the legal process."

"But the bill is almost three thousand dollars," Mr. Baldesi said. "I can't borrow money like that. My family and friends don't have it, and no bank would loan it to me without collateral."

"Then you'll just have to get a lawyer and get yourself declared bankrupt."

"But if I do that, I'll lose my business. My credit will be ruined, and I won't be able to get the materials I need from suppliers. Isn't there any other way?"

"I don't know of any," said Ms. Kearney. "But that's not really my problem. All I know is that Archway has to be paid. You received our services and we have to have the money for them."

Is Mr. Baldesi's situation possible in the U.S. today? If Sade's position is accepted, how should our society deal with cases like Mr. Baldesi's?

How might the health-care proposal outlined by Fried apply to such a case?

Archway Hospital (in the person of Ms. Kearney) is asserting its claim as a participant in a free-market economy. Why does Outka regard market considerations as irrelevant in determining the distribution of health care?

Suppose Mr. Baldesi's illness is connected with his failure to give up smoking and drinking, even though advised to do so by his physician. Would this lead you to view his situation any differently?

Decision Scenario 2 ....

"There's more than one way to get to Rome," Dr. Kenton said. "And we've got a couple of options to offer you."

"I'll take anything that will make the pain stay away," Mr. Czahz said.

"We can do a surgical procedure that we call a coronary-artery bypass. In your case, there are two arteries involved so it would be a double bypass."

"This is not something experimental, is it?"

"No, it's a well-established procedure with a pretty good safety record. Now something like 80 percent of the people who have the bypass get rid of their angina pains."

"I don't much like the idea of being cut, but I'd do most anything to stop those chest pains."

"Let me tell you the other option. We can treat you medically instead of surgically. That is, we can try you on some drugs and see how you do, put you on a diet, and keep a close watch on you. Now people we treat this way do a little bit better in terms of living longer than those treated surgically do. That's a little misleading, though, because those who have surgery usually have worse cases of the disease."

"What about the angina pains?" Mr. Czahz asked.

"There's the problem. Medical treatment can do something about the pains, but it's really not as effective as surgery."

"So I'll take the surgery."

"Aren't you on health stamps?" Dr. Kenton asked.

"That's right."

"We've got a problem then. You see, health stamps won't cover the cost of bypass surgery. It's an optional procedure under the HHS guidelines, and they won't kick in the extra money to pay for it."

"So I have to make up the difference myself?"

"That's right," Dr. Kenton said. "You're going to have to come up with about two thousand in cash."

"Dr. Kenton, there's no way I can do that."

"Okay, then. I just wanted you to know what the possibilities were. We can put you on a treatment program, and I'm sure you'll do just fine."

"But what about the angina pain?"

"We'll do what we can," Dr. Kenton said.

A health-stamp program might operate by granting a fixed amount of money to each person below a certain income level. This would permit someone to shop around for the best health-care bargain she or he could afford. What might be the advantages and disadvantages of such a program?

Would such a program be likely to provide the sort of equal access of health care argued for by Outka?

According to Fried's position, should Mr. Czahz be entitled to anything more than basic medical treatment for his heart condition?

Is such a program compatible with the form of medical individualism advocated by Sade?

Decision Scenario 3 ••

When the pain began, Alan Warfard was certain he was having a heart attack. The pain lasted over an hour, and when it was finally over, he was weak and exhausted. He knew there was something seriously wrong with him, and as soon as he was able, he called his next-door neighbor and asked her to drive him to Southwest Hospital.

"You have no insurance coverage, except for Medicare?" the man at the admitting desk asked Mr. Warfard. "No private insurance at all?"

"Just Medicare," Mr. Warfard said.

"Can you show us any financial records, such as savings-account passbooks, to establish that you are able to pay your charges here?"

"I live on my social security check, and I don't have a savings account."

"Do you have any relatives who would be willing to sign a statement assuming financial responsibility for your treatment here?"

"I'm afraid not," Mr. Warfard said. "But I don't see what the problem is. I told you, I'm covered by Medicare. Isn't that enough?"

The admitting clerk shook his head. "I'm afraid it's not. We don't know what your treatment is likely to cost, and we don't know whether Medicare would pay for all of it. You know, they pay only a certain amount, and you might run up bills above that. This is a private hospital, and I'm afraid without your being able to guarantee that you can pay us, I can't admit you for treatment."

"But I'm sick," Mr. Warfard said. "What am I supposed to do, just go home and die?"

"That's not really our concern," the clerk said. "But I suggest you see if you can get yourself admitted to a public hospital. Taking care of people like you is their responsibility."

The phrase "people like you" stung Mr. Warfard's pride. After all those years of paying his taxes and being a good citizen, how could he be dismissed so easily?

How does Mr. Warfard's case illustrate some of the drawbacks of the current prospective payment plan (DRGs) employed by Medicare? What are some of the other drawbacks of the plan?

Do private, for-profit hospitals pose particular difficulties for public hospitals and the public financing of health care?

How might it be argued that health care is such a special commodity that it should not be bought and sold on the open market the way that other goods are?

Decision Scenario 4 ••

"Let me see if I understand you correctly," Mrs. Burgone said. "I might be able to benefit from an operation to replace my hip, but you are not allowed to perform such an operation?"

"That's correct," Dr. Popp said. "The Department of Health and Human Services policy stipulates that total hip replacements cannot be performed on patients over the age of seventy."

Mrs. Burgone shook her head. "But I don't expect Medicare to pay for it. I'm able to pay for it myself."

"That doesn't matter. It's a matter of social policy, not medicine. The idea is that we can't afford, as a society, to do everything for every patient. You might be able to pay for such an operation, but not everybody can. The society would have to pay for those who can't afford it, and society can't afford to do that. Consequently, to be fair, the operation is denied to everyone above the age of seventy."

"That doesn't seem fair to me," Mrs. Burgone said. "How can it be fair to condemn someone to being a cripple, when the means to prevent that are available?"

"I didn't make the policy," Dr. Popp said.

According to Outka, the standard for determining who shall receive medical care is need alone. However, since resources are finite, he admits that access may have to be restricted and suggests that the principle of treating similar cases similarly might be used to limit access. Would the policy described above be a legitimate restriction on access? Is the age requirement relevant to determining whether the restriction is legitimate?

Is the policy compatible with the position taken by Fried? On Fried's view, is the policy one that

might legitimately be followed by Medicare and Medicaid?

Why might a "medical individualist" (represented here by Sade) object to such a policy?

Decision Scenario 5 ....

"Let me explain it to you, Mr. Faust," Charles Young said. "Although your wife is covered by Medicare, we cannot pay for the care she is receiving in the nursing home. As an Alzheimer's patient, she is receiving what we consider to be 'custodial' care, and that is explicitly excluded from Medicare coverage. Do you have any private insurance?"

"Yes, I do. But you're telling me exactly the same thing I heard from my insurance company. My policy doesn't cover long-term, chronic, or custodial care."

"I'm sorry to hear that," Charles Young said. "That means that you will have to pay the total cost of the care yourself."

"Where can I get that kind of money?" Mr. Faust said. "A nursing home will cost me thirty or forty thousand dollars a year. If I sell our house and use all our savings, I could pay for maybe a year, but then I wouldn't have anything to live on myself. Where could I live? How could I eat?"

"I understand. But the only alternative is to divest yourself of your assets so that you cannot be held legally responsible for paying for your wife's care. Then you and she can both get assistance under the Medicaid program."

"Then I have to literally bankrupt myself and become a pauper before I can get any help?"

"I'm sorry to say that's true."

Should Medicare be extended to pay for the sort of custodial care that is required by patients with Alzheimer's disease?

Should family members (adult children or grandchildren) be required by law to help pay the health-care expenses of other family members?

Should people with incomes or private insurance adequate to cover the cost of their health care be ineligible to receive Medicare payments?

We expect people to pay for the goods and services that they receive. Since Mrs. Faust is receiving goods and services in getting custodial care, why is it unfair to expect her husband to pay for them?

Decision Scenario 6 ....

"I've decided to do something that may cause me a lot of trouble," Dr. Miles Burgone said.

Alan Warfard took a sip of his drink and sat back in his chair. He had known Miles for a long time and knew he could be counted on to see most things in a novel way. Sometimes Miles could be annoying, but he always made you think.

"I'm not going to accept women as patients anymore," Burgone said. "I don't like dealing with them, and there's nothing that says I have to. From now on, I'm restricting my practice to men only."

"I don't think you can do that," Warfard said. "I suspect that involves civil rights violations of some sort. You know, discriminating on the basis of race or sex or something like that."

"Then I'll get a lawyer and show that the government can't force me to treat women without violating my own rights."

"I don't follow you."

"Look at it this way," Burgone said. "My medical knowledge and skills belong to me. I acquired them through the exercise of my own mind, and I have a constitutional right to privacy and freedom of expression. Therefore, I have a right to exercise my knowledge and skills in the way I see fit. Therefore, if I don't want to treat women, then I don't have to."

"That's an argument I've never heard," War-fard said.

"The government can't force me to do what I don't want to do without violating my rights and being despotic."

"I suspect you'll have to prove that in court."

"I'm prepared to," Burgone said.

State explicitly (and more fully if it seems necessary) the argument presented by Dr. Burgone.

Is the argument the same as Sade's argument? If not, how do the two differ?

Burgone's argument might be construed as one supporting what is sometimes called "medical individualism." Do the objections to medical individualism made by Outka also apply to Burgone's argument?

NOTES AND REFERENCES FOR INTRODUCTIONS, CASES, AND SCENARIOS

Ethical Theories, Moral Principles, and Medical Decisions: An Introduction

I learned much about medical ethics and about presenting it to a general audience from those who have gone before me. I have benefitted from the example (among others) of Samuel Gorovitz, et al., eds., *Moral Problems in Medicine* (Englewood Cliffs, N.J.: Prentice-Hall, 1976), Robert Hunt and John Arras, eds., *Ethical Issues in Modern Medicine* (Palo Alto, Calif.: Mayfield Publishing Co., 1977), and Richard W. Wertz, ed., *Readings on Ethical and Social Issues in Biomedicine* (Englewood Cliffs, N.J.: Prentice-Hall, 1973). All three have informative introductions, but the one by Hunt and Arras I found most helpful and most philosophically interesting.

My discussion of ethical theories is generally indebted to Richard B. Brandt, *Ethical Theory* (Englewood Cliffs, N.J.: Prentice-Hall, 1959) and William K. Frankena, *Ethics*, 2d ed. (Englewood Cliffs, N.J.: Prentice-Hall, 1973). My treatment of utilitarianism owes much to the excellent introductory essay by Paul Taylor in his *Problems of Moral Philosophy* (Belmont, Calif.: Dickenson Publishing Company, 1971), pp. 137–151. Mill's statement of the principle of utility is from *Utilitarianism* (Indianapolis: Bobbs-Merrill, 1971), p. 18; the second quotation is from p. 24. In the discussion of act and rule utilitarianism and their attendant difficulties, I am indebted to Michael D. Bayles and Kenneth Henley's introduction in their *Right Conduct* (New York: Random House, 1983), pp. 86–94, and to Carl Wellman, *Morals and Ethics* (New York: Scott, Foresman, 1975), pp. 39–42, 47–50. The quotation from Wellman is on p. 49.

The statements of Kant's categorical imperative are more paraphrases than literal translations. They are from his *Groundwork of the Metaphysics of Morals*, translated by H. J. Paton (New York: Harper and Row, 1964). Other translations and editions are easily available. Some of the criticisms of Kant are based on those of Brandt (*Ethical Theory*, pp. 27–35) and Frankena (*Ethics*, pp. 30–33).

The quotation from Ross is from his *The Right and the Good* (New York: Oxford University Press, 1930), p. 24. The prima facie duties are found on pp. 21–22 and the "rules" for resolving conflict on pp. 41–42. My exposition is indebted, in part, to G. J. Warnock, *Contemporary Moral Philosophy* (New York: St. Martin's Press, 1967) and to Fred Feldman, *Introductory Ethics* (Englewood Cliffs, N.J.: Prentice-Hall, 1978), pp. 149–160.

Rawls's theory is presented in *A Theory of Justice* (Cambridge, Mass.: Harvard University Press, 1971). The principles are quoted from p. 203; "natural duties" are discussed on pp. 340–350. My statement of the theory is indebted to Norman Daniels's introduction to his anthology *Reading Rawls* (New York: Basic Books, 1976). The first criticism is one made by Thomas Nagel, "Rawls on Justice" (Daniels, pp. 1–16) and Ronald Dworkin, "The Original Position" (Daniels, pp. 16–53). The second criticism is urged by R. M. Hare, "Rawls's Theory of Justice" (Daniels, 81–108) and David Lyons, "Nature and Soundness of the Contract and Coherence Arguments" (Daniels, 141–169). A relatively easy entrance into Rawls's theory is provided by the general reviews of the book that are listed in the Bibliography.

For Aquinas's view on "man," see his *Summa Theologica,* Part II (First Part), vol. 6, translated by Fathers of the English Dominican Province (London: Burns Oates and Washbourne, 1914). For his views on natural law and law in general, see vol. 8, "Treatise on Law." For an interpretation of Aquinas, see Frederick Copleston, *A History of Philosophy,* vol. 2, part 2 (New York: Doubleday, 1962), pp. 126–131, to which my account is indebted. For the presentation of the current Catholic natural law view I am indebted to Charles J. McFadden, *Medical Ethics,* 6th ed. (Philadelphia: F. A. Davis, 1967). The doctrine of double effect is treated on pp. 121–155; euthanasia, extraordinary means, and medical experimentation, pp. 239–270. The quotations from the Directives are from the appendix in McFadden: abortion, p. 441, euthanasia, p. 442.

My discussion of moral principles is indebted to Tom. L. Beauchamp and James F. Childress, *Principles of Biomedical Ethics* (New York: Oxford University Press, 1979), pp. 56–201, and to Beauchamp's and LeRoy Walters's introduction in *Contemporary Issues in Bioethics,* 2d ed. (Belmont, Calif.: Wadsworth Publishing Company, 1982), pp. 26–32. The discussion of liberty-limiting principles is based on Joel Feinberg, *Social Philosophy* (Englewood Cliffs, N.J.: Prentice-Hall, 1973), pp. 20–33, as is the discussion of principles of justice, pp. 98–119.

Chapter 1: Abortion

The Case Presentation has been fictionalized, but it is based on the case of an unnamed minor in the United Press Interna-tional story "Court Orders Abortion for a Rape Victim, 12" (Oklahoma City, 29 September 1981). The Social Context draws information from the following *New York Times* articles: "Abortion Stressed in Abduction Trial," 26 January 1983; Nadine Brozan, "Abortion Rights: New Tactics," 6 May 1985; Dudley Clendinen, "Abortion Choices Defended in Capital," 22 May 1985; Judy Llemesrud, "NOW Plans to Mount Campaign to Uphold the Right to Abortion," 21 July 1985. Information about the Akron decision is from Linda Greenhouse, "Justices Agree to Rule on Legality of Rules Impeding Abortion," *New York Times,* 25 May 1982, and George J. Annas, "*Roe* v. *Wade* Reaffirmed," *Hastings Center Report* 13 (1983): 21–22. The Justice Department's announcement that it would try for an appeal of the *Roe* v. *Wade* doctrine is reported in Leslie H. Gelb, "U.S. Set to Urge Court to Reverse Abortion Ruling," *New York Times,* 15 June 1985. The Supreme Court ruling in the Pennsylvania case is reported in Stuart Taylor, Jr., "Justices Uphold Abortion Rights by Narrow Vote," *New York Times,* 12 June 1986. Excerpts from the opinion are printed in the same issue.

Information on fetal development is found in Arthur J. Vender, J. H. Sherman, and D. S. Luciano, *Human Physiology,* chapter 15 (New York: McGraw-Hill, 1970).

The Finkbine Case Retrospective is based on Allen F. Guttmacher, *The Case for Legalized Abortion* (Berkeley, Calif.: Diablo Press, 1977), pp. 15–17. The Bishop Scenario is based on a case reported in the *New York Times,* 11 April 1982. The procedure described was developed at Mount Sinai Medical Center by Drs. Thomas Kerenyi and Usha Chitkara.

Chapter 2: Treating or Terminating: The Problem of Impaired Infants

"Social Context: The Baby Doe Cases" is based on information from the following sources: George J. Annas, "Disconnecting the Baby Doe Hotline," *Hastings Center Report* 13 (June 1983): 14–16, and "Baby Doe Redux," *Hastings Center Report* 13 (October 1983): 26–27; Bonnie Steinbock, "Baby Jane Doe in the Courts," *Hastings Center Report* 14 (February 1984): 13–19; Thomas H. Murray, "The Final Anticlimactic Rule on Baby Doe," *Hastings Center Report* 15 (June 1985): 5–9; *Time*, 14 November 1983, p. 107. Also the following articles from the *New York Times:* Marcia Chambers, "U.S. Suing for L.I. Records of Baby in Surgery Dispute," 3 November 1983, and "Letting Panels Decide the Fate of Defective Infants," 15 January 1984; Harold M. Schmeck, Jr., "Life, Death and the Rights of Handicapped Babies," 18 June 1985; Stuart Taylor, Jr., "High Court Upsets U.S. Intervention on Infants' Lives," 10 June 1986; Andrew H. Malcolm, "Ruling on Baby Doe: Impact Limited," 11 June 1986.

The Case Presentation is based on an actual case presented in James M. Gustafson, "Mongolism, Parental Desires, and the Right to Life," *Perspectives in Biology and Medicine* 16 (1973): 529–557, and in Milton D. Heifetz and Charles Mangel, *The Right to Die* (New York: G. P. Putnam's, 1975), pp. 59–60.

For a discussion of the medical and biological aspects of birth defects, see E. P. Volpe, *Human Heredity and Birth Defects* (New York: Pegasus, 1971). On prenatal diagnosis, see Theodore Friedman, "Prenatal Diagnosis of Genetic Disease," *Scientific American* 225 (November 1971): 34–42.

The R. S. Duff and A. G. M. Campbell article referred to is "Moral and Ethical Dilemmas in the Special-Care Nursery," *New England Journal of Medicine* 289 (1973): 75–78.

The "Juli" Decision Scenario is based on a case reported in B. D. Colen, *Karen Ann Quinlan: Dying in the Age of Eternal Life* (New York: Nash Publishing Company, 1976), pp. 130–137. The "Susan Roth" scenario is based on a case reported in Richard Trubo, *An Act of Mercy* (Los Angeles: Nash Publishing Company, 1973), pp. 149–150. The "Irene Towers" scenario is based on a Chicago case reported by the Associated Press, 18 May 1981.

The "Dr. Daniel McKay" Decision Scenario is based on information from E. R. Shipp, "Mistrial in Killing of Malformed Baby Leaves Town Uncertain about Law," *New York Times*, 18 February 1985.

The AMA policy decision is reported in Andrew H. Malcolm, "Reassessing Care of the Dying," *New York Times*, 16 March 1986.

The information about the Bartling case is drawn from the *New York Times*, 28 December 1984, and George J. Annas, "Prisoner in the ICU: The Tragedy of William Bartling," *Hastings Center Report* 14 (December 1984): 28–29.

The "Virginia Crawford" Decision Scenario is based on a Baltimore case reported by United Press International on 25 February 1979.

The facts in the Shick case are from a United Press International story of 8 February 1983; the Dohr-Engel case was reported in the *New York Times*, 20 March 1985; the Montigny case was reported by the Associated Press on 8 August 1985; the Gilbert case was reported by the *New York Times* on 9 August 1985 and the Associated Press on 26 August 1985. The policy endorsed by the Netherlands Supreme Court was outlined by a *New York Times* story, 27 November 1984.

Chapter 3: Euthanasia

For a discussion of covert and unilateral decisions made about euthanasia by physicians, see Milton D. Heifetz and Charles Mangel, *The Right to Die* (New York: G. P. Putnam's Sons, 1975). The information about and the criticisms of the California Natural Death Act are from Karen Lebacqz, "On 'Natural Death,' " *Hastings Center Report* 7 (1977): 14. An excellent discussion of the history and practice of euthanasia and of euthanasia legislation is O. Ruth Russell, *Freedom to Die: Moral and Legal Aspects of Euthanasia* (New York: Dell Publishing Company, 1976).

By far the most detailed account of the Karen Quinlan case is Joseph and Julia Quinlan with Phyllis Battelle, *Karen Ann Quinlan* (New York: Doubleday, 1977). The facts in the case presentation are mostly from Phyllis Battelle, "The Story of Karen Quinlan," *Ladies' Home Journal* 93 (September 1976): 69–76, 172–180. Direct quotations are from Battelle. I have also drawn from B. D. Colen, *Karen Ann Quinlan: Dying in the Age of Eternal Life* (New York: Nash Publishing Company, 1976), and *In the Matter of Karen Quinlan: The Complete Legal Briefs, Court Proceedings, and Decisions* (Arlington, Virginia: University Publications of America, 1975).

The "Elizabeth Bouvia" Case Presentation draws heavily upon George J. Annas, "When Suicide Prevention Becomes Brutality," *Hastings Center Report* 14 (April 1984): 20–21, 46. Additional information is from the United Press International article of 2 November 1983, the Associated Press article of 23 May 1985, and Robert Lindsy, "Ruling Is Upheld in Suicide Appeal," *New York Times*, 20 January 1983. More recent events are reported in the following *New York Times* articles: Marcia Chambers, "Woman Who Fought to Die Is Back in Court," 9 February 1986; "Winner of Right to Starve Faces New Fight at Hospital," 20 April 1986; "Quadriplegic Obtains Court Help on Morphine," 24 April 1986.

No philosophical or legal analysis has so far been made of the J. K. Collums case. The facts and quotations in the Case Presentation are from the account by William K. Stevens, *New York Times*, 9 December 1981. The facts and quotations about the punishment hearing are from a United Press International news story of 5 February 1982. Information about the sentencing is from a United Press International story of 5 March 1982.

Chapter 4: Paternalism, Truth Telling, and Confidentiality

The "AIDS" Case Presentation draws from the following sources: Susan West, "One Step Behind a Killer," *Science 83* 4 (March 1983): 36–46; Jacques Keibowitch, *A Strange Virus of Unknown Origin,* trans. Robert Howard (New York: Ballantine Books, 1985); *Newsweek,* 12 August 1985, pp. 20–27, and 23 September 1985, pp. 18–29. AIDS in the schools is reported in *New York Times* articles on 27 and 31 August 1985 and 1, 5, 8, 9, and 10 September 1985; screening by the military on 25 September 1985; proposed screening by insurers on 26 September 1985 and 2 October 1985; most recent statistics and five year projections on 12 June 1986 in Robert Pear, "Tenfold Increase in AIDS Death Toll Is Expected by '91"; the relative effectiveness of the drug AZT (azidothymidine) in the treatment of AIDS on 18 September 1986 in Eric Eckholm, "Test Results Are Due on Drug to Fight AIDS."

The quotations and facts in the "Gonzalez" Case Presentation are from Daniel Goleman, "Emergency Room Struggle: Deciding Who Is Dangerous," *New York Times,* 13 July 1986, and Frank Trippett, "The Madman on the Ferry," *Time,* 21 July 1986, p. 28.

For an account of the physician-patient relationship and the development of licensing procedures for physicians in the United States, see John Duffy, *The Healers: The Rise of the Medical Establishment* (New York: McGraw-Hill, 1977). Duffy also deals with American medical quackery, but the classic works in this area are James Harvey Young, *The Toadstool Millionaires: A Social History of Patent Medicines in America before Federal Regulation* (Princeton, N.J.: Princeton University Press, 1961), and *The Medical Messiahs* (Princeton, N.J.: Princeton University Press, 1971). An influential sociological account of the nature of the doctor-patient relationship as a social role is Talcott Parsons, "Illness and the

Role of the Physician: A Sociological Perspective," in Clyde Kluckhohn and H. A. Murray, eds., *Personality in Nature, Society, and Culture* (New York: Alfred A. Knopf, 1961).

The multiple sclerosis study is reported in *Hastings Center Report* 13 (June 1983): 2–3. The "Korin" Decision Scenario is based on information in Dudley Clendinen, "Therapist's Notes Issue in Fraud Case," *New York Times*, 17 March 1985. For an account of the V.D. inspection program mentioned, see Clyde Haberman, "New York Testing Prostitutes for V.D.," *New York Times*, 5 March 1982.

Chapter 5: Medical Experimentation and Informed Consent

"The Artificial Heart" Case Presentation draws from the following sources: for a discussion of the Cooley controversy, see Thomas Thompson, *Hearts* (New York: Fawcett Books, 1971), pp. 227–235; for current criticisms, see Philip M. Boffey, "Artificial Heart: Should It Be Scaled Back?" *New York Times*, 3 December 1985; for questions about terminating the experiment and DeVries's responses, see L. K. Altman, "The Ongoing Ordeal of a 'Human Experiment,' " *New York Times*, 14 May 1985.

The "Baby Fae" Case Presentation is based on information from the following *New York Times* stories: L. K. Altman, "Learning from Baby Fae," 18 November 1984, Philip M. Boffey, "Medicine Under Scrutiny," 20 November 1984, Sandra Blakeslee, "Baboon Implant in Baby Fae Assailed," 20 December 1985, and Erik Eckholm, "Baby Death Laid to Wrong Blood," 17 October 1985. The NIH report is summarized in the Associated Press story "Baby Fae's Survival Chances Overstated, U.S. Report Says," 14 March 1985, and in "NIH Approves the Consent for Baby Fae, or Does It?" *Hastings Center Report* 15 (April 1985): 2.

The "Kaimowitz" Case Presentation is based on the opinion of the Wayne County Circuit Court (references cited in the selection). (The quotation from the consent form is from the notes of the opinion.) But it is most indebted to the excellent account by Ronald S. Gass, "*Kaimowitz* v. *Department of Mental Health*," W. M. Gaylin and J. S. Meister, eds., *Operating on the Mind* (New York: Basic Books, 1975), pp. 73–87. Anyone seriously concerned with the Detroit case should read Gass's article. The full opinion is reprinted as an appendix to the book.

The details of the experiments in the "Willowbrook" Case Presentation are taken from Saul Krugman and Joan P. Giles, "Viral Hepatitis: New Light on an Old Disease," *Journal of the American Medical Association* 212 (1970): 1019–21.

The description of Nazi medical experiments is from the indictment in *United States* v. *Karl Brandt*, a selection from which is reprinted in *Hastings Center Report*, "Special Supplement: Biomedical Ethics and the Shadow of Nazism," 6 (August 1976): 5.

The description of drug testing is based on the account by Ross J. Baldessarini, *Chemotherapy in Psychiatry* (Cambridge, Mass.: Harvard University Press, 1977), pp. 4–11.

For a discussion of some of the problems of providing information, testing understanding, and getting consent I am indebted to William Shebar's unpublished paper "Understanding and Informed Consent in Psychiatric Research." The paternalistic view that physicians must decide because patients can never understand is expressed in Eugene G. Laforet, "The Fiction of Informed Consent," *Journal of the American Medical Association* 235 (12 April 1976): 1579–85. Problems with placebos are discussed in Sissela Bok, "The Ethics of Giving Placebos," *Scientific American* 231 (November 1974): 17–23. The discussion of research and children is indebted to Jean D. Lockhart, "Pediatric Drug Testing," *Hastings Center Report* 7 (June 1977):

8–10. Prisoners and research is discussed at length in Jessica Mitford, *Kind and Usual Punishment* (New York: Alfred A. Knopf, 1973). The historical cases of research on the poor are from M. H. Pappworth, *Human Guinea Pigs* (Boston: Beacon Books, 1961), pp. 61–62. The details of the Tuskegee case are from the "Final Report of the Tuskegee Syphilis Study Ad Hoc Advisory Panel," U.S. Public Health Service (Washington, D.C.: 1973), part of which is reprinted in S. J. Reiser, et al., *Ethics in Medicine* (Cambridge, Mass.: MIT Press, 1977), pp. 316–321. I am indebted to the letter by Jay Katz, in particular. In the discussion of fetal experimentation, I am indebted to "Individual Risks vs. Societal Benefits: The Fetus," a forum appearing in *Experiments and Research with Humans: Values in Conflict* (Washington, D.C.: National Academy of Sciences, 1975), pp. 59–90.

HHS regulations on using children as research subjects were published in the *Federal Register*, March 8, 1983. They are summarized in "Finally, Final Rules on Children Who Become Research Subjects," *Hastings Center Report* 13 (August 1983): 2–3.

The "Phoenix heart" Decision Scenario draws information and quotations from the following articles in the *New York Times:* Lawrence K. Altman, "Anguish, Hope, a Moment of Fame," 19 March 1985; Irvin Molotsky, "F.D.A. Ponders Action on Unsanctioned Implant," 8 March 1985. The questions raised reflect the doubts expressed by George J. Annas in "The Phoenix Heart: What We Have to Lose," *Hastings Center Report* 15 (June 1985): 15–16.

The "Boyd Rush" Decision Scenario is drawn from information cited in George J. Annas, "Baby Fae: The 'Anything Goes' School of Human Experimentation," *Hastings Center Report* 15 (February 1985): 15–17. The original source is Jurgen Thorwald, *The Patients* (New York: Harcourt Brace Jovanovich, 1972).

The case of Ms. Mink presented in the

Decision Scenario is based on a report in *Time*, 9 May 1977, p. 44, and on Marlene Cimons's article in the *Los Angeles Times*, 16 May 1977. The quotations are from these sources.

A report on the charges of so-called "guinea-pig" surgery involving mental patients in Chicago is to be found in the *New York Times*, 19 April 1979. Additional information is from *Time*, 23 April 1979.

Chapter 6: Genetics: Intervention, Control, and Research

The "Huntington's disease" Case Presentation relies heavily on information from Gina Kolata, "Closing in on a Killer Gene," *Discover* (March 1984): 83–87. See also Lawrence K. Altman, "Researchers Report Genetic Test Detects Huntington Disease," *New York Times*, 9 November 1983, and Albert Rosenfeld, "At Risk for Huntington's Disease," *Hastings Center Report* 14 (June 1984): 5–8.

The "gene therapy" Case Presentation is based on information from the following *New York Times* articles: 8 September 1981; Harold M. Schmeck, "Activity of Genes Reported Altered in Treating Man," 9 December 1982; Walter Sullivan, "Transplanting Cells into Brain Offers Promise as Therapy," 11 September 1984; Harold M. Schmeck, "Hereditary Disease: Therapies Are Closer," 28 January 1986. I am also indebted to the Anderson and Fletcher article reprinted here and to Clifford Grobstein and Michael Flower, "Gene Therapy: Proceed with Caution," *Hastings Center Report* 14 (April 1984): 13–17.

Other information relevant to the topic is drawn from these *New York Times* articles: Walter Sullivan, "Transplanting Cells into Brain Offers Promise as Therapy," 11 September 1984; Harold M. Schmeck, Jr., "U.S. Sets Guidelines on Using Gene Transplants in Humans," 23 September 1985.

For an account of diseases currently screened for and their relation to legal and social issues, see George Annas and B. Coyne, "Fitness for Birth and Reproduction: Legal Implications of Genetic Screening," *Family Law Quarterly* 9 (Fall 1975): 463–490, and Marc Lappé, "The Predictive Powers of the New Genetics," *Hastings Center Report* 14 (October 1984): 18–21. A review of recent diagnostic possibilities is offered by Harold M. Schmeck, Jr., "Fetal Tests Can Now Find Many More Genetic Flaws," *New York Times*, 11 March 1986. A critical look at Tay-Sachs screening is offered in Madeleine J. Goodman and Lenn E. Goodman, "The Overselling of Genetic Anxiety," *Hastings Center Report* 12 (October 1982): 20–27.

A general survey of the types of screening that are current and the ethical problems they pose is presented by Tabitha M. Powledge, "Genetic Screening," in Warrent T. Reich, ed., *Encyclopedia of Bioethics*, vol. 2 (New York: Free Press, 1978), pp. 567–573. The account of the experiences and problems (social and scientific) in PKU screening is found in National Academy of Sciences, *Genetic Screening: Programs, Principles, and Research* (Washington, D.C.: National Academy of Sciences, 1975). For an account of alpha-fetoprotein screening, see Barbara Gastel, et al., eds., *Maternal Serum Alpha-Fetoprotein: Issues in the Prenatal Screening and Diagnosis of Neural Tube Defects* (U.S. Department of Health and Human Services Publication HE 20.2: M41, 1981). For a discussion of social problems caused by PKU laws and sickle-cell screening, see Philip Reilly, "There's Another Side to Genetic Screening," *Prism* (January 1976): 55–57.

Genetic screening and the problems it poses for rights is considered by Susan West, "Genetic Testing on the Job," *Science 82* (September 1982): 16. See also Phillip M. Boffey, "Rapid Advances Point to the Mapping of All Human Genes," *New York Times*, 15 July 1986, and Morton Hunt, "The Total Gene Screen," *New York Times Magazine*, 19 January 1986.

For the controversy over genetic engineering guidelines, testing genetically altered substances, and the potential hazards of altered organisms, see the following *New York Times* articles (when no name is given, the author is Keith Schneider): "Field-Testing Permit for Genetic Concern Lifted for False Data," 26 March 1986; "U.S. Quietly Approved the Sale of Genetically Altered Vaccine," 4 April 1986; "Biology's Unknown Risks," 4 April 1986; "Release of a Gene-Altered Virus Is Halted by U.S. After Challenge," 8 April 1986; "Genetic Field Test Faces a Challenge," 7 April 1986; "U.S. Ends Curb on a Vaccine Using Altered Virus," 23 April 1986; " '84 Test of Altered Virus Stirs Concern," 29 April 1986; "Field Tests Backed for Gene-Altered Pesticide," 25 April 1986; "Another Inquiry Set for Gene-Altered Virus," 1 May 1986; William Dicke, "Gene Splicing Suit Dismissed," 8 May 1986; "President Weighs Easing of Controls for Gene-Splicing," 22 May 1986; "Tests Set for a Pesticide Made by Biotechnologists," 13 June 1986; "U.S. Unveils Rules on Biotechnology," 20 June 1986. See also *Time*, 21 April 1986, pp. 52–54. Jeremy Rifkin's views are stated in his book, written in collaboration with Nicanor Perlas, *Algeny* (New York: Viking Press, 1983).

For a review of some of the recent issues involving university research and its connection with private biotech industries, see Katherine Bouton, "Academic Research and Big Business: A Delicate Balance," *New York Times Magazine*, 11 September 1983. For both scientific and social issues, see G. V. Nossal, *Reshaping Life: Key Issues in Genetic Engineering* (New York: Cambridge University Press, 1985). Quite important and useful also is the report of the President's Commission for the Study of Ethical Problems in Medicine and Biomedical and Behavioral Research, *Splicing Life: The Social and Ethical Issues of Genetic*

Screening with Human Beings (Washington, D.C.: President's Commission, 1982).

Chapter 7: Reproductive Control: In Vitro Fertilization, Artificial Insemination, Surrogate Pregnancy, and Sterilization

The basic information for the "Louise Brown" Case Presentation is from *Newsweek*, 7 August 1978; *Time*, 7 August 1978; and *U.S. News and World Report*, 7 August 1978. For a discussion of the techniques and issues of in vitro fertilization, in addition to the popular accounts cited above, see R. G. Edwards, "Fertilization of Human Eggs In Vitro: Morals, Ethics, and the Law," *Quarterly Review of Biology* 49 (March 1974): 3–26. I am also indebted for information to George H. Kieffer, "Reproductive Technology: The State of the Art," in Thomas A. Mappes and Jane S. Zembaty, eds., *Biomedical Ethics* (New York: McGraw-Hill, 1981), pp. 485–490.

The "Unclaimed Infant" Case Presentation employs facts and quotations from the Associated Press story "Surrogate Infant Left Unclaimed," 22 January 1983, and from Iver Peterson, "Legal Snarl Developing Around Case of a Baby Born to Surrogate Mother," *New York Times*, 7 February 1983.

Information about sterility, the Norfolk clinic, and the moratorium on in vitro research in the U.S. is found in Michael Gold, "The Baby Makers," *Science 85* (April 1985): 26–38. The history of the moratorium and survey results about public attitudes is based on Susan Abramowitz, "A Stalemate on Test-Tube Baby Research," *Hastings Center Report* 14 (February 1984): 5–9. Abramowitz's analysis of present concerns and problems is highly recommended. For a general survey of all the issues in reproductive technology from a feminist perspective, see Gena Corea, *The Mother Machine* (New York: Harper and Row, 1985).

The historical background on artificial insemination is presented in R. Snowden and

G. D. Mitchell, *The Artificial Family* (London: George Allen and Unwin, 1981). The technical aspects of the process and the statistics mentioned are discussed in Ronald P. Goldstein, "Artificial Insemination by Donor— Status and Problems," in Aubrey Milunsky and George J. Annas, eds., *Genetics and the Law* (New York: Plenum Press, 1976), pp. 197–202. I am also indebted for information to Donald A. Goss, "Current Status of Artificial Insemination with Donor Semen," *American Journal of Obstetrics and Gynecology* 122 (May 1975): 246–249. For general objections to artificial insemination and other forms of reproductive technology, see Paul Ramsey, *Fabricated Man* (New Haven: Yale University Press, 1970), particularly Chapter 3.

Statistics and issues surrounding surrogate mothers are presented in Nadine Brozan, "Surrogate Mothers: Problems and Goals," *New York Times*, 27 February 1984. The nonsurgical technique of ova recovery is discussed in Walter Sullivan, "Clinic Offers Aid for Fertilization," *New York Times*, 30 January 1986. The "Rios" Case Presentation is based on information from the Associated Press story "Australians Reject an Effort to Destroy Frozen Embryos," 23 October 1984. For a general review of most of the issues in the current social context, see "Making Babies: The New Science of Conception," *Time Magazine*, 10 September 1984, pp. 46–56. The legal issues in reproductive technology are well reviewed by George Annas, "Surrogate Embryo Transfer" and "Redefining Parenthood and Protecting Embryos," *Hastings Center Report* 14 (June 1984): 25–26 and 14 (October 1984): 50–52. The Kim Cotton case is reported in the Associated Press story "Surrogate Mother's Child in English Court Custody," 9 January 1985.

The information about the Relf case and the federal sterilization guidelines prompted by it is from the *New York Times*, 4 December 1977. Additional information about the federal guidelines and the response to them is from Patricia Donovan, "Sterilizing the Poor and Incompetent," *Hastings Center Report* 6 (1976): 7–8. The account of *Buck* v. *Bell,* as well as the quotation from the opinion, is from "Eugenic Sterilization: A Biomedical Intervention," in Jonas Robitscher, ed., *Eugenic Sterilization* (Springfield, Ill.: Charles C. Thomas, 1973), pp. 10–12. The account of the Hartford sterilization case is based on information in the *New York Times,* 2 October 1978. Recent statistics and attitudes toward sterilization are from the Associated Press, "Sterilization for Birth Control Increases," 10 February 1985.

Information about the Baby M case is drawn from *The New York Times* articles of 4, 5, 6, 10, 26, 27 January 1987; 2, 3, 9, 10, 11, 17, February 1987; 5, 9, 10, 31 March 1987; 2 April 1987. Information about the Vatican "Instruction" and reaction to it is from *The New York Times,* 10, 11 March 1987.

Chapter 8: Allocating Scarce Medical Resources

The "Policy Decision" Case Presentation is based on a real incident. See the St. Louis *Post-Dispatch,* 5 July 1981, for an account of the policy at Tampa General Hospital.

There is no Brattle County, Texas, and the Case Presentation is wholly fictional. It does represent, however, the problem that was faced by some dialysis centers when programs were just starting. For a fine account of the workings of a real committee (the one at Swedish Hospital, Seattle, Washington, in 1961), see Shana Alexander, "They Decide Who Lives, Who Dies." The piece first appeared in *Life* magazine in 1962, but it is usefully reprinted in Robert Hunt and John Arras, eds., *Ethical Issues in Modern Medicine* (Palo Alto, Calif.: Mayfield Publishing Company, 1977), pp. 409–424.

Information in the Social Context section about organ transplants and the problems of allocation can be found in Susan Jacoby, "Lifesavers: The Drive for More Organ Donations," *New York Magazine,* 18 July 1983, pp.

39–43; Donald Sullivan, "New York to Require That Hospitals Seek Donation of Organs," *New York Times,* 14 August 1985; H. Tristram Engelhardt, Jr., "Allocating Scarce Medical Resources and the Availability of Organ Transplantation," *New England Journal of Medicine* 311 (5 July 1984): 66–71. The debate about means of increasing the supply is rehearsed in the following *Hastings Center Report* articles: Arthur L. Caplan, "Organ Transplants: The Costs of Success," 13 (December 1983): 23–32; George J. Annas, "Life, Liberty, and the Pursuit of Organ Sales," 14 (February 1984): 22–23; Alfred M. Sadler, Jr. and B. L. Sadler, "A Community of Givers, Not Takers," 14 (October 1984): 6–9; Arthur L. Caplan, "Organ Procurement: It's Not in the Cards," 14 (October 1984): 9–12; "In Minn. and Mass., No Transplants for the Sickest?" 15 (April 1985): 2–3.

The story of cyclosporine and its successful use in organ transplants is presented in Carol Bolotin, "Drug As Hero," *Science 85* (June 1985): 68–71. For the debate over the cost of the Medicare kidney program and relevant statistics, see Robert Reinhold, "Economics of Life and Death Arises in Debate over Kidney Therapy," *New York Times,* 28 May 1982.

For an account of how dialysis takes place and of what it is like from a personal point of view, see Lee Foster, "Man and Machine: Life without Kidneys," *Hastings Center Report* 6 (June 1976): 5–8. I have drawn heavily from Foster's account. The lifeboat analogy is discussed by Paul Ramsey in *The Patient as Person* (New Haven, Conn.: Yale University Press, 1970).

An important sociological study on dialysis and transplants is Renée C. Fox, "A Sociological Perspective on Organ Transplantation and Hemodialysis," *New Dimensions in Legal and Ethical Concepts for Human Research, Annals of the New York Academy of Sciences* 169 (1970): 406–428. A volume that concentrates on the transplant issue is G. W. Wostenholme and M. O'Connor, eds., *Ethics in Medical Progress:*

With Special Reference to Transplantation (Boston: Little, Brown, and Company, 1966). See also the relevant chapters in Paul Ramsey, *The Patient as Person* (New Haven, Conn.: Yale University Press, 1970). The ethical issues involved in transplants go beyond the question of distribution, of course.

Chapter 9: The Claim to Health Care

The "Mrs. Smith" Case Presentation is a fictionalized version of the woman described by Bruce Bernard, "Private Hospitals' Dumping of Patients," *New York Times*, 8 April 1985, using information from Robert Pear, "Study Examines Profit Role in Hospitals," *New York Times*, 4 June 1986.

The Social Context section is indebted to Stanley Hwang, "Dissecting the Health Care Beast," *Harvard Political Review* 6 (Fall 1977): 12–15, and Bernard Winter, "The Problem of Profits," *The Progressive* 41 (October 1977): 16–19. Statistics are from U.S. Health Care Financing Administration, *Health Care Financing Review* (Winter 1984). Information on DRGs and their difficulties is from Danielle A. Dolenc and Charles J. Dougherty, "DRGs: The Counterrevolution in Financing Health Care," *Hastings Center Report* 15 (June 1985): 20–29, and John K. Inglehart, "Medicare Begins Prospective Payment of Hospitals," *New England Journal of Medicine* 308 (9 June 1983): 1428–1432. Information about using DRGs to establish fee schedules for physicians can be found in Robert Pear, "Rx for Fees," *New York Times*, 24 August 1985. Problems caused public and teaching hospitals by DRGs and the increasing number of uninsured poor are discussed in Dudley Clendinen, "Meeting on Poor and Health Care," *New York Times*, 9 October 1985, and in Robert Pear, "White House Acting to End Rules Requiring Hospitals to Help Poor," *New York Times*, 4 November 1985. Problems associated with for-profit hospitals are discussed in Arnold S. Relman, "Investor-Owned Hospitals and Health-Care Costs," *New England Journal of Medicine* 309 (11 August 1983): 370–372, and Donald O. Nutter, "Access to Care and the Evolution of Corporate, For-Profit Medicine," *New England Journal of Medicine* 311 (4 October 1984): 917–919. The survey of public attitudes is found in Robert J. Blendon and Drew Altman, "Public Attitudes about Health-Care Costs," *New England Journal of Medicine* 311 (30 August 1984): 613–616.

The discussion of rights in the introduction is indebted to Joel Feinberg, "The Nature and Value of Rights," *Journal of Value Inquiry* 4 (1970): 243–257. For a discussion of the legal status of claims to health care, see Edward V. Sparer, "The Legal Right to Health Care: Public Policy and Equal Access," *Hastings Center Report* 6 (1976): 39–47.

For a discussion of the idea of health stamps or vouchers, see John Arras, "Health Care Vouchers and the Rhetoric of Equity," *Hastings Center Report* 11 (August 1981). A potential health-stamp plan is discussed by Gordon K. MacLeod, "Health Stamps, Maybe?" *New York Times*, 8 April 1980.

BIBLIOGRAPHY

The number of books and articles dealing with medical ethics is staggering, and it is growing larger at a rapid rate. The materials listed here are no more than a sample of those currently available. Thus, this bibliography is best thought of as a guide to further reading. The general and special bibliographies listed below—some book-length works—will provide guides for those who are looking for comprehensiveness.

I have tried to select works with substantial philosophical content. Thus, with a few exceptions, I have not listed publications that are primarily medical, biological, sociological, or otherwise scientific. Furthermore, I have not attempted to duplicate the references given in the selections or in the chapter introductions, and for the most part, I have restricted this bibliography to works that have appeared in the last five to ten years.

General Works and Anthologies

American Medical Association. *Current Opinions of the Judicial Council.* Chicago: American Medical Association, 1981.

Arras, John and Robert Hunt. *Ethical Issues in Modern Medicine.* 2d ed. Palo Alto, Calif.: Mayfield Publishing Company, 1983.

Augenstein, Leroy. *Come, Let Us Play God.* New York: Harper and Row, 1969.

Bandman, Elsie and Bertram Bandman, eds. *Bioethics and Human Rights: A Reader for Health Professionals.* Boston: Little, Brown, 1978.

Beauchamp, Tom L. and James F. Childress. *Principles of Biomedical Ethics.* New York: Oxford University Press, 1983.

Beauchamp, Tom L. and LeRoy Walters, eds. *Contemporary Issues in Bioethics.* 2d ed. Belmont, Calif.: Wadsworth Publishing Company, 1982.

Benjamin, Martin and Joy Curtis. *Ethics in Nursing.* New York: Oxford University Press, 1981.

British Medical Association. *Handbook of Medical Ethics.* London: British Medical Association, 1981.

Brody, Howard. *Ethical Decisions in Medicine.* Boston: Little, Brown, 1976.

Chapman, Carleton, B. "The Importance of Being Ethical." *Perspectives in Biology and Medicine* 24 (Spring 1981): 422–439.

Clouser, K. Danner. "Medical Ethics: Some Uses, Abuses, and Limitations." *Arizona Medicine* 33 (January 1976): 44–49.

Curran, William J. "The Proper and Improper Concerns of Medical Law and Ethics." *New England Journal of Medicine* 259 (4 November 1976): 1057–58.

Curtin, Leah and M. Josephine Flaherty. *Nursing Ethics: Theories and Pragmatics.* Bowie, Md.: Robert J. Brady Co., 1982.

Cutler, Donald R., ed. *Updating Life and Death.* Boston: Beacon Press, 1969.

Duncan, A. S. et al., eds. *Dictionary of Medical Ethics.* London: Darton, Longman, and Todd, 1975.

Engelhardt, H. Tristram, Jr., and Daniel Callahan, eds. *Science, Ethics and Medicine.* Hastings-on-Hudson, N.Y.: Institute of Society, Ethics and the Life Sciences, 1976.

Fletcher, Joseph. *Morals and Medicine.* Boston: Beacon Press, 1954. A classic book stating the "situation ethics" view of euthanasia, truth telling, contraception, etc.

Francoeur, Robert T. *Biomedical Ethics: A Guide to Decision Making.* New York: John Wiley & Sons, 1983.

Giles, James E. *Medical Ethics: A Patient-Centered Approach.* Cambridge: Schenkman Publishing Co., 1983.

Glover, Jonathan. *Causing Death and Saving Lives.* New York: Penguin Books, 1977.

Gorovitz, Samuel, et al., eds. *Moral Problems in Medicine.* Englewood Cliffs, N.J.: Prentice-Hall, 1976.

Gribetz, Donald and Moshe D. Tendler, guest editors. "Medical Ethics: The Jewish Point of View." *The Mount Sinai Journal of Medicine.* Special Issue 51 (January/February 1984).

Humber, James M. and Robert F. Almeder, eds. *Biomedical Ethics Reviews–1983.* Clifton, N.J.: Humana Press, 1983.

————. *Biomedical Ethics and the Law.* New York: Plenum Publishing Corporation, 1976.

Jonsen, Albert R., Mark Siegler, and William J. Winslade. *Clinical Ethics.* New York: Macmillan, 1982.

Labby, Daniel H., ed. *Life or Death: Ethics and Options.* Seattle: University of Washington Press, 1968.

Levine, Carol, ed. *Taking Sides: Clashing Views on Controversial Bio-Ethical Issues.* Guilford, Conn.: The Dushkin Publishing Group, Inc., 1984.

Mappes, Thomas A. and Jane S. Zembaty, eds. *Biomedical Ethics.* 2d ed. New York: McGraw-Hill, 1986.

McIntyre, Neil and Karl Popper. "The Critical Attitude in Medicine: The Need for a New Ethics." *British Medical Journal* 287 (24–31) December 1983): 1919–23.

Ostheimer, Nancy and John Ostheimer, eds. *Life or Death—Who Controls?* New York: Springer Publishing Company, 1976.

Peters, Karl E., ed. "Is Ethics a Science?" *Zygon* 15 (March 1980). Articles by Abraham Edel, R. B. Brandt, and Marcus Singer.

President's Commission for the Study of Ethical Problems in Medicine and Biomedical and Behavioral Research. *Summing Up.* Washington, D.C.: President's Commission, 1983.

Rachels, James. "Can Ethics Provide Answers?" *Hastings Center Report* 10 (1980): 32–40.

Ramsey, Paul. *Ethics at the Edges of Life: Medical and Legal Intersections.* New Haven: Yale University Press, 1978.

————. *The Patient as Person.* New Haven: Yale University Press, 1970. A classic work by a Christian theologian that presents influential views on experimentation, transplantation, allocation of resources, etc.

Reich, W. T., ed. *Encyclopedia of Bioethics.* New York: Macmillan, 1978. A wide-ranging collection of articles by many scholars. Good for a quick survey of major issues.

Reidy, Maurice. *Foundations for a Medical Ethic.* New York: Paulist Press, 1979.

Reiser, S. J., A. J. Dyck, and W. J. Curran, eds. *Ethics in Medicine: Historical Perspectives and Contemporary Concerns.* Cambridge, Mass.: M.I.T. Press, 1977. A large book, strong on historical writings and documents but not on philosophy.

Rivlin, Alice M., and P. Michael Timpane, eds. *Ethical and Legal Issues of Social Experimentation.* Washington, D.C.: The Brookings Institution, 1975. See in particular "Ethical Principles in Medical Experimentation" by Robert M. Veatch.

Shannon, Thomas A. and Jo Ann Manfra, eds. *Law and Bioethics.* Ramsey, N.J.: Paulist Press, 1982.

————. *Bioethics.* New York: Paulist Press, 1981.

Spicker, Stuart F. and H. Tristram Engelhardt, Jr., eds. *Philosophical Medical Ethics: Its Nature and Significance.* Boston: D. Reidel, 1977.

Thompson, Ian E., Kath M. Melia, and Kenneth M. Boyd. *Nursing Ethics.* New York: Churchill Livingstone, 1983.

Trial 16 (December 1980). An issue devoted to bioethical and biolegal issues.

Varga, Andrew C., S. J. *The Main Issues in Bioethics.* New York: Paulist Press, 1980.

Vaux, Kenneth. *Biomedical Ethics: Morality for the New Medicine.* New York: Harper and Row, 1974.

Veatch, Robert M. *Case Studies in Medical Ethics.* Cambridge Mass.: Harvard University Press, 1977.

————. *Death, Dying, and the Biological Revolution.* New Haven, Conn.: Yale University Press, 1976. Deals with dying patients, euthanasia, birth defects, defining death, and transplant organs. Contains much information.

————. *A Theory of Medical Ethics.* New York: Basic Books, 1981.

Wall, Thomas F. *Medical Ethics: Basic Moral Issues.* Lanham, Md.: University of America, 1980.

Wertz, Richard W., ed. *Readings on Ethical and Social Issues in Biomedicine.* Englewood Cliffs, N.J.: Prentice-Hall, 1973.

Williams, Granville. *The Sanctity of Life and the Criminal Law.* New York: Alfred Knopf, 1957.

Williams, Preston, ed. *Ethical Issues in Biology and Medicine.* Cambridge, Mass.: Schenkman Publishing Company, 1973. Original papers, several with a theological orientation.

Williams, Robert H.,ed. *To Live and to Die: When, Why, and How.* New York: Springer-Verlag, 1973.

Wojcik, Jan. *Muted Consent: A Case Book of Modern Medical Ethics.* West Lafayette, Ind.: Purdue University Press, 1978.

Yezzi, Ronald. *Medical Ethics: Thinking About Unavoidable Questions.* New York: Holt, Rinehart, and Winston, 1980.

Bibliographies

American Nurses' Association. *Ethics References for Nurses.* Kansas City, Mo.: American Nurses' Association, 1982.

American Nurses' Association, Committee on Ethics. *Ethics in Nursing: References and Resources.* Kansas City, Mo.: American Nurses' Association, 1979.

"Bioethics and the Law: A bibliography, 1974–1976." *American Journal of Law and Medicine* 2 (Winter 1976–1977): 263–281.

Calhoun, Cheryl. *Annotated Bibliography of Medical Oaths, Codes, and Prayers.* Washington, D.C.: Kennedy Institute, 1975.

Carmody, James. *Ethical Issues in Health Services: A Report and Annotated Bibliography.* Washington, D.C.: U.S. Department of Health, Education, and Welfare, 1974.

Clouser, K. Danner and Arthur Zucker. *Abortion and Euthanasia: An Annotated Bibliography.* Philadelphia: Society for Health and Human Values, 1974.

A Comprehensive Set of Bibliographies on Voluntary Sterilization. New York: The International Project of the Association for Voluntary Sterilization, January 1976.

Euthanasia: An Annotated Bibliography. New York: Euthanasia Educational Fund, 1970.

Goldstein, Doris M. *Bioethics: A Guide to Information Sources.* Detroit: Gale Research Company, 1982.

Kalish, Richard A. "Death and Dying: A Briefly Annotated Bibliography." In *The Dying Patient.* Edited by Orville G. Brim, Jr., et al. New York: Russell Sage Foundation, 1970, pp. 323–380.

Kutscher, A. *Bibliography of Books on Death, Bereavement, Loss, and Grief: 1955–1968.* New York: Health Sciences Publishing Corporation, 1969.

Lineback, Richard H., ed. *Philosopher's Index.* Vols. 1–. Bowling Green, Ohio: Philosophy Documentation Center, Bowling Green State University. Issued quarterly.

Nevins, Madeline M., ed. *Annotated Bibliography of Bioethics: Selected 1976 Titles.* Rockville, Md.: Information Planning Associations, 1977.

Pence, Terry. *Ethics in Nursing: An Annotated Bibliography.* New York: National League for Nursing, 1983.

Sollitto, Sharmon and Robert M. Veatch. Revised by Ira D. Singer. *Bibliography of Society, Ethics and the Life Sciences: 1979–1980.* Hastings-on-Hudson, N.Y.: Institute of Society, Ethics and the Life Sciences, 1978. This is the best general bibliography and also the best guide to philosophical articles on medical ethics. It is partially annotated and brought up to date periodically.

Sorenson, James R. *Social and Psychological Aspects of Applied Human Genetics: A Bibliography.* Washington, D.C.: Department of Health, Education, and Welfare, 1973.

Vernick, Joel J. *Selected Bibliography on Death and Dying.* Washington, D.C.: U.S. Department of Health, Education, and Welfare, National Institutes of Health, n.d.

Walters, LeRoy, ed. *Bibliography of Bioethics.* Vol. 9. Detroit: Gale Research Company, 1983.

Weiss, Gary B. and Harold Y. Vanderpool. *Ethics and Cancer: An Annotated Biography.* Galveston, Tex.: University of Texas Medical Branch, 1984.

Ethical Theories and Medical Decisions: An Introduction

A. General Works on Ethics

Beauchamp, Tom L. and Terry Pinkard, eds. *Ethics and Public Policy: An Introduction to Ethics.* Englewood Cliffs, N.J.: Prentice-Hall, 1983.

Brandt, Richard B. *Ethical Theory.* Englewood Cliffs, N.J.: Prentice-Hall, 1959.

Ewing, A. C. *Ethics.* New York: Free Press, 1965.

Feinberg, Joel. *Doing and Deserving: Essays in the Theory of Responsibility.* Princeton, N.J.: Princeton University Press, 1970.

————. *Social Philosophy.* Englewood Cliffs, N.J.: Prentice-Hall, 1973.

————. *Rights, Justice, and the Bounds of Liberty.* Princeton, N.J.: Princeton University Press, 1980.

Frankena, William K. *Ethics.* 2d ed. Englewood Cliffs, N.J.: Prentice-Hall, 1973.

Gert, Bernard. *The Moral Rules.* New York: Harper and Row, 1970.

Ladd, John. *Ethical Relativism.* Belmont, Calif.: Wadsworth Publishing Company, 1973.

MacIntyre, Alasdair. *After Virtue.* Notre Dame, Ind.: University of Notre Dame Press, 1981.

Rachels, James. *Understanding Moral Philosophy.* Encino, Calif.: Dickenson Publishing Company, 1976. A short, readable introduction.

Taylor, Paul W., ed. *The Moral Judgment: Readings in Contemporary Meta-Ethics.* Englewood Cliffs, N.J.: Prentice-Hall, 1963.

————, ed. *Problems of Moral Philosophy.* Belmont, Calif.: Dickenson Publishing Company, 1971. Clear and sophisticated introduction.

Warnock, Geoffrey James. *Contemporary Moral Philosophy.* New York: St. Martin's Press, 1967.

Wellman, Carl. *Morals and Ethics.* New York: Scott, Foresman, 1975.

White, Alan R. *Rights.* Oxford: Clarendon Press, 1984.

Williams, Bernard. *Morality: An Introduction to Ethics.* New York: Harper and Row, 1972.

B. Utilitarianism

Bayles, Michael D., ed. *Contemporary Utilitarianism.* New York: Doubleday, 1968.

Bentham, Jeremy. *A Fragment on Government and An Introduction to the Principles of Morals and Legislation.* Edited by Wilfried Harrison. Oxford: Blackwell, 1967.

Hodgson, D. H. *Consequences of Utilitarianism: A Study in Normative Ethics and Legal Theory.* Oxford: Clarendon Press, 1967.

Lyons, David. *Forms and Limits of Utilitarianism.* New York: Oxford University Press, 1965.

————. *In the Interest of the Governed: A Study in Bentham's Philosophy of Utility and Law.* Oxford: Oxford University Press, 1973.

Mill, John Stuart. *Utilitarianism: With Critical Essays.* Edited by Samuel Gorovitz. Indianapolis: Bobbs-Merrill, 1971.

Quinton, A. M. *Utilitarian Ethics.* New York: St. Martin's Press, 1973.

Regan, Donald H. *Utilitarianism and Co-operation.* New York: Oxford University Press, 1980.

Sen, Amartya and Bernard Williams, eds. *Utilitarianism and Beyond.* New York: Cambridge University Press. 1982.

Smart, J. J. C. and Bernard Williams. *Utilitarianism: For and Against.* New York: Cambridge University Press, 1973.

C. Kant

Beck, L. W. *Studies in the Philosophy of Kant.* Indianapolis: Bobbs-Merrill, 1965.

Kant, Immanuel. *Foundations of the Metaphysics of Morals: Text and Critical Essays.* Edited by Robert P. Wolff. New York: Bobbs-Merrill, 1969.

————. *Lectures on Ethics.* New York: Harper and Row, 1963.

Paton, H. J. *The Categorical Imperative: A Study of Kant's Moral Philosophy.* New York: Harper and Row, 1967.

Singer, Marcus G. *Generalization in Ethics: An Essay in the Logic of Ethics with the Rudiments of a System of Moral Philosophy.* New York: Atheneum, 1971.

Wolff, R. P., ed. *Kant: A Collection of Critical Essays.* Garden City, N.Y.: Doubleday, 1967.

D. Ross

Ross, W. D. *Foundations of Ethics.* Oxford: Oxford University Press, 1963. A reissue of the 1939 edition.

_____. *The Right and the Good*. Oxford: Clarendon Press, 1930. (For evaluations of Ross, see relevant sections of Frankena, Brandt, Ewing, Rachels, and Taylor listed above.)

E. Rawls

Barry, Brian. *The Liberal Theory of Justice*. New York: Oxford University Press, 1974. An exposition and criticism of Rawls.

Chen, Marshall. "The Social Contract Explained and Defended." *New York Book Review*, 16 July 1972, p. 1.

Daniels, Norman, ed. *Reading Rawls*. New York: Basic Books, 1976. This volume has a helpful introduction and contains some of the more important critical articles.

F. Aquinas and Natural Law

Copleston, F. C. *Aquinas*. Baltimore: Penguin Books, 1965.

Gilson, Etienne. *The Philosophy of St. Thomas Aquinas*. 3d ed. Translated by Edward Bullough. St. Louis: Herder Book Company, 1937.

Kelly, Gerald. *Medico-Moral Problems*. St. Louis: Catholic Hospital Association, 1958.

McFadden, Charles J. *Medical Ethics*. 6th ed. Philadelphia: F. A. Davis, 1967.

O'Connor, D. J. *Aquinas and Natural Law*. New York: St. Martin's Press, 1969.

Pegis, Anton, ed. *Basic Writings of St. Thomas Aquinas*. New York: Random House, 1945.

Tuck, Richard. *Natural Rights Theories: Their Origin and Development*. New York: Cambridge University Press, 1980.

Part I: Termination

Chapter 1: Abortion

Altman, Andrew. "Abortion and the Indigent." *Journal of Social Philosophy* 11 (1980): 5–9. Favors the Supreme Court decision that states need not fund abortions.

Annis, David. "Self-Consciousness and the Right to Life." *Southwestern Journal of Philosophy* 6 (1975): 123–128.

Bagley, C. "On the Sociology and Social Ethics of Abortion." *Ethics in Science and Medicine* 3 (1976): 21–32.

Becker, Laurence C. "Human Being: The Boundaries of the Concept." *Philosophy and Public Affairs* 4 (1975): 334–359. Attempts to develop a biological concept relevant to abortion and euthanasia.

Bok, Sissela. "Ethical Problems of Abortion." *Hastings Center Report* 2 (1974): 33–52.

_____. "Who Shall Count as a Human Being? A Treacherous Question in the Abortion Discussion." In **Robert L. Perkins, ed.** *Abortion: Pro and Con*. Cambridge, Mass.: Schenkman, 1974, pp. 91–105.

Bondeson, William B., H. Tristram Engelhardt, Jr., Stuart F. Spicker, and Daniel H. Winship, eds. *Abortion and the Status of the Fetus*. Boston: D. Reidel Publishing Company, 1983.

Brandt, R. B. "The Morality of Abortion." *Monist* 56 (1972): 503–526.

Brody, Baruch. *Abortion and the Sanctity of Human Life*. Cambridge, Mass.: MIT Press, 1975. Brody's several papers are embodied here.

_____. "Thomson on Abortion." *Philosophy and Public Affairs* 1 (1972): 335–340.

Callahan, Daniel. *Abortion: Law, Choice and Morality*. New York: Macmillan, 1970.

Callahan, Sidney and Daniel Callahan, eds. *Abortion: Understanding Differences*. New York: Plenum Press, 1984.

Camenisch, Paul F. "Abortion: For the Fetus's Own Sake?" *Hastings Center Report* 6 (1976): 38–41.

_____. "Abortion Analogies and the Emergence of Value." *Journal of Religious Ethics* 4 (1976): 131–158.

Chervenak, Frank A., et al. "When Is Termination of Pregnancy During the Third Trimester Morally Justifiable?" *New England Journal of Medicine* 310 (23 February 1984): 501–04.

Cohen, Marshall, et al., ed. *The Rights and Wrongs of Abortion*. Princeton: N.J.: Princeton University Press, 1974.

Connery, John R. *Abortion: The Development of the Roman Catholic Perspective*. Chicago: Loyola University Press, 1977.

Daniels, Charles B. "Abortion and Potential." *Dialogue* 18 (June 1979): 220–223.

Davis, Nancy. "Abortion and Self-Defense."

Philosophy and Public Affairs 13(3) (Summer 1984): 175–207.

Engelhardt, H. Tristram. "The Ontology of Abortion." *Ethics* 84 (April 1974): 217–234.

Feinberg, Joel. "Abortion." In **Tom Regan, ed.** *Matters of Life and Death.* New York: Random House, 1980, pp. 183–217.

————. "Is There a Right to Be Born?" In **James Rachels, ed.** *Understanding Moral Philosophy.* Belmont, Calif.: Dickenson Publishing Company, 1976.

————, ed. *The Problem of Abortion.* 2d ed. Belmont, Calif.: Wadsworth Publishing Company, 1984.

Finnis, John, Judith Thomson, Michael Tooley, and Roger Wertheimer. *The Rights and Wrongs of Abortion.* Princeton, N.J.: Princeton University Press, 1974. A collection of influential articles.

Fletcher, Joseph. "Four Indicators of Humanhood—The Enquiry Matures." *Hastings Center Report* 4 (December 1974): 4–7.

Foot, Phillippa. "The Problem of Abortion and the Doctrine of Double Effect." *Oxford Review* 5 (1967): 5–15.

Frohock, Fred M. *Abortion: A Case Study in Law and Morals.* Westport, Conn.: Greenwood Press, 1983.

Gerber, D. "Abortion: The Uptake Argument." *Ethics* 83 (1972): 80–83.

Gerber, R. J. "Abortion: Parameters for Decision." *Ethics* 82 (1972).

Gillespie, Norman C. "Abortion and Human Rights." *Ethics* 87 (April 1977): 237–243.

Goldman, Alan H. "Abortion and the Right to Life." *Personalist* 60 (October 1979): 402–406.

Goodrich, T. "The Morality of Killing." *Philosophy* 44 (1969): 127–139.

Gordon, Robert M. "The Abortion Issue." In **Eugene Freeman, ed.** *The Abdication of Philosophy: Essays in Honor of Paul A. Schilpp.* Chicago: Open Court, 1974, pp. 267–277.

Granfield, David. *The Abortion Decision.* New York: Doubleday, 1971. A Catholic point of view.

Hall, Robert E., ed. *Abortion in a Changing World.* New York: Columbia University Press, 1970.

Hare, R. M. "Abortion and the Golden Rule." *Philosophy and Public Affairs* 4 (1975): 201–222.

Harrison, Beverly Wildung. *Our Right to Choose: Toward a New Ethic of Abortion.* Boston: Beacon Press, 1983.

Harrison, S. M. "The Unwilling Dead." *Proceedings of the Catholic Philosophical Association* 46 (1972): 199–208. Argues that the concept of a person is central to the abortion issue and offers one based on C. S. Peirce.

Herbewick, Raymond M. "Remarks on Abortion, Abandonment, and Adoption Opportunities." *Philosophy and Public Affairs* 5 (Fall 1975): 98–104.

Humber, James M. "The Case against Abortion." *The Thomist* 39 (1975): 65–84. A criticism of major arguments.

Jaffee, Frederick, Barbara Lindheim, and Philip Lee. *Abortion Politics: Private Morality and Public Policy.* New York: McGraw-Hill, 1981.

Kohl, Marvin. "Abortion and the Argument from Innocence." *Inquiry* 14 (1971): 147–151.

————, ed. *Infanticide and the Value of Life.* Buffalo, N.Y.: Prometheus Books, 1978.

Langham, Paul. "Between Abortion and Infanticide." *Southern Journal of Philosophy* 17 (1979): 465–471.

Levy, Steven R. "Abortion and Dissenting Parents: A Dialogue." *Ethics* 90 (1980): 162–163.

Manier, Edward, William Liu, and David Solomon. *Abortion: New Directions for Policy Studies.* Notre Dame, Ind.: University of Notre Dame Press, 1977.

Margolis, Joseph. "Abortion." *Ethics* 84 (1973): 51–61.

Moore, E. C., et al. "Abortion: The New Ruling." *Hastings Center Report* 3 (1973): 4–7.

Moore, Harold F. "Abortion and the Logic of Moral Justification." *Journal of Value Inquiry* 9 (1975): 140–151.

Noonan, John T. *A Private Choice: Abortion in America in the Seventies.* New York: Free Press, 1979.

Petchesky, Rosalind Pollack. *Abortion and Woman's Choice: The State, Sexuality, and Reproductive Freedom.* New York: Longman, 1984.

Pole, Nelson. "To Respect Human Life." *Philosophical Context* 2 (1973): 16–22. Argues that a right to abortion promotes human dignity.

Regan, Tom. *Matters of Life and Death.* New York: Random House, 1980.

Rorty, Amelie O. "Persons, Policies, and Bodies." *International Philosophical Quarterly* 13 (March 1973): 63–80.

Schneider, Carl E. and Maris A. Vinouskis, eds. *The Law and Politics of Abortion.* Lexington, Mass.: D.C. Heath and Company, 1980.

Sher, George. "Hare, Abortion and the Golden Rule." *Philosophy and Public Affairs* 6 (Winter 1977): 185–190.

Sumner, L. W. *Abortion and Moral Theory.* Princeton, N.J.: Princeton University Press, 1981.

Talmage, R. S. "Utilitarianism and the Morality of Killing." *Philosophy* 47 (1972): 55–63.

Thomson, Judith Jarvis. "Rights and Deaths." *Philosophy and Public Affairs* 2 (1973): 146–159.

Tietze, Christopher. *Induced Abortion: A World Review, 1981* New York: The Population Council, 1981.

Tooley, Michael. *Abortion and Infanticide.* New York: Oxford University Press, 1983.

Vandever, Donald. "Justifying Wholesale Slaughter."*Canadian Journal of Philosophy* 5 (1975): 245–258.

Wade, Francis C. "Potentiality in the Abortion Discussion."*Review of Metaphysics* 29 (December 1975): 239–255.

Warren, Mary Anne. "Do Potential People Have Moral Rights?" *Canadian Journal of Philosophy* 7 (June 1977): 275–289.

Wasserstrom, Richard. "The Status of the Fetus." *Hastings Center Report* 5 (June 1975): 18–22.

Weiss, Roslyn. "The Perils of Personhood." *Ethics* 89 (October 1978): 66–75.

Werner, Richard. "Abortion: The Moral Status of the Unborn." *Social Theory and Practice* 3 (Fall 1974): 201–222.

————. "Abortion: The Ontological and Moral Status of the Unborn." In **Richard A. Wasserstrom, ed.** *Today's Moral Problems.* 2d ed. New York: Macmillan, 1979, pp. 51–74.

Wertheimer, Roger. "Understanding the Abortion Argument." *Philosophy and Public Affairs* 1 (1971): 67–95. A clear statement of issues.

Wicclair, Mark R. "The Abortion Controversy and the Claim That This Body Is Mine." *Social Theory* 7 (Fall 1981): 337–46.

Zaitchik, Alan. "Viability and the Morality of Abortion." *Philosophy and Public Affairs* 10 (Winter 1981): 18–26.

Chapter 2: Treating or Terminating: The Problem of Impaired Infants

Abrams, Natalie. "Defective Newborns: A Framework for a Case Analysis." *Westminister Institute Review* 2 (Winter 1983): 3–7.

American Academy of Pediatrics, ed. "Selected Readings on Infant Care Review Committees and Bioethical Issues in the Care of Seriously Ill and Disabled Newborns." May 1984.

Augenstein, Leroy. "Birth Defects, The Ethical Problem." *Humanist* 28 (1968): 18–20.

Coburn, Robert C. "Morality and the Defective Newborn." *Journal of Medicine and Philosophy* 5 (December 1980): 340–357.

Darling, Rosalyn Benjamin. "Parents, Physicians, and Spina Bifida." *Hastings Center Report* 7 (August 1977): 10–13.

Drane, James F. "The Defective Child: Ethical Guidelines for Painful Dilemmas." *Journal of Obstetric Gynecologic and Neo-Natal Nursing* 13 (January/February 1984): 42–48.

Duff, R. S. and A. G. M. Campbell. "Moral and Ethical Dilemmas in the Special Care Nursery." *New England Journal of Medicine* 289 (1973): 890–894.

Engelhardt, H. T. "Euthanasia and Children: The Inquiry of Continued Existence." *Journal of Pediatrics* 83 (1973): 170–171.

Fletcher, John C. "Abortion, Euthanasia, and Care of Defective Newborns." *New England Journal of Medicine* 292 (1975): 75–78.

————. "Attitudes toward Defective Newborns." *Hastings Center Studies* 2 (1974): 21–32.

————. "Choices for Life or Death in the Case of Defective Newborns." *Social Responsibility: Journalism, Law, Medicine.* Program on Society and the Professions: Studies in Applied Ethics. Lexington, Va.: Washington and Lee University, 1975, pp. 62–78.

Freeman, J. M. "To Treat or Not to Treat: Ethical Dilemmas of Treating the Infant with a Myelomeningocele." *Clinical Neurosurgery* 20 (1973): 134–146.

Gustafson, James M. "Mongolism, Parental Desires, and the Right to Life." *Perspectives in Biology and Medicine* 16 (1973): 529–557.

Hemphill, M., et al. "Ethical Aspects of Care of the Newborn with Serious Neurological Disease." *Clinical Perinatology* 4 (March 1977): 201–209.

Hetmann, Philip B. and Sara Holtz. "The Severely Defective Newborn: The Dilemma and the Decision Process." *Public Policy* 23 (Fall 1975): 381–418.

Horan, Dennis, J. and Melinda Delaboyde, eds. *Infanticide and the Handicapped Newborn.* Provo, Utah: Brigham Young University Press, 1982.

Johnson, Paul R. "Selective Nontreatment and Spina Bifida: A Case Study in Ethical Theory and Application." *Bioethics Quarterly* 3 (Summer 1981): 91–111.

Jonsen, A. R., et al. "Critical Issues in Newborn Intensive Care: A Conference Report and Policy Proposal." *Pediatrics* 55 (1975): 756–768.

_____ **and Michael J. Garland, eds.** *Ethics of Newborn Intensive Care.* Berkeley, Calif.: University of California, Institute of Governmental Studies, 1976.

Kelly, S., et al., eds. *Birth Defects.* New York: Academic Press, 1976.

Kelsey, Beverly. "Which Infants Shall Live? Who Shall Decide?" *Hastings Center Report* 5 (April 1975): 5–7.

Kohl, Marvin, ed. *Infanticide and the Value of Life.* Buffalo, N.Y.: Prometheus Books, 1978. See in particular papers by Richard Brandt and R. S. Duff.

Lorber, John. "Selective Treatment of Myelomeningocele." *Pediatrics* 53 (1974): 307–308.

McCormick, Richard A. "To Save or Let Die: The Dilemma of Modern Medicine." *Journal of the American Medical Association* 229 (1974): 172–76.

Paris, John J. and Anne B. Fletcher. "Infant Doe Regulations and the Absolute Requirement to Use Nourishment and Fluids for the Dying Infant." *Law, Medicine and Health Care* 11 (October 1983): 210–13.

Rhoden, Nancy K. "The New Neonatal Dilemma: Live Births from Late Abortions." *Georgetown Law Journal* 72 (June 1984): 1451–1509.

Shapiro, Robyn. "Medical Treatment of Defective Newborns: An Answer to the 'Baby Doe' Dilemma." *Harvard Journal on Legislation* 20 (1983): 137–52.

Shatten, Deborah A. and Robert S. Chabon. "Decision-Making and the Right to Refuse Lifesaving Treatment for Defective Newborns." *Journal of Legal Medicine* 3 (March 1982): 57–79.

Sherlock, Richard. "Selective Non-Treatment of Defective Newborns: A Critique." *Ethics in Science and Medicine* 7 (1980): 111–117.

Singer, Peter, et al. "The Treatment of Newborn Infants with Major Handicaps: A Survey of Obstetricians and Paediatricians in Victoria." *The Medical Journal of Australia* (17 September 1983): 274–78.

Smith, David H. "On Letting Some Babies Die." *Hastings Center Studies* 2 (1974): 37–46.

Smith, G. and E. D. Smith. "Selection for Treatment in Spina Bifida Cystica." *British Medical Journal* 27 (October 1973): 189–204.

Swinyard, Chester A., ed. *Decision Making and the Defective Newborn.* Springfield, Ill.: Charles C. Thomas, 1978.

Veatch, Robert M. "The Technical Criteria Fallacy." *Hastings Center Report* 7 (August 1977): 15–16.

Waldman, A. M. "Medical Ethics and the Hopelessly Ill Child." *Journal of Pediatrics* 88 (1976): 890–892.

Weir, Robert. *Selective Nontreatment of Handicapped Newborns.* New York: Oxford University Press, 1984.

Chapter 3: Euthanasia

Annas, George J. "In re Quinlan: Legal Comfort for Doctors." *Hastings Center Report* 6 (1976): 29–31. A criticism of the grounds of the New Jersey Supreme Court decision.

Arras, John. "The Right to Die on the Slippery

Slope." *Social Theory and Practice* 8 (Fall 1982): 285–328.

Battin, M. Pabst. *Ethical Issues In Suicide.* Englewood Cliffs: N.J.: Prentice-Hall, 1982.

Bayles, Michael D. "The Value of Life—By What Standard?" *American Journal of Nursing* 80 (December 1980): 2226–2230.

Baylor Law Review 27 (Winter 1975). Entire issue on euthanasia.

Beauchamp, Tom L. "The Moral Justification for Withholding Heroic Procedures." In Nora K. Bell, ed. *Who Decides? Conflicts of Rights in Health Care.* Clifton, N.J.: Humana Press, 1982.

————. "A Reply to Rachels on Active and Passive Euthanasia." In Wade L. Robinson and Michael S. Pritchard, eds. *Medical Responsibility.* Clifton, N.J.: Humana Press, 1979, pp. 182–195. See also Rachels below.

———— **and S. Perlin, eds.** *Ethical Issues in Death and Dying.* Englewood Cliffs, N.J.: Prentice-Hall, 1978.

Behnke, John A. and Sissela Bok. *The Dilemmas of Euthanasia.* New York: Doubleday Anchor, 1975.

Benjamin, Martin. "Moral Agency and Negative Acts in Medicine." In Wade L. Robinson and Michael S. Pritchard, eds. *Medical Responsibility.* Clifton, N.J.: Humana Press, 1979, pp. 170–181.

Bernat, James L., et al. "On the Definition and Criterion of Death." *Annals of Internal Medicine* 94 (March 1981): 389–394.

Black, Peter M. "Focusing on Some Ethical Problems Associated with Death and Dying." *Geriatrics* 31 (1976): 138–141.

————. "Three Definitions of Death." *Monist* 60 (January 1977): 136–146.

Bok, Sissela. "Personal Directions for Care at the End of Life." *New England Journal of Medicine* 295 (12 August 1976): 367–369.

Cahill, L. S. "A 'Natural Law' Reconsideration of Euthanasia." *Linacre Quarterly* 44 (February 1977): 47–63.

Cantor, Norman L. "A Patient's Decision to Decline Lifesaving Medical Treatment." *Rutgers Law Review* 26 (1973): 228.

Cassem, Ned. "When Illness Is Judged Irreversible: Imperative and Elective Treatments." *Man and Medicine* 5 (1980): 154–166.

Childress, James F. "To Live or Let Die." In his *Priorities in Biomedical Ethics.* Philadelphia: Westminster Press, 1981, pp. 34–50.

Cohen, Cynthia B. "Interdisciplinary Consultation on the Care of the Critically Ill and Dying: The Role of One Hospital Ethics Committee." *Critical Care Medicine* 10 (November 1982): 776–84.

Committee on Policy for DNR Decisions, Yale New Haven Hospital. "Report on Do Not Resuscitate Decisions." *Connecticut Medicine* 47 (August 1983): 477–83.

Devine, Philip E. *The Ethics of Homicide.* Ithaca, N.Y.: Cornell University Press, 1978.

Dimler, G. Richard, ed. *Thought* 47 (December 1982). Whole issue on "Issues of Life and Death."

Downing, A. B., ed. *Euthanasia and the Right to Die: The Case for Voluntary Euthanasia.* London: Peter Owen, 1969. See in particular the article by Anthony Flew.

Dyck, Arthur J. "Ethical Aspects of Care for the Dying Incompetent." *Journal of the American Geriatrics Society* 32 (September 1984): 661–64.

Eisendrath, Stuart J. and Albert R. Jonsen. "The Living Will: Help or Hindrance?" *Journal of the American Medical Association* 249 (15 April 1983): 2054–58.

Engelhardt, H. Tristram, Jr., and Michelle Malloy. "Suicide and Assisting Suicide: A Critique of Legal Sanctions." *Southwestern Law Journal* 36 (November 1982): 1003–37.

Feinberg, Joel. "Voluntary Euthanasia and the Inalienable Right to Life." *Philosophy and Public Affairs* 7 (Winter 1978): 93–123.

Fitzgerald, P. J. "Acting and Refraining." *Analysis* 27 (1974): 133–139.

Fletcher, Joseph. "Elective Death." In E. F. Torrey, ed. *Ethical Issues in Medicine.* Boston: Little, Brown, 1968.

————. "Ethics and Euthanasia." In Robert H. Williams, ed. *To Live and to Die: When, Why, and How.* New York: Springer-Verlag, 1973, pp. 113–122.

————. "The 'Right' to Live and the 'Right' to Die." *The Humanist* 34 (1974): 12–15.

Fried, Charles. "Terminating Life Support: Out of the Closet." *New England Journal of Medicine* 295 (12 August 1976): 390–391.

Gillick, Muriel. "The Ethics of Cardiopulmonary Resuscitation: Another Look." *Ethics in Science and Medicine* 7 (1980): 161–169.

Goodrich, T. "The Morality of Killing." *Philosophy* 44 (1969): 127–129. Ethanasia and abortion.

Green, Michael B. and Daniel Wikler. "Brain Death and Personal Identity." *Philosophy and Public Affairs* 9 (Winter 1980): 105–133.

Grisez, Germain and Joseph M. Boyle, Jr. *Life and Death with Liberty and Justice: A Contribution to the Euthanasia Debate.* Notre Dame, Ind.: University of Notre Dame Press, 1979.

Hare, R. M. "Euthanasia: A Christian View," *Proceedings of the Center for Philosophic Exchange* 2 (1975): 43–52.

Hausman, David B. "On Abandoning Life Support: An Alternative Proposal." *Man and Medicine* 2 (Spring 1977): 169–177. Also see 178–188 for commentaries.

Horan, Dennis J. and David Mall, eds. *Death, Dying, and Euthanasia.* Washington, D.C.: University Publications of America, 1977.

Human Life Review 2 (Spring 1976): 27–70. Three articles on euthanasia.

Institute of Society, Ethics and the Life Sciences, Task Force on Death and Dying. "Refinements in Criteria for the Determination of Death." *Journal of the American Medical Association* 221 (3 July 1972): 48–53.

Jonsen, Albert R. "Dying Right in California: The Natural Death Act." *Clinical Research* 26 (February 1978): 55–60.

Kamisar, Yale. "Some Non-Religious Views against Proposed 'Mercy-Killing' Legislation." *Minnesota Law Review* 42 (1958): 969–1042.

Kelly, Gerald. "The Duty of Using Artificial Means of Preserving Life." *Theological Studies* 11 (1950): 203–220.

Kohl, Marvin, ed. *Beneficent Euthanasia.* Buffalo, N.Y.: Prometheus Books, 1975. Contains several interesting philosophical articles.

⸻. "Beneficent Euthanasia." *The Humanist* 34 (1974): 9–11.

⸻. "Understanding the Case for Beneficent Euthanasia." *Science, Medicine and Man* 1 (1973): 111–121.

⸻. "The Word 'Mercy' and the Problem of Euthanasia." *The American Rationalist* 9 (1965): 5–7.

Kuhse, Helga. "A Modern Myth. That Letting Die Is Not the Intentional Causation of Death: Some Reflections on the Trial and Acquittal of Dr. Leonard Arthur." *Journal of Applied Philosophy* 1 (1984): 21–38.

Ladd, John, ed. *Ethical Issues Relating to Life and Death.* New York: Oxford University Press, 1979.

Levin, Donald L. and Nancy R. Levin. "DNR: An Objectionable Form of Euthanasia." *University of Cincinnati Law Review* 49 (1980): 567–79.

Lombardi, Joseph L. "Killing and Letting Die: What Is the Moral Difference?" *New Scholasticism* 54 (1980): 200–212.

Long, P. H. "On the Quantity and Quality of Life: Fruitless Longevity." *Physician* 6 (1960): 69–70.

Maguire, Daniel C. "A Catholic View of Mercy Killing." *The Humanist* 34 (1974): 16–18.

⸻. *Death by Choice.* New York: Doubleday, 1974.

Margolis, Joseph. "On Being Allowed to Die." *The Humanist* 36 (1976): 17–19.

McIntyre, R. V. "Voluntary Euthanasia: The Ultimate Perversion." *Medical Counterpoint* 2 (1970): 26–29.

Meilaender, Gilbert. "The Distinction between Killing and Allowing to Die." *Theological Studies* 37 (September 1976): 467–470.

Menzel, Paul T. "Are Killing and Letting Die Morally Different in Medical Contexts?" *Journal of Medicine and Philosophy* 4 (September 1979): 269–293.

Middleton, Carl L., Jr. "Principles of Life-Death Decision Making." *Linacre Quarterly* 42 (1975): 268–278.

Monagle, John F. "Living Will Does Not Resolve Medical-Ethical-Legal Dilemma." *Hospital Progress* 57 (1976): 76–79.

Moore, F. D. "Medical Responsibility for the

Prolongation of Life." *Journal of the American Medical Association* 206 (1968): 384–386.

Morrison, Robert and Leon Kass. "Death—Process or Event?" *Science* 173 (20 August 1971): 694–702.

Potter, Ralph B. "The Paradoxical Preservation of a Principle." *Villanova Law Review* 13 (1968): 874–892.

President's Commission for the Study of Ethical Problems in Medicine and Biomedical and Behavioral Research. *Deciding to Forego Life Sustaining Treatment.* Washington, D.C.: President's Commission, 1983.

Rachels, James. "Euthanasia." In Tom Regan, ed. *Matters of Life and Death.* New York: Random House, 1980, pp. 28–66.

————. "Euthanasia, Killing, and Letting Die," in Wade L. Robinson and Michael S. Pritchard, eds. *Medical Responsibility.* Clifton, N.J.: Humana Press, 1979, pp. 153–169. See also Beauchamp.

————. "Killing and Starving to Death." *Philosophy* 54 (1979): 159–171.

Ramsey, Paul. "The Two-Step Fantastic: The Continuing Case of Brother Fox." *Theological Studies* 42 (March 1981): 122–34.

Rhodes, Jonathan E. "The Right to Die and the Chance to Live." *Journal of Medical Ethics* 6 (1980): 53–54.

Robertson, John A. and Norman Fost. "Passive Euthanasia of Defective Newborn Infants: Legal Considerations." *Journal of Pediatrics* 88 (May 1976): 883–889.

Russell, O. Ruth. *Freedom to Die: Moral and Legal Aspects of Euthanasia.* New York: Human Sciences Press, 1975 (also New York: Dell Publishing Co., 1976). Contains a clear review of objections.

Saunders, Cicely and Mary Baines. *Living with Dying: The Management of Terminal Disease.* New York: Oxford University Press, 1983.

Showalter, J. Stuart and Brian L. Andrew. *To Treat or Not to Treat: A Working Document for Making Critical Life Decisions.* St. Louis: Catholic Health Association, 1984.

Strong, Carson. "Euthanasia: Is the Concept Really Nonevaluative?" *Journal of Medicine and Philosophy* 5 (December 1980): 313–325.

Suber, Daniel G. and William J. Tabor. "Withholding of Life-Sustaining Treatment from the Terminally Ill, Incompetent Patient: Who Decides?" Parts I and II. *Journal of the American Association* 248 (12 and 19 November 1982): 2250–51, 2431–32.

Suckiel, Ellen K. "Death and Benefit in the Permanently Unconscious Patient: A Justification of Euthanasia." *Journal of Medicine and Philosophy* 3 (March 1978): 38–52.

Sullivan, Thomas D. "Active and Passive Euthanasia: An Impertinent Distinction?" *Human Life Review* 3 (Summer 1977): 40–47.

Trammell, Richard L. "The Presumption Against Taking Life." *Journal of Medicine and Philosophy* 3 (March 1978): 53–67.

Vanderpool, H. Y. "The Ethics of Terminal Care." *Journal of the American Medical Association* 239 (27 February 1978): 850–852.

Veatch, Robert M. "An Ethical Framework for Terminal Care Decisions: A New Classification of Patients." *Journal of the American Geriatrics Society* 32 (September 1984): 665–69.

Walton, Douglas N. *Ethics of Withdrawing Life-Support Systems: Case Studies on Decision Making in Intensive Care.* Westport, Conn.: Greenwood Press, 1983.

————. "Omissions and Other Negative Actions." *Metamedicine* 1 (1980): 305–324.

————. *On Defining Death: An Analytic Study of the Concept of Death in Philosophy and Medical Ethics.* Montreal: McGill-Queen, 1979.

Weir, Robert F., ed. *Ethical Issues in Death and Dying.* New York: Columbia University Press, 1977.

Williams, Glanville. "Mercy-Killing Legislation—A Rejoinder." *Minnesota Law Review* 43 (1958): 1–12.

Williams, Peter C. "Rights and the Alleged Rights of Innocents to Be Killed." *Ethics* 87 (July 1977): 383–394.

Wolstenholme, Gordon, et al. "Euthanasia." *Proceedings of the Royal Society of Medicine* 63 (1970): 659–670.

Young, Robert. "Voluntary and Involuntary Euthanasia." *Monist* 59 (April 1976): 264–283.

Part II: Rights

Chapter 4: Paternalism, Truth Telling, and Confidentiality

Annas, George J. "Confidentiality and the Duty to Warn." *Hastings Center Report* 6 (December 1976): 6–8.

———— **and Joan E. Densberger.** "Competence to Refuse Medical Treatment: Autonomy vs. Paternalism." *The University of Toledo Law Review* 15 (Winter 1984): 561–96.

Barber, Barry, et al. "Some Problems of Confidentiality in Medical Computing." *Journal of Medical Ethics* 2 (June 1976): 71–73.

Bassford, H. A. "The Justification of Medical Paternalism." *Social Science and Medicine* 16(6) (1982): 731–39.

Basson, Marc, ed. *Rights and Responsibilities in Modern Medicine.* New York: Alan R. Liss, 1981.

Beauchamp, Tom L. and Lawrence B. McCullough. *Medical Ethics: The Moral Responsibilities of Physicians.* Englewood Cliffs, N.J.: Prentice-Hall, 1984.

Beigler, Jerome (American Psychiatric Association Committee on Confidentiality). "Statement of the American Psychiatric Association Before the Subcommittee on Government Information and Individual Rights." *New York State Journal of Medicine* 79 (December 1979): 2088–2092.

Bell, Nora K., ed. *Who Decides? Conflicts of Rights in Health Care.* Clifton, N.J.: Humana Press, 1982.

British Medical Association. "New Horizons in Medical Ethics: Confidentiality." *British Medical Journal* (23 June 1973): 700–705.

Brody, Howard. "The Physician-Patient Contract: Legal and Ethical Aspects." *Journal of Legal Medicine* 4 (1976): 25–29.

Byrn, Robert M. "Compulsory Life-Saving Treatment for the Competent Adult. *Fordham Law Review* 44 (1975): 1–36.

Cantor, Norman L. "A Patient's Decision to Decline Life-Saving Medical Treatment: Bodily Integrity vs. the Preservation of Life." *Rutgers Law Review* 26 (1972): 228–264.

Childress, James F. *Who Should Decide? Paternalism in Health Care.* New York: Oxford University Press, 1982.

Coleman, Lee. *The Reign of Error.* Boston: Beacon Press, 1984.

"Compulsory Medical Treatment: The State's Interest Re-evaluated." *Minnesota Law Review* 51 (1966): 293–305.

"The Confidentiality of Health Records." *Psychiatric Opinion* 12 (January 1975). Entire issue on confidentiality and society.

Cousins, Norman. "A Layman Looks at Truth-Telling in Medicine." *Journal of the American Medical Association* 244 (24 October 1980): 1929–1930.

Curran, W. J. "Ethical and Legal Problems in Medical Participation in Criminal Investigations." *New England Journal of Medicine* 249 (1976): 764–765.

————, **et al.** "Protection of Privacy and Confidentiality." *Science* 182 (1973): 797–802.

Davies, Edmund. "The Patient's Right to Know the Truth." *Proceedings of the Royal Society of Medicine* 66 (1973): 533–536.

Eck, Marcel. *Lies and Truth.* New York: Macmillan, 1970.

Ellin, Joseph S. "Lying and Deception: The Solution to a Dilemma in Medical Ethics." *Westminster Institute Review* 1(2) (May 1981): 3–6.

Everstine, Louis, et al. "Privacy and Confidentiality in Psychotherapy." *American Psychologist* 35 (September 1980): 828–840.

Ford, John C. "Refusal of Blood Transfusions by Jehovah's Witnesses." *Catholic Law* 10 (1964): 212–226.

Freedman, Alfred. "Threats to Confidentiality." *Journal of the American Academy of Psychoanalysis* 7 (January 1979): 1–5.

Fry, John. *A New Approach to Medicine: Principles and Priorities in Health Care.* Baltimore: University Park Press, 1978.

Gaylin, Willard and Daniel Callahan. "The Psychiatrist as Double Agent." *Hastings Center Report* 4 (February 1974):11–14.

Gazza, B. A. "Compulsory Medical Treatment and Constitutional Guarantees: A Conflict?"

University of Pittsburgh Law Review 33 (1972): 628–637.

Gewirth, Alan. "Human Rights and the Prevention of Cancer." *American Philosophical Quarterly* 17 (April 1980): 117–125.

Gibbs, R. F. "Money and Medical Ethics." *Journal of Legal Medicine* 4 (1976): 3–4.

Gilbert, Richard M. "Ethical Considerations in the Prevention of Smoking in Adults and Children." *Medicolegal News* 8 (June 1980): 4–7.

Gordis, Leon and Ellen Gold. "Privacy, Confidentiality, and the Use of Medical Records in Research." *Science* 207 (11 January 1980).

Grossman, M. "Confidentiality in Medical Practice." *Annual Review of Medicine* 28 (1977): 43–55.

Gurevitz, Howard. "Tarasoff: Protective Privilege Versus Public Peril." *American Journal of Psychiatry* 134 (March 1977): 289–292.

Journal of Medical Ethics 2 (1976): 28–33. "Limits of Confidentiality."

Kelman, Steven. "Regulation and Paternalism," *Public Policy* 29(2) (Spring 1981): 219–54.

Kelsey, Jennifer L. "Privacy and Confidentiality in Epidemiological Research Involving Patients." *IRB: A Review of Human Subjects Research* 3 (February 1981): 1–4.

Kleinig, John. *Paternalism.* Totowa, N.J.: Rowman and Allanheld, 1984.

Lasagna, Louis. "The Boston State Hospital Case (Rogers v. Okin): A Legal, Ethical and Medical Morass." *Perspectives in Biology and Medicine* 25 (Spring 1982): 382–403.

Litin, E. M. "Should the Cancer Patient Be Told?" *Postgraduate Medicine* 28 (November 1960): 470–475.

Lomasky, Loren E. and Michael Detlefsen. "Medical Paternalism Reconsidered." *Pacific Philosophical Quarterly* 62 (1981): 95–98.

Mahowald, Mary B. "Against Paternalism: A Developmental View." *Philosophy Research Archives* 6, no. 1386 (1980).

Marsh, Frank. "The 'Deeper Meaning' of Confidentiality within the Physician-Patient Relationship." *Ethics in Science and Medicine* 6 (1979): 131–136.

Merton, Vanessa. "Confidentiality and the 'Dangerous' Patient: Implications of Tarasoff for Psychiatrists and Lawyers." *Emory Law Journal* 31(2) (Spring 1982): 263–343.

Meyer, B. C. "Truth and the Physician." *Bulletin of the New York Academy of Medicine* 45 (January 1969): 59–71.

Nesbitt, Nancy A. "Tarasoff v. Regents of the University of California: Psychotherapist's Obligation of Confidentiality Versus the Duty to Warn." *Tulsa Law Journal* 12 (1977): 747–757.

Noll, John O. and Mark J. Hanlon. "Patient Privacy and Confidentiality at Mental Health Centers." *American Journal of Psychiatry* 133 (November 1976): 1286–1289.

Oken, Donald. "What to Tell Cancer Patients." *Journal of the American Medical Association* 175 (1961): 1120–1128.

Pemberton, L. B. "Diagnosis: Can/Should We Tell the Truth?" *Bulletin of the American College of Surgeons* (May 1971): 7–13.

Perr, I. N. "Confidentiality and Consent in the Psychiatric Treatment of Minors." *Journal of Legal Medicine* 4 (1976): 9–13.

Phillips, William R. "Patients, Pills, and Professionals: The Ethics of Placebo Therapy." *The Pharos* 44 (Winter 1981): 21–25.

Public Responsibility in Medicine and Research. *Privacy and Confidentiality: Can They Be Protected?* Boston: PRIM & R, 1982.

Roth, L. H., et al. "Dangerousness, Confidentiality, and the Duty to Warn." *American Journal of Psychiatry* 134 (March 1977): 508–511.

Samuels, Alec. "The Duty of the Doctor to Respect the Confidence of the Patient." *Medicine, Science, and the Law* 20 (January 1980): 58–66.

Sheldon, Mark. "Truth Telling Medicine." *Journal of the American Medical Association* 247 (5 February 1982): 651–54.

Sissons, P. L. "The Place of Medicine in the American Prison: Ethical Issues in the Treatment of Offenders." *Journal of Medical Ethics* 2 (1976): 173–179.

Stein, Eugene J. "Doctors and Patients: Partners or Adversaries?" *Bioethics Quarterly* 2 (Summer 1980): 118–122.

Standard, Samuel and Helmuth Nathan, eds. *Should the Patient Know the Truth?* New York: Springer, 1955.

Thomas, Judith J. "The Right to Privacy." *Philosophy and Public Affairs* 4 (1975): 295–314.

Van de Veer, Donald. "Autonomy Respecting Paternalism." *Social Theory Practice* 6 (Summer 1980): 187–208.

————. "The Contractual Argument for Withholding Medical Information." *Philosophy and Public Affairs* 9 (Winter 1980): 198–205.

————. "Paternalism and Subsequent Consent." *Canadian Journal of Philosophy* 9 (1979): 631–642.

Wangenstein, O. H. "Should Patients Be Told They Have Cancer?" *Surgery* 27 (1950): 944–947.

Weir, Robert. "Truthtelling in Medicine." *Perspectives in Biology and Medicine* 24 (Autumn 1980): 95–112.

Wexler, David B. "Patients, Therapists, and Third Parties: The Victimological Virtues of Tarasoff." *International Journal of Law and Psychiatry* 2 (1979): 1–28.

Whyman, Fran Lochan. "Laissez Faire in the Medical Marketplace—Recognition of a Constitutional Right to Un-Conventional Medical Treatment: Andrews v. Ballard. *New England Law Review* 18(1) (1982–83): 149–81.

Zimmerman, David R. "An Ethical Dilemma: Patient Privacy vs. His Insurability." *Modern Medicine* 42 (1974): 18–24.

Chapter 5: Medical Experimentation and Informed Consent

AAP Task Force on Pediatric Research, Informed Consent and Medical Ethics. "AAP Code of Ethics for the Use of Fetuses and Fetal Material for Research." *Pediatrics* 56 (August 1975): 304–305.

Abrams, Natalie. "Justice in Fetal Experimentation." *Journal of Value Inquiry* 13 (1979): 103–113.

Annas, George J. *Informed Consent to Human Experimentation: The Subject's Dilemma.* Cambridge, Mass.: Ballinger Publishing Company, 1977.

————. "Report on the National Commission: Good as Gold." *Bioethics Quarterly* 2 (Summer 1980): 84–93. On the protection of human subjects.

————. *The Rights of Hospital Patients.* New York: Avon Books, 1975.

Berber, Bernard. "The Ethics of Experimentation with Human Subjects." *Scientific American* 234 (1976): 25–31.

————, **et al.** *Research on Human Subjects: Problems of Social Control in Medical Experimentation.* New York: Russell Sage Foundation, 1973 (reprinted New Brunswick, N.J.: Transaction Books, 1979).

Bartholome, William G. "Parents, Children, and the Moral Benefits of Research." *Hastings Center Report* 6 (December 1976): 44–45.

Beauchamp, Tom L. and Ruth R. Faden. "Decision-Making and Informed Consent: A Study of the Impact of Disclosed Information." *Social Indicators Research* 7 (1980): 313–336. An empirical and normative study.

Beecher, H. K. "Ethics and Clinical Research." *New England Journal of Medicine* 274 (1966): 1354–1360.

————. "Experimentation in Man." *Journal of the American Medical Association* 169 (1959): 461–478.

————. *Research and the Individual: Human Studies.* Boston: Little, Brown, 1970.

Bloomberg, Seth Allan and Leslie Wickins. "Ethics of Research Involving Human Subjects in Criminal Justice." *Crime and Delinquency* (October 1977): 435–444.

Bogomolny, Robert L., ed. *Human Experimentation.* Dallas: Southern Methodist University Press, 1976.

British Medical Association. "New Horizons in Medical Ethics: Research Investigation and the Fetus." *British Medical Journal* (26 May 1973): 464–468.

Capron, Alexander. "Informed Consent in Catastrophic Disease Research." *University of Pennsylvania Law Review* 123 (1974): 340–438.

————. "Medical Research in Prisons." *Hastings Center Report* 3 (1973): 4–6.

Case Western Reserve Law Review 24 (Spring 1975). A symposium on human experimentation.

Childress, James. "A Response to 'Conferred Rights and the Fetus.' " *Journal of Religious Ethics* 2 (1974): 27–33.

Cooke, Robert E. "An Ethical and Procedural Basis for Research on Children." *Journal of Pediatrics* 90 (April 1977): 681–682.

Cowles, Jane. *Informed Consent.* New York: Coward, McCann and Geoghegan, 1976.

Curran, W. J. "The Tuskegee Syphilis Study." *New England Journal of Medicine* 289 (4 October 1973): 730–731.

Eisenberg, Leon. "The Social Imperatives of Medical Research." *Science* 198 (December 1977): 1105–1110.

Experiments and Research with Humans: Values in Conflict. Washington, D.C.: National Academy of Sciences, 1975.

Faden, Ruth R., Carol Lewis, Catherine Becker, Alan I. Faden, and John Freeman. "Disclosure Standards and Informed Consent." *Journal of Health Politics, Policy and Law* 6 (Summer 1981): 255–84.

Federal Proceedings 36 (September 1977): 2344–2364. Special section on drugs and human research.

Fletcher, John. "Human Experimentation: Ethics in the Consent Situation." *Law and Contemporary Problems* 32 (1967): 620–649. A good general review.

Forssman, Werner. *Experiments on Myself: Memoirs of a Surgeon in Germany.* New York: St. Martin's Press, 1974. An experimenter who used himself as a research subject for cardiac catheterization.

Freund, Paul A. "Ethical Problems in Human Experimentation." *New England Journal of Medicine* 273 (1965): 687–692.

————, ed. *Experimentation with Human Subjects.* New York: George Braziller, 1970. An influential collection of twenty articles.

Fried, Charles. *Medical Experimentation: Personal Integrity and Social Policy.* New York: American Elsevier, 1974.

Gardner, E. Clifton. "Ethical Issues in the Testing of New Drugs in Man." *Journal of Drug Issues* 7 (Summer 1977): 275–286.

Gaylin, Williard and Ruth Macklin, eds. *Who Speaks for the Child: The Problems of Proxy Consent.* New York: Plenum Press, 1982.

———— and Marc Lappé. "Fetal Policies: The Debate on Experimenting with the Unborn." *Atlantic Monthly* 235 (May 1975): 66–71.

Goldiamond, Israel. "Protection of Human Subjects and Patients: A Social Contingency Analysis of Distinctions between Research and Practice and Its Implications." *Behaviorism* 4 (1976): 1–41.

Graham, John B. "Ethical and Social Issues Posed by Genetic Studies of Cardiovascular Disease." *Perspectives in Biology and Medicine* 20 (Winter 1977): 260–270.

Guttentag, O. E. "Ethical Problems in Human Experimentation." In E. F. Torrey, ed. *Ethical Issues in Medicine.* Boston: Little, Brown, 1968.

Halper, Thomas. "Ethics and Medical Experimentation: Some Unconfronted Problems." *Connecticut Medicine* 40 (1976): 267–268.

Hastings Center Report 5 (June 1975): 13–46. Special issue on fetal research.

Hatfield, Frank. "Prison Research: The View from Inside." *Hastings Center Report* 7 (February 1977): 11–12.

Heller, P. "Informed Consent and the Old-Fashioned Conscience of the Physician-Investigator." *Perspectives in Biology and Medicine* 20 (Spring 1977): 434–438.

Hilton, Bruce and Daniel Callahan, eds. *Ethical Issues in Human Genetics: Genetic Counseling and the Use of Genetic Knowledge.* New York: Plenum Publishing Corporation, 1976.

Hubbard, Ruth. " 'Fetal Rights' and the New Eugenics." *Science for the People* 16(2) (March/April 1984): 7–9, 27–29.

The Human Life Review 1 (Fall 1975). "A Symposium: Fetal Research."

Katz, Jay. *Experimentation with Human Beings.* New York: Russell Sage Foundation, 1972.

Kidd, Alexander M. "Limits of the Right of a Person to Consent to Experimentation on Himself." *Science* 117 (1953): 211–212.

Ladimer, Irving, ed. "New Dimensions in Legal and Ethical Concepts for Human Research. *Annals of the New York Academy of Sciences* 169 (1970): 293–593.

———— and R. W. Newman, eds. *Clinical Investigation in Medicine: Legal, Ethical and Moral Aspects.* Boston: Boston University Press, 1963.

Laforet, Eugene G. "The Fiction of Informed Consent." *Journal of the American Medical Association* 235 (12 April 1976): 1579–1585.

Langer, E. "Human Experimentation: New York Verdict Affirms Patients' Rights." *Science* 151 (1966): 663–666. On the Sloan-Kettering case.

Lebacqz, Karen and Robert Levine. "Respect for Persons and Informed Consent to Participate in Research." *Clinical Research* 25 (April 1977): 101–107.

Lewis, Melvin. "Comments on Some Ethical, Legal, and Clinical Issues Affecting Consent in Treatment, Organ Transplants, and Research in Children." *Journal of the American Academy of Child Psychiatry* 20 (1981): 581–96.

Lipsett, Mortimer B. "On the Nature and Ethics of Phase I Clinical Trials of Cancer Chemotherapies." *Journal of the American Medical Association* 248 (27 August 1982): 941–42.

Lower, Charles U., et al. "Nontherapeutic Research on Children: An Ethical Dilemma." *Journal of Pediatrics* 84 (April 1974): 468–473.

Ludlum, James E. *Informed Consent.* Chicago: American Hospital Association, 1978.

Luker, Kristin. *Abortion and the Politics of Motherhood.* Berkeley, Calif.: University of California Press, 1984.

Macklin, Ruth. "Some Problems in Gaining Informed Consent from Psychiatric Patients." *Emory Law Journal* 31(2) (Spring 1982): 345–74.

_____. "Consent, Coercion, and Conflicts of Rights." *Perspectives in Biology and Medicine* 20 (Spring 1977): 360–371.

_____ **and Susan Sherwin.** "Experimenting on Human Subjects: Philosophical Perspectives." *Case-Western Reserve Law Review* 25 (1975): 434–471. A good review of issues with respect to Mill, Kant, and Rawls. Part of a symposium on human experimentation.

Margolis, Joseph. "Conceptual Aspects of a Patient's Bill of Rights." *Journal of Value Inquiry* 11 (Summer 1977), 126–135.

Martin, Michael M. "Ethical Standards for Fetal Experimentation." *Fordham Law Review* 43 (1975): 548–570.

McCormick, Richard A. "Proxy Consent in the Experimentation Situation." *Perspectives in Biology and Medicine* 18 (Autumn 1974): 2–20.

_____. "A Reply to Paul Ramsey—Experimentation in Children: Sharing in Socialty." *Hasting Center Report* 6 (December 1976): 41–46.

McKinley, Sonja M., ed. "Experimental Evidence and Social Policy." *Milbank Memorial Fund Quarterly/Health and Society* (Summer 1981). Special issue.

Meisel, Alan. "Informed Consent—The Rebuttal." And Mills, Don Harper. "Informed Consent—The Rejoinder." *Journal of the American Medical Association* 234 (1975): 615–616.

_____ **and Lisa Kabnick.** "Informed Consent to Medical Treatment: An Analysis of Recent Legislation." *University of Pittsburgh Law Review* 41 (Spring 1980): 407–564.

_____ **and Loren H. Roth.** "Toward an Informed Discussion of Informed Consent: A Review and Critique of the Empirical Studies." *Arizona Law Review* 25(2) 1983.

_____ **and Loren H. Roth.** "What We Do and Do Not Know About Informed Consent." *Journal of the American Medical Association* 246 (27 November 1981): 2473–77.

Meyers, David W. *The Human Body and the Law.* Chicago: Aldine Publishing, 1970.

Miller, Leslie J. "Informed Consent: I, II, III, IV." *Journal of the American Medical Association* 244 (7 November 1980–12 December 1980): 2100–2103, 2347–2350, 2556–2558, 2661–2662.

Mills, D. H. "Whither Informed Consent?" *Journal of the American Medical Association* 229 (1974): 305–310.

Montange, C. H. "Informed Consent and the Dying Patient." *Yale Law Journal* 83 (1974): 1632–1664.

Murphy, Jeffrie G. "Therapy and the Problem of Autonomous Consent." *International Journal of Law and Psychiatry* 2 (1979): 415–430.

_____. "Total Institution and the Possibility of Consent to Organic Therapies." *Human Rights* 5 (Fall 1975): 25–45.

Norton, Martin L. "When Does an Experimental/Innovative Procedure Become an Accepted Procedure?" *Pharos* 38 (October 1975): 161–165.

President's Commission for the Study of Ethical Problems in Medicine and Biomedical and

Behavioral Research. *Implementing Human Research Regulations.* Washington, D.C.: President's Commission, 1983.

_____. *Making Health Care Decisions: Empirical Studies of Informed Consent.* Volume Two: Appendices. Washington, D.C.: President's Commission, 1982.

_____. *Making Health Care Decisions: The Ethical and Legal Implications of Informed Consent in the Patient-Practitioner Relationship.* Washington, D.C.: President's Commission, 1982.

_____ . *Protecting Human Subjects: First Biennial Report on the Adequacy and Uniformity of Federal Rules and Policies, and Their Implementation, for the Protection of Human Subjects in Biomedical and Behavioral Research.* Washington, D.C.: President's Commission, 1981.

Ramsey, Paul. "Children as Research Subjects—A Reply." *Hastings Center Report* 7 (April 1977): 40–41.

_____. "A Reply to Richard McCormick—The Enforcement of Morals: Nontherapeutic Research on Children." *Hastings Center Report* 6 (August 1976): 21–30.

_____. "The Enforcement of Morals: Nontherapeutic Research on Children." *Hastings Center Report* 6 (1975): 21–30.

_____. "The Ethics of a Cottage Industry in an Age of Community and Research Medicine." *New England Journal of Medicine* 284 (1971): 700–706.

_____. *The Ethics of Fetal Research.* New Haven: Yale University Press, 1975.

Robinson, Wade L. and Michael S. Pritchard, eds. *Medical Responsibility: Paternalism, Informed Consent, and Euthanasia.* Clifton, N.J.: Humana Press, 1979. See in particular articles by Abrams, Browne, and Toulmin.

Schreiner, G. E. "The Ethics of Human Experimentation." *Pharos* 29 (1966): 78–83.

Science 198 (18 November 1977): 677–705. "Medical Research: Statistics and Ethics."

Smith, Richard. "Prison Doctors: Ethics, Invisibility, and Quality." *British Medical Journal* 288 (10 March 1984): 781–83.

Varley, A. B. "Protection of Human Research Subjects: Are Ethics Necessary?" *Journal of Legal Medicine* 4 (1976): 23–26.

Veatch, Robert M. "Human Experimentation: The Crucial Choices Ahead." *Prism* 2 (1974): 58ff.

_____. " 'Experimental' Pregnancy." *Hastings Center Report* 1 (1971): 2–3. About the Goldzieher experiment, in which placebos were used instead of contraceptive pills.

Visscher, Maurice B. *Ethical Constraints and Imperatives in Medical Research.* Springfield, Ill.: Charles C. Thomas, 1975.

Walters, LeRoy. "Ethical Issues in Experimentation on the Human Fetus." *Journal of Religious Ethics* 2 (1974): 33–54.

_____. "Some Ethical Issues in Research Involving Human Subjects." *Perspectives in Biology and Medicine* 20 (Winter 1977): 193–211.

Wecht, C. H. "Medical, Legal and Moral Considerations in Human Experiments Involving Minors and Incompetent Adults." *Journal of Legal Medicine* 4 (1976): 27–30.

Welt, L. G. "Reflections on the Problems of Human Experimentation." *Connecticut Medicine* 25 (1961): 75–78.

White, L. P. "Biomedical Experimentation on Prisoners." *Western Journal of Medicine* 124 (1976): 514–516.

Willis, David P., ed. "The Problem of Personhood: Biomedical, Social, Legal, and Policy Views." *Milbank Memorial Fund Quarterly* 61(1) (Winter 1983).

Wolfenberger, W. "Ethical Issues in Research with Human Subjects." *Science* 155 (1967): 47–51.

Part III: Controls

Chapter 6: Genetics: Intervention, Control, and Research

The Ann Arbor Science for the People Editorial Collective. *Biology as a Social Weapon.* Minneapolis: Burgess Publishing Company, 1977.

Annas, George J. and Brian Cogne. "Fitness for the Birth and Reproduction: Legal Implications of Genetic Screening." *Family Law Quarterly* 9 (Fall 1975): 463–489.

Applebaum, Eleanor Gordon and Stephen K. Firestein. *A Genetic Counseling Casebook.* New York: Free Press, 1983.

Ausubel, F., J. Beckwith, and K. Janssen. "The Politics of Genetic Engineering: Who Decides Who's Defective." *Psychology Today* 7 (June 1974): 30–43. The authors are members of Science for the People.

Baker, Robert. "Protecting the Unconceived." In John W. Davis, Barry Hoffmaster, and Sarah Shorten, eds. *Contemporary Issues in Biomedical Ethics.* Clifton, N.J.: Humana Press, 1978, pp. 89–100.

Bass, I. Scott. "Governmental Control of Research in Positive Eugenics." *Journal of Law Reform* 8 (Spring 1974): 615–630.

Bayles, Michael D. *Reproductive Ethics.* Englewood Cliffs, N.J.: Prentice-Hall, 1984.

————. "Harm to the Unconceived." *Philosophy and Public Affairs* 5 (Spring 1976): 292–304.

Beckwith, Jon and Jonathan King. "The XYY Syndrome: A Dangerous Myth." *New Scientist* 14 (November 1974): 474–476.

Beers, Roland F., Jr., and Edward G. Bassett, eds. *Recombinant Molecules: Impact on Science and Society.* New York: Raven Press, 1977.

Berg, Paul, et al. "Asilomar Conference on Recombinant DNA Molecules." *Science* 188 (1975): 991–994.

Breyer, Stephan and Richard Zeckhauser. "The Regulation of Genetic Engineering." *Man and Medicine* 1 (Winter 1976): 1–9.

Buckley, John J., Jr., ed. *Genetics Now: Ethical Issues in Genetic Research.* Washington, D.C.: University Press of America, 1978.

Capron, Alexander. *Genetic Counseling: Facts, Values and Norms.* New York, Alan R. Liss, 1979.

————. "Reflections on Issues Posed by Recombinant DNA Molecule Technology." *Annals of the American Academy of Sciences* 265 (1976): 71–81. Entire issue is devoted to genetic issues.

Curran, William J. "The Questionable Virtues of Genetic Screening Laws." *American Journal of Public Health* 64 (1974): 1003–1004.

Daedalus 90 (1961). "Evolution and Man's Progress." See in particular the articles by Muller and Crow.

Danielli, James F. "Industry, Society, and Genetic Engineering." *Hastings Center Report* 2 (December 1972): 5–7.

Davidson, Michael D. "First Amendment Protection for Biomedical Research." *Arizona Law Review* 19 (1977): 893–918.

Davis, Bernard D. "Prospects for Genetic Intervention in Man." *Science* 170 (1970): 1279–1283.

Edwards, Robert G. "Fertilization of Human Eggs in Vitro: Morals, Ethics, and the Law." *Quarterly Review of Biology* 49 (March 1974): 3–26.

Ellison, Craig, W., ed. *Modifying Man.* Washington, D.C.: University Press of America, 1978. A "Christian evangelical" view.

Etzioni, Amitai. "Amniocentesis: A Case Study of the Management of 'Genetic Engineering.' " *Ethics in Science and Medicine* 2 (May 1975): 13–24.

————. *Genetic Fix: The Next Technological Revolution.* New York: Harper and Row, 1975.

————. "Sex Control, Science and Society." *Science* 161 (1968): 1107–1112.

Ferguson, James R. "Scientific Inquiry and the First Amendment." *Cornell Law Review* 64 (April 1979): 639–665.

Fletcher, John C. "Ethics and Trends in Applied Human Genetics." *Birth Defects* 19(5) (1983): 143–58.

————. "Moral Problems and Ethical Issues in Prospective Human Gene Therapy." *Virginia Law Review* 69(3) (April 1983): 515–46.

————. "Ethical Issues in Genetic Screening and Antenatal Diagnosis." *Clinical Obstetrics and Gynecology* 24 (December 1981): 1151–68.

————. "Ethics and Amniocentesis for Fetal Sex Identification." *Hastings Center Report* 10 (1980): 15–17.

————. "Moral and Ethical Problems of Pre-Natal Diagnosis." *Clinical Genetics* 8 (1975): 251–257.

Fletcher, Joseph. "Ethical Aspects of Genetic Controls." *New England Journal of Medicine* 285 (1971): 776–783.

Frankel, Charles. "The Specter of Eugenics." *Commentary* 57 (1974): 25–33.

Frankel, Mark S. "The Application of Genetic Technology: Ethics and Pitfalls." *Impact of Science on Society* 25 (1975): 85–90.

Friedman, Theodore. "The Future of Gene Therapy: A Reevaluation." *Annals of the American Academy of Sciences* 265 (1976): 141–152.

Fudenberg, H. Hugh and Vijaya Melnick, eds. *Biomedical Scientists and Public Policy.* New York: Plenum Press, 1978.

Gastel, Barbara. *Maternal Serum Alpha-Fetoprotein: Issues in the Prenatal Screening and Diagnosis of Neural Tube Defects.* Washington, D.C.: Government Printing Office, 1981.

Gaylin, Willard. "Genetic Screening: The Ethics of Knowing." *New England Journal of Medicine* 286 (22 June 1972): 1361–1362.

Georgia Law Review II (Summer 1977): 785–878. "Recombinant DNA and Technology Assessment." Special issue.

Golding, Martin. "Obligations to Future Generations." *The Monist* 56 (January 1972): 85–99.

Goodfield, June. *Playing God: Genetic Engineering and the Manipulation of Life.* New York: Random House, 1977.

Green, Harold P. "The Boundaries of Scientific Freedom." *Newsletter on Science, Technology, and Human Values* 20 (June 1977): 17–21.

Grobstein, Clifford. *A Double Image of the Double Helix: The Recombinant-DNA Debate.* San Francisco: W. H. Freeman, 1979.

Harris, Maureen, ed. *Early Diagnosis of Human Genetic Defects: Scientific and Ethical Considerations.* Fogarty International Center Proceedings, no. 6, 1972.

Harzanyi, Zsolt and Richard Hutton. *Genetic Prophecy: Beyond the Double Helix.* New York: Rawson, Wade Publishers, Inc. 1981.

Hilton, Bruce, et al., eds. *Ethical Issues in Human Genetics: Genetic Counseling and the Use of Genetic Knowledge.* New York: Plenum Press, 1973.

Hoffman, John C. *Ethical Confrontation in Counseling.* Chicago: University of Chicago Press, 1979.

Holton, Gerald, ed. "Limits of Scientific Inquiry." *Daedalus* 107 (Spring 1978): 1–234. Special issue.

Hull, R. T. "Philosophical Considerations in the Growing Potential for Human Genetic Control." *Annals of the American Academy of Sciences* 265 (1976): 118–126.

Humber, James M. and Robert F. Almeder, eds. *Biomedical Ethics and the Law.* New York: Plenum Press, 1976.

Ingle, D. J. "Ethics of Genetic Intervention." *Medical Opinion Review* 3 (1967): 54–61.

Institute of Society, Ethics and the Life Sciences: Research Group on Ethical, Social and Legal Issues in Genetic Counseling and Genetic Engineering. "Ethical and Social Issues in Screening for Genetic Disease." *New England Journal of Medicine* 286 (25 May 1972): 1129–1132.

Jackson, David A. and Stephen P. Stich, eds. *The Recombinant DNA Debate.* Englewood Cliffs, N.J.: Prentice-Hall, 1979.

Kass, Leon. "Implications of Prenatal Diagnosis for the Human Right to Life." In Bruce Hilton, et al., eds. *Ethical Issues in Human Genetics.* New York: Plenum Press, 1973.

————. "Making Babies: The New Biology and the 'Old' Morality." *Public Interest* 26 (1972): 18–56.

————. "New Beginning in Life." In Michael Hamilton, ed. *The New Genetics and the Future Man.* Grand Rapids, Mich.: Eerdmans, 1972, pp. 15–63. On in vitro fertilization.

Kelly, Patricia T. *Dealing with Dilemma: A Manual for Genetic Counselors.* New York: Springer-Verlag, 1977.

Klein, David. "Genetic Manipulations." *Impact of Science on Society* 23 (1973): 21–27.

Kolata, Gina B. "Prenatal Diagnosis of Neural Tube Defects." *Science* 209 (12 September 1980): 1216–1218.

Kopelman, Loretta. "Genetic Screening in Newborns: Voluntary or Compulsory?" *Perspectives in Biology and Medicine* 22 (Autumn 1978): 83–89.

Lakoff, Sanford A. "Moral Responsibility and the 'Galilean Imperative.'" *Ethics* 91 (October 1980): 100–116.

Lappé, Marc and Robert S. Morrison, eds. "Ethical and Scientific Issues Posed by Human Uses of Molecular Genetics." *Annals of the New York Academy of Sciences* 265 (1976): 1–208.

Lappé, Marc, et al. "Ethical and Social Issues in Screening for Genetic Disease." *New England Journal of Medicine* 286 (1972): 1129–1132. Problems and guidelines in social programs.

————. *Genetics Politics: The Limits of Biological Control.* New York: Simon and Schuster, 1979.

————. "Moral Obligations and the Fallacies of Genetic Control." *Theological Studies* 33 (1972): 411–427.

———— **and Peter Steinfels.** "Choosing the Sex of Our Children." *Hastings Center Report* 4 (1974): 1–4.

Lederberg, Joshua. "DNA Splicing: Will Fear Rob Us of Its Benefits?" *Prism* 2 (November 1975): 33–37.

————. "Experimental Genetics and Human Evolution." *American Naturalist* 100 (1966): 519–531.

————. "Orthobiosis: The Perfection of Man." In Nicholas Rescher, ed. *The Place of Value in a World of Facts.* New York: John Wiley, 1970.

Leiser, Burton M. "The New Genetics and Lives Not Worth Living." In John J. Buckley, Jr. ed. *Genetics Now: Ethical Issues in Genetic Research.* Washington, D.C.: University Press of America, 1982, pp. 41–58.

Leonard, C. O., et al. "Genetic Counseling: A Consumer's View." *New England Journal of Medicine* 287 (1972): 433–449. An empirical survey of consumer attitudes and information.

Lenzer, Gertrud. "Gender Ethics." *Hastings Center Report* 10 (1980): 18–19.

Lipkin, Mack, Jr., and P. T. Rowley, eds. *Genetic Responsibility: On Choosing Our Children's Genes.* New York: Plenum Press, 1974.

Ludmerer, Kenneth M. *Genetics and American Society.* Baltimore: Johns Hopkins University Press, 1972. A history of the eugenics movement.

Man and Medicine 2 (Winter 1977): 78–132. Special issue on recombinant DNA.

McCormick, Richard. "Genetic Medicine: Notes on the Moral Literature." *Theological Studies* 33 (September 1972): 531–532.

Mercola, Karen and Martin Cline. "The Potentials of Inserting New Genetic Information." *New England Journal of Medicine* 303 (27 November 1980): 1297–1300.

Milunsky, A. and G. J. Annas, eds. *Genetics and the Law.* New York: Plenum Press, 1976.

Muller, H. J. "The Guidance of Human Evolution." *Perspectives in Biology and Medicine* 3 (1959):1–43.

————. "What Genetic Course Will Man Steer?" In J. F. Crow and J. V. Neel, eds. *Proceedings of the Third International Congress of Human Genetics.* Baltimore: Johns Hopkins University, 1967.

National Academy of Sciences. *Genetic Screening: Programs, Principles, and Research.* Washington, D.C.: National Academy of Sciences, 1975.

————. *Research with Recombinant DNA: An Academy Forum, 7–9 March 1977.* Washington, D.C.: National Academy of Sciences, 1977.

National Research Council, Committee for the Study of Inborn Errors of Metabolism. *Genetic Screening: Programs, Principles, and Research.* Washington, D.C.: National Academy of Sciences, 1975.

Neville, Robert. "Gene Therapy and the Ethics of Genetic Therapeutics." *Annals of the New York Academy of Sciences* 265 (1976): 153–161.

Omenn, Gilbert. "Genetics and Epidemiology: Medical Interventions and Public Policy." *Social Biology* 26 (Summer 1979): 117–125.

Osborn, Frederick. "The Emergency of a Valid Eugenics." *American Scientist* 61 (1973): 425–429.

Panel on Bioethical Concerns, National Council of Churches of Christ/U.S.A. *Genetic Engineering: Social and Ethical Consequences.* New York: The Pilgrim Press, 1984.

Powledge, Tabitha. "The New Ghetto Hustle." *Saturday Review of the Sciences* (February 1973): 38–47.

————. "There's Another Side to Genetic Screening." *Prism* 3 (1976): 55–57.

Powledge, Tabitha and John Fletcher. "Guidelines for the Ethical, Social, and Legal Issues in Prenatal Diagnosis." *New England Journal of Medicine* 300 (January 1979): 168–172.

President's Commission for the Study of Ethical Problems in Medicine and Biomedical and Behavioral Research. *Screening and Counseling for Genetic Conditions: The Ethical, Social, and Legal Implications of Genetic Screening, Counseling, and Education Programs.* Washington, D.C.: President's Commission, 1983.

————. *Splicing Life: The Social and Ethical Issues of Genetic Engineering with Human Beings.* Washington, D.C.: President's Commission, 1982.

Ramsey, Paul. *Fabricated Man: The Ethics of Genetic Control.* New Haven: Yale University Press, 1970.

————. "Genetic Engineering." *Bulletin of the Atomic Scientists* 29 (December 1972): 14–17.

Reed, Sheldon. *Counseling in Medical Genetics.* New York: Alan R. Liss, 1980.

Reilly, Philip. *Genetics, Law and Social Policy.* Cambridge, Mass.: Harvard University Press, 1977.

Richards, John, ed. *Recombinant DNA: Science, Ethics and Politics.* New York: Academic Press, 1978.

Robertson, John A. "Procreative Liberty and the Control of Conception, Pregnancy, and Childbirth." *Virginia Law Review* 69(3) (April 1983): 405–64.

————. "The Right to Procreate and in Utero Fetal Therapy." *Journal of Legal Medicine* 3 (September 1982): 333–66.

Robitscher, Jonas. *Eugenic Sterilization.* Springfield, Ill.: Charles C. Thomas, 1973.

Rogers, Michael. *Biohazard.* New York: Alfred A. Knopf, 1977.

Ruse, Michael. "Genetics and the Quality of Life." *Social Indicators Research* 7 (January 1980): 419–441.

Sinsheimer, Robert. "An Evolutionary Perspective for Genetic Engineering." *New Scientist* 73 (20 January 1977): 150–152.

————. "Troubled Dawn for Genetic Engineering." *New Scientist* 68 (1975): 148–151. An excellent review of problems.

Sorenson, James R., Judith P. Swazey, and Norman A. Scotch. *Reproductive Pasts, Reproductive Futures: Genetic Counseling and Its Effectiveness.* New York: Alan R. Liss, 1982.

Southern California Law Review 51 (September 1978): 969–1573. "Biotechnology and the Law: Recombinant DNA and the Control of Scientific Research." Special issue.

Stetten, DeWitt. "Freedom of Enquiry." *Genetics* 81 (November 1975): 415–425.

Sylvester, Edward J. and Lynn C. Klotz. *The Gene Age: Genetic Engineering and the Next Industrial Revolution.* New York: Charles Scribner's Sons, 1983.

Thomas, Lewis. "The Hazards of Science." *New England Journal of Medicine* 296 (10 February 1977): 324–328.

Tormey, Judith F. "Ethical Considerations of Prenatal Genetic Diagnosis." *Clinical Obstetrics and Gynecology* 19 (1976): 957–963.

Tsuang, Ming T. and Randall VanderMey. *Genes and the Mind: Inheritance of Mental Illness.* New York: Oxford University Press, 1980.

Twiss, S. B., Jr. "Ethical Issues in Priority Setting for the Utilization of Genetic Technologies." *Annals of the New York Academy of Sciences* 265 (1976): 22–45.

Ulrich, Lawrence P. "Reproductive Rights and Genetic Disease." In James M. Humber, ed. *Biomedical Ethics and the Law.* New York: Plenum Press, 1976, pp. 351–360.

Veatch, Robert M. "Ethical Issues in Genetics." Arthur G. Steinberg and Alexander G. Bearn, eds. *Progress in Medical Genetics*, vol. X. New York: Grune and Stratton, 1974.

Wade, Nicholas. "Genetics: Conference Sets Strict Controls to Replace Moratorium." *Science* 187 (1975): 931–935.

————. *The Ultimate Experiment.* New York: Walker and Company, 1977.

Walters, LeRoy. "Genetics, Reproductive Biology, and Bioethics." In Marguerite Neumann, ed. *The Tricentennial People: Human Applications of the New Genetics.* Ames, Iowa: Iowa State University Press, 1978, pp. 66–80.

Wautz, Jon R. and Carol R. Thigpen. "Genetic Screening and Counseling: The Legal and Ethical Issues." *Northwestern University Law Review* 68 (September–October 1973): 696–767.

Watson, James D. "Moving toward Clonal Man: Is That What We Want?" *Atlantic Monthly* 227 (1971): 50–53.

Westoff, Charles F. and R. R. Rindfuss. "Sex Preselection in the U.S.: Some Implications." *Science* 184 (1974): 633–636.

Yoxen, Edward. *The Gene Business: Who Should Control Biotechnology?* New York: Oxford University Press, 1983.

Zimmerman, Burke K. *Biofuture Confronting the Genetic Era.* New York: Plenum Press, 1984.

Chapter 7: Reproductive Control: In Vitro Fertilization, Artificial Insemination, Surrogate Pregnancy, and Sterilization

Amicus, 2 (February 1977): 33–47. "Society's Right to Sterilize: What Are the Limits?" A special issue.

Annas, George J. and Sherman Elias. "In Vitro Fertilization and Embryo Transfer: Medicolegal Aspects of a New Technique to Create a Family." *Family Law Quarterly* 17(2) (Summer 1983): 199–223.

Beck, William, W., Jr. "A Critical Look at the Legal, Ethical, and Technical Aspects of Artificial Insemination." *Fertility and Sterility* 27 (January 1976): 1–8.

Bellotis, Raymond A. "Morality and *In Vitro* Fertilization." *Bioethics Quarterly* 2 (1980): 6–19.

Burgdorf, Robert and Marcia Burgdorf. "The Wicked Witch Is Almost Dead: Buck vs. Bell and the Sterilization of Handicapped Persons." *Temple Law Quarterly* 50 (1977): 995–1034.

Burt, Robert and Monroe E. Price. "Sterilization, State Action and the Concept of Consent." *Law and Psychology Review* (Spring 1975): 57–78.

Callahan, Daniel, et al. "In Vitro Fertilization: Four Commentaries." *Hastings Center Report* 8 (October 1978): 7–14.

Cushan, Anna Marie, ed. *Adoption and A.I.D.: Access to Information?* Melbourne: Monash Centre for Human Bioethics, 1984.

Davis, Morris E. "Involuntary Sterilization: A History of Social Control." *Journal of Black Health* 1 (August-September 1974).

Deroulin, Judy. "In re Guardianship of Eberhardy: The Sterilization of the Mentally Retarded." *Wisconsin Law Review* 6 (1982): 1199–1227.

Donovan, Patricia. "Sterilization and the Poor: Two Views on the Need for Protection from Abuse." *Family Planning/Population Reporter* 5 (April 1976): 28–30.

Edwards, Robert G. "Fertilization of Human Eggs in Vitro: Morals, Ethics, and the Law." *Quarterly Review of Biology* 49 (March 1974): 3–26.

_____ **and D. J. Sharpe.** "Social Values and Research in Human Embryology." *Nature* 231 (14 May 1971): 87–91.

Flynn, Eileen P. *Human Fertilization In Vitro: A Catholic Moral Perspective.* Lanham, Md.: University Press of America, 1984.

Frankel, Mark S. "Human Semen Banking: Social and Public Policy Issues." *Man and Medicine* 1 (Summer 1976): 289–309.

Hellegers, Andre and Richard A. McCormick. "Unanswered Questions on Test-Tube Life." *America* 139 (August 1978): 74–78.

Holder, A. R. "Voluntary Sterilization." *Journal of the American Medical Association* 225 (24 September 1973): 1743–1744.

Horne, Herbert, Jr. "Artificial Insemination Donor: An Issue of Ethical and Moral Values." *New England Journal of Medicine* 293 (23 October 1975): 873–874.

Kass, Leon R. "Babies by Means of In Vitro Fertilization: Unethical Experiments on the Unborn?" *New England Journal of Medicine* 285 (18 November 1971): 1174–1179.

_____. "Making Babies: The New Biology and the Old Morality." *Public Interest* 26 (Winter 1972): 18–56.

Keane, Noel P. with Dennis L. Breo. *The Surrogate Mother.* New York: Everest House Publishers, 1981.

Law and Ethics of A.I.D. and Embryo Transfer. CIBA Foundation Symposium 17. New York: Associated Scientific Publishers, 1973.

Macklin, Ruth and William Gaylin, eds. *Mental Retardation and Sterilization: A Problem of Competency and Paternalism.* New York: Plenum Press, 1981.

Marsh, Frank H. and Donnie L. Self. "In Vitro Fertilization: Moving from Theory to Therapy." *Hastings Center Report* (10 January 1980): 5–6.

Marx, Jean L. "Embryology: Out of the Womb—Into the Test Tube" and "In Vitro Fertilization of Human Eggs: Bioethical and Legal Considerations." *Science* 182 (23 November 1973): 811–814.

McGarrah, Robert E., Jr., and Susan L. Peck. "Voluntary Female Sterilization." *Hastings Center Report* 4 (June 1974): 5–10.

Meyers, David. *The Human Body and the Law.* Chicago: Aldine Publishing Company, 1970.

Peckins, David M. "Artificial Insemination and the Law." *Journal of Legal Medicine* (July–August 1976): 17–22.

Perrin, J. C., et al. "A Considered Approach to Sterilization of Mentally Retarded Youths." *American Journal of Diseases of Children* 130 (March 1976): 288–290.

Ramsey, Paul. "Shall We Reproduce?" *Journal of the American Medical Association* 220 (5 June 1972): 1346–1350.

Reilly, Philip. "The Surgical Solution: The Writings of Activist Physicians in the Early Days of Eugenical Sterilization." *Perspectives in Biology and Medicine* 26 (Summer 1983): 637–53.

Robitscher, Jonas, ed. *Eugenic Sterilization.* Springfield, Ill.: Charles C. Thomas, 1973.

Rosoff, Jennie. "Sterilization: The Montgomery Case." *Hastings Center Report* 3 (September 1973): 6.

Schima, Marilyn and Ira Lumbell, eds. *Advances in Voluntary Sterilization.* New York: Elsevier, 1974.

Smith, George P., II. "Through a Test Tube Darkly: Artificial Insemination and the Law." *Michigan Law Review* 67 (1968): 127–150.

Snowden, R., G. D. Mitchell, and E. M. Snowden. *Artificial Reproduction: A Social Investigation.* Winchester, Mass.: Allen and Unwin, Inc., 1983.

———— **and Peter Singer, eds.** *Test-Tube Babies.* New York: Oxford University Press, 1982.

Veatch, Robert M. "Sterilization: Its Socio-Cultural and Ethical Determinants." In Marilyn E. Schima and Ira Lumbell, eds. *Advances in Voluntary Sterilization.* New York: Elsevier, 1974, pp. 138–150.

Wadlington, Walter. "Artificial Insemination: The Dangers of a Poorly Kept Secret." *Northwestern University Law Review* 64 (January–February): 777–807.

Walters, LeRoy. "Human In Vitro Fertilization." *Hastings Center Report* 9 (August 1979): 23–43.

Walters, William and Peter Singer, eds. *Test-Tube Babies.* New York: Oxford University Press, 1982.

Working Party Council for Science and Society. *Human Procreation: Ethical Aspects of the New Techniques.* Oxford: Oxford University Press, 1984.

Zaner, Richard M. "A Criticism of Moral Conservatism's View of In Vitro Fertilization and Embryo Transfer." *Perspectives in Biology and Medicine* 27(2) (Winter 1984): 201–12.

Part IV: Resources

Chapter 8: Allocating Scarce Medical Resources

Aaron, Henry J. and William B. Schwartz. *The Painful Prescription: Rationing Hospital Care.* Washington, D.C.: The Brookings Institution, 1984.

American Medical Association Judicial Council. "Ethical Guidelines for Organ Transplantation." *Journal of the American Medical Association* 25 (1968): 341–342.

Anscombe, G. E. M. "Who Is Wronged?" *Oxford Review* 5 (1967): 16–17. A general argument relating to distribution.

Beecher, Henry K. "Scarce Resources and Medical Advancement." In Paul Freund, ed. *Experimentation with Human Subjects.* New York: George Braziller, 1970.

Bermant, Gordon, Peter Brown, and Gerald Dworkin. "Of Morals, Markets, and Medicine." *Hastings Center Report* 5 (1975): 14–16.

Caplan, Arthur L. "Kidneys, Ethics, and Politics: Lessons of the ESRD Program." *Journal of Health Politics, Policy and Law* 6(3) (Fall 1981): 488–503.

Coward, Howard and Donald E. Larsen, eds. *Ethical Issues in the Allocation of Health Care Resources.* Calgary: University of Calgary, 1982.

Daniels, Norman. "Am I My Parents Keeper?" *Midwest Studies in Philosophy* VII (1982): 517–40.

————. "Cost-Effectiveness and Patient Welfare." In Marc Basson, ed. *Rights and Responsibilities in Medicine.* New York: Alan R. Liss, 1981, pp. 159–170.

Dukeminier, J., Jr., and D. Sanders. "Organ Transplantation: A Proposal for Routine Salvaging of Cadaver Organs." *New England Journal of Medicine* 279 (22 August 1968): 413–419.

Engelhardt, H. Tristram, Jr., "Shattuck Lecture: Allocating Scarce Medical Resources and the Availability of Organ Transplantation: Some Moral Presuppositions." *The New England Journal of Medicine* 331(1) (5 July 1984): 66–71.

Evans, Roger W. "Health Care Technology and the Inevitability of Resource Allocation and Rationing Decisions." Parts I and II. *Journal of the American Medical Association* 249 (15 and 16) (15 and 22/29 April 1983): 2047–53, 2208–19.

Ezorsky, Gertrude. "How Many Lives Shall We Save?" *Metaphilosophy* 3 (1972): 156–162. Includes a criticism of Anscombe's "Who Is Wronged?"

Fellner, Carl H. "Altruism in Disrepute." *New England Journal of Medicine* 284 (1973): 589–592.

————. "Kidney Donors—The Myth of Informed Consent." *American Journal of Psychiatry* 126 (1970): 9.

————. "Organ Donation: For Whose Sake?" *Annals of Internal Medicine* (October 1973): 589–592.

Fox, R. C. and J. P. Swazey. *The Courage to Fail: A Social View of Organ Transplants and Dialysis.* Chicago: University of Chicago Press, 1974.

Gorovitz, Samuel. "Ethics and the Allocation of Medical Resources." *Medical Research Engineering* 5 (1966): 5–7.

Hanink, J. G. "On the Survival Lottery." *Philosophy* 51 (1976): 223–225. Criticism of John Harris's "The Survival Lottery."

Harris, John. "The Survival Lottery." *Philosophy* 50 (1975): 81–87. Argues that perfection of transplants would make it right to sacrifice a healthy person chosen by lottery to save lives of several people needing organs.

Havighurst, Clark C. "The Ethics of Cost Control in Medical Care." *Soundings* 60 (Spring 1977): 22–39.

Hiatt, H. "On the Distribution of Resources." *New England Journal of Medicine* 293 (1975).

Kaplan, M. B. "The Case of the Artificial Heart Panel." *Hastings Center Report* 5 (1975): 41–48.

Katz, Jay and Alexander Morgan Capron. *Catastrophic Diseases: Who Decides What? A Psychological and Legal Analysis of the Problems Posed by Hemodialysis and Organ Transplantation.* New York: Russell Sage Foundation, 1975.

Kilner, John F. "A Moral Allocation of Scarce Lifesaving Medical Resources." *Journal of Religious Ethics* 9 (Fall 1981): 245–85.

Knutson, A. L. "Body Transplants and Ethical Values." *Social Science and Medicine* 2 (1968–1969): 393–414.

Leake, C. D. "Technical Triumph and Moral Muddle." In T. E. Sturzl, ed. *Experience in Renal Transplantation.* Philadelphia: W. B. Saunders Company, 1964.

Leenen, H. J. J. "The Selection of Patients in the Event of a Scarcity of Medical Facilities—An Unavoidable Dilemma." *International Journal of Medicine and Law* (1980): 161–180.

Lyons, Catherine. *Organ Transplants: The Moral Issues.* Philadelphia: Westminister Press, 1970.

Mack, Eric. "Bad Samaritanism and the Causation of Harm." *Philosophy and Public Affairs* 9 (Spring 1980): 230–259.

Mechanic, David. *Future Issues in Health Care: Social Policy and the Rationing of Medical Sources.* New York: Free Press, 1979.

Miller, George W. *Moral and Ethical Implications of Human Organ Transplants.* Springfield, Ill.: Charles C. Thomas, 1971.

Mooney, Gavin. "Cost-Benefit Analysis and Medical Ethics." *Journal of Medical Ethics* 6 (December 1980): 177–179.

Plant, Raymond. "Gifts, Exchanges and the Political Economy of Health Care." Part 1: "Should Blood Be Bought and Sold?" *Journal of Medical Ethics* 3 (December 1977): 166–173; and Part 2: "How Should Health Care Be Distributed?" (March 1978): 5–11.

Ramsey, Paul. "Choosing How to Choose: Patients and Sparse Medical Resources." In *The Patient as Person*. New Haven: Yale University Press, 1980, chapter 7.

Rhoads, Steven E. "How Much Should We Spend to Save a Life?" *Public Interest* 51 (Spring 1978): 74–92.

"The Sale of Human Body Parts." *Michigan Law Review* 72 (1974): 1182–1264.

"Scarce Medical Resources." *Columbia Law Review* 69 (1969): 620–692.

Schiffer, R. M. and Benjamin Freedman. "Case Studies in Bioethics: The Last Bed in the ICU." *Hastings Center Report* 7 (December 1977): 21–22.

Shapiro, M. H. "Who Merits Merit? Problems in Distributive Justice and Utility Posed by the New Biology." *California Law Review* 48 (1974): 318–370.

Simmons, Roberta G., et al. *Gift of Life: The Social and Psychological Impact of Organ Transplantation*. New York: John Wiley and Sons, 1977.

Smith, Harmon L. "Distributive Justice and American Health Care." In W. M. Finnin, Jr., ed. *The Morality of Scarcity*. Baton Rouge: Louisiana State University Press, 1977, pp. 67–80.

Taurek, John M. "Should the Numbers Count?" *Philosophy and Public Affairs* 6 (Summer 1977): 293–316.

Westervelt, B., Jr., "The Selection Process Viewed from Within: A Reply to Childress." *Soundings* 53 (1970): 154–158.

Chapter 9: The Claim to Health Care

Alford, Robert R. *Health Care Politics: Ideological Interest Group Barriers to Reform*. Chicago: University of Chicago Press, 1975.

Anderson, Gerald and Earl Steinberg. "To Buy or Not to Buy: Technology Acquisition Under Prospective Payment." *New England Journal of Medicine* 311(3) (19 July 1984): 182–85.

Arrow, Kenneth J., et al. "Government Decision Making and the Preciousness of Life." In Lawrence R. Ranoredi, ed. *Ethics of Health Care*. Washington D.C.: National Academy of Sciences, 1974, pp. 33–64.

Bayer, Ronald, Arthur Caplan, and Norman Daniels, eds. *In Search of Equity: Health Needs and the Health Care System*. New York: Plenum Press, 1983.

Bayles, Michael D. "National Health Insurance and Non-Covered Services." *Journal of Health Politics, Policy and Law* 2 (Fall 1977): 335–348.

Birnbaum, Morton. "The Right to Treatment." *American Bar Association Journal* 46 (1960): 499–505.

Black, M. M. and C. Riley. "Moral Issues and Priorities in Biomedical Engineering." *Science, Medicine and Man* 1 (1973): 67–74.

Blackstone, William T. "On Health Care as a Legal Right: Philosophical Justifications, Political Activity, and Adequate Health Care." *Georgia Law Review* 10 (Winter 1976): 391–418.

Brown, Lawrence D. "The Scope and Limits of Equality as a Normative Guide to Federal Health Care Policy." *Public Policy* 26 (Fall 1978): 481–532.

Buxton, M. J. and R. R. West. "Cost-Benefit Analysis of Long-Term Hemodialysis for Chronic Renal Failure." *British Medical Journal*, 17 (May 1975): 376–379. A caution about instituting similar programs for other diseases.

Cairl, R. E. et al. "National Health Insurance Policy in the United States: A Case of Non-Decision-Making." *International Journal of Health Services* 7 (1977): 167–178.

Callahan, Daniel. "How Much Is Enough? A National Perspective." *Alabama Journal of Medical Sciences* 17 (January 1980): 76–80.

————— and Bruce Jennings, eds. *Ethics, the Social Sciences, and Policy Analysis*. New York: Plenum Press, 1983.

Childress, James F. *Priorities in Biomedical Ethics*. Philadelphia: Westminster Press, 1981.

Cleverly, W. "Cost Containment in the Health Care Industry." *Topics in Health Care Financing* 3 (Spring 1977): 1–17.

Curran, William J. "The Right to Health in National and International Law." *New England Journal of Medicine* 284 (1971): 1258.

Devries, Andre. "Health Care Responsibility." *Metamedicine* 1 (Fall 1980): 95–106.

Daniels, Norman. "Equity of Access to Health Care: Some Conceptual and Ethical Issues."

Milbank Memorial Fund Quarterly: Health and Society 60(1) (1982): 51–81.

Dougherty, Charles J. "The Right to Health Care: First Aid in the Emergency Room." *Public Law Forum* 4(1) (1984): 101–28.

"Due Process in the Allocation of Scarce Lifesaving Medical Resources." *Yale Law Journal* 84 (1975): 1734–1749.

Edwards, Marvin Henry. *Hazardous to Your Health: A New Look at the "Health Care Crisis" in America.* New York: Arlington House, 1972.

Ehrenreich, Barbara and John Ehrenreich. *The American Health Empire: Power, Profits and Politics.* New York: Random House, 1970.

Falk, I. S. "Proposals for National Health Insurance in the USA: Origins and Evolution, and Some Perceptions for the Future." *Milbank Memorial Fund Quarterly: Health and Society* (Spring 1977): 161–191.

Fein, Rashi. "On Achieving Access and Equity in Health Care." *Milbank Memorial Fund Quarterly* 50 (1972): 157–190.

Feldstein, Paul J. "National Health Insurance: An Approach to the Redistribution of Medical Care." In *Health Care Economics.* New York: John Wiley and Sons, 1979, chapter 19.

Freedman, Benjamin. "The Case for Medical Care: Inefficient or Not." *Hastings Center Report* 7 (April 1977): 31–39.

Fried, Charles. "Rights and Health Care—Beyond Equity and Efficiency." *New England Journal of Medicine* 293 (31 July 1975): 241–245.

Fromer, Margot Joan. *Ethical Issues in Health Care.* St. Louis: C. V. Mosby Company, 1981.

Fuchs, Victor. *Who Shall Live?* New York: Basic Books, 1974.

Garfield, Sidney. "The Delivery of Medical Care." *Scientific American* 222 (1970): 15–23.

Ginzberg, Eli. *The Limits of Health Reform: The Search for Realism.* New York: Basic Books, 1977.

———— **and Miriam Ostow.** *Men, Money and Medicine.* New York: Columbia University Press, 1969.

Greenberg, Selig. *The Quality of Mercy.* New York: Atheneum, 1971.

Gutmann, Amy and Dennis Thompson, eds. *Ethics and Politics: Cases and Comments.* Chicago: Nelson-Hall, 1984.

Halberstam, Michael. "Liberal Thought, Radical Theory and Medical Practice." *New England Journal of Medicine* 284 (1971): 1180–1185.

Hiatt, Howard H. "Protecting the Medical Commons: Who Is Responsible?" *New England Journal of Medicine* 293 (31 July 1975): 235–241.

Hodgson, Godfrey. "The Politics of American Health Care." *Atlantic* (October 1973): 45–61.

Illich, Ivan. *Medical Nemesis.* New York: Pantheon, 1976.

Journal of Medicine and Philosophy 4 (1979). Special issue on the right to health care.

Kass, Leon R. "Reading the End of Medicine and the Pursuit of Health." *The Public Interest* 40 (1975): 11–42.

Kelman, Steven. "Cost-Benefit Analysis: An Ethical Critique." *Regulation* 5 (January/February 1981): 33–40.

Knowles, John H., ed. *Doing Better and Feeling Worse: Health Care in the United States.* New York: Norton, 1977.

Krizay, John and Andrew Wilson. *The Patient as Consumer: Health Care Financing in the United States.* Lexington, Mass.: D. C. Heath and Company, 1974.

Lesser, Paul B. "A Right to Health?" *Forum on Medicine* 3 (October 1980): 667–669.

Lewis, Charles E. et al. *A Right to Health—The Problem of Access to Medical Care.* New York: John Wiley and Sons, 1976.

Lomasky, Loren E. "Medical Progress and National Health Care." *Philosophy and Public Affairs* 10 (Winter 1981): 65–88.

MacLeon, Gordon and Jeffrey A. Prussin. "Continuing Evolution and Health Maintenance Organizations." *New England Journal of Medicine* 288 (1973): 439–443.

McCreadie, Claudine. "Rawlsian Justice and Financing of the National Health Service." *Journal of Social Policy* 5 (April 1976): 113–130.

Mechanic, David. "Approaches to Controlling the Costs of Medical Care: Short-Range Alternatives." *New England Journal of Medicine* 298 (2 February 1978): 249–254.

_____. *The Growth of Bureaucratic Medicine: An Inquiry into the Dynamics of Patient Behavior and the Organization of Medical Care.* New York: John Wiley and Sons, 1976.

_____. "Rationing Health Care: Public Policy and the Medical Marketplace." *Hastings Center Report* 6 (1976): 34–37.

Mistichelli, Judith. "Diagnosis Related Groups (DRGs) and the Prospective Payment System: Forecasting Social Implications." *Scope Note* 4 (June 1984).

Morison, Robert S. "Rights and Responsibilities: Redressing the Uneasy Balance." *Hastings Center Report* 4 (1974): 1–4.

Navarro, Vicente. "Justice, Social Policy, and the Public's Health." *Medical Care* 15 (May 1977): 363–370.

New England Journal of Medicine 293 (31 July 1975). A large part of this issue is devoted to health-care delivery. See, in particular, the articles by Hiatt and Fried.

Northwestern University Law Review 70 (1975). "Current Problems in Health Care: A Symposium."

Omenn, Gilbert S. and Douglas A. Conrad. "Implications of DRGs for Clinicians." *New England Journal of Medicine* 311 (15 November 1984): 1314–317.

Outka, Gene. "Social Justice and Equal Access to Health Care." *Journal of Religious Ethics* 2 (1974): 11–32.

Pilpel, Harriet F. "Minors' Rights to Medical Care." *Albany Law Review* 36 (1972): 462–487.

President's Commission for the Study of Ethical Problems in Medicine and Biomedical and Behavioral Research. *Securing Access to Health Care: The Differences in the Availability of Health Services.* Washington, D.C.: President's Commission, 1982.

Review of Radical Political Economics 9 (Spring 1977). A special issue entitled "The Political Economy of Health."

Sade, R. "Concepts of Rights: Philosophy and Application to Health Care." *Linacre Quarterly* 46 (November 1979): 330–344.

Schwartz, William B. "Policy Analysis, Politics and the Problems of Health Care." *New England Journal of Medicine* 286 (1972): 1057–1058.

Seham, Max. *Blacks and American Medical Care.* Minneapolis: University of Minnesota Press, 1973.

Shelp, Earl, ed. *Justice and Health Care.* Boston: D. Reidel, 1981.

Slaby, Andrew E. and Laurance R. Tancredi. "The Economics of Moral Values: Policy Implications." *Journal of Health Politics, Policy, and Law* 2 (Spring 1977): 20–31.

Soble, Alan. "On Health Care as a Right: More on the Right to Health Care." *Georgia Law Review* 10 (Winter 1976): 525–544.

Sparer, Edward V. "The Legal Right to Health Care: Public Policy and Equal Access." *Hastings Center Report* 6 (October 1976): 39–47.

Stevens, Rosemary. *American Medicine and the Public Interest.* New Haven: Yale University Press, 1971.

Steiner, Hillel. "The Just Provision of Health Care: A Reply to Elizabeth Telfer." *Journal of Medical Ethics* 2 (December 1976): 185–189.

Taylor, Vincent. "How Much Is Good Health Worth?" *Policy Sciences* 1 (1970): 49–72.

Tancredi, Laurence, ed. *Ethics of Health Care.* Washington, D.C.: National Academy of Sciences, 1975.

Telfer, Elizabeth. "Justice, Welfare and Health Care." *Journal of Medical Ethics* 2 (September 1976): 107–111.

Veatch, R. M. and Roy Branson, eds. *Ethics and Health Policy.* Cambridge, Mass.: Ballinger Publishing Company, 1976.

Weaver, Jerry L. *National Health Policy and the Underserved: Ethnic Minorities, Women, and the Elderly.* St. Louis: C. V. Mosby Company, 1976.

Yaggy, Duncan and William G. Anlyan, eds. *Financing Health Care: Competition Versus Regulation.* Cambridge, Mass.: Ballinger Publishing, 1982.

INDEX

Abortion
  and concept of a person, 55–56, 59–60, 61, 62, 65–67, 68–71, 72, 81, 83–85, 87, 88–92, 94*ff*
  definition of, 54
  and development, 53–54, 66–67, 70, 71, 73
  and duty to fetus, 57, 61, 62, 96*ff*
  and eugenics, 349–350, 371–379
  and Kant's ethics, 59–60
  and the law, 51, 52, 53, 58–59, 60, 62–63, 94, 102
  methods of, 54, 63
  and natural law ethics, 29, 31, 59–60, 66
  and potentiality, 55
  and principle of double effect, 29, 31, 59–60
  and privacy, 64–65
  and Rawls's theory of justice, 59–60
  and Ross's ethics, 59–60
  selective, 349–350, 371–379
  and self-defense, 28–29, 63, 71, 74*ff*
  therapeutic, 57–58, 63
  and utilitarianism, 59–60
  and women's rights, 56–57, 61, 62, 64–75, 74*ff*
Acquired Immune Deficiency Syndrome. *See* AIDS
AIDS
  discovery of, 195–197
  and paternalism, 231–233
  and prejudice, 228–229
  and quarantine, 233–236, 253
  and social issues, 198, 214, 226*ff*, 253
  statistics about, 198
  transmission and risks of, 197, 229–231
Akron *v.* Akron Center for Reproductive Health, 51
Allocation of scarce resources. *See* Scarce resources, allocation of
Alphafetoprotein test, 116, 349. *See also* Birth impairments; Genetic screening
American Medical Association, 162, 166, 170, 240, 278
Amniocentesis, 116, 348–349
Anencephaly, 117. *See also* Birth impairments
Aquinas, St. Thomas, 27, 28, 31, 32

Artificial heart
  criticisms of, 286, 321, 324
  and informed consent, 260–261
  and Phoenix heart case, 334–335
  and priorities, 324, 539
  risks as therapy, 260, 286, 321–323
  social context of, 258–261
Artificial insemination
  and donor responsibility, 445–449
  moral issues about, 416–417, 444, 458–462
  reasons for, 414–415
  and surrogate pregnancy, 411, 427*ff*, 432*ff*, 434
  techniques of, 414
  types of, 415
Autonomy
  and abortion, 58
  and euthanasia, 164
  and Kant's ethics, 14, 15, 16, 59
  and paternalism, 207, 209, 216*ff*, 243
  and prisoners, 277–278, 308–309
  and Ross's ethics, 212
Autonomy, principle of
  and actions, 42
  and decision making, 43
  and options, 43
  restrictions on, 44–46, 216*ff*
  stated, 41

Baby Doe cases, 110–111
Baby Doe regulations, 112–113. *See also* Birth impairments
Baby Fae, 261–262, 286, 325–326. *See also* Heart transplants; Experimentation and children
Baby M case, 438–440. *See also* Surrogate mothers
Bartling, William, case, 190. *See also* Euthanasia
Beneficence, principle of, 19, 35–37, 240
Bentham, Jeremy, 3, 4
Birth impairments
  and best-interest standard, 141–142, 145*ff*